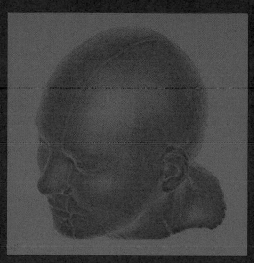

Figure 2.18 **(Chapter 2)**

Three-dimensional geometric alignment of scalp surface. (Courtesy
Dorota Kozinska, Ph.D., University of Warsaw, Warsaw, Poland.)

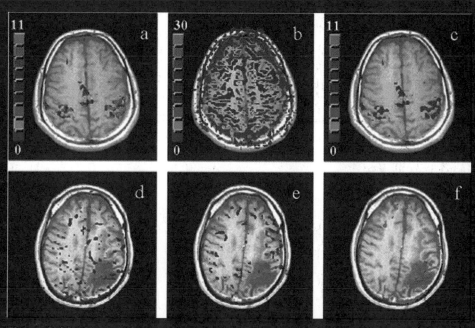

Figure 2.19 **(Chapter 2)**

Functional magnetic resonance imaging signal response (percentage change)
from normal adult (a–c) and patient with severe traumatic brain injury (TBI) (d–f).
(a, d) Motor response (i.e., finger tapping): note focal activation in healthy subject
and disorganization activation in TBI patient. (b, e) Normal cerebral blood flow:
note diminished cerebral blood flow in patient. (c, f) Corrected motor response
based on baseline cerebral blood flow: note less organized activation in patient.
(Courtesy Frank Hillary, Ph.D., Pennsylvania State University.)

Second Edition

PRINCIPLES OF NEUROPSYCHOLOGY

Eric A. Zillmer

Drexel University

Mary V. Spiers

Drexel University

William C. Culbertson

Drexel University

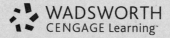
WADSWORTH
CENGAGE Learning™

Australia • Brazil • Japan • Korea • Mexico • Singapore • Spain • United Kingdom • United States

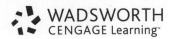
WADSWORTH
CENGAGE Learning™

**Principles of Neuropsychology,
Second Edition**

Eric A. Zillmer, Mary V. Spiers,
William C. Culbertson

Acquisitions Editor: Erik Evans

Assistant Editor: Gina Kessler

Editorial Assistant: Christina D. Ganim

Technology Project Manager: Lauren Keyes

Marketing Manager: Sara Swangard

Marketing Assistant: Melanie Cregger

Senior Marketing Communications Manager:
    Linda Yip

Content Project Manager: Christy Krueger

Creative Director: Rob Hugel

Senior Art Director: Vernon Boes

Senior Print Buyer: Rebecca Cross

Permissions Editor: Robert Kauser

Production Service: Graphic World Inc.

Photo Researcher: Terri Wright

Copy Editor: Graphic World Inc.

Illustrator: International Typesetting and
    Composition

Cover Designer: Denise Davidson

Cover Image: © UHB Trust/Getty Images

Compositor: International Typesetting and
    Composition

For product information and technology assistance, contact us at
Cengage Learning Customer & Sales Support, 1-800-354-9706

For permission to use material from this text or product,
submit all requests online at **www.cengage.com/permissions**
Further permissions questions can be emailed to
permissionrequest@cengage.com

Library of Congress Control Number: 2007920598

ISBN-13: 978-0-495-00376-2

ISBN-10: 0-495-00376-X

Wadsworth
10 Davis Drive
Belmont, CA 94002-3098
USA

Cengage Learning is a leading provider of customized learning solutions with office locations around the globe, including Singapore, the United Kingdom, Australia, Mexico, Brazil, and Japan. Locate your local office at: **www.cengage.com/global**

Cengage Learning products are represented in Canada by Nelson Education, Ltd.

To learn more about Wadsworth, visit **www.cengage.com/wadsworth**

Purchase any of our products at your local college store or at our preferred online store **www.ichapters.com**

Printed in the United States of America
3 4 5 6 7 13 12 11 10

This book is dedicated to the memory of
Carl R. Pacifico
Drexel Alumnus, Class of '44
Friend, Mentor, Benefactor
E.A.Z.

This book is dedicated to my father.
His guidance as a psychologist and his personal struggle with Parkinson's disease
have brought some of my greatest lessons.
M.V.S.

This book is dedicated to
my wife and daughter, my greatest gifts.
W.C.C.

BRIEF CONTENTS

CONTENTS

Chapter 15   Subcortical Dementias   423

Chapter 16   Alterations of Consciousness   443

PREFACE

How can behavior make neuropsychological sense? That is the question we try to answer when we teach neuropsychology to our students. Like many teachers, we have had the experience of observing instructors and examining books on the topic of neuropsychology that presented the material in an esoteric manner removed from real-life situations. Neuropsychology is an exciting and dynamic field that readily stimulates and inspires students and teachers alike. It was with this goal in mind that we have written a progressive and accessible text on the study of neuropsychology.

The goal of *Principles of Neuropsychology* was to write an undergraduate or beginning graduate-level psychology textbook that teaches brain function in a clear, interesting, and progressive manner. The guiding thesis of *Principles of Neuropsychology* is that all interactions in daily life, whether adaptive or maladaptive, can be explained neuropsychologically. Thus, the text challenges the reader to consider behavior from a broader biological perspective. This, in turn, leads to the conceptualization of a more neuropsychologically oriented discipline within psychology. In this respect, the text covers the role of the brain in behavior as simple as a reflex and as complex as personality. *Principles of Neuropsychology* stresses the following specific ideas:

1. An emphasis on human neuropsychology, experimental and clinical

Human neuropsychology is most appealing to psychology students, given that approximately half of all professional psychologists identify with a clinical or counseling specialty. A major focus of *Principles of Neuropsychology* is to integrate the relatively new field of human clinical neuropsychology and compare it with what is known about the normal brain.

Rather than focus on a purely cognitive organization, which characterizes brain functioning and behavior according to specific aspects or components such as memory, attention, or executive functioning, we chose to focus on disorders. Because neurologic disorders are multifaceted and usually involve overlapping and interacting cognitive

components, we believe it is most useful for aspiring practitioners and researchers to obtain a comprehensive view of each neurologic disorder with its multiple cognitive components.

2. An emphasis on integrating theory and research

The integration of theory with studies of neuroanatomic structure and functioning is central to a dynamic understanding of neuropsychology. In this respect, *Principles of Neuropsychology* reviews general theories of brain function and specific theories of higher cortical functioning. A conceptual understanding of brain function is important because it provides a foundation on which to base the study of complex behavioral syndromes as they correspond to brain regions and neuronal networks. Otherwise, nothing more than the memorization of brain anatomy and corresponding behavioral correlates is achieved, and an integrated understanding of neuropsychology remains out of reach.

3. An emphasis on behavioral function

We give special attention to presenting the function of specific neuroanatomic structures. Students often do not absorb the tremendous amount of information presented in similar texts because the material is presented in isolation, out of a psychological context. In this text, we present basic neurobiology as it relates specifically to behavior. Using such a functional approach facilitates both the absorption and comprehension of the material.

4. A focus on presenting real-life examples

To facilitate the reader's understanding of complex material and to augment specific points, *Principles of Neuropsychology* includes numerous examples of clinical and normal cases, procedures, and classic research findings at strategic places in the text. Like many other teachers, we find that didactic information is better understood when "real-life" situations are used. Many of the cases and procedures draw on our clinical and research experiences, which we accumulated in a variety of settings and services including state psychiatric hospitals, sleep centers, psychiatry departments, rehabilitation hospitals, and neurology and neurosurgery services. Throughout the text, we feature case examples and Neuropsychology in Action boxes, written by prominent neuropsychologists, that focus on interesting current issues related to brain functioning.

5. The presentation of didactic aids

Principles of Neuropsychology differs from other texts on the didactic dimension, because it uses unique aids to facilitate learning. These aids include an *Instructor's Manual,* which provides outlines, class exercises, additional reference materials, and didactic information; Web support, which includes practice examinations, exercises, and additional reference materials; more than 200 illustrations in the text; color illustrations; boldfaced Key Terms throughout the text, which are listed at the end of each chapter and again in the Glossary at the end of the text; a Keep in Mind section at the beginning of each chapter and Critical Thinking Questions at the end of each chapter; and annotations on Web sites, called Web Connections, at the end of each chapter.

The companion Web sites for students and instructors have been updated and expanded for the new edition with a format that is easier to navigate. Now you will find chapter-by-chapter glossaries and interactive flash cards, plus videos and more practice exercises. To access these features and more, visit www.cengage.com/psychology/zillmer. For instructors, the Instructor's Manual with Test Bank has been updated for the new edition and contains even more sample test items. Many of the figures and tables from the book are available for instructors as PowerPoint® electronic transparencies.

This second edition was revised related to the many suggestions that we have received. Specifically, the authors have integrated the latest studies and research to give students the most up-to-date information in this dynamic and expanding field. Furthermore, this edition includes an increased emphasis on neuroscience coverage to provide empirical data in support of the discussions of neuropsychology. Clinical examples throughout the text are updated in support of the new research in the developing field of neuropsychology. This second edition also provides additional chapters and coverage on topics of Somatosensory, Chemical and Motor Systems, Vision and Language, and Memory, Attention, and Executive Functioning. A reorganization of the material now places assessment methods of the brain, both medical and psychological, at the beginning of the text to introduce students to this area early in their studies.

In summary, the intent of *Principles of Neuropsychology* is to discuss brain functions, neurophysiology, and neuroanatomy in an integrated and accessible format. An in-depth discussion on the relation among neuroscience, anatomy, and behavior is emphasized. Numerous examples of clinical and real-life examples of neuropsychology are provided, as is a focus on relevant scientific and theoretical contributions in the field of neuropsychology. Unique to the study of neuropsychology is an organization of the material from history, assessment, neuroanatomy, to clinical assessment that makes intuitive and didactic sense. To facilitate a dynamic understanding of the field, the text emphasizes theory, functional process, case examples, and research, related to what has been learned about normal and neuropathological functioning. Approaching the field from this perspective challenges students to examine the field of neuropsychology as a framework for behavior.

ABOUT THE AUTHORS

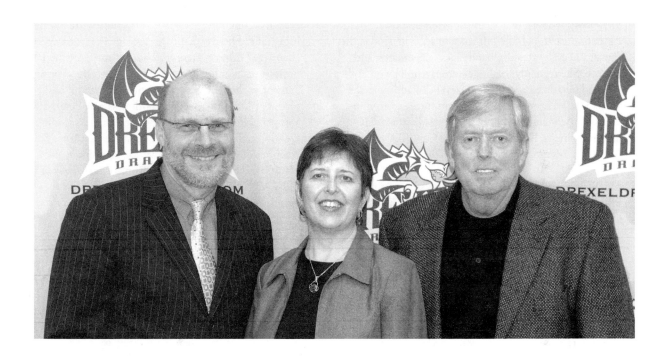

Dr. Eric A. Zillmer, a licensed Clinical Psychologist, received his Doctorate in Clinical Psychology from Florida Tech in 1984 and was subsequently awarded the Outstanding Alumnus Award in 1995. Dr. Zillmer completed internship training at Eastern Virginia Medical School and a postdoctoral fellowship in clinical neuropsychology at the University of Virginia Medical School. A member of Drexel University's faculty since 1988, Dr. Zillmer is a Fellow of the College of Physicians of Philadelphia, the American Psychological Association, the Society for Personality Assessment, and the National Academy of Neuropsychology, for which he has also served as President. He has written extensively in the area of sports psychology, neuropsychology, and psychological assessment, having published more than 100 journal articles, book chapters, and books, and he is a frequent contributor to the local and national media on topics ranging from sports psychology, forensic psychology, to the psychology of terrorism. *The Quest for the Nazi*

Personality, published in 1995, has been summarized as the definitive psychological analysis of Third Reich war criminals. He is the coauthor of the d2 Test of Attention and the Tower of London test. Dr. Zillmer serves on the editorial boards of *Journal of Personality Assessment* and *Archives of Clinical Neuropsychology.* His most recent book is entitled *Military Psychology— Clinical and Operational Applications* (2006). Dr. Zillmer currently serves as the Director of Athletics at Drexel University.

Dr. Mary V. Spiers is Associate Professor of Psychology in the Department of Psychology at Drexel University and is a licensed Clinical Psychologist specializing in Neuropsychology. She earned her Ph.D. in Clinical Psychology from the University of Alabama at Birmingham, where she specialized in medical psychology and neuropsychology. Dr. Spiers's research and clinical expertise is in two areas. The first area is neuropsychological assessment with a focus on everyday problems of memory. She has developed tests to assess memory and cognitive problems in daily medication taking. Recently, she has focused on the development of ecologically valid spatial memory tests within a virtual reality environment. Dr. Spiers's second area of focus relates to cognitive performance and strategy differences related to sex and gender. She leads the Women's Cognitive Health Research Group at Drexel University, whose aim is to investigate variation in brain functioning through the influence of sex and gender, the menstrual cycle, genetics/handedness, experience, and culture. She regularly teaches Neuropsychology on both the undergraduate and graduate levels. In addition, she has taught a variety of graduate courses related to clinical assessment and memory, including Neuropsychological Assessment, Neuropsychological Case Analysis, and Models of Memory in Neuropsychology.

Dr. William C. Culbertson is in private practice as a Clinical Neuropsychologist who specializes in the assessment and treatment of childhood and adolescent disorders, particularly those with attention-deficit/hyperactivity disorder. He received his doctorate degree from Rutgers University and completed a postdoctoral fellowship in neuropsychology at Drexel University. Dr. Culbertson's research interests are in the assessment of higher order problem-solving ability, specifically as it relates to assessing frontal lobe damage, and executive functioning deficits. Dr. Culbertson has published in the field of neuropsychology (e.g., *Assessment, Archives of Clinical Neuropsychology*) and presented at professional conferences. He is an Associate Visiting Scholar at the University of Pennsylvania and has taught at Drexel University, both at the undergraduate and graduate level, including Counseling Psychology, Developmental Psychology, Cognitive Psychology, Theories of Personality, and various Seminars in Neuropsychology. He is a coauthor of the *Tower of London^{DX},* now in its second edition, which is a neuropsychological measure of executive function.

ACKNOWLEDGMENTS

This book could not have been written without the cooperation, assistance, and support of numerous individuals. Many students, scholars, and friends listened to us, offered suggestions, and provided encouragement along the way. Many reviewers helped shape the book from beginning to end. We are most grateful to the following reviewers for their generous contributions to this second edition: Joan Ballard, SUNY Geneseo; Jody Bain, University of Victoria; Robert Deysach, University of South Carolina; Kenneth Green, California State University Long Beach; Julian Keenan, Montclair State University; Ann Marie Leonard-Zabel, Curry College; Jim Nelson, Valparaiso University; Elizabeth Seebach, Saint Mary's University of Minnesota; Pamela Stuntz, Texas Christian University; Benjamin Walker, Georgetown University; Arthur Wingfield, Brandeis University; Nancy Zook, Purchase College SUNY. We would also like to thank those who contributed to the previous edition: Timothy Barth, Texas Christian University; Richard Bauer, Middle Tennessee State University; Gary Berntson, Ohio State University; Thomas Fikes, Westmont College; Michael R. Foy, Loyola Marymount University; Kenneth F. Green, California State University Long Beach; Gary Hanson, Francis Marion University; Barbara Knowlton, University of California Los Angeles; Paul Koch, St. Ambrose University; Mark McCourt, North Dakota State University; James Rose, University of Wyomong; Lawrence Ryan, Oregon State University; Bennett Schwartz, Florida International University; Michael Selby, California Polytechnic Institute; Frank Webbe, Florida Institute of Technology; and finally, the many reviewers who did not wish to be named. We would also like to acknowledge those scholars who have contributed Neuropsychology in Action boxes to this text. All of them are prominent neuropsychologists who have, going beyond the call of duty, given valuable time to make *Principles of Neuropsychology* "come alive."

Drexel University psychology students played an important role in this project. They read initial chapters and provided feedback, were willing to use early versions of the manuscript as their textbook in class, and provided important research assistance. Simply put, this project could not have been accomplished without their diligent efforts. Psychology undergraduate and graduate students who provided valuable research support on the first edition included Barbara Holda, Priti Panchal, Dan Rosenberg, Holly Giordano, Stephanie Cosentino, Carrie Kennedy, Melissa Lamar, and Cate Price. Drexel University students in Dr. Spiers's undergraduate and graduate neuropsychology classes provided valuable comments on both the structure and content of this second edition. Special thanks go to Karen Friedman, who coordinated reference updating in this second edition; to Heather McNiece, who coordinated the Key Terms and Glossary; and to Maiko Sakamoto, who assisted with the question bank.

Appreciation also goes to our colleagues Sepp Zihl and Karin Muenzel, both from the Ludwig-Maximilians University, Institute für Neuropsychologie, in Munich, Germany. Sepp and Karin allowed Dr. Zillmer to teach neuropsychology in an international forum. Our discussions on neuropsychology have been most stimulating and inspiring and have provided a springboard for many issues discussed in this text. We also want to acknowledge our colleagues Mark Chelder and Joelle Efthimiou, who have assisted us in the development of the Assessment of Impairment Measure (AIM), which we have used extensively throughout the text to demonstrate the principles of neuropsychological assessment.

Our friend Carl Pacifico played a special role in this venture. He reminded us of how important it is to think about brain-behavior functioning within the context of evolution. Carl, ever the pragmatist, also shaped our thinking about the functional and applied aspects of neuropsychology. We especially welcomed the occasions when we discussed neuropsychology and its relation to culture, religion, and philosophy.

Special recognition goes to key administrators at Drexel University. Former Dean of the College of Arts and Sciences Thomas Canavan provided encouragement for our doctoral program in neuropsychology at Drexel and assistance for the successful APA accreditation process. Constantine "Taki" Papadakis, President of Drexel University, is acknowledged for revitalizing our university and, most importantly, making Drexel an exciting and fun place to teach and to do research.

Our department faculty served as an important discussion group, "think tank," and sounding board; whether it was around the copying machine, in the hallways, or over lunch, they allowed us to argue over the role of the brain and its relation to behavior. Thanks to Doug Porpora, David Kutzik, Tom Hewett, Elizabeth Petras, Arthur Shostak, Doug Chute, Lamia Barakat, and Anthony Glascock. Dorota Kozinska, at the University of Warsaw, Poland, taught us the three-dimensional imaging of brains and provided state-of-the-art brain electrical activity mapping pictures. Erin D. Bigler, Professor of Psychology at Brigham Young University, and Frank Hillary, Assistant Professor at Penn State University, generously provided three-dimensional images of the brain. Frank Ruben C. Gur and his research group at the Department of Psychiatry, University of Pennsylvania, allowed us to use cerebral blood flow study pictures.

Any scholar with a family knows what it means to write a book and attempt to maintain a normal family life. Dr. Zillmer is grateful to his wife, Rochelle, and his daughter, Kanya, for their support. Dr. Spiers thanks her husband, Sean, for his patience and understanding. Dr. Culbertson acknowledges his wife, Nancy, who provided countless hours of critical readings, tolerated his absences during those periods when he needed to write, and was unwavering in her support.

We cannot think of having had better editors for this project. We thank the production editor, Dan Fitzgerald, and the psychology editor, Erik Evans, assistant editor, Gina Kessler, and editorial assistant, Christina Ganim. They took our project seriously and forced us to focus on finishing a product of the highest quality. The assistance of many individuals has enabled us to publish this second edition. We are grateful to all of them and have benefited from their understanding, criticism, and advice. Thank you.

Eric A. Zillmer
Mary V. Spiers
William C. Culbertson

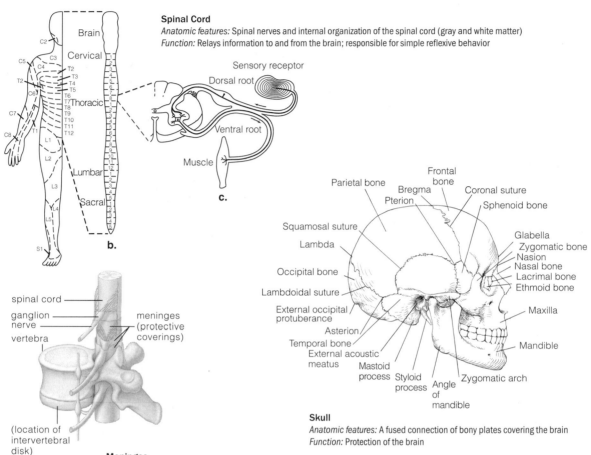

Spinal Cord

Anatomic features: Spinal nerves and internal organization of the spinal cord (gray and white matter)
Function: Relays information to and from the brain; responsible for simple reflexive behavior

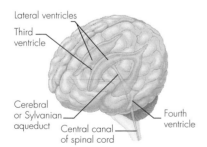

Meninges

Anatomic features: Dura mater, arachnoid membrane, and pia mater
Function: Protective covering of the central nervous system, location of venous drainage, and cerebrospinal fluid absorption

Skull

Anatomic features: A fused connection of bony plates covering the brain
Function: Protection of the brain

Ventricular System

Anatomic features: Lateral (1st and 2nd), 3rd, and 4th ventricles, choroid plexus, cerebral aqueduct, and arachnoid granulations
Function: Balancing intracranial pressure, cerebrospinal fluid production, and circulation

Vascular System

Anatomic features: Arteries, veins, circle of Willis
Function: Arteries: nourishment; supply of oxygen and nutrients
Veins: carrying away waste products

(continued)

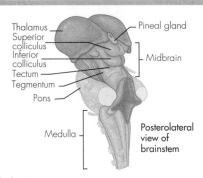

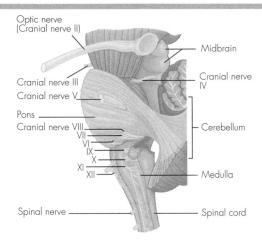

Lower Brainstem

Anatomic features:

Hindbrain: medulla oblongata (myelencephalon),
pons (metencephalon)

Midbrain: tectum and tegmentum, cranial nerves, reticular
activating system

Function: Relays information to and from the brain;
responsible for simple reflexive behavior

Cranial Nerves

Anatomic features: Located within the brainstem

Function: Conducting specific motor and sensory information

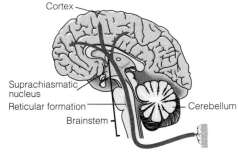

Reticular Formation

Anatomic features: Neural network within the lower brainstem
connecting the medulla and the midbrain

Function: Nonspecific arousal and activation, sleep and wakefulness

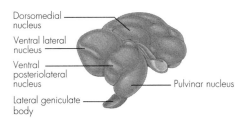

Thalamus

Anatomic features: Thalamic nuclei and thalamocortical
connections

Functions: Complex relay station—major sensory and
motor inputs to and from the ipsilateral cerebral
hemisphere

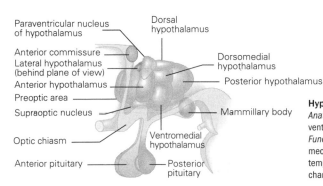

Hypothalamus

Anatomic features: Hypothalamic nuclei, major fiber systems, and third
ventricle

Function: Activates, controls, and integrates the peripheral autonomic
mechanisms, endocrine activity, and somatic functions, including body
temperature, food intake, and the development of secondary sexual
characteristics

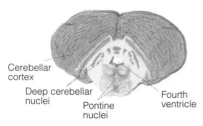

Cerebellum

Anatomic features: Cerebellar cortex, cerebellar white matter, and glia

Function: Coordination of movements, posture, antigravity, balance, and gait

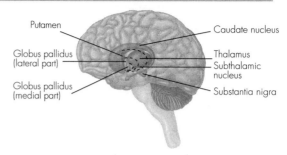

Basal Ganglia

Anatomic features: Structures of the caudate nucleus, putamen, globus pallidus, substantia nigra, and subthalamic nuclei

Function: Important relay stations in motor behavior (such as the striato-pallido-thalamic loop); connections form part of the extrapyramidal motor system (including cerebral cortex, basal nuclei, thalamus, and midbrain) and coordinate stereotyped postural and reflexive motor activity

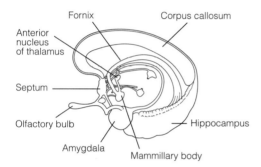

Limbic System

Anatomic features: Structures of the amygdala, hippocampus, parahippocampal gyrus, cingulate gyrus, fornix, septum, and olfactory bulbs

Function: Closely involved in the expression of emotional behavior and the integration of olfactory information with visceral and somatic information

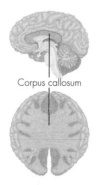

Corpus Callosum

Anatomic features: A large set of myelinated axons connecting the right and left cerebral hemispheres

Function: Information exchange between the two hemispheres

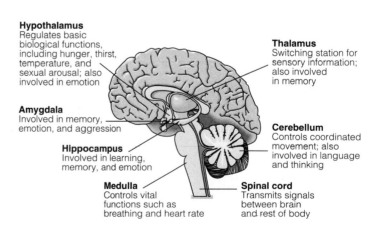

Hypothalamus
Regulates basic biological functions, including hunger, thirst, temperature, and sexual arousal; also involved in emotion

Amygdala
Involved in memory, emotion, and aggression

Hippocampus
Involved in learning, memory, and emotion

Medulla
Controls vital functions such as breathing and heart rate

Thalamus
Switching station for sensory information; also involved in memory

Cerebellum
Controls coordinated movement; also involved in language and thinking

Spinal cord
Transmits signals between brain and rest of body

Cerebral Hemispheres

Anatomic features: Structures of the frontal, parietal, occipital, and temporal lobes

Function: Higher cognitive functioning, cerebral specialization, and cortical localization

Part One

INTRODUCTION

Chapter 1

A HISTORY OF NEUROPSYCHOLOGY

I think, therefore I am.

—*René Descartes,* Discourse on Method

There is no ghost in the machine.

—*Gilbert Ryle,* The Concept of Mind

Overview

All the preceding questions concern the functions of the brain. The brain has evolved to play a particularly significant role in the human body, not only in sustaining life, but also in all thought, behavior, and reasoning. It is the only organ completely enclosed by protective bony tissue, the skull, and it is the only organ that cannot be transplanted and still maintain the person's self. But how exactly does brain tissue generate and constrain mental events?

Efforts to understand mind–body relationships and their relative contributions to health and well-being extend back at least to the philosophies of Plato, Descartes, and Kant. Like many other sciences, neuropsychology has evolved from related fields, most notably psychology, neurology, neuroscience, biology, and philosophy. **Psychology** is the study of behavior; specifically, it seeks to describe, explain, modify, and predict human and animal behavior. **Neuropsychology,** a subspecialty of psychology, is the study of how complex properties of the brain allow behavior to occur. Neuropsychologists study relationships between brain functions and behavior; specifically, changes in thought and behavior that relate to the brain's structural or cognitive integrity. Thus, neuropsychology is one way to study the brain by examining the behavior it produces.

Humans read and write, compose music, and play sports. You would expect an organ that coordinates and mediates all activity to have a huge number of components. And, in fact, the brain contains billions of cells, or **neurons,** and an *infinite* number of possible connections among individual neurons, allowing us to exchange complex information. This amazing pattern of connections determines how and what the brain does. Understanding this network of neurons is the central focus of neuropsychology.

Neuropsychology has grown tremendously since the 1970s, and in the 1990s, it was the fastest growing subspecialty within psychology. Neuropsychologists lead the study of brain–behavior relationships and are involved in the design and development of technologies to treat diseases of the brain. They are involved in patient care and research on the brain and work in universities, research institutes, medical and psychiatric hospitals, correctional facilities, the armed forces, and private practice.

The study of neuropsychology currently is shaping our understanding of all behavior. But this has not always been true. Many previous ideas about how the brain functions did not derive from scientific evidence. In general, two doctrines have emerged. The first doctrine, **vitalism,** suggests that many behaviors, such as thinking, are only partly controlled by mechanical or logical forces—they are also partially self-determined and are separate from chemical and physical determinants. Extreme proponents of vitalism argue that spirits or psychic phenomena account for much observable behavior. Sigmund Freud's psychoanalysis would be a good example of this doctrine. The second doctrine, **materialism,** suggests that logical forces, such as matter in motion, determine brain–behavior functions. Materialism, in its simplest form, favors a mechanistic view of the brain (as a machine). Walter Freeman's lobotomies embraced this idea. The history of neuropsychology is shaped by these two opposing principles.

This introductory chapter provides grounding in the historical, theoretical, and philosophical aspects of neuropsychology. By charting the work of noted scholars, this chapter traces the development of neuropsychology from antiquity to the present.

The Brain in Antiquity: Early Hypotheses

Evidence from as long ago as the time of cave drawings shows that people have long been aware of brain-behavior relationships. The earliest neuropsychological investigations recognized how diseases and blows to the brain affect behavior. For example, **trephination** is an ancient surgical operation that involves cutting, scraping, chiseling, or drilling a pluglike piece of bone from the skull. This procedure relieves pressure related to brain swelling. Archaeologists have recovered several thousand such skulls worldwide. Many who underwent trephination clearly survived the operation, because many of the skulls show evidence of healing (new callus tissue); other skulls show no signs of healing, so the patients died during or shortly after the operation. In some cases, the same skull was trephined more than once. One recovered skull was found with seven boreholes, at least some of which were made on separate occasions.

Why did our ancestors perform trephination (Figure 1.1)? Did they have a reasonable understanding of the brain and its relationship to behavior? Did they use this procedure for medical reasons, such as trauma with swelling, or for other reasons? Did practitioners avoid certain areas of the brain because they knew that permanent behavioral problems or death were likely to follow?

Much debate focuses on the reason for trephinations. Researchers have suggested that some cases may have involved a medical reason, such as a skull fracture. Such injuries presumably occurred during hand-to-hand fighting with stone-headed war clubs or perhaps as a result of a fall unconnected with warfare. On some skulls, however, trephination was performed on intact crania with no sign of violence. Thus, some investigators suggest that trephination was a "magical" form of healing, perhaps for displays of bizarre behaviors, including what we would now recognize as epilepsy or schizophrenia (Lisowski, 1967) (Figure 1.2).

Similar operations are important in modern neurosurgery (Figure 1.3). Surgeons widely use two procedures. The first procedure, similar to the ancient Peruvian

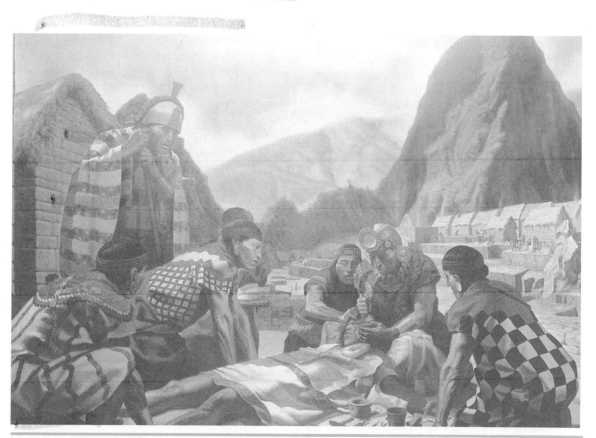

Figure 1.1 Trephination scene in Peru. (Image reprinted with permission from Department of Anthropology, National Museum of Natural History, Smithsonian Institution, Washington, D.C. Photo courtesy of the San Diego Museum of Man.)

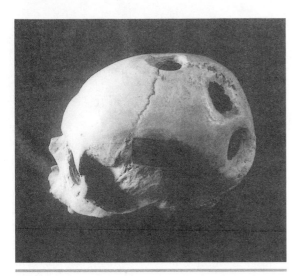

Figure 1.2 Adult male skull showing multiple trephinations by the scraping method. Evidence of inflammation indicates temporary survival. (Courtesy Mütter Museum, College of Physicians of Philadelphia.)

technique of drilling a number of small holes, involves drilling a hole next to a depressed skull fracture to facilitate the elevation and removal of depressed bone fragments. Incidentally, modern neurosurgeons still use manual drills, which allow them more control during the operation. The second surgical procedure drains internal bleeding after a blow to the head. With a special drill bit, the surgeon makes a hole over the site of the bleed. Then the surgeon screws a precisely machined bolt into the skull, allowing excessive blood to drain from within the cranium. This procedure reduces the intracranial pressure that is a major cause of death after a head injury (see Chapter 13).

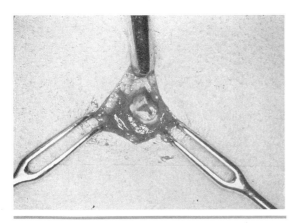

Figure 1.3 Modern trephination. A surgical hole is opened in the skull to relieve the intracranial pressure often associated with consequences of head trauma. (Courtesy Jeffrey T. Barth, PhD, University of Virginia.)

That surgeons today use an ancient surgical technique that even modern doctors once thought controversial underscores that people have often misinterpreted the historical context in which ancient scientists proposed certain ideas about the brain or performed specific procedures. Most ideas about the brain make more sense when considered within the societal and cultural context in which they were originally developed.

ANCIENT GREEK PERSPECTIVES

Classical Greeks wrote the first accounts of brain–behavior relationships. **Heraclitus,** a philosopher of the sixth century B.C., called the mind an enormous space with boundaries that we could never reach. A group of scholars, including the geometer **Pythagoras** (about 580–500 B.C.), was the first to suggest that the brain is at the center of human reasoning and plays a crucial role in the soul's life. They described what is now called the **brain hypothesis:** the idea that the brain is the source of all behavior.

Hippocrates (460–377 B.C.), a Greek physician honored as the founder of modern medicine (Figure 1.4), also believed the brain controls all senses and movements. He was the first to recognize that paralysis occurs on the side of the body opposite the side of a head injury, following the areas governed by the right and left hemispheres of the brain. Hippocrates suggested that pleasure, merriment, laughter, and amusement, as well as grief, pain, anxiety, and tears, all arise from the brain (Haeger, 1988). Furthermore, Hippocrates argued that epilepsy, once considered the "sacred disease" (because people thought the patient was possessed by gods or spirits), is, in fact, no more divine or sacred than any other disease, but has specific characteristics and a definite medical cause. These were bold propositions at a time when people thought behavior was mostly under divine control. Hippocrates and his associates could not, however, discuss exactly how such brain–behavior relationships arose, perhaps because it was then sacrilegious to dissect the human body, especially the brain.

Plato (420–347 B.C.) suggested in *The Republic* that the soul has three parts: appetite, reason, and temper. This may have served as the model for Freud's psychoanalytic subdivision of the psyche into the id, ego, and superego (see later discussion). Plato believed the rational part of the tripartite soul lay in the brain, because it is the organ closest to the heavens. Plato also discussed the idea that health is related to harmony between body and mind. Thus, historians credit Plato as being the first to propose the concept of mental health.

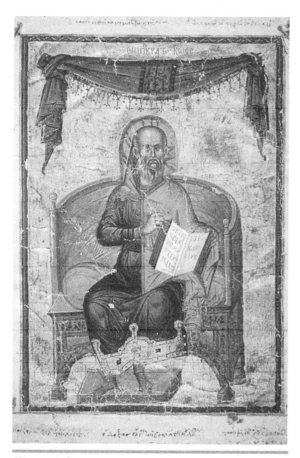

Figure 1.4 Hippocrates suggested that all thoughts and emotions originated in the brain, not the heart, as Aristotle had believed. Here, the ancient Greek physician opens his book to one of his favorite axioms, "Life is short, and the art is long." (© Snark/Art Resource, NY.)

Not all ancient philosophers believed in the importance of the brain to behavior. Aristotle (384–322 B.C.), a disciple of Plato, was a creative thinker in fields as varied as ethics, logic, psychology, poetry, and politics, and he founded comparative anatomy. Aristotle, however, erroneously believed the heart to be the source of all mental processes. He reasoned that because the heart is warm and active, it is the locus of the soul. Aristotle argued that because the brain is bloodless, it functions as a "radiator," cooling hot blood that ascends from the heart. The influence of Aristotle's so-called cardiac hypothesis proposing the heart as the seat of such emotions as love and anger can still be seen in words such as *heartbroken*. Nevertheless, Aristotle's view of nature and his anatomic findings dominated medical thinking and methods for the next 500 years.

THE CELL DOCTRINE

In Egypt, during the third and fourth centuries B.C., the so-called Alexandrian school reached its height. Well-known scientists worked in physiology and anatomy. They gained considerable knowledge of the nervous system and neuroanatomy from performing public dissections, which the Ptolemaic rulers encouraged. Reports exist of scientists actually vivisecting subjects—condemned criminals were at the scientists' disposal. These dissections allowed scientists to notice different anatomic details, and they hypothesized that specific parts of the brain control different behaviors. Furthermore, they broke new ground by distinguishing between ascending (sensory) and descending (motor) nerves, and demonstrating that all nerves connect with the central nervous system.

An interesting development during this time was the erroneous suggestion that ventricular cavities within the brain control mental abilities and movement. The **ventricular localization hypothesis** postulated that mental as well as spiritual processes reside in the ventricular chambers of the brain. Indeed, gross dissection of the brain shows that the lateral ventricles are the most striking features. Thus, brain autopsies might have led investigators to conclude that these cavities contain animal spirits and are in large part responsible for mental faculties. This hypothesis subsequently became known as the **cell doctrine** ("cell" meaning a small compartment or ventricle), a notion that endured for 2000 years. **Leonardo da Vinci** (1452–1519), an Italian painter, sculptor, architect, and scientist, was a keen observer of anatomy. However, many of his early drawings were not guided by his keen scientific acumen, but instead by the inaccurate medieval conventions of his times. For example, Figure 1.5 shows one of his drawings based on a common, but inaccurate belief about spherical ventricles. According to the cell doctrine, foremost was the cell of common sense, where people thought the soul resided and that connected to nerves leading to the eyes and ears.

Today, people know that the cell doctrine is entirely inaccurate. The ventricles are actually the anatomic site through which cerebrospinal fluid passes. This fluid protects the brain and facilitates the disposal of waste material. It plays no role in thinking; in fact, a neurosurgeon friend of ours conceptualizes it poetically as "the urine of the brain." The cell doctrine was scientifically important precisely because it was in error, and thus presented an obstacle to further inquiry that people did not overcome until centuries later. However, it did focus the medical community on the brain and stimulated discussion of how behavior, thought processes, and brain anatomy may be related.

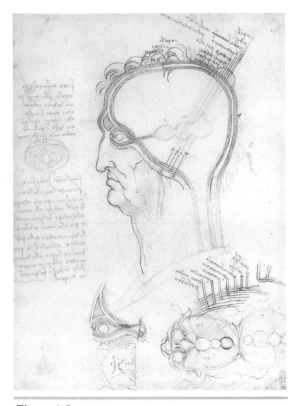

Figure 1.5 Drawing by Leonardo da Vinci demonstrating, inaccurately, the placement of three spherical ventricles in accordance with the cell doctrine. (The Royal Collection © 2007, Her Majesty Queen Elizabeth II.)

Together with Hippocrates, Galen (A.D. 130–201), a Roman anatomist and physician, stands out as a supreme figure in ancient medicine (Figure 1.6). Galen was undoubtedly the greatest physician of his time. By significantly advancing the anatomic knowledge of the brain, Galen distinguished himself as the first experimental physiologist and physician. He identified many of the major brain structures and described behavioral changes as a function of brain trauma. It was Galen's misfortune, however, that during his life the Roman authorities forbade autopsies. He therefore based much of his clinical knowledge on his experience as a surgeon appointed to treat gladiators; he remarked that war and gladiator games were the greatest school of surgery. Contemporary neuropsychologists have also made significant advances during periods of war, including World Wars I and II and the Korean and Vietnam conflicts, by studying the behavioral effects of wounds to the brain.

Galen suggested that the brain is a large clot of phlegm from which a pump forced the psychic pneuma out into the nerves. Perhaps he was comparing the brain to a major

technologic achievement of his time, the Roman system of aqueducts, which relied on hydraulic principles. Although Galen believed the frontal lobes (Figure 1.7) are the location of the soul, he supported the ventricular localization hypothesis, describing in detail how he imagined human ventricles to look and function, based on his studies of the pig and the ox. Galen believed that all physical function, including the brain, as well as the rest of the body, depends on the balance of bodily fluids of **humors,** specifically blood, mucus, and yellow and black bile, which he related to the four basic elements—air, water, fire, and earth, respectively. Given that people thought the agent that causes sickness resides in blood, doctors often bled patients as a curative procedure. Galen's view of humors became so ingrained in Western thought that physicians barely elaborated on the role of the brain and other organs, which remained largely unquestioned for nearly the next thousand years. We still say "good humor" or "bad humor" to describe someone's mental disposition. Terms such as *melancholic* (having frequent spells of sadness) and *choleric* (having a low threshold for angry outbursts) also remain in our vocabulary (Figure 1.8).

ANATOMIC DISCOVERIES AND THE ROLE OF THE SPIRITUAL SOUL

During the thirteenth century, scientists began to take initial steps away from the ventricular theory. For example, **Albertus Magnus,** a German Dominican monk, theorized that behavior results from a combination of brain structures that includes the cortex, midbrain, and cerebellum (Figure 1.9).

Not until scientific inquiry by **Andreas Vesalius** (1514–1564), however, were Galen's anatomic mistakes corrected, particularly those related to the role of the ventricles and their effect on behavior. Galen had initially demonstrated the similar relative size of the ventricles in animals and humans, whereas Vesalius placed more emphasis on the relatively larger overall brain mass of humans as responsible for mediating mental processes. Through continual dissections and careful scientific observations, Vesalius demonstrated that Galen's views were inaccurate. Vesalius also pioneered the anatomic theater—a sort of performance dissection, where medical students and doctors could watch from a circular gallery. Despite a climate of political and religious restrictions, Vesalius performed the first systematic dissections of human beings in Europe. Clearly, many opposed and objected to his experimental predilections. After all, the church retained authority over the soul, which was not subject to direct investigation. But Vesalius proceeded to revolutionize

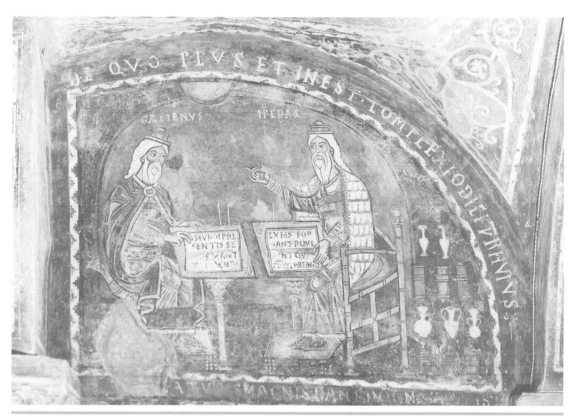

Figure 1.6 Galen learned from Hippocrates. Later, however, he was rather cynical about Hippocrates's writings, stating that they "have faults, and lack essential distinctions his knowledge of certain topics is insufficient, and he is often unclear as the old tend to be. In sum: he prepared the way, but I have made it passable" (Haeger, 1988, p. 59). (© Scala/Art Resource, NY.)

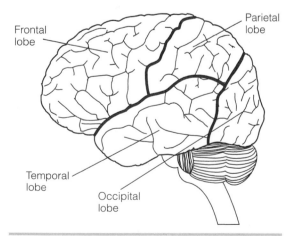

Figure 1.7 The lobes of the brain. (Adapted from Heller, K. W. [1996]. *Understanding physical, sensory, and health impairments* [p. 51, Figure 4.5]. Pacific Grove, CA: Brooks/Cole.)

medicine through precise drawings of human anatomy (Figure 1.10). For the first time, surgeons could see what they were dealing with.

By the seventeenth century, scientists were looking for a single component of the brain as the site of mental processes. **René Descartes** (1596–1650), for example, proposed a strict split or schism between mental processes and physical abilities. He hypothesized that the mind and body are separate, but interact with each other. Descartes theorized that mental processes reside in a small anatomic feature, the pineal gland. He reasoned that because the pineal gland lies in the center of the brain and is the only structure not composed of two symmetric halves, it was the logical seat for mental abilities. It is also close to the ventricular system; thus, the "flow of the spirits" might influence it. Today, the function of the pineal gland is something of a mystery and is perhaps related to light–dark cycles and the production of sleep-enhancing melatonin.

Descartes has had an important philosophic influence on the study of the brain, precisely because dualist thinking

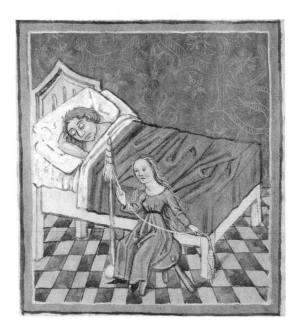
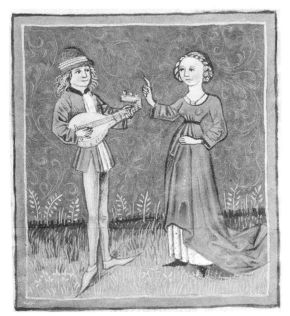
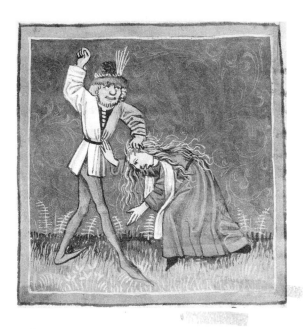
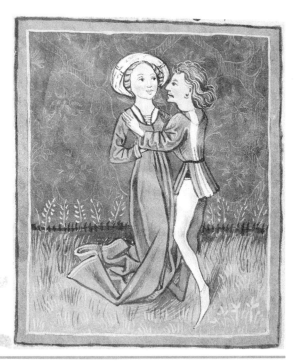

Figure 1.8 Ancient physicians took interest in humors, which served medieval notions of health and disease. (Clockwise) Excess black bile was responsible for a patient suffering from melancholy (depression); blood impassioned a lutist to play; phlegm is responsible for a slow response to a lover; and yellow bile results in anger. (Courtesy Zentralbibliothek Zürich.)

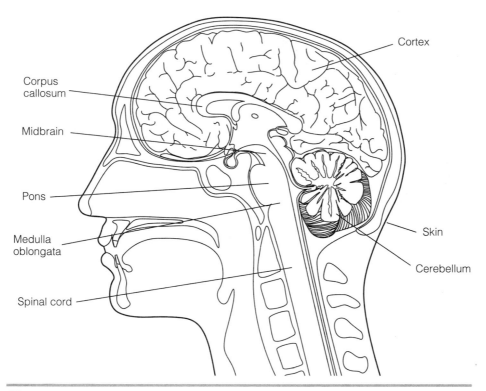

Figure 1.9 Basic anatomy of the brain. (Reproduced from Heller, K. W. [1996]. *Understanding physical, sensory, and health impairments* [p. 50, Figure 4.4]. Pacific Grove: Brooks/Cole.)

opposes the idea that we can explain psychological states and processes for physical phenomena. In fact, historians often call Descartes the founder of body–mind dualism. If he had been correct, it would be hopeless to search for an explanation of mental processes for brain states. However, people have sometimes misunderstood Descartes. He proposed a concept of bodily movement, such as the eye blink, that reflected the mechanistic concepts of his time, such as the functioning of clockworks and water fountains (Figure 1.11). He generally believed the body to be a machine. Reflexes stem not from the intervention of the soul, but from nerves or message cables to and from the brain. Voluntary actions require a rational, nonmaterial soul and the free exercise of will. The church, however, steadfastly endorsed the idea that animal spirits and vital forces are nonmaterial, and that all nervous activity requires such vital forces. Descartes, a devoted Catholic, barely remained respectable in the scientific community because of his constant warnings that he was probably incorrect. His work *Treatise on Man* (1664) (from which Figure 1.11 is taken) was not published until 14 years after his death because he feared being charged with heresy.

By the seventeenth and eighteenth centuries, more precise models of the brain became possible. This advance was related, in part, to the conviction that people could explain everything by mechanics. English anatomist **Thomas Willis** (1621–1675), best known for his work on blood circulation in the brain, theorized that all mental faculties reside in the corpus striatum, a structure deep within the cerebral hemispheres. Others suggested that most mental faculties reside in the white matter of the cerebral hemispheres. **Giovanni Lancisi** (1654–1720), an Italian clinician who contributed greatly to our knowledge of the aneurysm (an abnormal, blood-filled ballooning of an artery in the brain), selected the corpus callosum, a band of fibers that joins the left and right cerebral hemispheres, as the seat of mental functions.

Early investigators were preoccupied with identifying the one precise part of the brain that was the seat of the mind, but they based their discussions primarily on speculation and, in fact, conducted relatively little experimentation. Nevertheless, they were part of a movement that would become stronger in the centuries to come.

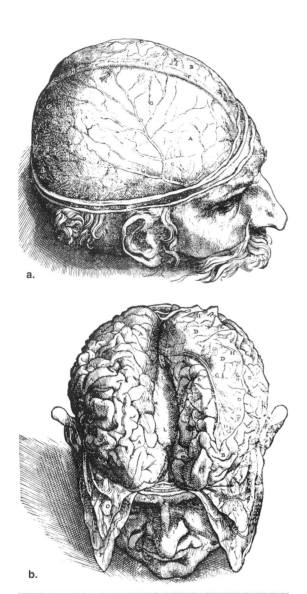

a.

b.

Figure 1.10 Vesalius's drawings of the human brain. In his attempt to learn about anatomy, Vesalius initially depended on the work of others. Later, he wanted to see for himself, performing the first systematic dissections of human beings done in Europe. (National Library of Medicine.)

NON-WESTERN ATTITUDES

Although Western ideologies predominantly shaped the behavioral sciences, non-Western cultures also developed theories to explain behavior. Although some of these theories certainly must have involved the role of the brain, we know little about how advanced people such as the Egyptians and Eastern cultures approached the brain, because we lack detailed written accounts.

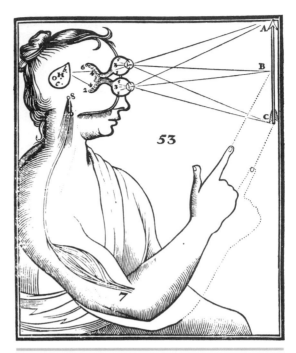

Figure 1.11 Seventeenth-century philosopher René Descartes's illustration of the mechanistic view of how light transmits images to the retina, stimulating nerves in the arm to produce movement. Descartes proposed, erroneously, that the mind interacts with the brain at the pineal gland. (National Library of Medicine.)

Common to eastern Mediterranean and African cultures was the belief that a god or gods sent diseases. For example, Egyptians viewed life as a balance between internal and external forces. As a result, they treated many mental disorders as integrating physical, psychic, and spiritual factors (Freedman, Kaplan, & Sadock, 1978). They conceptualized the brain as different from the mind. As in Aristotelian theory, they considered the heart the center of mind, sensation, and consciousness. In India, one of the earliest and most important medical documents, the **Atharva-Veda** (700 B.C.), proposed that the soul is nonmaterial and immortal.

During the Middle Ages, Arab countries demonstrated a humanist attitude toward the mentally ill, partly because of the Muslim belief that God loves the insane person. Because of this, the same treatments were available for the rich and poor. The treatment of mental patients was humanist and emphasized diets, baths, and even musical concerts especially designed to soothe the patient.

Ancient Chinese medical texts also discussed psychological concepts and psychiatric symptoms. For example, Chinese medical practitioners endorsed a mechanistic view of mental processes. They conceptualized many mental health disorders as illnesses or vascular disorders, as opposed to the prevailing European belief in demonic possession. The ancient Chinese medical textbook *The Yellow Emperor's Classic of Internal Medicine* (ca. 1000 B.C.) includes references to dementia, convulsions, and violent behavior. Confucian writings reflected early Chinese philosophical thought in proposing that mental functions are not distinct from physical functions and do not reside in any part of the organism, although these writings give the heart special importance as a guide for the mind. Surgeons practiced trephination in eastern Mediterranean and North African countries as early as 4000 to 5000 B.C. There is no evidence of trephination in ancient Japan, China, or Egypt. Because contributions to the development of neuropsychology by non-Western scholars remain unknown, we are left to wonder whether there may have been great discoveries or, alternatively, many of the same fallacies that Western cultures endorsed about the role of the brain on behavior.

Localization Theory

PHRENOLOGY AND FACULTY PSYCHOLOGY

Not until the nineteenth century did modern neuropsychological theories on brain function begin to evolve. Thinkers formulated them, in part, from a need not only to recognize the brain as responsible for controlling behavior, but more importantly, to demonstrate precisely how the brain organizes behavior. Early in the century, Austrian anatomist **Franz Gall** (1758–1828), borrowing perhaps from the concept of geography (the notion of borders, at a time when people were discovering and mapping new continents), postulated that the brain consists of a number of separate organs, each responsible for a basic psychological trait such as courage, friendliness, or combativeness. Gall, a distinguished Viennese physician and teacher, suggested that mental faculties are innate and depend on the topical structures of the brain. His theory sought to describe differences in personality and cognitive traits by the size of individual brain areas. He hypothesized that the size of a given brain area is related to the amount of skill a person has in a certain field. Craniology is the study of cranial capacity in relation to brain size, which indicated intelligence.

Gall's work, however, was severely limited by faculty psychology, the predominant psychological theory of that time, which held that such abilities as reading, writing, or intelligence were independent, indivisible faculties. Such

---

Table 1.1 *Definition of the Organs*

Selected "interpretations" corresponding to specific locations on the skull:

1. **Amativeness:** love between the sexes, desire to marry

2. **Parental love:** regard for offspring, pets, and so on

3. **Friendship:** adhesiveness, sociability, love of society

4. **Inhibitiveness:** love of home and country

5. **Continuity:** one thing at a time, consecutiveness

6. **Combativeness:** resistance, defense, courage, opposition

7. **Destructiveness:** executiveness, force, energy

8. **Alimentiveness:** appetite, hunger, love of eating

9. **Acquisitiveness:** accumulation, frugality, economy

10. **Secretiveness:** discretion, reserve, policy, management

Source: Wells, S. (1869). *How to read character: New illustrated hand-book of phrenology and physiognomy* (p. 35). New York: Fowler & Wells.

---

specific brain functions, therefore, were performed in isolation from functional systems in other parts of the brain. Gall also lacked statistical or methodologic theory that would have let him reliably measure the basic skills of interest to him. By assigning specific functions to particular places in the cerebral cortex, Gall formulated the basis of the **localization theory** of brain function (Table 1.1). Although Gall was wrong on most counts, he did help shape how we currently perceive brain–behavior relationships. For example, Gall correctly suggested that because their complexity is greatest in humans, the most intellectual parts of the brain are the frontal lobes. He also argued that the brain is the organ of the mind and functions are grouped within it.

From Gall's basic theory of localization, the "science" of **phrenology** was born. This theory holds that if a given brain area is enlarged, then the corresponding area of the skull will also be enlarged. Conversely, a depression in the skull signals an underdeveloped area of the cortex. It is generally accurate that skull configurations closely follow brain configurations. Phrenology, in its most popular form, involves feeling the cranial bumps to ascertain which cerebral areas are largest (Figure 1.12). Sophisticated mechanical equipment was developed, such as the phrenology cap (Figure 1.13), to accurately identify bumps and indentations on the skull to make "precise" predictions about psychological strengths and weaknesses.

Although Gall made remarkable discoveries in neuroanatomy, the theory of phrenology was entirely inaccurate. In Vienna and Paris, critics accused Gall of materialism

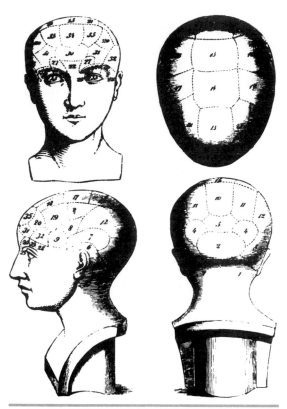

Figure 1.12 Phrenology head. Specific locations on the skull were thought to correspond to specific abilities. (National Library of Medicine.)

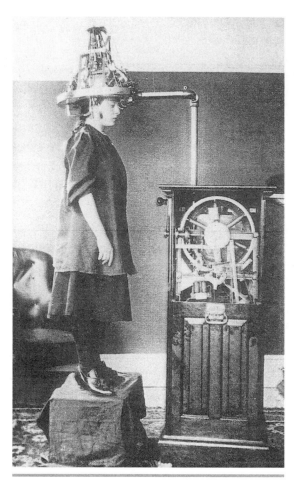

Figure 1.13 Phrenology machine (ca. 1905) was intended to measure "bumps" on the skull and correlate those with specific human attributes. (Copyright © Museum of Questionable Medical Devices.)

and ultimately forced him to leave teaching. His student **Johann Spurzheim** (1776–1832) carried on his phrenology teachings, lecturing extensively on phrenology in the United States. As a result, phrenology societies sprang up in the United States, and the movement became increasingly popular. To this day, people sometimes make attributions about an individual solely from specific physical characteristics.

Gall also played an important role in developing deterministic thought about the functions of the brain and the mind; but in the final analysis, his critics accused him of having made the most absurd theories about the faculties of human understanding. Phrenology in its simplistic form had followers who made sweeping statements about the brains and minds of men and women. Men, they suggested, have larger brain areas in the social region, with a predominance of pride, energy, and self-reliance, compared with women, whose brains reflect "inhabitiveness" (love of home) and a lack of firmness and self-esteem. Phrenologists also attempted cross-cultural comparisons, suggesting that the skulls of races and nations differ

widely in form (Neuropsychology in Action 1.1). Erroneously, phrenologists (largely white individuals) suggested that the skulls of white people were superior, indicating great intellectual power and strong moral sentiment. The skulls from "less advanced races" did not fare as well, because those virtues were thought to be almost invariably small in "savage" and "barbarous tribes" (Wells, 1869).

The promise of finding anatomic differences that could explain even complex social and intellectual behaviors is, for some scientists, still quite tempting. Controversy exists whether the brains of murderers and geniuses are indistinguishable or different. Scientists in the former Soviet Union preserved and studied the brains of famous communists to identify their "intellectual superiority." In the United States, Albert Einstein has been

Neuropsychology in Action 1.1

The Brain of a Nazi

by Eric A. Zillmer

Borrowing on ideas of Gall and Spurzheim, the Nazi propaganda leadership suggested that natural biological traits decide the total being of a person, and they challenged those who sought to explain personality on any basis other than a biological or racial one. Of course, the Nazis erred in refusing to recognize complex contributing environmental and social influences that also shape and determine behavior and individual differences. But U.S. armed forces leadership was also invested in the same fallacy, trying to demonstrate that there may be something biologically wrong with the Nazis. For example, in 1945, the U.S. Army ordered a postmortem autopsy of Robert Ley's brain, a high-ranking Nazi Labor Front boss, after he had committed suicide while waiting to stand trial at the International Military Tribunal in Nuremberg. Allied doctors argued that deterioration in Ley's frontal lobes as a result of an old head injury explained his criminal behavior, which included violent anti-Semitism. Army pathologists concluded that "the [brain] degeneration was of sufficient duration and degree to have impaired Dr. Ley's mental and emotional faculties and could well account for his alleged aberrations in conduct and feelings" ("Dr. Robert Ley's Brain," 1946, p. 188).

That the U.S. Army and the American public had an investment in the pathology of Ley's brain is ironic, because the Nazis themselves expended much effort to demonstrate, through pseudomedical research using principles based on phrenology, that the skulls of *Untermenschen* ("subhumans") were biologically inferior. In a morbid display of unethical medicine, Nazi doctors at concentration camps routinely sent postmortem specimens of the targeted groups to Berlin to exhibit and demonstrate inferiority (Lifton, 1986). In the same mode, the American public and media were invested in viewing the Nuremberg gang as biologically and psychologically abnormal. After World War II, British and U.S. psychiatrists went so far as to suggest that one could detect a Nazi by phrenology. They argued that Rudolf Hess, Hitler's deputy, had specific anatomic features, including an "extreme primitive skull formation and misshapen ears," that could serve as possible warning signals in spotting future Nazis (Rees, 1948).

The neuropathologic evidence that Ley's brain was abnormal actually turned out to be weak and undoubtedly distorted by the significant external pressure to find something wrong with the Nazis at Nuremberg. Interestingly, after the execution of the 11 high-ranking Nazi leaders at Nuremberg, scientists asked to perform additional autopsies, particularly histologic studies of the Nazis' brains (Zillmer, Harrower, Ritzler, & Archer, 1995). The authorities denied this request, however, because the bodies were to be cremated at the Dachau concentration camp and the ashes disposed of secretly. Currently, the remains of Ley's brain are kept at the U.S. Army Institute of Pathology in Washington, DC.

Although a variety of functional and organic disturbances may lead to aggression and violent behavior, most violence (e.g., domestic violence) is committed by people with no diagnosable brain impairment. Phrenology has always been a tempting theory, because it reduces complex racial views to simple physical observations. For example, when my mother studied physics at the University of Vienna during the early 1940s, the Nazi authorities did not have much interest in the study of individual differences. A required course during the Nazi occupation was Rassenkunde (Racial Theory), which replaced psychology and philosophy.

The final analysis of the Nazi data suggested that the Nazis could not plead "brain damage" in the court of universal justice. There was no specific biological or even psychological inclination found toward violence, aggression, or sadism. The Nazis were not deranged in a clinical sense. Crazy was not the answer. The Nazis came in a variety of stripes. Hitler's men were more different from each other than they were alike (Kennedy & Zillmer, 2006).

---

preserved in storage for later analysis. Einstein's brain, the focus of several studies, may be anatomically larger in strategic areas that may partly explain his uncommon ability for conceptual and multidimensional thinking (Witelson, Kigar, & Harvey, 1999). Most neuroscientists, however, agree that the idea of explaining a person's personality and abilities from neuroanatomic evidence is premature (Figure 1.14.)

Faculty psychology and discrete localization theory continued to develop for a century. Many factors were erroneous and simplistic, but three major developments represented significant progress. First, scientists were reluctant to accept a single part or component of the brain as responsible for all behavior, as had proponents of earlier theories. Second, they placed more emphasis on the role of the cortex, which until then had not been seen as functioning neural tissue but as relatively unimportant protective "bark" ("cortex" in Latin). Third, and perhaps most important, scientists focused on the brain for their study of behavior and the mind.

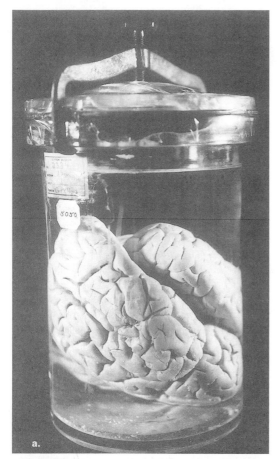

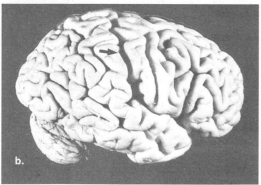

Figure 1.14 (a) Preserved brain of murderer John Wilson. In a widely publicized case in 1884, Wilson admitted to killing Anthony Daly in a fit of rage. Wilson attacked the former butcher with a cleaver to the forehead and then dismembered him. Phrenologists argued that murderers "generally have the forehead villainously low." (b) Brain of Albert Einstein. Much controversy exists whether the physicist's brain is in any way superior anatomically to the brain of a "normal" person. (a: Courtesy Mütter Museum, College of Physicians of Philadelphia; b: Reproduced from Witelson, S. F., Kigar, D. L., & Harvey, T. [1999]. The exceptional brain of Albert Einstein. *Lancet, 353,* 2149–2153, by permission.)

THE ERA OF CORTICAL LOCALIZATION

Before the nineteenth century, people knew little about the cortex of the brain. Almost completely unexplored as to their functions, cerebral convolutions were not considered the least bit interesting. Scientific evidence supporting a localization position was not available until 1861, when **Paul Broca** (1824–1880) announced to the medical community that motor speech was specifically located in the posterior, inferior region of the left frontal lobe. Before Broca's time, what he called this "grotesquely shaped, fast-decaying, and unmanageable organ" had attracted few investigators (Schiller, 1982).

Broca's accomplishments in his 56 years of life are impressive. Even nonhistorians know about his work in surgery, neuroanatomy, neurophysiology, and neuropathology. Broca, who was sympathetic to Charles Darwin's concept of evolution by natural selection (*On the Origin of Species,* 1859), was also the founder of French anthropology. In fact, because of his stature in that field, he was one of the first to have been presented with a trephined skull recovered from a Peruvian burial site. Broca dismissed the evidence, however, as merely a "hole in the head," because he was biased about "primitive" cultures and their ability for intellectual thought.

Broca's landmark contribution was in understanding the origins of **aphasia** (Neuropsychology in Action 1.2). In Paris, he was a professor of surgery, but contributed most to advancing the field of brain anatomy. Broca presented two clinical cases to support his proposal for the locus of speech. Both individuals had fairly extensive injuries, involving lesions in the left posterior frontal lobe, corresponding paralyses on the right side, and motor speech deficits; but in other respects, they appeared to be intelligent and normal. From his investigations, Broca described the condition of aphasia (often called *Broca's aphasia* or *nonfluent aphasia*), an inability to talk because the musculature of speech organs do not receive appropriate brain signals. Broca's announcement, hailed by many as a major breakthrough, led to numerous investigations into the localization of other higher cognitive functions. Broca, of course, supported other localizationists by proposing that behavior, in this case, expressive speech, is controlled by a specific brain area. It was also one of the first discoveries of a separation of function between the left and right hemispheres of the brain. But most important, it was one of the first indications that specific brain functions exist in particular locales in the brain. There is a connection, or so it seemed, between the anatomy of the brain and what the brain does.

Contemporary research methodology proposes that to attribute a precise cognitive function to a specific anatomic

Neuropsychology in Action 1.2

Paul Broca: A Manner of Not Speaking

by Eric A. Zillmer

Paul Broca identified a specific area on the convoluted surface of the human brain, approximately 1 cubic centimeter (cm³) in size, as the central organ for expressive speech. Broca's famous discovery came at a time when he viewed the convolutions of the brain as distinct organs. The evidence for this, however, was particularly weak, and phrenology was receiving some criticism. Thus, it was not a coincidence that Broca made such a discovery. He had been searching for some time for a patient just like Monsieur Leborgne. In May 1861, Broca presented the brain of Leborgne, alias "Tan," a 51-year-old man who had died the previous day under Broca's care:

> "I found one morning on my service a dying patient who 21 years ago had lost the faculty of articulate speech. I gathered his case history with the greatest care because it seemed to serve as a touchstone for the [localization] theory of my colleague. The patient died on April 17 [1861] at 11 A.M. The autopsy was performed as soon as possible, that is to say within 24 hours. The brain was shown a few hours later in the Société d'Anthropologie, then immediately put in alcohol." (Schiller, 1982, pp. 177–178)

"The abolition of speech is a symptom of sufficient importance, that it seems useful to designate it by a special name. I have given it the name aphemia [the term was later changed to *aphasia* by a colleague of Broca's, Professor Trousseau]. For what is missing in these patients is only the faculty to articulate words." (Schiller, 1982, pp. 180)

"Although I believe in the principle of localization, I have been and still am asking myself, within what limits may this principle apply? If it were demonstrated that the lesions, which abolish speech constantly, occupy the same convolution then one could hardly help admitting that this convolution is the seat of articulated speech." (Schiller, 1982, pp. 182)

Probably no other single preserved human brain has aroused more attention than the one Broca was describing. Some criticized the manner of its preservation (in an unorthodox vertical position) and the damage to the brain involving chronic and progressive softening of the second and third left frontal convolutions, as well as the specimen's unavailability for examination (Figure 1.15). Broca responded to his critics, "I have refrained from studying the deeper parts (of the brain), in order not to destroy the specimen, which I thought should be deposited in the (Dupuytren) museum" (Schiller, 1982, p. 180).

Tan's history has often been told, but his basic disease has never been satisfactorily diagnosed. Broca's acquaintance with this patient lasted barely a week. Neither the history nor the appearance and description of the brain allow a confi-

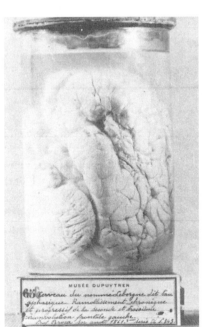

Figure 1.15 Leborgne's brain. Note atrophy in Broca's area. (Courtesy Museé Dupuytren.)

dent clinical and pathologic interpretation in modern terms. Leborgne had been epileptic since his youth and became aphasic at the age of 30. He showed progressive weakening on his right side since the age of 40, first in the arm. He became hemiplegic and was bedridden for 7 years. Leborgne deteriorated gradually, losing his intellect and vision, and finally died at 51 of cellulitis with gangrene of the paralyzed right leg. His early history of epilepsy arouses the suspicion that successive thrombotic infarcts might not have been the correct diagnosis, and that perhaps a form of degenerative disease may be more plausible. He was also known to have cursed when he was disturbed, which may also suggest that aphasia was the least of his problems (however, as we discuss in later chapters, cursing and grunts may be actually controlled by the right hemisphere, which does not dominate speech). In retrospect, Leborgne's history suggests that many other symptoms accompanied his aphasia. It now appears that Leborgne was a poor choice as the prototype for Broca's aphasia. If Broca had had a statistical consultant, he would have been advised not to make such sweeping conclusions based on only one subject!

Just as Broca preserved Leborgne's brain for safekeeping, he would have been pleased to know that his own brain also has been stored in the Museum de l'Homme (Museum of Man) in Paris. There, deep in the museum in a remote, musty corner among abandoned cabinets and shelves hidden from the public, is a collection of gray convoluted objects stored in formaldehyde. Among them is the brain of Paul Broca. If you look closely, you can detect the small region in the third convolution on the left frontal lobe of the cerebral cortex that made him famous—Broca's area!

section of the brain, research must meet two conditions. The first condition, which Broca did demonstrate, is that destruction of a localized brain site impairs a specific function, in this case, articulate speech. The second condition, which Broca did not demonstrate, relates to that damage to any other area of the brain—for example, the patient's right frontal lobe—should not result in the same deficit. This second condition is called **double dissociation** (Teuber, 1950) and requires that "symptom A appear in lesions in one structure but not with those in another, and that symptom B appear with lesions of the other but not of the one" (Teuber, 1959, p. 187). Nevertheless, although Broca may not have followed the standards of modern science, to an important extent, articulate speech is, in fact, localized in and controlled by Broca's area.

A decade after Broca's discovery, **Carl Wernicke** (1848–1904) announced that the understanding of speech was located in the superior, posterior aspects of the temporal lobe (Wilkins & Brody, 1970). Wernicke noted that no motor deficit accompanied a loss of speech comprehension caused by damage in this area; only the ability to understand speech was disrupted. That is, the patient was still able to talk, but his speech made no sense and sounded like some unknown foreign language. Such speech was called **fluent aphasia** (Geschwind, 1965). Although Wernicke, who like Broca has an area of the brain named after him (Figure 1.16), supported localizationists by locating a specific area important for word comprehension, he also demonstrated that language is not strictly localized. Broca's area, or expressive speech, is in the frontal

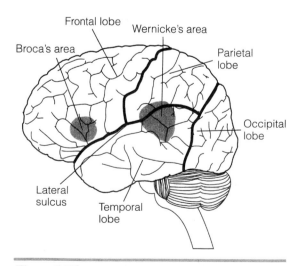

Figure 1.16 Broca's area and Wernicke's area. (Adapted from Heller, K. W. [1996]. *Understanding physical, sensory, and health impairments* [p. 52, Figure 4.7]. Pacific Grove, CA: Brooks/Cole.)

lobes, and Wernicke's area, or receptive speech, is posterior to that, in the temporal lobe. As a result of Wernicke's work, theories of strict localization have become less feasible because speech is not located in one specific location of the cortex, but rather in two distinct cortical areas.

CRITICS OF CORTICAL LOCALIZATION

Sigmund Freud (1856–1938) is best known as the founder of psychoanalysis. Yet Freud's initial love was for investigating the secrets of the central nervous system (Neuropsychology in Action 1.3). Freud, who made significant discoveries in the area of brain-behavior relationships, never gained the respect that he deserved for his work as a neurologist. In *Zur Auffassung der Aphasien* (An Understanding of Aphasia) (1891), Freud criticizes Wernicke's and Broca's localization doctrine of aphasia. At the time of Freud's publication, many neurologists confronted the task of explaining the many partial and mixed varieties of aphasias. We now know that aphasia comes in a variety of "flavors," including the inability to speak spontaneously, the inability to repeat words, the inability to read words yet being able to read letters, and so on. Wernicke proposed that for each different syndrome there was one corresponding specific lesion in the connections between Wernicke's and Broca's areas that would account for the disturbance. The more combinations of aphasic disturbances that he observed, however, the more complicated became Wernicke's diagrams. To simplify Wernicke's diagrams, Freud suggested that various aphasias could be explained by subcortical lesions in less localized association pathways. Freud pointed out, quite correctly, that the Broca and Wernicke centers are little more than nodal points in a general and complicated network of neurons. Freud proposed that Broca's and Wernicke's areas were not self-acting agencies and their significance was simply due to their anatomic location (in the former case, to the motor areas of the brain, and in the latter, to the entry of the fibers from the acoustic nuclei). Freud also described the distinction between the ability to recognize an object and the inability to name it, **agnosia;** this term remains in use today.

Is the whole greater than the sum of its parts? Clinical observation did not validate the idea that each skill is controlled by a circumscribed part of the brain. Localizationists could not explain findings, reported by numerous physicians, that lesions in widely disparate parts of the brain, not one specific area, impaired the same skill. Moreover, many patients with lesions in a specific brain area could still perform a skill assigned exclusively to that area.

Pierre Flourens (1794–1867) was the foremost early advocate of an alternative to localization theories (Krech,

Neuropsychology in Action 1.3

Sigmund Freud: The Neurologist

by Eric A. Zillmer

Freud entered the University of Vienna in the autumn of 1873, at the early age of 17, and graduated with a medical degree in 1881. Considering an academic research career in physiology, he went to work in the laboratory of the Brücke Institute. There he enjoyed laboratory work and, initially, harbored an aversion to the clinical practice of medicine. Beset by financial difficulties, in May 1883, he began working under Meynert, a neurosurgeon and psychiatrist, to gain additional practical experience. During this time, Freud came closer to disorders of the brain, but he restricted his laboratory work to dissecting the nervous system. At first, Freud investigated the cells of the spinal cord, the part of the nervous system that held his chief interest. For the next 2 years, he concentrated on a specific area of the brainstem, the medulla, that resulted in three published articles. From October 1885 to February 1886, Freud visited Paris to study with the great neurologist Jean-Martin Charcot. Charcot was then at the zenith of his fame. No one, before or since, had so dominated the world of neurology, and for Freud to have been a pupil of his was a passport to distinction.

When Freud went to Paris, his anatomic interests were still more in his mind than any ambition as a clinician. On his return to Vienna, he researched topics of visual field deficits, hemianopsia, in children and its localization. From correspondence, it is also known that in 1887 and 1888 Freud was working on a book on the anatomy of the brain, which he never finished (Jones, 1981). His next publication in 1891 was his first book *Zur Auffassung der Aphasien* (An Understanding of Aphasia). Freud thought this text the most valuable of his neurologic writings, although it proved not to be the one by which neurologic circles remembered his name. Despite Freud's critical and speculative monograph on aphasia, which ultimately achieved acceptance, he did not have much luck with his book. Of the 850 copies printed, only 257 had sold after 9 years, and Freud was paid only $62 in royalties (Jones, 1981). The neurologic community was not yet ready for his insights, and all historical writings on aphasia omit any reference to the book. Yet his neurologic achievements were remarkable, especially for a young student, and they illustrate his biological and genetic outlook.

In retrospect, Freud's psychoanalytic model can be loosely related to brain processes. For example, Freud's id, the unconscious "beast in the basement" that operates on the pleasure principle, might have developed out of the reptilian brain, a product of presocial evolutionary history. Freud's superego, our conscience, is an evolutionarily more recent invention, conceptualized within prefrontal lobe processes that are involved in forming such abstract concepts as morality, guilt, planning, and inhibition. At this highest, most complex level of brain structure, a major function is to inhibit the spontaneous expression of the more biologically programmed patterns of behavior that arise from lower and evolutionary older structures of the brain such as the id. The ego, based on the reality principle, is perhaps related to complex brain processes in the "middle," that is, the cortex, excluding the prefrontal lobes (Wright, 1994). It is often difficult to trace threads between Freud's subsequent focus on unobservable, intrapsychic events and his early investigation of the nervous system. He never did, however, venture too far away from his neurologic roots, as demonstrated in his work *On Narcissism* (1959), in which he suggested that all provisional ideas on psychology will one day be explained by organic substrates.

1962). Through an extensive number of experiments and logical arguments, Flourens attempted to disprove Gall's localization theory. To support his beliefs, Flourens developed the **ablation experiment,** in which removing any part of the brain in birds led to generalized disorders of behavior. From his experiments, he reached several general conclusions. Sensory input at an elementary level is localized, but the process of perception involves the whole brain. Loss of function depends on the extent of damage, not on the location. All cerebral material is **equipotential;** that is, if sufficient cortical material is intact, the remaining material will take over the functions of any missing brain tissue. Flourens suggested that the brain operated in an integrated fashion, not in discrete faculties, and that mental functions depend on the brain functioning as a whole. Thus, the size of the injury, rather than its location, determines the effects of brain injury.

Flourens, however, was criticized on a number of different points. First, he used animals with brains so small that any ablation would invade more than one functional area. Second, he observed only motor behavior—that is, behaviors such as eating or wing flapping—whereas the localizationists were mostly interested in more complex faculties such as friendship or intellect. Flourens also erroneously suggested that humans use only 10% of the brain, an idea that laypeople still commonly hold today. Despite these scientific problems, many accept Flourens as having refuted localization theory. Nevertheless, the work of Broca and other localization theorists was the predominant view of brain–behavior relationships and was in large part accepted by the scientific community. Consequently, few people supported Flourens's work until the early 1900s, when equipotentialists again began to develop evidence and research to support their position.

Localization versus Equipotentiality

Pierre Marie (1906) challenged Broca's findings by examining the preserved brains of the patients Broca had used to support his hypothesis of localization. Marie found that Leborgne had widespread damage, not a specific lesion, as Broca had suggested. Marie attacked Broca's theory, indicating that the patient could not speak because the extensive lesion had caused a general loss of intellect, rather than a specific inability to speak. Other researchers soon expressed support for the equipotentiality position. In general, these researchers proposed that, although basic sensorimotor functions may be localized in the brain, higher cortical processes were too complex to confine to any one area.

Two important neuropsychological findings also challenged strict localization theory. In 1881 (cited by Blakemore, 1977), **Hermann Munk** (1839–1912) found that experimental lesions in the association cortex of a dog produced temporary **mind-blindness:** The animal could see objects but failed to recognize their significance (e.g., as objects of fear). In the experiment, Munk first had the dogs learn to associate the shape of a triangle with fear by pairing them together with an electric shock. After the dogs learned the association, Munk lesioned parts of the cortex that were not primarily involved with vision. Afterward, the dogs could see the object but could not perceive the meaning of the stimuli to which they were conditioned before the surgery. In 1914, **Joseph Babinski** (1857–1932), the founder of neurology, introduced the term *anosognosia,* which means "no knowledge of the disease," to describe an inability or refusal to recognize that one has a particular disease or disorder, thereby introducing the phenomenon of unawareness (Babinski & Joltran, 1924). Babinski observed patients who had lesions, most often in the association cortex of the right hemisphere. These patients were capable of seeing and hearing, but denied that anything was wrong with them even when they had severe neurologic damage such as hemiplegia.

Karl Lashley (1890–1958), a student of the famous behaviorist John Watson, was a great exemplar of experimental neuropsychology and, according to Hebb (1983),

practically its founder. He was one of the first to combine behavioral sophistication in experiments with neurologic sophistication. Lashley become America's most eminent early neuropsychologist, highly respected for his ingenuity in devising ways of disclosing the effects of brain operations (Popplestone & McPherson, 1994). Although Lashley accepted the localization of basic sensory and motor skills, he supported equipotential views with experiments on rats similar to those of Flourens on birds (Lashley, 1929). Lashley found that impairment in maze running in the rat was directly related to the amount of cortex removed. He stated that the specific area removed made little difference. From his experiments, Lashley formulated his famous principle of **mass action:** The extent of behavioral impairments is directly proportional to the mass of the removed tissue. Lashley also emphasized the multipotentiality of brain tissue: Each part of the brain participates in more than one function (Teuber, Battersby, & Bender, 1960). Lashley believed that his results were highly compatible with a view that brain tissue is equipotential and can be involved in tasks other than those assigned by the localizationists.

In one form or another, localization and equipotentiality have dominated U.S. psychology, although neither approach has enjoyed universal acceptance because neither can encompass all the collected scientific data and clinical observations. Clinical observers of medical patients with very small lesions have often reported marked behavioral deficits, even though the lesion may be microscopic. Thus, equipotentiality theory fails to account for the specific deficits often seen in the absence of general impairment in intellect, abstract attitude, perception, or other global ability.

Integrated Theories of Brain Function

JACKSON'S ALTERNATIVE MODEL

Unable to accept either the localization or equipotentiality models of brain function, psychologists and neurologists have searched for other alternative models. The creation of one such model has been credited to the English neurologist **Hughlings Jackson** (1835–1911), whose primary work was written during the second half of the nineteenth century, but was not published in the United States until the 1950s. Jackson, a London neurologist, devoted his research to the investigation of epileptic seizures and the study of connections between limb movements and specific areas in the brain. Jackson observed that higher mental functions are not unitary abilities, but consist of simpler and more basic skills. He suggested that one does not have a speech center; rather, one has the ability to combine certain basic skills, such as hearing, discrimination of speech sounds, and fine-motor and kinesthetic control of the speech apparatus, to create more complex higher skills (Hebb, 1959). Consequently, the loss of speech can be traced to the loss of any one of a number of basic abilities or functional systems. It can be related to, for example, the loss of motor control, the loss of adequate feedback from the mouth and tongue, a defect in the understanding and use of the basic parts of speech, or the inability to decide to speak.

Thus, the loss of a specific area of the brain causes the loss or impairment of all higher skills dependent on that one area. Furthermore, a lesion that causes the loss of speech does not necessarily indicate that the brain area responsible for speech has been found. Jackson proposed that localizing damage that destroys speech and localizing speech are two different things. Jackson also believed that behavior can exist on many different levels within the nervous system. Thus, a patient may be unable to repeat the word "no" when asked to repeat it, even though the patient is capable of saying, in exasperation, "No, Doctor, I can't say no!" (Luria, 1966). In the first instance, the patient cannot say the word voluntarily. When the word is given as an automatic response, however, the patient is able to say it. The ability to say "no" exists as two separate skills: one voluntarily and one automatic. Each ability can be impaired independently of the other. Because of this, Jackson noted, behavior rarely is lost completely unless the damage to the brain is severe (Golden, Zillmer, & Spiers, 1992).

Jackson suggested that, given his observations, behavior results from interactions among all the areas of the brain. Even the simplest motor movement requires the full cooperation of all the levels of the nervous system, from the peripheral nerves and the spinal cord to the cerebral hemispheres. In this regard, Jackson pointed toward a more holistic, nearly equipotential view of brain function. But Jackson also argued that each area within the nervous system had a specific function that contributed to the overall system. Thus, his views also had a localizationist flavor. In actuality, of course, Jackson's views were those of neither school but reflected an integration of significant empirical data. Jackson's influence can first be seen in British neurology of the early twentieth century, although many people overlooked the essential nature of what Jackson had proposed. They interpreted his work as more supportive of an equipotentiality

view of higher mental functions than it actually was. Since World War II, many major theorists have presented views compatible with Jackson's. For example, Harlow (1952) concluded from his experimental monkey studies that no cognitive ability is completely destroyed by any limited lesion, although there appears to be some localization, a view entirely consistent with Jackson's beliefs. After reviewing much of the literature, Krech (1962) also reached two similar conclusions (Chapman & Wolff, 1959). First, no learning process or function depends entirely on any one area of the cortex. Second, each area within the brain plays an unequal role in different kinds of functions. These conclusions, although contrary to either the localization or equipotentiality views, were also in accordance with Jackson's alternative approach.

LURIA'S FUNCTIONAL MODEL

The most detailed adaptation of the principle first suggested by Jackson has appeared in the work of Russian neuropsychologist **Alexander Luria** (1902–1977). Luria was responsible for the most profound changes in our approach to understanding the brain and the mind. Luria, who earned doctoral degrees in psychology, medicine, and education, was the most significant and productive neuropsychologist of his time, and during the 1960s, he raised the field to a level that could not have been imagined. Luria realized that a viable brain–behavior theory must not only explain data that fit both the localization and equipotentiality hypothesis but also must account for findings inconsistent with either theory. Luria—building on the work of his mentor and arguably the founder of cognitive psychology, Vygotsky (1965) as well as on Jackson's alternative approach (Hebb, 1959)—conceived each area in the central nervous system as being involved in one of three basic functions, which Luria labeled *units*. The first unit, roughly defined as the brainstem and associated areas, regulates the arousal level of the brain and the maintenance of proper muscle tone. The second unit, including posterior areas of the cortex, plays a key role in the reception, integration, and analysis of sensory information from both the internal and external environments. The third unit, the frontal and prefrontal lobes, is involved in planning, executing, and verifying behavior (Luria, 1964, 1966).

All behavior requires the interaction of those three basic functions. Consequently, all behavior reflects the brain operating as a whole. At the same time, each area within the brain has a specific role in forming behavior. The importance of any one area depends on the behavior to be

Neuropsychology in Action 1.4

The Walter Freeman Lobotomies: Mind over Matter?

by Eric A. Zillmer

Freeman saw his mission as severing the fibers of a sick mind. He believed that most psychiatric patients' mental illnesses were related to "confused" neurologic processes, and that an appropriate surgical cut would free the patient of that confusion (Freeman & Watts, 1950). Over the span of 20 years, Freeman performed more than 3,500 lobotomies across the United States and pioneered the transorbital lobotomy. Freeman recommended lobotomies for any patient who had been institutionalized for more than 2 years, regardless of the patient's diagnosis or response to other therapy. The actual transorbital procedure consisted of initially anesthetizing the patient, typically achieved by electroconvulsive shock, with which the psychiatrist was familiar. Next, the patient's frontal lobes were pierced with an ice pick–like surgical instrument, a leukotome, inserted through the orbital cavity and passed through the orbital plate into the prefrontal region of the cortex, often "accompanied by an audible crack" (El-Hai, 2005, p. 185). The psychiatrist swung the handle of the surgical instrument laterally and medially, "windshield wiper fashion," to sever the

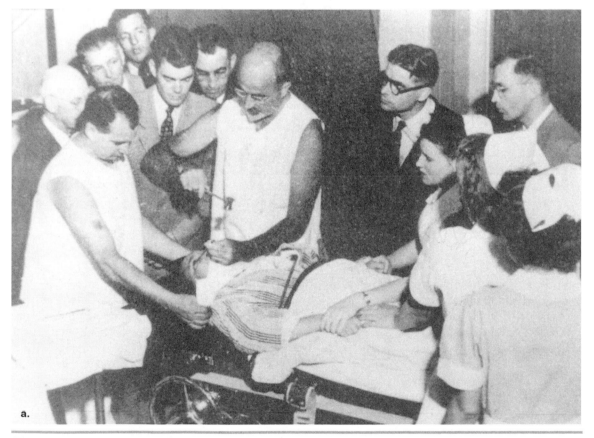

a.

Figure 1.17   (a) Dr. Freeman performing a lobotomy. According to Freeman, lobotomies should be performed in every patient if conservative therapy fails. (b) Lobotomy leukotome with Freeman's name engraved at the handle. Freeman suggested that, even though the risk for infections was low, different leukotomes be used for the two frontal lobes because of hygienic reasons. (c) Electroconvulsive shock apparatus (ca. 1950s). Lobotomy patients were anesthetized using electroconvulsive shock to the brain. After an induced seizure, the patient was typically in a dazed and confused state, during which the lobotomy was performed. (a: © Bettmann/CORBIS; b, c: Courtesy Mütter Museum, College of Physicians of Philadelphia.)

fibers at the base of the frontal lobe (Valenstein, 1973). The complete procedure took less than 10 minutes and could be performed in an office by a psychiatrist and one assistant (Figure 1.17).

Between 1940 and 1954, approximately 40,000 to 50,000 psychiatric patients, most diagnosed as schizophrenic, underwent prefrontal orbital lobotomies in their doctors' efforts to decrease inappropriate behavior whereas increasing ease of patient management. Although doctors claimed that many of these patients subjected to prefrontal lobotomies were "cured," some patients died and a large number showed dangerous side effects, including confusion, flat affect, impulsive-

ness, continued psychotic episodes, and deteriorated intellectual functioning (Glidden, Zillmer, & Barth, 1990). Furthermore, because a major function of the frontal lobes is to inhibit behavior, many lobotomized patients actually developed new symptoms (such as incontinence, inappropriate affect, violent behavior, and so forth). When I was a fellow in neuropsychology, I once evaluated an elderly schizophrenic woman. In reviewing the medical chart, I was surprised to learn that Freeman had operated on the same patient more than 30 years earlier. Freeman's medical note was still in the patient's medical chart, detailing the more gruesome aspects of this so-called treatment:

July 2, 1953 PRE-LOBOTOMY EXAMINATION: This patient looks quite a bit younger than her given age of 42. She stands with her head bowed and relatively little change of expression on her face. For the most part, she answers questions with a nod of her head, or a very silent yes, and even though conflicting statements are given, she nods just the same. At times she moves her lips in a way that suggests that she is continuously hallucinating. A story of a long psychotic illness with difficult behavior and brief furloughs since 1929 indicates that the problem is a very tough one. A proposal is made in this case to accompany the transorbital operation with an injection of 10cc. blood on each side into the inferior

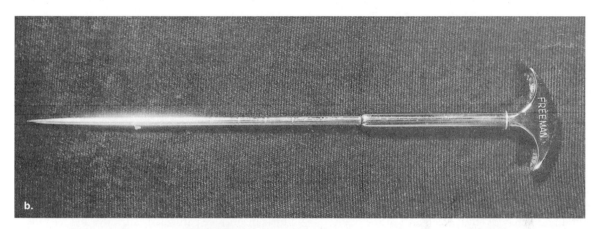

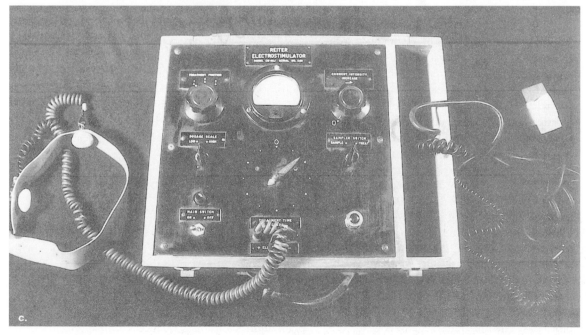

Figure 1.17   (Cont.)

(continued)

performed. For example, picking up the receiver when the phone rings—a simple, well-practiced act—requires little arousal, planning, or evaluation. A more complex behavior, such as telling a caller what you will be doing next Tuesday evening, however, requires attention and arousal, as well as planning and evaluation. An injury that has little effect on the first behavior might be disastrous for the second, more complex one.

For each behavior, Luria formulated the concept of **functional systems,** which represent the pattern of interaction among the various areas of the brain necessary to complete a behavior. Each area in the brain can operate only in conjunction with other areas of the brain. Furthermore, no area of the brain is singly responsible for any voluntary human behavior; thus, each area of the brain may play a specific role in many behaviors. As with the equipotentiality theory, Luria regards behavior as the result of interaction among many areas of the brain. As with the localization theory, Luria assigns a specific role to each area of the brain. The multifunctional role of the brain is called **pluripotentiality;** any given area of the brain can be involved in relatively few or many behaviors.

Luria suggested that behavior results from several functions or systems of brain areas, rather than from unitary or discrete brain areas. A disruption at any stage is enough to immobilize a given functional system. For example, an individual without injury to what localizationists would call the "reading center" is unable to read if there is damage to any of a number of parts of the functional systems involved in reading. Each functional system, however, has some plasticity and can change spontaneously or through retraining. For example, sensory feedback is necessary for continually knowing the location of one's fingers and arm to direct motor movement. A person who loses sensory feedback from the arm loses an important link in completing fine-motor tasks. The functional system, however, can be altered by using visual feedback to locate the fingers of

the hand, something not previously needed. The patient can thus reestablish fine-motor skills, despite the disruption of the old functional system. Luria's concept of alternative functional systems accounts for the ability of higher level brain skills to compensate for lower level skills in brain injury. This concept was demonstrated clearly in an interesting case of ours. At age 3 months, the patient had undergone a complete left hemispherectomy (removal of a hemisphere). When we saw him at age 7, not only could he walk, but he also spoke fluently. This was undoubtedly related to the plastic nature of the patient's brain, in which the right side of the brain developed the organization necessary to execute behaviors, such as speech and controlling the right side of the body.

Luria's theories are particularly attractive and relevant to clinical neuropsychologists because they can account for most observations of patients with brain injuries. The theory also explains the observation that certain lesions generally yield consistent deficits. In addition, through the concept of reorganization, Luria's theory can account for individuals who recover from brain trauma. Finally, the theory suggests ways to establish rehabilitation and treatment programs for the brain-injured patient and provides a strong theoretical basis for understanding clinical neuropsychology.

Modern Neuropsychology

Herman Ebbinghaus (1850–1909) proposed that psychology has a long past but a short history. This is true for modern neuropsychology as well. Since Broca made his momentous discovery in the 1860s, a number of major achievements and influential concepts led to the evolution of neuropsychology as a discipline as we know it today. In 1933, Kleist published his monumental work on wartime brain injuries. Although his localization approach was accepted in Germany, it was largely unknown outside that country. In the United States and Britain, the findings and conclusions of Lashley, Marie, and Jackson set up a general antilocalization bias. In particular, the field of aphasia remained divided between the "holists" and "diagram makers" such as Wernicke (Benton, 1994). The birth of modern psychosurgery was in 1935, when Moniz and Lima first attempted to alleviate mental suffering by operating on the human frontal lobes. The novelty of his concept and the "quality" of Moniz's results earned him a controversial Nobel Prize in medicine in 1949. In the 1940s, the apparently favorable effects of the surgery on the majority of severely disturbed patients led to its introduction in the United States by psychiatrist Walter Freeman and his surgical colleague James Watts. Currently, however, treating psychiatric patients with lobotomies is regarded as a step backward (Neuropsychology in Action 1.4).

Clinical neuropsychology originally emerged in the medical setting within traditional neurosurgery and neurology services. Early research was primarily concerned with the cortical functioning of patients with penetrating missile wounds or the diagnosis of neurologic disorders such as brain tumors or strokes. For example, a famous neurosurgeon who was advancing an understanding of the relationship between brain anatomy and behavior was **Wilder Penfield** (1891–1976). Penfield was educated at Princeton, Johns Hopkins, and Oxford universities and was the founder and director of the renowned Montreal Neurological Institute. He pioneered direct electrical stimulation of the brain during surgery by systematic mapping of the brain as a technique for finding damaged areas of the brain. He also used the services of psychologists as consultants to help him with the diagnosis of neurologic behavioral conditions. In the 1930s, psychologists played a large role in diagnosing brain lesions, including stroke and tumor. For example, a friend and mentor of ours, Molly Harrower, a professor emeritus at the University of Florida and inventor of the Group Rorschach, was routinely asked in the 1930s to evaluate "organic patients." In her autobiographical essay "Inkblots and Poems" (1991), she describes how as a research fellow of noted neurologist Wilder Penfield at the Montreal Neurological Institute, she was asked to perform regular diagnostic workups using the Rorschach test: "I was assigned to examine all incoming patients suspected of tumor, with re-testing 14 days postoperatively" (Harrower, 1991, p. 141). Currently, neuropsychologists play a smaller role in diagnosing neurologic disorders but an important part in evaluating functional impairment, prognosis, and recovery.

In the late 1930s, neuropsychology engaged the interest of only a few neurologists, psychiatrists, and psychologists. Neuropsychology was loosely organized, and no journals reflected a focused interest in this area. But a number of scholars were working on issues that in time made decisively important contributions to the field and shaped neuropsychology as we know it today.

The first neuropsychology laboratory in the United States was founded in 1935 by Ward Halstead at the University of Chicago. Halstead worked closely with neurosurgery patients and developed assessment devices that differentiated between patients with and without brain damage (Figure 1.18). Together with Ralph Reitan, Halstead later developed the popular **Halstead-Reitan Neuropsychological Battery,** an empirical approach to assessing brain damage (Halstead, 1947; Reitan & Wolfson, 1993).

The term *neuropsychology* itself is of recent origin and was most likely first coined by Sir William Osler in 1913, when he used the word in an inaugural address for a new psychiatric clinic at Johns Hopkins Hospital in Baltimore, Maryland (Bruce, 1985). In 1936, Karl Lashley also used the term when he addressed the Boston Society of Psychiatry and Neurology (Bruce, 1985). **Hans-Leukas Teuber** (1916–1977) is credited for first using the term in a national forum during a presentation to the American Psychological Association in 1948, during which he described different aspects of brain–behavior relationships in war veterans with penetrating brain wounds (Teuber, 1950). Then, in 1949, Canadian **Donald Hebb** published his classic, *The Organization of Behavior: A Neuropsychological Theory.* Neuropsychology has enjoyed tremendous growth ever since. The study of neuropsychology has drawn information and knowledge from many disciplines, including anatomy, biology, physiology, biophysics, and even philosophy. Thus, many interdisciplinary professionals, including neurologists, neuropsychiatrists, linguists, neuroscientists, speech pathologists, and school psychologists, are interested in the field of brain–behavior relationships and have contributed to its development.

Nevertheless, until the 1960s and Luria's writings, there was no unifying theory of brain–behavior relationships. In fact, before the 1960s, few neuropsychology practitioners existed. Those that did were primarily researchers in what is now considered experimental neuropsychology.

Between 1960 and 1990 neuropsychology was characterized by a movement from the laboratory to the clinic and the establishment of distinct neuropsychological organizations (e.g., The International Neuropsychological Society in 1967; The National Academy of Neuropsychology in 1975; and the American Psychological Association, Division 40 of Clinical Neuropsychology, in 1980). This phase also marked the creation of many scientific journals that focused exclusively on advancing the science of neuropsychology (Table 1.2).

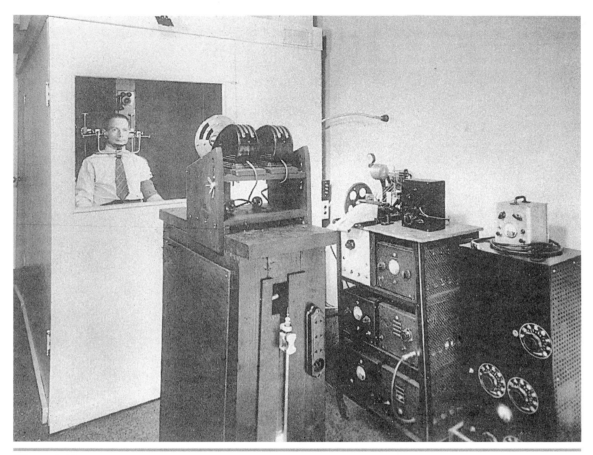

Figure 1.18 Ward C. Halstead is recording eye movements (summer, 1940). (Courtesy Archives of the History of American Psychology, David P. Boder Museum Collection, Encyclopaedia Britannica.)

Henry Hécaen (b. 1912) founded the journal *Neuropsychologia*. Hécaen, who earned his M.D. degree, made important contributions to brain–behavior relationships in health and disease. One of his discoveries, which earned him an enduring place in the history of neuropsychology,

---

Table 1.2 *Major Neuropsychology Journals*

Applied Neuropsychology

Archives of Clinical Neuropsychology

Behavioral Brain Research

Brain and Cognition

Cortex

Journal of Clinical and Experimental Neuropsychology

Neuropsychology

Neuropsychologia

---

was his demonstration of the functional properties of the right hemisphere. In the 1940s and 1950s, most scientists believed that the left hemisphere dominated the brain, because it plays an important role in the mediation of language. Hécaen and his coworkers generated an irrefutable mass of evidence that the right, supposedly minor, hemisphere played a crucial role in mediating visuoperceptual and visuoconstructional processes. Much of Hécaen's work was not translated into English from French until the 1970s (e.g., see Hécaen & Albert, 1978), and as recently as the early 1960s, scientists seldom discussed or researched issues regarding the role of the right cerebral hemisphere. The U.S. neuropsychologist **Arthur Benton** continued to explore the role of the right cerebral hemisphere in behavior (Benton, 1972). In the 1940s, Benton established one of the first neuropsychology laboratories in the Neurology Department at the University of Iowa School of Medicine, which still carries his name; he also supervised dissertations in the new field of neuropsychology and authored numerous books and neuropsychological testing instruments, including the Benton Visual Retention Test (BVRT).

Oliver Zangwill (b. 1913) founded neuropsychology in Great Britain. Zangwill, who received his M.A. from Cambridge University and saw no necessity to work for the Ph.D. degree, transformed into a clinical neuropsychologist while working in the Edinburgh Injury Unit of the British military services during World War II. There he was called on to evaluate hundreds of patients with traumatic brain lesions. Zangwill was also among the first investigators to show that hemispheric specialization for speech in left-handers did not conform to the then-accepted rule of right hemisphere dominance (Zangwill, 1960). He also contributed significantly to understanding of the nature of neuropsychological deficits associated with unilateral brain disease or injury.

Norman Geschwind (1926–1984) is another important neuropsychologist who helped to shape his profession's focus and development. Geschwind received his M.D. degree at Harvard and later single-handedly founded behavioral neurology. In 1958, he joined the staff of the neurologic service of the Boston Veterans Administration Hospital, where he made many significant contributions to neuropsychology. Among his contributions was his proposal that behavioral disturbances are based on the destruction of specific brain pathways that he called *disconnections.* He presented his idea in his now classic article "Disconnexion Syndromes in Animals and Man" (1965), which was largely responsible for reemphasizing the important role of neuroanatomy in neuropsychology. Based on his faith that anatomy must play a central role for the description and operation of many complex mental functions, Geschwind set out to prove that the dominance of the left hemisphere for speech must have an anatomic basis. He and a young colleague set out to study the morphologic features of 100 brains and determined that, indeed, there was a strong trend toward a larger auditory association cortex in the left hemisphere (Geschwind & Levitsky, 1968). This finding led to a continuing search for anatomic disparities that might be correlated with functional differences. His premature death at the age of 58 deprived behavioral neurology of its preeminent figure.

The most recent phase of modern neuropsychology, the 1990s to the present, has enjoyed unprecedented growth, and clinical neuropsychology has made important professional and theoretical contributions during the 1990s; in fact, the U.S. Congress recognized the 1990s as the "Decade of the Brain." **Muriel Lezak** is one of several neuropsychologists who pioneered the assessment approach in clinical neuropsychology. Since the late 1980s, neuropsychological assessment has played a major role in the development of clinical neuropsychology. Neuropsychological evaluations have become an important procedure, allowing the generation of useful behavioral,

Table 1.3 *Professionals Who Study the Brain*

Psychologists study behavior. Education includes an undergraduate degree in psychology and a doctoral degree (Ph.D. or Psy.D.) in an area of psychology.

Neuropsychologists are psychologists who study brain–behavior relationships. Education includes a doctoral degree in psychology and specialty (postdoctoral) training in neuropsychology.

Neurologists identify and treat clinical disorders of the nervous system, emphasizing the anatomic correlates of disease. Training includes a premed major at the college level, a doctoral degree from a medical school (M.D.), and residency training in neurology.

Neuropsychiatrists are medical doctors who have had residency training in psychiatry and are mostly concerned with the organic aspects of mental disorders, such as schizophrenia or bipolar disorder.

Neurosurgeons are medical doctors who have specialized in the surgery of nervous structures, including nerves, brain, and spinal cord.

Neuroscientists are researchers and/or teachers who have completed doctoral training in biology or related fields. They are primarily interested in the molecular composition and functioning of the nervous system.

cognitive, and clinical information about diagnosis and the impact of a patient's limitations on educational, social, and vocational adjustment. In addition to the development of new testing methods to meet special needs in diagnostic evaluation, there has been a steady increase in the use of neuropsychological assessment techniques in neurology and psychiatry and an expansion of their scope of application into other fields such as education, behavioral medicine, and gerontology. Lezak proposed that neuropsychological testing is clinically relevant and suggested a flexible approach to assessing the individual patient. She also reminded those neuropsychologists who became interested in a rather narrow subspecialty within psychology that clinical neuropsychology is firmly rooted in clinical psychology. Her classic text *Neuropsychological Assessment,* originally published in 1976, is now in its fourth edition (Lezak, Howieson, & Loring, 2004).

The popularity of neuropsychology did not occur in isolation, but was directly related to developments in other fields, including clinical (e.g., behavioral neurology, biological psychiatry, and radiology) and experimental sciences (such as neurosciences and neurochemistry) (Table 1.3).

Emerging Research Areas in Neuropsychology

Many research areas of neuropsychology in which neuropsychologists and neuropsychology students can participate are emerging. Three such areas are at the forefront of applied neuropsychological science: forensic neuropsychology; sports neuropsychology; and the neuropsychology of terrorism, law enforcement, and the military (Zillmer, 2004).

FORENSIC NEUROPSYCHOLOGY

Forensic assessment is one of the fastest growing areas in the field of clinical psychology, with an increasing number of neuropsychologists presenting and/or evaluating assessment results in the courtroom setting. Because of the expertise of neuropsychologists in psychological assessment, they have been at the forefront of performing evaluations relative to the determination of damages in personal injury cases and assistance in criminal cases. Most often, these have included the bread and butter of forensic neuropsychology, an assessment of brain injury.

Neuropsychologists have become increasingly more involved in evaluating the emotional sequelae of injury, custody evaluations, and the complex appraisal of deception and malingering in assessments performed in the forensic domain. In fact, it has become a common occurrence that a neuropsychologist is eventually confronted with some sort of forensic issue in his or her clinical work. Research in forensic neuropsychology is important because it provides the practicing clinician with scientific data and a scientific process that allows neuropsychologists to pursue his or her work with increased precision. Also, as a scientist, the forensic expert must keep abreast of new scientific techniques and research in the field of neuropsychology. The sophistication of forensic neuropsychology attests to its emergent maturity (Zillmer, 2003a). Examples of emerging research areas in forensic neuropsychology include the neuropsychology of comprehending an individual's Miranda rights; the evaluation and detection of attempts to deceive or malinger in evaluations performed in the forensic domain; and the assessment of competency to stand trial, of criminal responsibility, and of insanity (Zillmer & Green, 2006).

SPORTS NEUROPSYCHOLOGY

Much attention has been given to the study of sports-related concussions, and great strides have been made in understanding this health concern, including the cultivation of neuropsychological assessment tools to diagnose concussions and the refinement of recovery curves after injury. Concussion injuries are now thought of as significant neuropsychological events with real long-term consequences. Nevertheless, many issues related to the diagnosis, assessment, and management of concussions are akin to putting a complex puzzle together. What is the effect of age and sex in concussions? What neuropsychological tests are best suited for assessing concussions? What is the gold standard

for grading concussions? What return-to-play guidelines are most practical? Most often, the neuropsychologist's role in the area of sports-related concussions is that of a consultant (Zillmer, 2003b).

Participation in competitive sports has increased worldwide, and sports-related concussions represent a significant potential health concern to all of those who participate in contact sports. Given that there are approximately 300,000 sports-related concussions reported each year, the neuropsychologist's role in testing for concussions for purposes of diagnosis and symptom resolution is one that our profession should embrace. Moreover, for those neuropsychologists who love sports, it provides a unique opportunity to merge one's professional skills with one's affinity for sports. The neuropsychologist's training and expertise uniquely prepares him or her to play an important and rewarding role in this growing field. Examples of current research interests in this area include the return to play decisions after concussive injuries in sports (Zillmer, Schneider, Tinker, & Kaminaris, 2006), the neuropsychology of performance enhancement in competitive athletics, and the relationship between cognitive and personality factors related to sports injury and rehabilitation.

TERRORISM, LAW ENFORCEMENT, AND THE MILITARY

The surprise terrorist attacks against the United States and the devastating effects of hurricane Katrina have changed the collective psychology of our nation. Thus, there is an increased opportunity for the neuropsychology community to conduct behavioral research and consultation in law enforcement, disaster relief, and the armed forces.

Neuropsychologists have expertise that allows them to provide insight into the cognitive operations of terrorism; they can play an important role in using research in the cognitive sciences to assist in understanding the psychology of terrorism and the mindset of terrorists. In addition, neuropsychologists are in a unique position to study how the brain reacts in a crisis to investigate the optimal form of comprehending verbal information during a catastrophe, to examine the effects of anxiety among law-enforcement officials on their decision-making ability during a calamity, to understand the psychological impact of first responders, and to develop means for treating victims of terrorist attacks.

The most recent terrorism attacks and threats of chemical and biological warfare have also brought a new perspective to the psychologist's role in the military, in law enforcement (e.g., in the search for the Washington, D.C., sniper), and in the military's role in enforcing peace (e.g., Iraq, Bosnia, and Korea). The armed forces can provide some real-life experience, responsibility, and exposure for military neuropsychologists that are seldom available for their civilian counterparts. For example, each operating U.S. Navy aircraft carrier has a "resident" psychologist onboard. Neuropsychologists are also deployed as part of combat stress units in Iraq, where they evaluate and manage combat stress "on site."

Neuropsychologists are experts in the science of human decision making, and we believe that neuropsychological science can be put to good use in counterterrorism endeavors, law enforcement, and the military. Advancing neuropsychological science directly and indirectly in these areas benefits the security of our nation, as well as the discipline of neuropsychology. Research examples include military fitness for duty evaluations, preparing military members for the demands of captivity, the neuropsychology of terrorists, the neuropsychological effects of weapons of mass destruction, and the assessment and selection of operational personnel for high-risk assignments (Kennedy & Zillmer, 2006).

Table 1.4 *Time Line of Significant Developments in Neuropsychology*

2000 B.C.: Early Brain Hypotheses

Peruvian and central European cultures practice trephination

Sixth to Fourth Centuries B.C.: Ancient Greek Influences

Heraclitus (sixth century B.C.): The mind is an unreachable, enormous space

Pythagoras (580–500 B.C.): The brain is the center of human reasoning

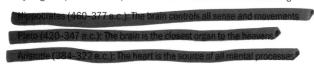

Hippocrates (460–377 B.C.): The brain controls all sense and movements

Plato (420–347 B.C.): The brain is the closest organ to the heavens

Aristotle (384–322 B.C.): The heart is the source of all mental processes

Third Century B.C. to Middle Ages: The Cell Doctrine

Alexandrian school (third to fourth century B.C.): Made advances in physiology and anatomy

Galen (Italian, A.D. 130–201): Suggested ventricular hypothesis and role of humors in health

Medieval and Renaissance Europe: Anatomic Discoveries and the Spiritual Soul

Albertus Magnus (German, ca. 1200): Deemphasized the role of the ventricles

Andreas Vesalius (Italian, 1514–1564): Corrected many historical mistakes about brain anatomy

René Descartes (French, 1596–1650): Proposed a strict split between mental and physical processes

Thomas Willis (English, 1621–1675): Made contribution to understanding the brain's vascular structure

Giovanni Lancisi (Italian, 1654–1720): Highlighted the role of the corpus callosum

Eighteenth and Nineteenth Centuries: Phrenology

Franz Gall (Austrian, 1758–1828): Personality is related to different sizes of specific brain areas

Johann Spurzheim (Austrian, 1776–1832): Intellectual capacity is related to brain size

Nineteenth-Century Europe: The Era of Cortical Localization

Paul Broca (French, 1824–1880): Motor speech is located in a small region of the left, frontal lobe.

Carl Wernicke (German, 1848–1904): Understanding of speech is located in the temporal lobe.

Nineteenth- and Twentieth-Century Critics of Cortical Localization

Sigmund Freud (Austrian, 1856–1938): Coined the term *agnosia*

Pierre Flourens (French, 1794–1867): Early advocate of an alternative tolocalization theories.

Hermann Munk (German, 1839–1912): Coined the term *mind-blindness*

Joseph Babinski (English, 1857–1932): Introduced the term *anosognosia*

Karl Lashley (American, 1890–1958): Formulated the principle of mass action in equipotentiality

Late Nineteenth- and Twentieth-Century Theories of Brain Function

Hughlings Jackson (English, 1835–1911): Claimed behavior exists on different levels in the nervous system

Alexander Luria (Russian, 1902–1977): Formulated the concept of functional systems of behavior.

Modern Neuropsychology

Karl Kleist (German, 1879–1960): Refined localization approach to neuropsychology

Wilder Penfield (Canadian, 1891–1976): Neurosurgeon who discovered direct electrical stimulation of the brain

Ward Halstead and Ralph Reitan (American, ca. 1940s): Pioneered neuropsychological testing

Donald Hebb (Canadian, 1904–1985): Published classic *The Organization of Behavior*

Henry Hécaen (French, ca. 1950s): Pioneered the role of the right hemisphere in neuropsychology

Arthur Benton (American, b. 1909): Continued to advance the role of the right hemisphere

Oliver Zangwill (British, ca. 1960s): Examined neuropsychology with traumatic brain injury

Norman Geschwind (American, 1926–1984): Founded behavioral neurology

Edith Kaplan (American, 1970s): Pioneered the process approach

Muriel Lezak (American, 1970s): Refined clinical assessment in neuropsychology

Summary

Neuropsychology has had a particularly rich history (Table 1.4), and the future is promising as well. Philosophical thought, medical practice, and religious dogma have shaped human's beliefs about the brain. Understanding "where we came from" and "where we are" shows how neuropsychology has evolved as a discipline. Furthermore, recognizing different viewpoints encourages the neuropsychology student to compare and contrast different theories. Knowledge of brain–behavior relationships is a developing science, rather than an absolute fact. In addition, we propose that neuropsychology is a paradigm of how to explain and research behavior, not just a body of knowledge. Neuropsychology is also not a separate area of research to be pursued in isolation from other models of psychology. It is distinct from physiology, however, because its direct concern is not with synapses but with behavior. In 1983, Donald Hebb suggested: "[The] neuropsychologist of the future must be a psychologist as well as a neurologist. The complexities of psychology and the complexities of neurology are the same complexities" (p. 7). We propose that neuropsychology is a natural part of psychology. We still know relatively little about the 3-pound organ that defines us, but many significant advances in recent years have brought the field to a new threshold of knowledge that has allowed researchers to identify many of the anatomic areas and functional systems within the brain that help determine behavior. The next chapter examines procedures for investigating the brain.

Critical Thinking Questions

- How does localization brain theory differ from equipotentiality brain theory? What are the lasting contributions of each theory?
- Has the quest for the search of the organ of the soul been completed?
- Why is Luria's functional model of the brain such an important step in understanding brain functions?

Key Terms

Psychology	Cell doctrine	Double dissociation	Functional systems
Neuropsychology	da Vinci, Leonardo	Wernicke, Carl	Pluripotentiality
Neurons	Galen	Fluent aphasia	Penfield, Wilder
Vitalism	Humors	Freud, Sigmund	Halstead–Reitan
Materialism	Magnus, Albertus	Agnosia	Neuropsychological Battery
Trephination	Vesalius, Andreas	Flourens, Pierre	Teuber, Hans-Leukas
Heraclitus	Descartes, René	Ablation experiment	Hebb, Donald
Pythagoras	Willis, Thomas	Equipotential	Hécaen, Henry
Brain hypothesis	Lancisi, Giovanni	Munk, Hermann	Benton, Arthur
Hippocrates	Atharva-Veda	Mind-blindness	Zangwill, Oliver
Plato	Gall, Franz	Babinski, Joseph	Geschwind, Norman
Aristotle	Localization theory	Anosognosia	Lezak, Muriel
Cardiac hypothesis	Phrenology	Lashley, Karl	
	Spurzheim, Johann	Mass action	
Ventricular localization hypothesis	Broca, Paul	Jackson, Hughlings	
	Aphasia	Luria, Alexander	

Web Connections

http://nanonline.org
National Academy of Neuropsychology—The official home page of the National Academy of Neuropsychology (NAN). This site includes information on doctoral programs in neuropsychology, annual meetings, membership information, and more.

http://www.the-ins.org
International Neuropsychological Society—The International Neuropsychological Society is a multidisciplinary organization dedicated to enhancing communication among the scientific disciplines that contributes to the understanding of brain-behavior relationships.

http://www.apa.org
American Psychological Association—The official site of the American Psychological Association (APA) provides links to student information, membership information, PsychNET, and career-planning information.

http://www.psychologicalscience.org
American Psychological Society—The American Psychological Society is dedicated to the advancement of scientific psychology and its representation at the national level. The Society's mission is to promote, protect, and advance the interests of scientifically oriented psychology in research, application, teaching, and the improvement of human welfare.

Chapter 2

METHODS OF INVESTIGATING THE BRAIN

The most important advancement in the clinical neurosciences is the imaging of the living human brain.

—Erin Bigler

The brain is the last and greatest biological frontier.

—James Watts

Neurohistology Techniques

Radiologic Procedures

Electrophysiologic Procedures

Imaging of Brain Metabolism

Magnetic Imaging Procedures

Cerebrospinal Fluid Studies: Lumbar Puncture

Behavioral Examinations

New Advances in Imaging Techniques: Mapping
   the Brain

Neuropsychology in Action

2.1 Case Example of Brainstem Auditory-Evoked
   Response

2.2 Undergoing a Magnetic Resonance Imaging
   Procedure

2.3 New Frontiers in Functional Magnetic Resonance
   Imaging

2.4 Diagnostic Neuroimaging and Neuropsychology

Keep in Mind

- What is the difference between a CT scan and an MRI?
- What does an EEG measure?
- What is functional imaging?
- What is the difference between an invasive and a noninvasive procedure?
- Are modern imaging techniques dangerous to the brain? Explain.

Overview

The primary constraint in unlocking the secrets of the brain has been the limit of available techniques and examination procedures for investigating the brain. This was certainly true for early scientists, who struggled with how inaccessible the living brain is to direct visualization. Short of performing in vivo neurosurgical procedures or postmortem examinations immediately after death, early scientists simply could not examine the living brain. As a result, study of the brain was largely speculative and inferential, and researchers have made many errors (see Chapter 1). Because of such difficulties, many famous psychologists, including William James and B. F. Skinner, insisted that the brain is not the province of psychologists. They suggested that the brain is like a "black box"—researchers cannot study the brain itself, but can associate certain inputs with specific outputs of behavior.

Since the 1970s, an explosion in technology has allowed more precise examination of the brain. During the end of the nineteenth century, researchers developed staining techniques by which they could visualize neurons. In the early part of the twentieth century, X-ray technology and pneumoencephalography allowed scientists to visualize the skull and the ventricles. The brain, however, remained elusive. This all changed in the 1970s when researchers introduced computed transaxial tomography (CT), and then magnetic resonance imaging (MRI) in the mid-1980s. These two procedures, although crude in their initial stages of development, were soon refined so that visualizing specific and detailed brain structures became possible, including visualizing asymmetries in the living brain. At the same time, other technologies, including electroencephalography (EEG), single-photon emission computed tomography (SPECT), and positron emission tomography (PET) advanced, allowing clinicians to view the brain from structural, metabolic, and electrophysiologic perspectives. For example, using PET, scientists can now measure, with three-dimensional (3-D) resolution, biochemical and physiologic processes in the human brain. More recently, the structural imaging of brain anatomy has been correlated with functional parameters of the brain, which created a new direction in brain research, namely, that of functional imaging.

These recent advances in neuroimaging dramatically changed how scientists investigate neural correlates of human behavior. These spectacular new developments are akin to changing filters in a camera, resulting in new and different images of the same picture. A "window to the brain" has opened, and so has our understanding of the brain.

This chapter summarizes the major technologic methods of examining the brain, and Chapter 3 examines neuropsychological techniques of studying the brain. We discuss advantages and disadvantages for each procedure, particularly as they relate to understanding brain–behavior relationships and disease processes. This chapter provides the neuropsychology student with background on the various investigational procedures he or she will likely encounter in the literature, research laboratory, or in clinical practice. Neuropsychologists should familiarize themselves with the basic information these techniques can provide. In fact, neuropsychologists play an important role in advancing this technology and are working side by side with radiologists and neurologists to unlock the secrets of the brain.

Neurohistology Techniques

On visual inspection of brain tissue under a microscope, one can find order to the anatomic arrangement of neurons. For example, pyramidal cell bodies in the cerebral cortex and hippocampal tissue "line up" to process neural information. For neuroscientists, the key to understanding the structures that make up the brain lies in technology that facilitates visualization of different aspects of neural tissue. One of the first ways to study neural processes involves stains; stains are chemicals that attach to specific cell structures, thereby making it possible for researchers to examine the cells visually and even count them. For more than a century, neuroscientists have developed several staining techniques to help visualize mapping fiber connections. Initially, the light microscope, invented in the 1890s, gave birth to the pioneering works of Cajal (1937) and Brodmann (1909) in cellular neuroanatomy. The introduction of the powerful electron microscope in the 1950s made it possible to analyze in detail the synaptic contacts between individual neurons. Next, we outline this remarkable progress for several classic histologic techniques.

GOLGI STAIN

One of the most remarkable developments in the neurosciences came with a discovery made by **Camillo Golgi** (1843–1926). Golgi, an Italian physician, discovered in the early 1870s that silver chromate stained dead neurons black. This remarkable breakthrough allowed, for the first time, visualization of individual neurons (Figure 2.1). The Golgi method enabled detailed study of cell process, often allowing a 3-D view of the cell and its processes. Practically overnight, the basic building blocks of the nervous system became visible. More recently, researchers have even been able to stain single neurons in a Golgi-like fashion and visualize many of the different cells that make up the brain. Using this method, they found that Purkinje cells reside in the cerebellum and have a remarkably differentiated dendritic tree (see Chapter 4). The Golgi method also led to the classification of neurons based on the length of their axon. Golgi type I neurons, for example, have long axons that transfer information from one region of the brain to another. In contrast, Golgi type II neurons are those with short axons. The Golgi method has remained in use for more than 100 years to characterize specific cell types in different regions of the nervous system.

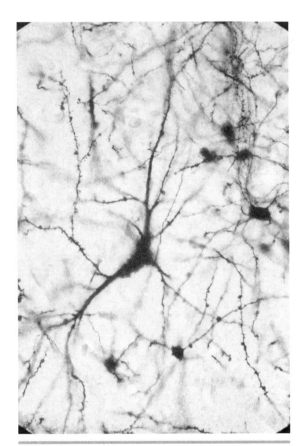

Figure 2.1 Golgi-stained neurons at 400 × magnification. (Reproduced from Kalat, J. W. [1998]. *Biological psychology,* [6th ed., p. 104]. Pacific Grove, CA: Brooks/Cole, by permission. © Martin Rotker/Photo Researchers.)

NISSL STAIN

One drawback of the Golgi stain is that it provides little information about the number of neurons in a specific brain region, because it only affects a few neurons. It also permits a view only of neural tissue in silhouette and does not allow visualization of the inner structure of the neuron. In the 1880s, **Franz Nissl** (1860–1919), a German histologist, discovered that a simple dye will selectively stain cell bodies in neurons. As a result, researchers adapted several different stains, originally developed for dyeing cloth, for histologic purposes. Methylene blue, for example, is a neural stain that has an affinity for the inner structures of neural cell bodies. One of the most popular dyes is cresyl violet, a cell body stain that is not selective for neural cell bodies, but stains all central nervous system cells. Cresyl violet facilitates the differentiation of fiber bundles, which appear lighter, and nuclei, which appear darker. Using the Nissl stain technique, scientists could then count the number of Nissl-stained dots that represented neurons in any area of the brain.

The Nissl method has become the classic microscopic method for studying the cell body and one of the most valuable techniques for studying neurons in both normal and pathologic states. The Nissl stain outlines all cell bodies and selectively stains the nucleus but not the axon. Furthermore, Nissl patterns vary among different types of neurons. For example, motor neurons have larger Nissl bodies, and sensory neurons have smaller ones. The appearance of the Nissl substance also varies with cell activity; that is, Nissl bodies disintegrate when the axon of the neuron is injured.

OTHER STAINING TECHNIQUES

The Nissl and Golgi methods are selective in their affinity for specific characteristics of neurons. The Nissl method shows the cell body, specifically the cell nucleus. Thus, it maps cell density. The Golgi method is particularly useful for investigating the distribution of dendrites and axons in individual neurons, which appear pitch-black. Scientists have developed other staining procedures specifically for studying axons. For example, **myelin staining** selectively dyes the sheaths of myelinated axons. As a result, white matter, which consists of myelinated axons, is stained black, whereas other areas of the brain that consist primarily of cell bodies and nuclei are not (Figure 2.2).

Since the 1970s, researchers have introduced new tracing methods based on the principle of axonal transport to chart previously unexplored regions and circuits of the brain. For example, the **horseradish peroxidase (HRP)** method (HRP is an enzyme found in horseradish roots) was introduced. Researchers inject HRP into a region of the nervous system, and surrounding cell bodies and axon terminals take it up. In neurons that have incorporated HRP, axonal transport carries the enzyme to other interconnected cell bodies, where researchers can detect it with a simple staining procedure. Using the axonal transport technique, neuroscientists can study the tracing of pathways in the brain. Staining remains a viable method for studying the cellular function of the nervous system and helps neuroscientists in studying the specialized contacts among neurons and their complex and often puzzling arrangements. Table 2.1 summarizes the different staining techniques used in neuroscience.

Radiologic Procedures

From the initial X-ray of the head and the practically extinct air encephalogram to sophisticated CT, the rapid progress of radiology has made a significant impact on the

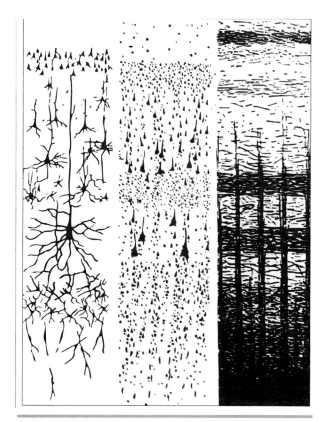

Figure 2.2 Different staining techniques of the human cortex highlight different aspects of nerve structures. (left) A Golgi stain visualizes individual cortical cells. In the middle, a Nissl-stained section shows only the cell bodies. (right) A myelin-stained section of the human brain shows the myelin coating of the axon of neurons. (Adapted from Brodal, A. [1981]. *Neurological anatomy in relation to clinical medicine* [3rd ed., p. 25, Figure 2.7]. New York: Oxford University Press, by permission.)

field of clinical neurology and neuropsychology. This section discusses the techniques involved in neuroradiology, with special emphasis on computed tomography and angiography.

Table 2.1 *Different Staining Techniques*

Nissl stain: A dye that stains the cell body of the neuron; this method is particularly useful for detecting the distribution of cell bodies in specific regions of the brain

Golgi stain: A method of staining brain tissue that marks a few selected individual cells, differentiating the cell body, as well as its extensions

Myelin stain: Shows the myelin coating of axons, rendering it useful for mapping pathways in brain tissue

Horseradish peroxidase: Allows mapping of neuronal pathways using axonal transport mechanisms; this technique works in both directions, that is, from the axon back to the cell body, and vice versa

SKULL X-RAY

Physicist **Wilhelm Conrad Röntgen** (1845–1923) made a remarkable discovery that changed the science of medicine forever and earned him the 1901 Nobel Prize in physics. Röntgen (or Roentgen, to transliterate the German *ö* into English) quite serendipitously produced an invisible ray that, unlike heat or light waves, could pass through wood, metal, and other solid materials. This ray, also called the **X-ray,** created the field of radiology. The principle of X-ray technology is the generation of Roentgen rays, electromagnetic vibrations of very short wavelength that can penetrate biological tissue and can be detected on a photographic plate. At the basis of its medical application was the principle that the diagnostic rays travel through the body at different rates according to the density of organs. The resulting picture would show clear contrast between bones and, to a lesser degree, soft parts. Researchers discovered that X-rays pass easily though low-density tissue (water) but are absorbed by high-density tissue (bone). In addition, they found that the possible harmful effects of X-rays could destroy diseased tissue, a discovery that led to radiotherapy.

Diagnostic X-ray films are useful for clinical work on various parts of the body, because they demonstrate the presence and position of bones, fractures, and foreign bodies. A clinical disadvantage of X-ray films, specifically of the head, is that they are two-dimensional (2-D). Thus, positive diagnosis of a 3-D clinical pathology is difficult. Second, an X-ray film of the head shows little differentiation between brain structures and cerebrospinal fluid (CSF), making clinical use of this procedure ineffective, with the exception of large and vascularized brain tumors or massive bleeds. Furthermore, X-rays are potentially dangerous, because they are cumulatively absorbed by high-density tissue. Thus, X-ray exposure entails a minor risk. The advantage of X-raying the head is that it uses universally available technology, is inexpensive, and provides good visualization of the skull. Thus, if there is the possibility of a skull fracture, X-ray technology remains a useful diagnostic tool (Figure 2.3).

AIR ENCEPHALOGRAPHY (PNEUMOENCEPHALOGRAPHY)

An **air encephalogram,** or **pneumoencephalogram,** is the radiographic visualization of the fluid-containing structures of the brain, the ventricles, and spinal column. It is similar to X-ray visualization, but it involves withdrawing CSF by lumbar puncture (see later); the CSF is then replaced with a gas such as air, oxygen, or helium. The gas rises and enters the ventricular system, specifically the four interconnecting cavities of the brain. Once

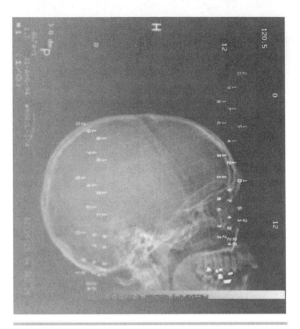

Figure 2.3 X-ray film of the head. (Courtesy Eric Zillmer.)

the gas has filled the ventricles, a technician takes a standard X-ray film of the head. Because the gas is of much lower density than the surrounding brain, the ventricles appear as a dark shadow on the X-ray film and clearly outline the surrounding brain tissue. Using this approach, a clinician can make a clinical diagnosis. The air encephalogram represented an advance on the standard X-ray film because it allowed visualization of the ventricular system.

However, patients did not tolerate the procedure well. Attendants had to turn patients in various positions, often awkwardly, and invert them in 3-D space to advance the gas to a specific ventricle before the technician could take an X-ray film. Because gas had replaced the CSF, the cushioning aspects of the CSF had been compromised, which often resulted in excruciating headaches that could last for several days before the gas was reabsorbed. Today, the more modern CT scan has replaced both the traditional X-ray image and the pneumoencephalogram.

COMPUTED TRANSAXIAL TOMOGRAPHY

Computed transaxial tomography (CT) is based on the same principle as the X-ray examination. The medical community has widely embraced CT, making it the standard technology for examining the brain.

History

CT scanning was invented in Great Britain in 1971 and introduced to the United States in 1972 (Haeger, 1988). Physicists developed the first model of transaxial tomography in part by building on dramatic advances in computer technology. Since its development, CT technology has progressed from detecting only gross brain features to visualizing highly refined structural features. Before this technology, precise neuropathologic diagnosis was difficult.

Technique

After placing the patient's head in the center of the CT scanner, the technician revolves an X-ray source around the head as detectors monitor the intensity of the X-ray beam passed through the brain. The technician does not take the images at a perfect horizontal perspective of the head. Rather, he or she slightly tilts the images at a 20-degree angle to avoid scanning the air-containing sinuses, which produce distortion because of the combination of low (air) and high (bone) density (Figure 2.4). The first (lowest) image selected is usually at the level of the foramen magnum, the base of the brain. Multiple sequential images show the ventricles, basal ganglia, thalamus, and cerebral cortex. Multiple transaxial images of the brain are obtained from many different angles. This requires a large apparatus or X-ray tube, which can rotate 360 degrees around the patient's head (Figure 2.5). The detectors, which either rotate with the X-ray scanner or are placed in a circle around the patient, are more sensitive than the traditional X-ray film. For comparison, X-ray film can detect difference of 10% to 15% in the density of soft tissue, whereas CT can measure variations as small as 1%, often pinpointing density changes as small as 2 mm in diameter.

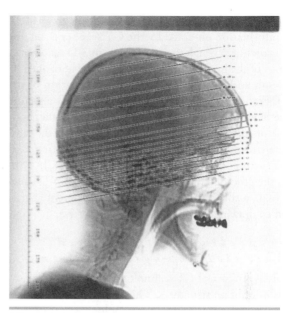

Figure 2.4 X-ray image of the head demonstrating the various "slices" of which the images are calculated. Note the absence of any differentiation of this patient's brain using X-ray technology. The 20-degree angle of the cuts is implemented to avoid rays passing through the brain sinuses at the front of the brain, which often causes distortion. (Courtesy Eric Zillmer.)

In contrast with the traditional X-ray visualization, in CT, the head is scanned using a very narrow beam. This allows for the segmentation of the brain into many different slices. Depending on the nature of the study, the slices of

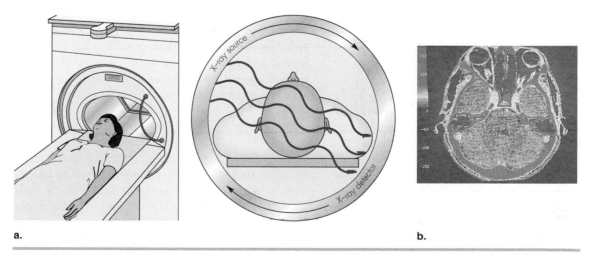

a.   **b.**

Figure 2.5 Computed transaxial tomography scanner. (a) The subject's head is placed in the scanner, which is then subjected to a rotating source of X-rays that pass through the brain at various angles. (b) A computer constructs the final image of the brain. (Reproduced from Kalat, J. W. [1998]. *Biological psychology* [6th ed., p. 106, Figure 4.28]. Pacific Grove, CA: Brooks/Cole, by permission. Photo by Dan McCoy/Rainbow.)

the brain range from thin (2 mm) to thick (up to 13 mm). The information obtained by the CT scanner is entered into a computer, which then calculates, in 3-D space, cross sections of the brain within the plane of the horizontal X-ray beam and the available density information of the brain. From these data, the computer generates a picture of the brain that can be in any orientation (sagittal, horizontal, or coronal). The complicated calculations the computer performs use the mathematics for computing solid 3-D structures based on data from a 2-D source. In principle, the procedure is similar to examining any 3-D structure (e.g., a soft drink can) from many different angles, and then drawing it from a different perspective.

Interpreting the Computed Transaxial Tomography Scan

The final product of CT technology is to produce a visualization of brain structures. This can take any form, including numbers or colors, but radiologists, not surprisingly, have favored an end result similar to the familiar X-ray film, with black-and-white shadings that reflect structure density. Accordingly, bone (high density) is white and CSF (low density) is dark. Dense collections of cell bodies, gray matter, and nuclei look darker. In contrast, myelinated pathways or white matter look lighter. Neuroradiologists complete the interpretation of CT images, which they relate to their examination of the general symmetry of the brain. Marked asymmetries of brain structures typically signal a pathologic process. Neuroradiologists also closely examine the scans for sites of abnormal densities, both **hypodensity** (associated with low density and perhaps an old lesion) and **hyperdensity** (typically signaling an abnormal density such as a tumor or a bleed). In this way, they examine the general distribution of white versus gray matter (Figure 2.6).

Enhanced Computed Transaxial Tomography

Soon after the introduction of CT, researchers realized that the brain could be X-rayed more clearly by using a contrast material that would better absorb the rays. Thus, the **enhanced CT** scan, which involves intravenously injecting an iodinated contrast agent, shows more contrast of brain structures. In the intact cardiovascular system, the contrast agent does not enter the brain because it remains contained in the vascular system. But if there is a lesion, increased vascularization (as in an arteriovenous malformation or a tumor), or a defect in the blood–brain barrier, that area shows increased contrast.

The refinement of the CT scan has made available a new generation of brain images that previously were possible

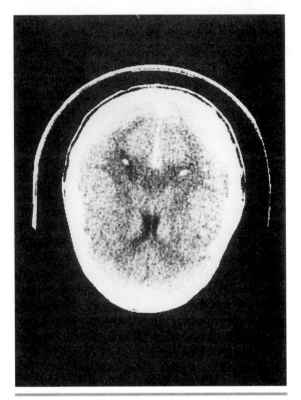

Figure 2.6 Early-generation computed transaxial tomography scan (horizontal). (Courtesy Eric Zillmer.)

only on autopsy. The CT scan has become a useful diagnostic tool because alterations caused by pathologic processes or deformation of brain structures are easily visible, even to the untrained eye. The routine availability of CT has also increased, almost overnight, the diagnosis of specific disorders. For example, small strokes, previously undetectable with X-ray technology, were all of a sudden easily diagnosed, which increased the prevalence of diagnosed multi-infarct dementia.

ANGIOGRAPHY

Angiography is the roentgenographic visualization (X-raying) of blood vessels in the brain after introducing contrast material into the arterial or venous bloodstream. Consistent and sufficient blood supply is essential for a healthy brain, and angiography has become a standard procedure for examining the integrity of the vascular system of the brain. Because the blood vessels of the brain reflect the surrounding brain tissue, angiography is a technique based on the X-ray procedure of examining the brain through its vascular system. Angiography is particularly important in diagnosing structural abnormalities in the blood vessels themselves or in their arrangement. As a result, angiography has become a useful tool in the early identification of aneurysms (a ballooning of an artery; see Chapter 12) and the subsequent prevention of stroke. To a lesser extent, clinicians can also identify other pathologies such as tumor, because they depend on increased vascularization or blood supply. Angiography also can detect shifts in cerebral arteries, which may indicate a mass-occupying lesion.

Technique

Femorocerebral angiography, developed in the mid-1950s, introduces a catheter into the arterial system. Previously, physicians injected the contrast material directly into an artery, such as the internal carotid artery, but it is safer to insert a catheter via the femoral artery. The specialist passes the preshaped, semirigid catheter through a needle inserted in the femoral artery, and then guides it up the aorta to the aortic arch with the assistance of X-ray and television monitoring. The specialist can then place the catheter into any of the three major arteries arising from the aortic arch; the brachiocephalic artery, which leads to the common right carotid artery or the right vertebral artery; the left common artery, which leads to the left internal and external carotid artery; or the left subclavian artery, which connects to the left vertebral artery (see Chapter 12 for a more detailed discussion of the vascular system of the brain). Using this technique, the specialist can position or "park" the catheter tip at various strategic places of blood supply to the brain, to examine anterior or posterior cerebral arteries. Next, an automatic injector sends an iodinated contrast agent through the catheter. At the same time, a technician takes rapid, serial X-ray films of the head over an 8- to 10-second interval in the frontal and lateral planes, providing visualization of the injected vessels and their complex intracranial branches.

Digital subtraction angiography, compared with conventional film angiography, is particularly effective in enhancing visualization of blood vessels, including the morphologic and physiologic states of the arterial, capillary, and venous phases of the cerebral circulation (Figure 2.7). In this procedure, after the images of the contrast material have been acquired, the computer stores and subtracts the X-ray image of the brain. The resulting visualization of the vascular system is easily distinguished from that of brain tissue.

Intravenous angiography is somewhat more complicated than femorocerebral angiography; therefore, clinicians do not use it as routinely. In intravenous angiography, the specialist inserts the catheter in the patient's arm but must pass it through the heart, then the lungs, and then to the left side of the heart before it reaches the aortic arch. Thus, larger amounts of contrast medium must be used, which increases the patient's risk for renal toxicity.

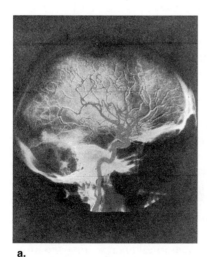

a.

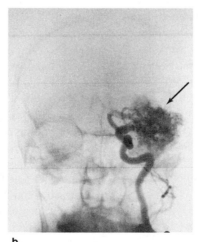

b.

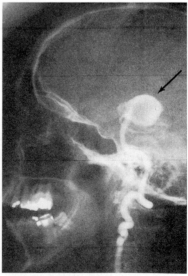

c.

Figure 2.7 Examples of angiography: (a) normal lateral view angiogram; (b) arteriovenous malformation from coronal perspective; and (c) aneurysm from lateral perspective. (a: SPL/Custom Medical Stock Photo; b: English/Custom Medical Stock Photo; c: English/Custom Medical Stock Photo.)

Clinical Use

Angiography allows, from the puncture of a single artery, the maximum radiographic detail for diagnosing intracerebral lesions. Angiography is an invasive procedure, yet it is relatively safe and well tolerated by the patient, who is awake but slightly sedated. The risk from the procedure is related to the possibility of the catheter loosening plaques in the arteries that may then separate and travel to a smaller location in the arterial system, where they can block the flow of blood, leading to an embolism. This is a concern in patients with arteriosclerotic vascular disease. Few patients are allergic to the contrast medium, but the procedure is contraindicated for these patients. In general, for initial diagnosis, clinicians prefer noninvasive techniques, including CT scan and ultrasound (see Chapter 12 for a description of ultrasound used to examine the carotid arteries). Angiography is, however, the most accurate diagnostic procedure for evaluating vascular anatomy and its abnormalities. Thus, it is particularly useful in diagnosing cerebrovascular disorders.

SODIUM AMYTAL INJECTIONS (WADA TECHNIQUE)

The **Wada technique,** named after its developer, is similar to the angiogram in that the examiner places a catheter, typically in the left or right internal carotid artery. Then, a barbiturate sodium amytal is injected, which temporarily anesthetizes one hemisphere. Only one hemisphere is affected, even though vascular structures connect the two hemispheres (Wada & Rasmussen, 1960). This difference relates to that the pressure gradients along cerebral arteries in both hemispheres are the same; thus, there is no cross-filling (or crossover) of blood from one hemisphere to the other, except if there is a stroke or other damage to the vascular system. In this way, neuropsychologists can study the precise functions of one hemisphere while the other "sleeps" (see Chapter 16 for a detailed discussion of the Wada technique). Table 2.2 provides an overview of the radiologic procedures discussed in this section.

▉ Electrophysiologic Procedures

ELECTROENCEPHALOGRAPHY

One of the most widely used techniques in neurology is **electroencephalography (EEG).** The electroencephalogram is a recording of the electrical activity of nerve cells

---

Table 2.2 *Overview of Radiologic Procedures*

Skull X-ray: Two-dimensional representation of the head. Disadvantages include low resolution of brain anatomy; advantages include low cost, availability, and its use in the diagnosis of skull fractures, which are easily seen using this technique.

Air encephalography (pneumoencephalography): The radiographic visualization of the fluid-containing structures of the brain, which have been filled with gas. An improvement over the skull X-ray, but because of its invasive nature and side effects, it is not used in contemporary medicine.

Computed transaxial tomography (CT scan): CT renders an anatomic image of brain density based on multiple X-ray images of the brain. CT, which is readily available and can be used with almost anyone, provides a three-dimensional perspective of the brain with acceptable differentiation of brain structures. Its disadvantages include the use of penetrating radiation and that CT does not provide as much spatial resolution as does magnetic resonance imaging.

Enhanced CT: A CT scan that involves injecting a contrast agent to provide better visualization of brain structures, particularly bleeds. Disadvantages are it is invasive and some patients may not tolerate the contrast agent well.

Angiography: The roentgenographic visualization of blood vessels in the brain after introducing contrast material into the arterial or venous bloodstream. Angiography is the most useful technique for examining the blood supply to and from the brain. One disadvantage is that a catheter must be inserted into the patient's bloodstream, which requires an invasive medical procedure.

Sodium amytal injections (Wada technique): The injection of sodium amytal temporarily anesthetizes one hemisphere. This is primarily a research technique. It is used clinically to determine the lateralization of language before temporal lobectomy is performed. It is a complicated medical procedure that requires placing an arterial catheter.

---

of the brain through electrodes attached to various locations on the scalp. The Austrian psychiatrist Hans Berger first discovered in 1924 that patterns of electrical activity can be recorded using metal electrodes placed on the human head (Brazier, 1959). Initially, Berger was interested in finding physiologic evidence for telepathy, the scientifically unverified phenomenon of a mind communicating with another by extrasensory means. Berger was, however, frustrated in his search to find support of mental telepathy, but he discovered that the electrical activity of the sleeping brain differed fundamentally from that of the awake brain. Researchers have used the resulting electroencephalogram ("electrical brain writing") to investigate distinct patterns of electrical activity in both the normal and pathologic brain. Its potential use for identifying EEG correlates of behavior and personality have made it a popular research tool among behavioral scientists. Thus, EEG became the first dynamic way to measure brain function.

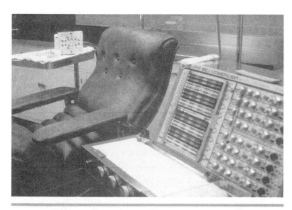

Figure 2.8 Electromechanical electroencephalographic recorder of the type used in the mid-1980s. (Courtesy Jeffrey T. Barth, University of Virginia.)

Technique

To record an EEG, the technician places small metal electrodes, or leads, on the scalp and connects them via wires to the electroencephalograph machine (Figure 2.8), which amplifies the electrical potential of neurons recording their activity on moving paper, a polygraph. Previously, electrodes were small needles that were inserted just below the skin of the scalp. Modern electrodes used with conductive gel have proved to be just as effective. In principle, each pair of electrodes can act as its own recording site, measuring the electrical activity of millions of neurons close to the scalp. The neuronal activity of deeper, subcortical structures is not easily evaluated using EEG. Also, surface electrodes are placed at electrically inactive sites on the head, such as the mastoid bone behind the ear (electrode placement A1 and A2), which act as ground leads. The EEG itself is generated primarily by neuronal activity immediately below the cortex. Pyramidal nerve cells, which have somewhat conical cell bodies, make up about 80% of neurons in that region and exist in all areas of the cerebral cortex. Thus, EEG is mostly a measure of cortical nerve cells of the pyramidal type.

The electrical signal of a neuron must penetrate through different tissues to reach the electrodes, including the meninges, CSF, blood, the skull, and the scalp, to be measured. The electrical contribution of each neuron is tiny, and it takes many thousands of neurons firing in concert to generate an electrical signal large enough for EEG to detect. Thus, the most easily visible EEG wave patterns depend on the synchronicity of millions of neurons.

In general, brain wave patterns are either rhythmic or arrhythmic. Neurons typically fire in a rhythmic or synchronous pattern, leading to alpha, beta, theta, and delta waveforms. In epilepsy, however, many neurons fire at once, or in a burst or "spike" that corresponds with the amplitude that the EEG record shows. In principle, each electrode measures the summed signal of electrical activity of groups of neuronal dendrites. EEG can be thought of as analogous to holding a microphone over New York City to estimate the traffic by measuring the amount of noise from automobiles. Thus, EEG is a diagnostic tool more sensitive to the "forest" than to the individual "tree."

Overview of Brain Wave Activity

Brain wave activity may differ in polarity, shape, and frequency. The amplitude typically ranges from 5 to 100 microvolts and is a measure of the signal strength of neural activity. The EEG records frequency of the waveforms from 1 to 100 Hz (signal frequency per second), meaning that neural activity oscillates in a particular frequency. The specific shape of the waveform also interests the electroencephalographer. For example, during light sleep, the EEG shows a characteristic spindle activity and vertex (V) waves. Researchers have established a system of dividing brain wave activity that is based on its frequency and amplitude. To the neuropsychology student, frequency subdivisions of the EEG may appear somewhat arbitrary, but in general, they correlate with distinct divisions of subjective experience of attention and arousal. Several different basic types have been established that vary according to whether a person is alert, wakeful, drowsy, or sleeping (Table 2.3).

Table 2.3 *Brain States and Associated Subjective Experience*

Gamma activity (35+ Hz) is a low-amplitude, fast-activity wave. Gamma rhythms are the fastest and are often associated with peak performance states and hyperarousal.

Beta is a low-amplitude, fast-activity wave with a frequency of more than 12 Hz. Beta is often divided into high beta (18–35 Hz), typically associated with a narrow focus, overarousal, and anxiety; mid-beta (15–18 Hz), often correlated with being active, alert, excited, or focused; and low beta (12–15 Hz), which has been associated with relaxed, external attention.

Alpha activity (8–12 Hz) is the predominant background activity in wakeful persons. Alpha is most often associated with quiet, passive, resting, but wakeful states.

Theta activity ranges from 4 to 7 Hz and is most indicative of drowsiness, deeply relaxed states, and inwardly focused states.

Delta activity is the slowest frequency (<0.5–4 Hz). High-voltage, slow-frequency delta waves are never present in a wakeful, healthy person, but mostly occur during non-rapid eye movement (nondream) deep stage 4 sleep.

The pursuit of a specific brain state is a goal in itself. Because alpha and theta waves are characteristic of a person being relaxed, isolation floatation tanks and relaxation audio cassette tapes, among other tools, have proved effective in helping achieve such brain states. In athletics, researchers have demonstrated that peak performance is associated with specific cortical arousal levels (Van Raalte & Brewer, 1996). Alpha waves, in contrast, are incompatible with being alert and focused. Thus, it is advantageous for the competitive athlete to be in mid-beta rhythm when a difficult task is required, such as in ice hockey when the goalie faces a breakaway or in baseball when the batter steps to the home plate to face a pitch. During beta waves, the cortex is most actively engaged via complex sensory input and external processing. The activity rate of cortical neurons should be high, but also unsynchronized, because neurons may be involved in different aspects of complex neuropsychological tasks. During beta waves, neurons fire rapidly, but not in concert with each other. However, it is difficult to sustain beta rhythm for long periods; thus, successful athletes are skilled in switching from alpha to beta rhythm and back "on command."

Seizures and Electroencephalography

Neurons can organize their rate of electrical activity in two fundamental ways. First, groups of neurons can fire in synchronized oscillations by taking cues from other cells, also known as *pacemaker cells* or *k neurons* (k for constant). Cortical neurons also take cues from other brain structures such as the thalamus, which can act as a powerful pacemaker, even when there is no external sensory input. For example, during non–rapid eye movement (NREM, or nondream sleep), the thalamus generates rhythmic, self-sustaining discharge patterns that prevent organized information from reaching the cortex. Thus, one's brain is asleep, demonstrating large, rhythmic delta waves. Second, neurons may fire in a consistent rhythmic pattern in response to collective behavior, such as a large group of people clapping in a synchronized way without a cheerleader being present.

Seizures are the most extreme form of synchronous brain activity, during which the whole brain (as in a grand mal seizure) or large portions of the brain (as in a partial seizure) fire with a defined and pronounced synchrony that never occurs during normal behavior (Figure 2.9).

Grand Mal Epilepsy

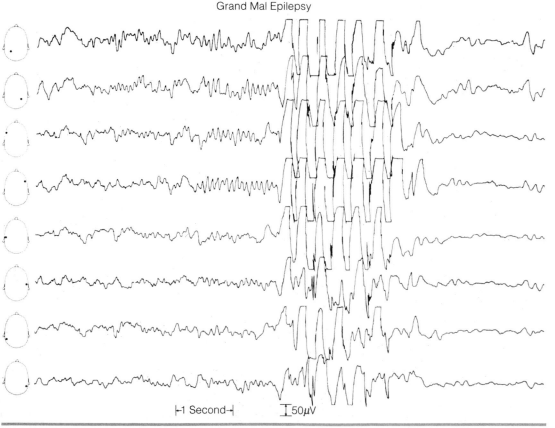

|-1 Second-| I 50μV

Figure 2.9 Electroencephalogram example of spiking activity that accompanies epilepsy. (Courtesy Eric Zillmer.)

During seizures, most, if not all, cortical neurons participate in excitation. Behavior is disrupted, and often consciousness is lost. Seizures themselves are best conceptualized as a symptom, not unlike a fever, and may be triggered by dozens of different causes. It is unlikely that seizures have one underlying cause. The lifetime prevalence for a single seizure is high, approximately 10%. Drugs that block gamma-aminobutyric acid (GABA) receptors increase the possibility of a seizure. GABA has strong inhibitory properties and plays a major role in the basic type of neuronal transmission that depends on rapid communication among neurons. Conversely, drugs that prolong the inhibitory action of GABA (barbiturates or benzodiazepines, e.g., Valium) suppress the possibility of seizures. The brain is potentially always close to having a seizure, because runaway excitation is possible given the redundant feedback circuitry of the brain and its delicate balance between inhibitory and excitatory potentials. Multiple seizures, however, are typical of a disorder known as *epilepsy* (see Chapter 16 for a detailed discussion of epilepsy).

In patients with intractable (incurable) epilepsy, one intervention is neurosurgery to remove, if possible, the precise site or origin of the pathologic electric discharge. In such cases, a more precise EEG measurement is needed, which can be obtained by placing electrodes directly on the surface of the brain. This form of EEG, known as **electrocorticography (ECoG),** often is performed during temporal lobectomy surgery to isolate a precise location of brain pathology. In addition, a surgeon can place depth electrodes in the brain close to the projected area of interest while the patient is awake and being monitored via 24-hour closed-circuit television. This is usually done to correlate seizure activity with EEG data. Depth electrodes and ECoG are invasive techniques and entail risks, including infection. These methods are used only when the medical benefits greatly outweigh the risks to the patient. Thus, surface scalp electrode placement is the first and least invasive electrophysiologic study of the brain. EEG is also relatively inexpensive compared with CT and MRI procedures and is readily available.

Clinical Use of Electroencephalography

The primary referral for a clinical EEG is to help with diagnosis of a seizure disorder, sleep disorder, level of coma, or presence of brain death. In fact, EEG is the primary tool in diagnosing epilepsy and can often pinpoint the type and location of seizure disorder. EEG is also useful in diagnosing sleep disorders, because specific sleep states are associated with particular forms of electrical activity. The primary abnormality seen on EEG recordings is a slowing of activity, as well as the presence of epileptiform activity. For example, it is abnormal to find delta activity in a wakeful person. Typically, the slower the frequency in an awake patient, the more severe its abnormality. People with partial seizures often have EEG activity that slows to 3 Hz. Epileptiform EEG activity consists of sharp waves (spike-and-wave discharge), which indicate a seizure disorder. EEG diagnosis of epilepsy, however, produces frequent type II errors (misses). Thus, a normal EEG may not indicate a normal brain.

Unfortunately, the EEG also demonstrates type I errors (false positive or false hits). That is, a mildly abnormal EEG may not necessarily reflect an abnormal brain unless the EEG indicates the specific profile of epilepsy, which, if present, has few false positives. Interpreting the EEG recording is something of an art because so many different variables are introduced. These variables include amplitude configuration of the polygraph, speed of recording paper, different electrode montages, a high incident of artifact caused by muscle movement that contributes to electrical activity, and inadequate electrical shielding of the examination room. Thus, different electroencephalographers often disagree on interpreting borderline abnormal EEGs, although they easily diagnose the more definite epileptic EEG patterns.

When a diagnostician suspects seizure disorder, several techniques can provoke epileptic discharges during the EEG recording, which is the absolute positive sign of epilepsy. These methods include administering an EEG during the patient's sleep or when sleep deprived; that is, after the patient stays awake for one night, the diagnostician administers the EEG in the morning. Other activation techniques that provoke epileptic discharges during the EEG recording include hyperventilation and photic stimulation. The latter is the presentation of a strobe light, right in front of closed eyes, that is set at different frequencies to influence the base-rate activation pattern of occipital neurons. Diagnosticians also use serial EEGs and 24-hour EEG recordings to monitor brain wave patterns over time. Once epilepsy is identified, doctors most commonly treat it with anticonvulsant medication to reduce spiking activity.

Electroencephalography and Neuropsychology

EEG is a safe, painless, and relatively simple procedure. Its use in neuropsychology has been disappointing and limited historically by a lack of relationship between EEG parameters and behavior, specifically indices of higher cortical functioning. In fact, complex EEG waveforms do not change much during different kinds of sensory input, but appear to be most sensitive to the general arousal level of the brain (Penfield & Jasper, 1954). This lack of convergence between EEG activity and behavior is probably caused by the fact that the EEG is a relatively nonspecific measure of the underlying brain activity. Thus, using the traditional eight-channel EEG, researchers have established only general relationships related to right versus left hemisphere differences, or to posterior and anterior regions of the cortex.

EEG does not give an account of *what* a person is thinking; rather, it tells us *if* the person is thinking. Over recent years, more sophisticated recording equipment and computer analysis have refined the EEG. Investigators have been using increased numbers of electrodes (64, 128, and even up to 256) placed over the patient's entire head to correlate specific neural networks involved in a particular neuropsychological task. Such enhanced EEGs have greatly improved signal quality and localization.

One invention that examines the more dynamic aspects of electrophysiologic activity in the brain is brain electrical activity mapping (BEAM) (Duffy, 1989). CT shows the structure of brain tissue, and PET scans (see later) let researchers and clinicians examine the pattern of brain biochemistry and metabolism. BEAM, in contrast, uses computer technology to provide color-coded mapping of the brain's electrical activity in real time, that is, as quickly as it is occurring in the patient's brain. In general, BEAM is nothing more than a way of enhancing the amount of information available on a standard EEG. Using an automated, integrated approach to EEG, the computer can calculate color-coded maps of electrical brain activity (Figure 2.10). Then it codes computed EEG parameters as topographic displays showing neuroelectric activity across the cortex while the patient is performing a neuropsychological task. BEAM is much more sensitive to electrical correlates of cognitive tasks than the traditional EEG. Quantitative EEG analysis also has shown some promise in the diagnosis of clinical disorders such as dyslexia, a reading disorder.

Other improvements in EEG technology entail merging the temporal resolution of EEG with the anatomic detail of MRI or the ability of PET to localize function. Such coregistration of different approaches to represent the functioning brain has resulted in multimodal approaches to neuroimaging, often providing new insights, as well as corroborating established findings. For example, schizophrenics show abnormal, less active BEAMs and PET scans (less metabolism) in the frontal regions of the brain.

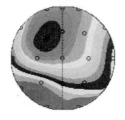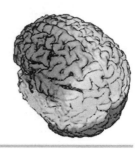

Figure 2.10 Schizophrenic subject with history of seizures was examined by electroencephalography and magnetic resonance imaging (MRI) to observe extent of abnormal activity during a seizure (left). Color-coded brain electrical activity mapping (BEAM) presentation, with red indicating increased neuronal activity in the left frontal lobe (right). Results from BEAM superimposed over three-dimensional MRI cortex indicate abnormal discharge in left frontal lobe; note also widening sulci. See inside covers for color image. (Courtesy Dorota Kozinska, Ph.D., University of Warsaw, Warsaw, Poland.)

EVOKED POTENTIAL

A further electrophysiologic diagnostic test is **evoked potential** (**EP;** also called *event-related potential [ERP]*). EP involves artificial stimulation of sensory fibers that, in turn, generate electrical activity along the central and peripheral pathways, as well as the specific primary receptive areas in the brain. In contrast with EEG, EP is dependent on a stimulus and is most useful for assessing the integrity of the visual, auditory, and somatosensory pathways at specific regions of the brain. EEG technology can record the electrical activity in response to a stimulus or event. During the traditional EEG, the overall background activity of the cerebral cortex hides specific sensory stimuli. In EP, a computer makes it possible to visualize the changes in EEG responses to a specific stimulus (visual, auditory, or somatosensory), canceling out random electrical activity, but displaying electrical activity related to the potential evoked by the stimulus. The resulting EP consists of a series of positive and negative changes lasting for about 500 milliseconds after the stimulus ceases. The diagnostician analyzes the EP according to amplitude, latency, and the location of the specific brain region where the stimulus is processed.

Brainstem Auditory-Evoked Response

In brainstem auditory-evoked response (BAER), the examiner presents clicks to each ear of the patient individually via headphones. In response to the auditory stimulus, the auditory pathways generate an electrical signal along

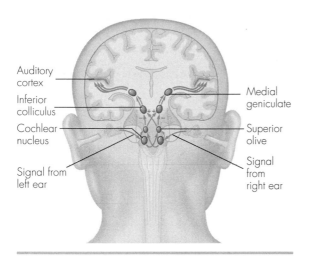

Figure 2.11   Auditory pathways from receptors in the ear to the auditory cortex. Note the different nuclei along the pathways that form the basis for measuring integration delays, which can be measured and amplified using evoked potential and electroencephalographic technology. (Reproduced from Kalat, J. W. [1998]. *Biological psychology* [6th ed., p. 184, Figure 7.6]. Pacific Grove, CA: Brooks/Cole, by permission.)

the central auditory pathways. EEG recording consists of five distinct waves that represent different latencies related to five nuclei groups where the auditory signal is being integrated. Although this delay is short, the examiner can measure and amplify it. Abnormal delays in responses, measured in milliseconds, often can pinpoint specific lesions, but only along the pathways measured. The BAER can diagnose a malfunction of the auditory nerve at the cochlear nucleus, the superior olive, the lateral lemniscus, and the inferior colliculus (Figure 2.11).

In BAER, five characteristic waves are recorded. Wave I reflects activity of the vestibular nerve; wave II, the cochlear nucleus; wave III, the superior olivary complex; and waves IV and V, the pons or lower midbrain. Decreased amplitudes, the absence of a wave, or prolonged interwave latencies may point to abnormal brainstem responses.

Approximately 50% of patients with multiple sclerosis demonstrate a pathologic BAER typically at the level of the brainstem. BAER has also aided in diagnosing patients with acoustic neuromas (tumors). Research using EP indicates that schizophrenics, compared with healthy subjects, demonstrate an abnormality that may indicate a deficit in the "sensory gating" at the brainstem level, which may result in impaired attention (Cullum et al., 1993). Researchers can then confirm the finding using neuropsychological measures of attention, sustained concentration, and digit vigilance (e.g., digit cancelation). As with many of the other

imaging techniques featured in this chapter, there are interesting implications and a promising future in the interrelationships between neurophysiologic and neuropsychological indices of brain function. Neuropsychology in Action 2.1 reviews a case example using BAER technology.

Visual-Evoked Response

Similar to the auditory-evoked response procedure, in visual-evoked response (VER), the examiner presents a visual stimulus separately to each eye of the patient. An alternating light/dark reversing checkerboard pattern provides the visual stimulus. EEG responses are recorded from electrodes over the parietal and occipital regions. One wave originates in the receptive visual cortex and is measured using EEG technology. A normal delay from the presentation of the visual stimulus to the registration of the electrodes over the occipital cortex is about 100 milliseconds. Lesions along the visual nerve pathways result in abnormal delays, decreased amplitude of the recorded response, or both.

Somatosensory-Evoked Response

In somatosensory-evoked response (SER), the examiner stimulates peripheral nerves via an electrode placed over the median nerve at the patient's wrist. In addition, the examiner places three electrodes for purposes of measurement, with the first two measuring peripheral electrical activity of sensory pathways at the level of the patient's arm and spinal cord. The third electrode is placed over the patient's contralateral somatosensory cortex. Abnormalities in amplitude or latencies at the first two points of measurement suggest peripheral nerve involvement. Delays at the third wave suggest central sensory pathway involvement.

Figure 2.12 shows the graphic results of an SER examination to evaluate somatosensory pathways in three dimensions. The technician delivers pulses transcutaneously via a cup electrode to the median nerve at the patient's wrist. He or she adjusts the intensity of the stimulus to determine a painless muscle twitch of the thumb. Collected data are then transmitted to a computer for analysis.

ELECTRICAL STIMULATION

Historically, the electrical stimulation of nerve tissue is one of the oldest ways of investigating the living brain. Initially, scientists hoped that use of this technique could chart a precise map of the cortex that would outline, akin to phrenology, the behavioral and cognitive properties of the brain, specifically the topography of the cortex.

The patient is a 38-year-old man who was employed as a mechanic. Previously, he had worked as a tile layer for 6 months, during which he reported he was exposed to epoxy, alcohol, and other possibly toxic solvents.

in milliseconds at slow rate of 11.4 clicks/sec for waves I, III, and V were as follows: Note that the delays in milliseconds increase the further the signal is measured from its initial detection in the ear (e.g., at

rates. The audiologist measured interpeak delays at waves I to III for the slow and fast rates, and waves III to V and I to V for the fast rate. Interear absolute and interpeak latency differences are within normal limits. Even though

	I	III	V	I–III	III–V	I–V
RIGHT	1.50	3.90	5.87	2.40	1.97	4.37
LEFT	1.60	4.14	6.10	2.54	1.87	4.42

Since then, he has reported dizziness and short-term memory loss. Physicians subsequently diagnosed him with chronic solvent intoxication. An audiogram showed normal hearing bilaterally. An audiologist performed brainstem auditory-evoked response (BAER) testing. Specifically, the tester presented monaural click stimulation in each ear at 70 dB using click rates of 11.4 and 57.7 clicks/sec, with 2000 and 4000 repetitions, respectively. Absolute and interpeak latencies

nuclei I, the vestibular nerve, the latency is 1.5 milliseconds for the right ear; but at nuclei III, the superior olive, the signal was measured 3.9 milliseconds after it was introduced to the right ear). Also, note the symmetry between right and left auditory processing routes. BAER testing showed normal absolute and interpeak latencies at slow and fast rates in the right ear for waves I through III. Findings for the left ear demonstrated delayed absolute latencies for waves III and V at the fast and slow

there were minor variations among the brain wave recordings, the audiologist concluded that the test results suggested a normal BAER not consistent with brainstem dysfunction. Subsequent neuropsychological testing did show neuropsychological impairment on various tasks of new learning and memory. BAER, however, ruled out the possibility that those cognitive deficits were related to brainstem impairment, and they were thus most likely related to cortical dysfunction.

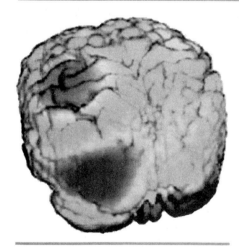

Figure 2.12 Sensory-evoked responses were averaged in a group of 10 healthy volunteers and superimposed onto the surface of a healthy brain. Images show electroencephalographic distribution of sensory-evoked potential to right median nerve, computed 18 milliseconds after stimulus presentation. See inside covers for color image. (Courtesy Dorota Kozinska, Ph.D., University of Warsaw, Warsaw, Poland.)

Surprisingly, this technique, which has been largely confined to the primary and sensory areas of the cortex, has elicited few positive responses (the generation of a measurable behavior). However, scientists have found a great number of negative responses (disruption of function) as a result of electrical stimulation of the cortex.

For example, researchers easily demonstrated aphasia, a disruption of language functions, by numerous stimulations in different locations of the left hemisphere (Ojemann, 1980). More recently, neurologists have introduced electrical stimulation in the treatment of Parkinson's disease, based on the advances of stereotaxic operations and knowledge of specific associations between electrical stimulation and subcortical regions of the brain. Obviously, because of its invasive nature, direct electrical stimulation of the brain is not a routine diagnostic procedure. Primarily, researchers use it experimentally in clinical cases for whom other interventions have not been successful. It can, however, provide great theoretical and clinical value in understanding the functions of the brain.

ELECTROMYOGRAPHY

Electromyography (EMG) is the electrical analysis of muscles. In EMG, diagnosticians perform a nerve conduction study of a specific muscle to diagnose neuromuscular disorders. Patients undergoing EMG receive deepneedle stimulation of a muscle, which the technician measures electrophysiologically ventral (closer to the spinal cord) to the stimulation. The technician delivers an electrical potential to a muscle, using a wire inserted within a hollow needle. The electrical activity is amplified and displayed graphically via an oscilloscope. At the basis of EMG is that a relaxed muscle is electrically silent. During voluntary contraction, muscle action potentials are present.

EMG is an important medical diagnostic technique that aids in diagnosing peripheral nerve damage, because it can isolate the dysfunction to a specific sensorimotor unit, including a motor or sensory neuron, neuromuscular transmission, or the muscle cell itself. The procedure also helps substantiate the presence of intact sensorimotor pathways—for example, when hysteria or malingering is suspected. If Sigmund Freud had had this diagnostic test available, he could have proved that Anna O., the patient of his first famous published case study, was truly hysterical and did not suffer from a neuromuscular disorder as she complained. Anna O. actually was treated by Freud's mentor Breuer, but Freud wrote up her case. Anna O.'s motor functioning was normal, even though she complained of partial paralysis. Freud suspected this normality anyway and concluded that Anna produced the paralysis of the arm hysterically, because of her unconscious wish to remain in the role of a patient and to receive daily visits by famous doctors. Nevertheless, using EMG technology, he could have diagnosed this much more efficiently, without needing to develop elaborate psychoanalytic theories.

A variation on the preceding techniques is recording an electric shock stimulus of a peripheral nerve and measuring the subsequent muscle contraction. This technique can test both motor and sensory nerves. Results assist in the differential diagnosis of muscle disease and peripheral nerve damage. For example, in carpal tunnel syndrome, a relatively common peripheral nerve disorder with accompanying sensory deficits in the first three digits and weakness of the thumb, there is a characteristic latency of muscle and nerve action potentials. Although most patients tolerate this procedure well, EMG is mildly uncomfortable because pain accompanies the insertion of the needle into the muscle. Table 2.4 reviews the most popular electrophysiologic procedures currently in use.

Table 2.4 *Electrophysiologic Procedures*

Electroencephalography (EEG): EEG is one of the oldest brain-monitoring techniques. It measures the general electrical activity of the cortex. It is most useful in assessing, in real time, the overall arousal state in a person. Increased electrode placements and computer integration capabilities have resulted in high-resolution EEG and BEAM (brain electrical activity mapping), a promising assessment and research tool of the electrical activity of neurons.

Evoked potential (EP): EP, or event-related potential (ERP), is similar to EEG in that it assesses an electrical signal, but is related to a specific auditory (brainstem auditory-evoked response), visual (visual-evoked response), or sensory event (somatosensory-evoked response). Evoked potential assessment provides not an evaluation of general brain activity, but a millisecond-by-millisecond record of a specific sensory process.

Electrical stimulation: Researchers have used electrical stimulation of nerve tissue to empirically map pathways of the cortex. More recently, clinicians have introduced electrical stimulation in the treatment of Parkinson's disease. Direct electrical stimulation of the brain, an invasive medical procedure, is used only in those cases for whom other interventions or diagnostic procedures have not succeeded.

Electromyography (EMG): EMG is the electrical analysis of muscles, a diagnostic procedure useful in diagnosing peripheral nerve damage. The procedure, however, is uncomfortable because it requires insertion of a needle into the muscle.

Imaging of Brain Metabolism

Since the 1980s, researchers have developed techniques for analyzing the brain that focus on measuring parameters of regional brain physiology. Such techniques are related to the biological fact that neurons have an active metabolism that the cerebral blood supply provides. Specifically, the delivery of oxygen and glucose to neurons depends on cerebral blood flow (CBF). If the metabolic needs of the active neurons are high, the rate of CBF is correspondingly higher. In this manner, neurologists can study regional blood flow while the patient is performing neuropsychological tasks. In contrast with CT, which provides a static representation of brain structures, measuring regional blood flow provides dynamic data on CBF and metabolic activity. The imaging of brain metabolism, therefore, permits a completely different approach to examining the brain.

REGIONAL CEREBRAL BLOOD FLOW

Blood flow in the cerebral hemispheres varies with metabolism and activity. It can be a sensitive index of the changes in cellular activity in response to cognitive tasks

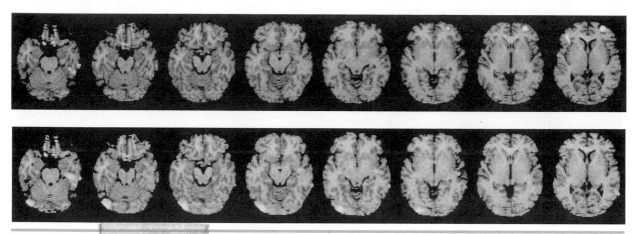

Figure 2.13 Verbal encoding using positron emission tomography cerebral blood flow. Brain images show differences in regional blood flow between word encoding and averaged baseline for 23 healthy volunteers (top) and 23 patients with schizophrenia (bottom). Note activation in left and right prefrontal cortex for healthy volunteers and in right temporal and left occipital cortex for patients. Deactivation is visible in left precentral and occipital areas for healthy volunteers and in left precentral area for patients. The inability to activate prefrontal regions during encoding may underlie learning difficulties in patients with schizophrenia. See inside covers for color image. (Reproduced from Ragland, J. D., Gur, R. C., Raz, J., Schroeder, L., Smith, R. J., Alavi, A., et al. [2000]. Hemispheric activation of anterior and inferior prefrontal cortex during verbal encoding and recognition: A PET study of healthy volunteers. *NeuroImage, 11,* 624–633, by permission.)

(Andreasen, 1988). The amount of blood flowing through different regions of the brain can indicate the relative neural activity of that region. In the 1940s, researchers introduced a technique in which the patient inhaled nitrous oxide (N_2O), which circulates through the brain. Using this technique, scientists were able to measure total CBF per unit weight of brain per minute. The procedure, however, had disadvantages: It was invasive and could provide only a measure of overall CBF (Kety, 1979).

Lassen and Ingvar pioneered regional cerebral blood flow (rCBF) in living and awake subjects (Haeger, 1988). These researchers developed a special radioactive isotope known as xenon 133 (^{133}Xe), which emits a low gamma radiation and stays in the bloodstream for approximately 15 minutes. Isotopes are a form of chemical element with the same atomic number and position in the periodic table and nearly identical chemical behavior, but with differing atomic mass numbers and different physical properties. Thus, isotopes are highly unstable. Initially, researchers injected this tracer intra-arterially into the bloodstream (via the internal carotid artery). The blood supply then carried the ^{133}Xe to either hemisphere, over which researchers placed special scintillation detectors that recorded the number of gamma rays the tracer emitted. In this manner, scientists could determine the rate of clearance of ^{133}Xe from various regions of the brain. From this information, they could quantify the rCBF with considerable accuracy. CBF studies corroborate many brain–behavior relationships established in the literature

(Figure 2.13). Occipital areas are more involved when a subject examines moving stimuli, and auditory areas are involved when speech is initiated. The most interesting aspects are anteroposterior comparisons of blood flow in the brain, rather than right–left differences. For example, the ^{133}Xe technique reliably showed that the anterior brain regions have an increased rCBF in the resting subject (Gur et al., 1982).

One of the findings regarding rCBF relates to an absence of measurable information in the deepest regions of the brain. Furthermore, the ^{133}Xe technique can measure only one hemisphere at a time. In the 1970s, researchers developed a special noninvasive technique in which subjects inhaled an air-xenon mixture through a face mask. Using this technique, researchers can study both hemispheres at the same time. The amount of detail for measuring specific brain region blood flow depends on the number of detectors. Initially, this number was 8, then 16, and more recently, 254 detectors. A computer then analyzes the data and provides a color-coded visualization of the findings (Figure 2.14).

SINGLE-PHOTON EMISSION COMPUTED TOMOGRAPHY

A technique for the 3-D imaging of rCBF is **single-photon emission computed tomography (SPECT).** SPECT is similar to PET, which uses radionuclides, but unlike

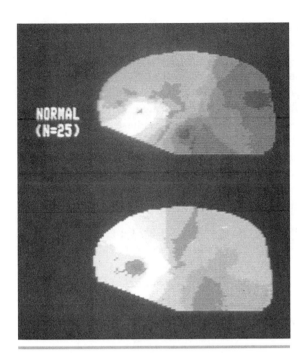

Figure 2.14 Topographic display of resting regional cerebral blood flow (rCBF) using an early system. Darker areas signal high rCBF; lighter areas suggest low rCBF. (Reproduced from Kalat, J. W. [1998]. *Biological psychology* [6th ed., p. 109, Figure 4.33]. Pacific Grove, CA: Brooks/Cole. Courtesy Karen Berman and Daniel Weinberger, National Institute of Mental Health.)

positron emission, SPECT does not require an expensive cyclotron (a device that can generate radioactive chemicals with a short half-life, also known as *radioactive isotopes*) for their production. Radiologists can label biochemicals of interest with a radioactive compound whose gamma rays can be picked up by detectors surrounding the brain. Using SPECT, it is possible to three-dimensionally image the distribution of a radioactively labeled contrast agent. As in CT, a computer analyzes the data and reconstructs a 3-D cross section of the emissions pattern. The tracer is injected intravenously and crosses into the brain tissue based on CBF. Using this technique, analysts can estimate CBF and blood volume. Researchers can study subjects undergoing SPECT while they are engaged in a neuropsychological task; however, the tracer has a long half-life, and it is difficult to keep a subject in the same mental state for a long period. A further limitation is that the tracer takes approximately 2 days to clear from the brain; thus, it is possible to obtain only a single exposure of the brain using SPECT. An advantage of SPECT is that it is relatively inexpensive (it is referred to as "the poor person's PET"). A further advantage is that

individuals can be imaged while they are sleeping or sedated, a useful option with young children or unmanageable patients. Thus, imaging studies that require multiple conditions typically are investigated by using the more costly **positron emission tomography (PET)** technique.

POSITRON EMISSION TOMOGRAPHY

Emission tomography is a new visualization technique that detects a diverse range of physiologic parameters, including glucose and oxygen metabolism, in addition to blood flow, by distributing a radioactively labeled substance in any desired cross section of the head. The method of PET technology is intravenous injection of a radioactive tracer (specifically positron-emitting substances) and subsequent scanning of the brain for radioactivity. In contrast with SPECT, the radioactive isotopes injected with the PET procedure have a short half-life and can attach to specific agents, such as glucose. Glucose, the body's fuel, mixes with blood to reach the brain. As mentioned earlier, the metabolism of the human brain varies in relation to its activity. The more active a specific area of the brain is, the more glucose it uses. Thus, the resting brain differs metabolically from the active brain. PET is the only procedure by which researchers can examine three-dimensionally the regional cerebral glucose use and oxygen metabolism in the living brain. PET analysts do not view the brain as a static structure, but investigate the dynamic properties of the brain (Raichle, 1983).

Technique

In the PET procedure, technicians administer radionuclides intravenously that the subject's brain tissue takes up. The radionuclei are unstable, because they have an excess positive charge. When the radioactive tracer decays, it emits a positron that then travels a short distance (a few millimeters) before colliding with an electron. This collision results in the emission of two photons traveling in opposite directions, generating energy that detectors around the scalp can measure (Figure 2.15). When two detectors calculate photon absorption at the same approximate time, the computer assumes they originate from the same collision and can then calculate the exact position showing neural "hotspots." PET functions by calculating millions of counts from detectors and estimating their origin. Using a subtraction technique, investigators can isolate blood flow patterns related to specific mental tasks. Computed tomography allows researchers to calculate a count and the locations of these collisions (depending on the type of radionuclide used, such as carbon 11, nitrogen 13, oxygen 15, or fluorine 18) to generate a visual

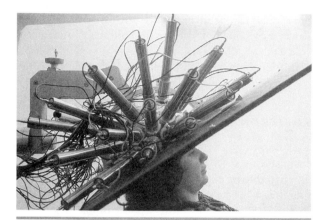

Figure 2.15   An early version of a position emission tomography scanner in which detectors around the scalp measure energy caused by the emission of photons. (© Burt Glinn/Magnum.)

representation of radionuclide uptake. In this manner, researchers can obtain varied physiologic parameters, including glucose and oxygen metabolism, blood flow, and receptor density of neurotransmitters for specific anatomic regions of interest (ROIs). For example, PET has shown different glucose uptake during various cognitive tasks (Figure 2.16). The major disadvantage of using PET clinically is the cost involved, principally related to the need for an expensive cyclotron, which can produce the short-lived radioactive isotopes. As a result, PET technology often is available only in large medical centers associated with research institutes.

Positron Emission Tomography and Neuropsychology

Can PET technology detect changes that occur during cognitive activity? Or are the changes in metabolic activity

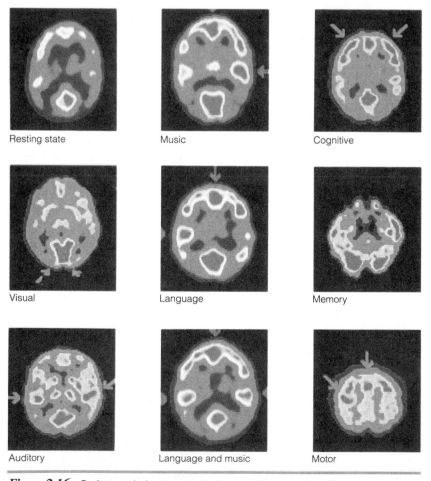

Figure 2.16   Positron emission tomography images obtained during different cognitive tasks. Regions of highest metabolism are gray. (Reproduced from Kalat, J. W. [1998]. *Biological psychology* [6th ed., p. 108, Figure 4.31]. Pacific Grove, CA: Brooks/Cole. Courtesy E. Phelps and John C. Mazziota, UCLA School of Medicine.)

too small to be detected? Measuring glucose metabolism rate is a more direct measure of neuron function than is CBF. New tracers with a shorter half-life (such as positron-labeled oxygen, O^{15}) have led to investigations of neuropsychological functions using PET, often with remarkable findings. Researchers use O^{15}, which readily crosses the blood–brain barrier, as a reference point for approximate blood intake of various regions in the brain. PET research demonstrates that the effects of cognitive effort on regional brain activity can be detected and measured (e.g., a verbal task corresponds to the left hemisphere and a spatial task to the right hemisphere). PET is also sensitive to individual differences, such as sex, that affect the direction and degree of hemispheric specialization for specific neuropsychological abilities. Thus, studies using imaging technology indicate that there is a relationship between brain activity and behavior, and that PET can detect these associations (Gur, Levy, & Gur, 1977).

A major finding using PET technology is that metabolic activity is suppressed in patients with a history of head trauma, brain tumors, and stroke, even though structural representation of the brain, using MRI or CT, suggests intact brain anatomy. Thus, metabolic imaging of the brain can lead to a clearer understanding of the functioning brain, specifically where the pathology is unclear, as in schizophrenics or epileptics. Although PET remains primarily a research tool because of its cost, it has proved to be an important technique in measuring physiologic activity in the normal and damaged brain at rest or while engaging in behavior.

One of the most interesting research aspects of PET concerns subjects performing various mental activities. Experimenters have taken PET scans of female and male adult brains when subjects were either resting or solving a rotating figure problem, a rather difficult spatial puzzle (Gur et al., 1982). Female subjects not only scored lower than male subjects, but there was a sex difference on the PET results. Even though the PET scans were not different while subjects were resting, when subjects were solving the rotating figure problem, male brains showed maximum neural activity in the right frontal area, whereas female brains demonstrated maximum activity in the right parietotemporal lobe. This suggests that men outperform women on the rotation problem, and that there may be a neural reason for this. There are, of course, tasks at which women outperform men. For example, women are generally faster on tests that require perceptual speed and score higher than men on a test of verbal fluency in which one must list as many words as one can that begin with the same letter (Lezak, Howieson, & Loring, 2004).

Table 2.5 *Imaging of Brain Metabolism*

Single-photon emission computed tomography (SPECT): SPECT measures blood flow, a correlate of brain activity. Because the radioactive tracer takes almost 2 days to be eliminated from the body, researchers cannot use SPECT to monitor the brain's mental activity "moment to moment."

Positron emission tomography (PET): PET tracks blood flow, which is associated with brain activity. It is primarily used to assess brain physiology, including glucose and oxygen metabolism, and the presence of specific neurotransmitters. The disadvantages of PET are that it is expensive, involves radiation, and renders low spatial resolution and data must be averaged over time (PET is not based on real time). The most promising use of PET has been its combined application with structural imaging techniques, which can provide a remarkable tool for mapping brain location and function.

PET studies have generated much controversy regarding sex differences in the brain. Are there really functional differences in the brain that arise from being male or female? The most recent studies indicate there are. Some theorists suggest an evolutionary perspective by which sex differences in the brain might have come from different skills needed by early humans. Male individuals with good spatial skills, they argue, had an advantage in hunting, and female individuals with good communication skills had an advantage in child rearing (Springer & Deutsch, 1993).

But researchers have not established whether sex differences are related to differences in socialization and learning experiences that are different for male and female individuals, or whether the brains of female and male individuals are organized differently and, therefore, function differently. This controversy is not easily decided, but PET may shed light on this puzzle. Table 2.5 reviews the most frequently used imaging techniques based on brain metabolism.

Magnetic Imaging Procedures

MAGNETIC RESONANCE IMAGING

Magnetic resonance imaging (MRI) is based on the work of Felix Bloch and Edward Purcell, who won the Nobel Prize in physics in 1952 for their development of a new method of nuclear magnetic precision measurement. This led to the medical application of this technology called MRI during the early 1970s. Whereas CT uses penetrating X-ray radiation and PET uses radioactive

Neuropsychology in Action 2.2

Undergoing a Magnetic Resonance Imaging Procedure

by Eric A. Zillmer

"Eric, your brain looks OK!" announces Dr. Jonathan "Yoni" Nissanov, Research Professor of Biomedical Engineering and Science at Drexel University. It is 11:30 P.M., and I am lying in a magnetic resonance imaging (MRI) scanner at Drexel College of Medicine in Philadelphia. Yoni has reserved the million-dollar diagnostic tool for research he is conducting on functional imaging. I have agreed to be one of his test subjects. Because using the machine is expensive, research time is allotted only at night.

MRI is a relatively new diagnostic procedure that has been available for routine brain imaging only since the mid-1980s. Therefore, I am not surprised by the up-to-date, modern look of the facility, a space age–like control station. Yoni and his research assistant, who are operating the complex computerized machinery, greet me. My brain will be exposed to a strong magnetic field, so I must remove all metals that are on me, including my credit cards. The procedure is completely safe, I am being reassured. Yoni goes through his protocol: "You don't have a pacemaker? You don't have an aneurysm clip? Is there any shrapnel in your head or metal plates in your skull?" Finally, Yoni asks, "You know the risks?" Yes, as a neuropsychologist I know them all too well. The risks relate to the possibility that I may find out something about my brain that I do not necessarily want to know. The MRI will produce textbook-quality anatomy pictures of my brain. Although the probability is small, there is the outside chance that the diagnostic procedure may reveal a tumor or some other abnormality of my brain. Just a month ago, one of my research colleagues learned that she had a malformation of her venous system in her brain. She was also one of Yoni's research participants. I repress these thoughts as I enter the imaging suite. The layout of the MRI scanner consists of two rooms, which are connected via intercom. The first one is the control room, which features a rectangular window overseeing the second larger room, where an oversize, doughnut-shaped machine is placed. The control room has an assortment

of electronic gadgetry, the centerpiece being a large TV-type console that controls the imager and provides immediate visual feedback of the results. This is where Yoni and his assistant will remain during the procedure.

I lie on a stretcher-like surface, and at the push of a button I am whisked via electrical motors headfirst into the center of the large electromagnet. Yoni asked me earlier whether I was claustrophobic, and now I understand why. There is only about an inch of space around my head, which is placed approximately 4 feet within the center of the imager.

The small confines of the MRI machine are a significant problem for patients who suffer from claustrophobia. I have been told that in the past such people were referred to the animal MRI at the Philadelphia Zoo, which can accommodate large animals, before "open" MRI was developed. I am grateful there is a small mirror positioned in an oblique angle right over my head, which gives me the illusion of space, because I can look out through the narrow opening toward my feet. I can see Yoni behind the window in the control room. "OK, we're ready to start." His voice reverberates through the intercom as a loud clicking noise begins.

For clinical diagnostic studies, the procedure takes about 15 minutes, during which the patient must remain as stationary as possible. But Yoni wants to go through a series of experiments during which I, on command, will clench my fists, right and left alternately, to see how the MRI machine detects functional activity in my brain. Yoni will then superimpose the functional MRI data, which reflect changes in blood oxygenation in my motor cortex, over the structural images of my brain. So I must keep my head still all the time. Yoni constantly reminds me of this over the intercom. I've agreed to be in the imager for more than 90 minutes. Given the confines of the space and the incredibly loud, jackhammer-like, staccato noise, all of a sudden this does not seem like such a good idea, after all. The first task for Yoni is to establish a traditional MRI

study of my brain, a baseline. The loud clicks I hear are bombardments of radiofrequency (RF) on my brain, which has been placed under a high magnetic field. The radio frequencies realign the magnetic fields of billions of hydrogen protons in my brain. The MRI machine is tuned into the frequencies that the water molecules in my brain emit after the external RF stops. The deflection or realignment of this hydrogen map to the magnetic field can be detected, amplified, and recorded, and is the basis of the MRI process. Amazingly, I do not feel anything.

To be honest, I've thought about my MRI results for some time. As a neuropsychologist, I know that my personality, my intellect— essentially who I am—depends on the integrity of my brain. What if they find something wrong? Wouldn't a small change in the organization of my brain almost guarantee an altered sense of my reality? Haven't I been acting rather eccentric lately? How would they break the news to me? Would a team of summoned doctors rush in to announce, "There is a problem with your brain"? I find myself wondering how much training in psychology physicians receive for sharing diagnostic test results with patients and their families.

After 15 minutes, Yoni steps into the imaging room to deliver his personal analysis of my brain. Although Yoni is a biomedical engineer, I am greatly relieved when he announces that my brain, on visual inspection, looks "OK." I have to remain in the increasingly uncomfortable same position for the next 75 minutes as Yoni goes through a series of studies. But now I am excited about the thought of actually seeing anatomic pictures of my brain for the first time. I can hardly wait until the procedure is over and Yoni shows me the coronal images on the control screen. Yes, everything is there, lateral ventricles, brainstem, cerebellum, and most importantly, my frontal lobes! I am a happy neuropsychologist as I leave the hospital at 1:30 A.M. with memory stick in hand, on which Yoni loaded an electronic copy of my brain images.

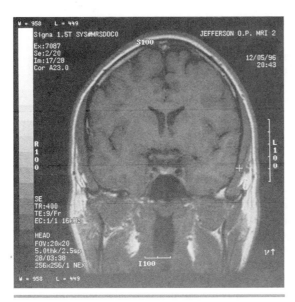

Figure 2.17 Normal magnetic resonance image (coronal view). Note the symmetry of the lateral ventricles and density differences between white and gray matter in the cortex. (Courtesy Eric Zillmer.)

isotopes, MRI is based on a fundamentally different process, namely, that the hydrogen nucleus, which is present in high concentration in biological systems, generates alterations in a small magnetic field, which can be measured (Neuropsychology in Action 2.2). MRI provides pictures of anatomy superior to CT (Figure 2.17), particularly for diagnosing underlying pathologic disorders.

Technique

The principal technique involved in MRI is based on patterns similar to the pattern a magnet makes on surrounding metal flakes. The metal flakes align themselves according to the magnetic field. Similarly, when the head is subjected to a strong magnetic field, hydrogen protons magnetize and align in the direction of the magnetic field. A proton, which is an elementary particle present in all atomic nuclei, has a positive charge equal to the negative charge of an electron. A strong radio-frequency (RF) signal applied at a right angle to the magnetic field can alter the alignment of the hydrogen protons. This radio wave sets the aligned hydrogen atom oscillating. The RF specifically selects only aligned hydrogen atoms; other atoms will not react. Once the RF ceases, the hydrogen "spins back" to its original

orientation as determined by the magnetic field, which remains active.

The emission of a small RF signal accompanies this deflection, or spin back to equilibrium. That is, the return of the hydrogen atoms to their previous orientation generates a magnetic field, which researchers can amplify, measure, and record. Computer analysis can then present a visualization of hydrogen density in various regions throughout the brain. Because water is present in most biological tissue, this procedure can generate a strikingly accurate picture of the brain, or any other anatomy.

The principle of MRI is that the hydrogen atom resonates as a result of the combined effect of the radio waves and the magnetic field. This frequency is specific for a given nuclear species in a magnetic field and allows scientists to determine the origin of a given RF signal in space. For example, one measure of RF signal amplitude is hydrogen density. Thus, variation of number of protons returning the RF signal is unique for different biological molecules, including fat, brain tissue, bone, and blood. This variation contributes to the MRI contrast, allowing spatial detection of signal data in 3-D space. As a result, researchers can accurately calculate brain tissue densities and can generate a computer-constructed image, which is so spatially precise that it can visualize structures as small as 1 mm.

There is one more major determinant of signal amplitude, namely, the magnetic relaxation times, also known as T1 and T2. These are the time intervals necessary for a nucleus to magnetize when placed in a magnetic field and the delay before returning to its original equilibrium. Protons with short T1 values (solids) emit higher signal intensities and appear white on the MRI, whereas those with longer T1 values (fluids) appear dark. T2 measures the loss of the magnetic orientation (or spin) after RF perturbation. On T2-weighted images, nuclei with relatively long T2 values retain their signal strength, emit a higher intensity signal, and appear brighter. Sometimes, the difference in T1 and T2 values may provide additional visual information, such as differentiating tumors and surrounding edema (swelling). More recently, 3-D images of the brain have been produced, based on MRI technology. MR images are used as a starting point, specifically, MRI pixels in the X-Y plane resolution of the subject's original images. Using mathematic algorithms, a computer can generate a surface model of the scalp, as well as the brain. The algorithms assume that a rigid body transformation of objects can be matched. In this way, it is suitable to align MRI data sets into one whole object. The result is an exact model of the brain in three dimensions (Figure 2.18).

Neuropsychology in Action 2.3

New Frontiers in Functional Magnetic Resonance Imaging

by Frank Hillary Ph.D., Pennsylvania State University

Blood oxygen level dependent (BOLD) magnetic resonance imaging (MRI) has become synonymous with functional MRI (fMRI) and, largely because of its accessibility, has grown to be the most widely used functional neuroimaging technique in the examination of human behavior. Put simply, fMRI is the measurement of blood flow in response to neural firing. The fMRI signal is based primarily on the ratio of oxyhemoglobin to deoxyhemoglobin expressed as a hemodynamic response function, and this signal is influenced by multiple factors including blood flow, blood volume, and vessel size. fMRI provides excellent spatial resolution (on the order of millimeters) and good temporal resolution (about 2000 milliseconds). It is important to emphasize that fMRI measures neither oxygen perfusion nor neural firing, but the hemodynamic response function that it does measure is reliable and well characterized.

Since the advent of fMRI, neuropsychology has been shaped and guided by noninvasive means of accessing information about the brain. Understanding brain and behavior relationships has profited greatly from continued MRI advancements, including novel sequences that provide information about the structural, neurometabolic, and functional status of the brain. The development of neuroimaging methods that integrate information about both structural and functional brain organization in many ways has served to emphasize the role of neuropsychology in the clinical and cognitive neurosciences. An important reason for the integration of neuropsychology and neuroimaging is that information about brain status achieved through various imaging techniques is often difficult to interpret without a behavioral reference point; that is, the critical dependent variable is, and always has

been, human behavior. In functional imaging work, the role of the neuropsychologist is to provide expertise for the cognitive, motor, or sensory paradigm development, as well as the out-of-the-scanner interview and assessment. These assessment components are critical to linking information about the cerebral substrate to human behavior. For these reasons, the neuropsychologist has become an important figure within many multidisciplinary teams using neuroimaging techniques to better understand the effect of pathophysiology on human behavior. Moreover, although many novel imaging techniques, such as fMRI, are only beginning to be used clinically, to date, the field of neuropsychology has played an important role in the application and validation of these techniques in neurologically impaired samples (Figure 2.19).

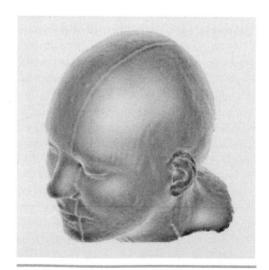

Figure 2.18 Three-dimensional geometric alignment of scalp surface. See inside covers for color image. (Courtesy Dorota Kozinska, Ph.D., University of Warsaw, Warsaw, Poland.)

Clinical Use

MRI of the central nervous system has provided behavioral scientists and neuroradiologists with revolutionary quality of brain images in all planes (coronal, sagittal, and horizontal). As a result, MRI has become an important diagnostic tool for detecting disease processes. This usefulness is related to that MRI is sensitive to tissue alteration, including those seen in diseases associated with demyelination (such as multiple sclerosis), hemorrhage (bleeding), and tumor. Because of its increased clinical use, MRI has become readily available, and mobile units have even been built that travel to remote hospitals.

MRI is a complex procedure based, in part, on molecular physics and mathematics of imaging 3-D objects in space. The principles underlying MRI sound complicated, and they are. Its scientific basis lies in physics and computer science; thus, an exact understanding of the procedure is not necessary for the neuropsychology student. But

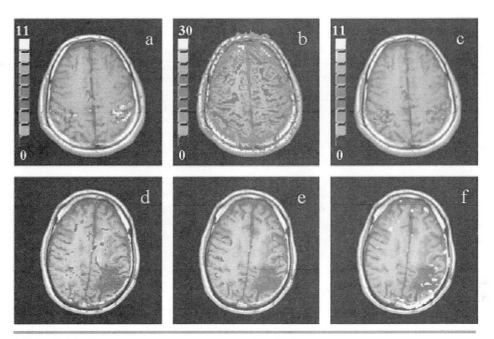

Figure 2.19 Functional magnetic resonance imaging signal response (percentage change) from normal adult (a–c) and patient with severe traumatic brain injury (TBI) (d–f). (a, d) Motor response (i.e., finger tapping): note focal activation in healthy subject and disorganization activation in TBI patient. (b, e) Normal cerebral blood flow: note diminished cerebral blood flow in patient. (c, f) Corrected motor response based on baseline cerebral blood flow: note less organized activation in patient. See inside covers for color image. (Courtesy Frank Hillary, Ph.D., Pennsylvania State University.)

neuropsychologists are participating in the research using this technology because of their expertise in the functional aspects of neuroanatomic structures, their knowledge of neuropsychological tests, and their background in scientific methodology and design.

Functional Magnetic Resonance Imaging

Traditional MRI measures the frequencies of magnetically perturbed water molecules and provides a structural representation of the brain. More recent advances have focused on detecting frequencies emitted from other molecular species associated with cerebral metabolism. Efforts have concentrated on reconstructing images from glucose metabolism and changes in blood oxygenation. A recent finding is that oxygenated blood has slightly different magnetic properties that special-sequence MRI scans can detect. In this manner, researchers can measure motor activity and neuropsychological tests. The data from functional MRI (fMRI) can then be superimposed (cross-sectioned

or co-registered) over the structural MRI for a precise mapping of structure and function. This combined use of MRI and fMRI may revolutionize the study of the activated brain, because it can provide almost continuous real-time data on cerebral activity (Cohen, Noll, & Schneider, 1993).

The advantage of fMRI over SPECT, PET, and CT is that there is no radiation exposure. Therefore, fMRI is less invasive. However, scientists do not completely know the effects of exposure of the brain to high magnetic fields, which is higher in fMRI because molecules other than hydrogen are assessed. Furthermore, resolution of fMRI is better than in PET images, which are reconstructed from thousands of calculations averaged over 90 seconds, the half-life of the tracer. In contrast, fMRI can provide independent images every few seconds or as frequently as the RF is turned on and off. This capability gives investigators a better picture-by-picture account of the neural correlates involved in specific tasks (Neuropsychology in Action 2.3).

MAGNETOENCEPHALOGRAPHY

Magnetoencephalography (MEG) involves measurement of changes in magnetic fields that are generated by underlying electrical activity of active neurons. Neuronal activity generates not only electrical fields but also magnetic fields. When neurons fire, the magnetic changes resulting from the electrical fields, which reflect neural activity, can be measured. Recording the magnetic fields that accompany the electrical activity of neurons is known as MEG. MEG is the magnetic equivalent of EEG. The magnetic field of neurons is small, and it requires special superconducting coils, housed in elaborate magnetically shielded rooms, to detect and measure the weak magnetic fields. This specialized detector is called the *superconducting quantum interference device (SQUID),* which is capable of measuring tiny magnetic fields of the brain. MEG traditionally has used systems with one to seven SQUID sensors, although recent technology has made larger sensor arrays possible. The response of the brain to different stimuli, similar to the EP technique, results in measurable alterations in the magnetic field. A computer then can calculate a 3-D location based on the source of the magnetic field in the brain. The physical location of the magnetic source can be improved by projecting the MEG onto MR images. MEG is more elaborate than EEG, but it can better localize the source of activity using isocontour maps of magnetic fields.

MEG is expensive and relies on complex technology; the SQUID is immersed in liquid helium to keep the system at a low temperature, which is necessary for superconductivity. Currently, MEG is experimental and is not used for routine clinical diagnostic studies, although MEG is an added diagnostic tool in epilepsy, because it provides more accurate seizure diagnosis than EEG technology (Hari, 1994). Table 2.6 reviews current magnetic imaging procedures.

Cerebrospinal Fluid Studies: Lumbar Puncture

The **lumbar puncture,** or spinal tap, is a medical technique to collect a sample of CSF surrounding the spinal cord for diagnostic study. The patient lies on his or her side in a fetal position, and the physician administers a local anesthetic. A long (3- to 3.5-inch) puncture needle is inserted perpendicular between the third and fourth (or fourth and fifth) lumbar vertebrae. The needle penetrates the dura and enters the spinal canal. Then the physician collects CSF and checks CSF pressure (normal

---

Table 2.6 *Magnetic Imaging Procedures*

Magnetic resonance imaging (MRI): MRI can provide the most detailed images of brain structures. The obtained images are of excellent clarity, but individuals who have metal in their bodies are contraindicated for the procedure. Recent research focuses on the functional mapping of blood flow or oxygenation using MRI. The advantage of functional MRI over other functional procedures such as positron emission tomography is that it provides good spatial resolution and images in short time periods or "real time."

Magnetoencephalography (MEG): MEG is the magnetic equivalent of electroencephalography, in which a computer can calculate a three-dimensional magnetic field of the brain. Superconducting quantum interference devices detect the small magnetic fields in the brain that are a marker of neural activity. A disadvantage of MEG is that it is expensive and not readily available for clinical applications.

---

range = 100 mm). In some cases, the physician administers radiopaque material or medication through the needle, in which case, the CSF withdrawn is equal to the volume of fluid introduced. At the end of the procedure, the physician withdraws the needle quickly. The lumbar puncture is a relatively easy and routine way by which to obtain a CSF sample. Yet, lumbar puncture is invasive and painful, requiring a local anesthetic, and infection is always a concern.

On visual inspection, normal CSF is colorless and does not coagulate. After a subarachnoid hemorrhage (for example), the CSF may be stained with blood. Technicians typically examine the CSF sample in a laboratory for cell count, glucose levels, and protein content to detect CSF abnormalities. The lumbar puncture is a useful diagnostic aid for a variety of neurologic conditions in which the CSF has been "contaminated," including acute and subacute bacterial meningitis, viral infections, brain abscess or tumor, multiple sclerosis, and hemorrhage.

Behavioral Examinations

NEUROLOGIC EXAMINATION

The **neurologic examination** is a routine, introductory evaluation that a neurologist performs. A neurologist is a physician who has specialized in evaluating and treating neurologic disorders. Although there are many variations, in principle, the neurologic examination involves a detailed history of the patient's medical history and a careful assessment of the patient's reflexes, cranial nerve functioning, gross movements, muscle tone, and ability to perceive sensory stimuli. The neurologic examination typically includes a number of brief cognitive procedures. These include language function, memory (e.g., remembering digits or memory for words), visuospatial function (drawing), attention (reverse counting), and mental status (i.e., an assessment of the patient's understanding of where he or she is, what time it is, who he is, and why he is there). The neurologic examination is not as detailed as a neuropsychological evaluation, because it is difficult to obtain an accurate comprehensive assessment of higher cortical function during a brief examination. More recently, a special focus in neurology, on behavior and higher cortical function (behavioral neurology), has overlapped more with neuropsychology. In general, the domains previously held by neurologists and by neuropsychologists are getting much closer, and both disciplines have much to learn from each other.

NEUROPSYCHOLOGICAL EVALUATION

Whereas neurologists are interested in changes in the nervous system that occur within the clinical context (such as lesions, disease, and trauma), neuropsychologists are primarily interested in higher cognitive functioning. Luria (1990) suggests that neuropsychology is the most complex and newest chapter in neurology, without which modern clinical neurology would be unable to exist and develop. The **neuropsychological evaluation** provides additional information about the patient's health and is used, in conjunction with other pertinent information, for diagnosis, patient management, intervention, rehabilitation, and discharge planning. Chapter 3 gives a detailed account of the role of the neuropsychological evaluation, its purpose, and its applications.

After reading this chapter, the student may wonder whether modern imaging technology will soon replace neuropsychology. We strongly suggest that imaging technologies and neuropsychology are compatible. In fact, we are now in an era in which data from CT, for example, should be used routinely with neuropsychology information. Note that even though modern imaging technology has had spectacular success in depicting the brain's anatomy, neuropsychological findings appear more sensitive to the progression of degenerative diseases than either CT or MRI. Modern imaging technology is most useful in concert with neuropsychological studies. For example, consider a CT scan that shows a large, marble-size tumor in the patient's right parietal hemisphere. From a neurobehavioral view, we may make certain assumptions about what cognitive functions may be compromised, based on the CT data. Such assumptions, however, would be only hypothetical, and one would need to assess the precise neurobehavioral sequelae using

neuropsychological techniques. In addition, no imaging tool yet developed can indicate how patients will adapt with a specific neurologic disorder, whether they will be able to work, or what quality of life they will have.

New Advances in Imaging Techniques: Mapping the Brain

SUBTRACTION PROCEDURES

Researchers often use the subtraction technique in imaging studies to isolate brain characteristics that are relevant during a specific neuropsychological task. In principle, the procedure uses two sets of data. The first set is obtained using the control condition. For example, to use PET in studying the neuronal aspects of a calculus task in the control condition, researchers would ask subjects to recite numbers that have no meaningful relationship to each other. In the task condition, researchers obtain brain images while subjects are performing calculus problems. The logic behind reciting numbers in the control task is that both tasks involve the neural mechanism of using numbers, but only one condition uses numbers in a meaningful way. After researchers subtract the image of the noncalculus condition from the second image they obtained during the calculus condition, the new picture should show brain regions involved in the mathematical effort of using numbers in meaningful relationship to each other.

IMAGE ANALYSIS AND QUANTIFICATION (THREE-DIMENSIONAL)

Recent advances in computer software have allowed 3-D computer reconstruction of specific brain structures. Because of recent advances in calculating volumetric analysis of specific brain structures, scientists applied segmentation methods to construct 3-D images, to visualize a specific structure of the brain (such as ventricles) or a known pathology (such as hemorrhage). Such 3-D images advance the understanding of pathologic conditions, as well as brain structures, because scientists can now visualize the site of the lesion from any angle or perspective. The ventricular system is difficult to appreciate in a 2-D perspective, but in a 3-D model, it can be easily visualized. More recent quantitative imaging techniques have automated the evaluation of definable ROIs throughout the brain. Because normative data are not yet available, serial quantitative image examinations of individual cases have proved useful. The correlation between quantitative neuroimaging findings and neuropsychological indices of brain function has been only moderate.

One procedure focuses on using volumetric MRI analyses to estimate brain volume and ventricle-to-brain ratio (VBR). A normal VBR is approximately 1.5%; that is, about 1.5% of a normal, healthy, adult brain is dedicated to CSF. Increased VBR has been particularly consistent in subjects after traumatic brain injury, who have much higher VBR ratios, up to 4% (Johnson, Bigler, Burr, & Blatter, 1994). This increase is related to brain atrophy after the injury to the brain, with a corresponding increase of its ventricular space.

Furthermore, researchers can now digitize and superimpose serial MRI sections to create a 3-D picture of the entire head or brain or specific brain structures. This current technology can use 3-D representation of any isolated brain structure (Bigler, 1996). Other methods, including SPECT, PET, quantitative EEG, and MEG, can also be used to generate 3-D images.

After establishing image analysis and quantification, the next step was to address the interfacing of different imaging technologies to further explore structure and function in brain-behavior relationships. For example, the high detail of MRI-based images of the brain can be superimposed over images derived from those obtained by PET. In this way, researchers can examine both structure and function simultaneously. As technology develops further, it will be possible to increase the combination and integration of imaging techniques. Thus, one key focus in current imaging research is integrating multifaceted data to understand regional brain function. In this manner, topographic information from CT and MRI about the integrity of brain regions can complement information on regional brain physiologic activity derived from EEG, SPECT, and PET (Figure 2.20). However, as with any research, neuropsychological theory is needed to guide explorations of how brain activity relates to behavior (Neuropsychology in Action 2.4).

FUTURE DIRECTIONS

One of the greatest uncharted territories before the human species is the functional mapping of its own brain. Cartographers are scientists who use powerful technology to examine the living brain right through the skull. The task is formidable: 100 billion neurons with a seemingly infinite number of interconnections. The human brain is the most complex structure known in the entire universe. To make sense of this 3-pound "jungle" of cells, will it be enough to take pictures of the brain? Any new approach to brain mapping must move beyond simply visualizing structure. The challenge before the cartographers of the new millennium is to map function; that is, what brain structures do what, and when. It is true that neuropsy-

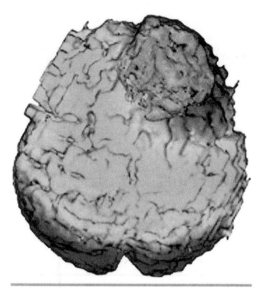

Figure 2.20 Sensory-evoked response examination with magnetic resonance imaging. With this technique, electrical activity and anatomic detail can be co-registered for clinical analysis. Image includes visualization of right frontal tumor. See inside covers for color image. (Courtesy Dorota Kozinska, Ph.D., University of Warsaw, Warsaw, Poland.)

chologists have identified many regions that specialize in particular cognitive jobs, but they have gained much of this knowledge from people with brain pathology or injury. The new imaging technologies are capable of examining the normal, healthy, functioning brain. We stand on the brink of learning how the living, normal brain performs sophisticated mental functions.

The most exciting use of neuroimaging, we propose, is in combination with neuropsychological procedures. That neuroimaging measures and neuropsychological studies depend on shared neuroanatomy needs to be studied further. Thus, it is likely that scientists will combine measures of neurophysiology and neuropsychology to unlock the secrets of how the human brain functions. Furthermore, imaging technologies will continue to be refined, with specific regard to the functional and structural aspects of the brain. It will soon be possible to perform biochemical dissections on the human brain, to pinpoint the concentration of a neurotransmitter receptor within the brain of a living subject. It will be possible to examine the effects of treatment of diseases known to be associated with disturbances in neurotransmitters or its receptors (e.g., schizophrenia, Parkinson's disease, and Huntington's chorea).

New advances will also demonstrate brain activity from moment to moment in real time with precise localization.

Neuropsychology in Action 2.4

Diagnostic Neuroimaging and Neuropsychology

by Erin D. Bigler Ph.D., Professor of Psychology, Brigham Young University

Contemporary neuroimaging represents a remarkable scientific breakthrough. Before the advent of computed transaxial tomography (CT) scanning around 1975, there was no way to visualize actual brain structure except during neurosurgery or in cases in which skull trauma exposed the brain. In one technique, pneumoencephalography, technicians would remove cerebrospinal fluid (CSF) from the brain, replace it with air, and take a standard X-ray image. But that method only outlined the ventricular system (internal cavity) of the brain and did not provide any actual direct image of brain tissue. Also, radioisotope scans would

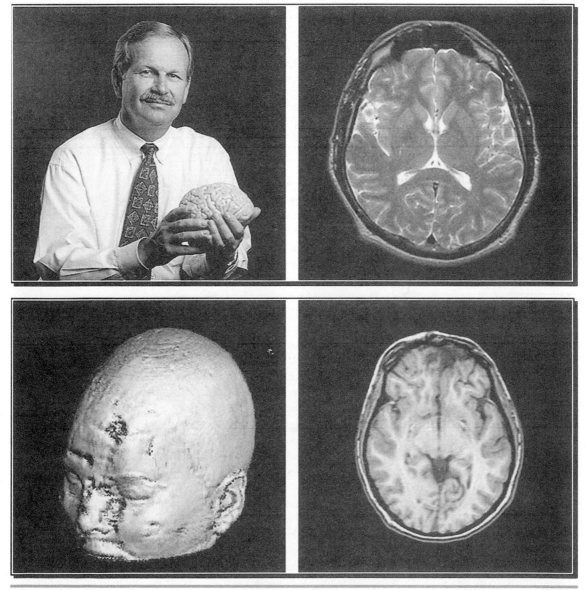

Figure 2.21 Dr. Erin D. Bigler and imaging examples. (Courtesy Erin Bigler, Brigham Young University.)

(continued)

(*continued*)

measure uptake of a radiopharmaceutical, but could not visualize actual tissue. Thus, in the early history of neurology and neuropsychology, the clinician had to rely on the powers of inference to make conclusions about underlying brain pathology and neurologic disorders, because the brain could not be viewed directly. Before the current state of neuroimaging, knowing the patient's history, an in-depth knowledge of brain anatomy and pathology, and examining the patients on standard neurologic and neuropsychological tests allowed clinicians to make an inference about particular brain regions that might be involved (damaged) or what type of disease process might be present. All this changed radically with the advent of modern brain imaging techniques. The CT scan was the forerunner for the development of magnetic resonance imaging (MRI), which uses an entirely different technology. In scanning with CT technology, an X-ray beam passes through the head and various computer computations

create an index of tissue density. These tissue density values are then used to form an image of the brain on a gray scale. MRI uses radiofrequency waves that permit a reconstruction of the brain, essentially mimicking gross anatomy. The beauty of MRI is that scientists can use it to acquire images of the brain in any plane and in any angle or orientation.

For example, the first set of images in Figure 2.21 (top right) are of my brain (that's me, holding a brain, in the top left). Viewing my brain in the horizontal (axial) position, you can see that the brain is a symmetric organ; therefore, a view of one side should mirror the other side. In comparison, just below my MRI scan is one from a patient who sustained severe traumatic brain injury (TBI) in a motor vehicle accident, with penetrating damage to the frontal lobe. The lower left-hand quadrant shows the three-dimensional MRI reconstruction of the person's head. You can see the residual scars about the face and nose and the indentation that is in the frontal

region where the rearview mirror stand penetrated the skull and brain. Looking at the horizontal (axial) view of this individual's brain in the bottom right-hand corner and applying the principle of symmetry, you can see the frontal (top) region of the brain, and on the right-hand side of the picture (the left side of the patient), a large area of degeneration in the frontal pole (areas in black). This indicates necrosis or wasting of the brain. From the neuropsychological standpoint, because the patient has predominantly a frontal injury, you would expect difficulties with complex reasoning, decision making, change in temperament and personality, as well as alterations in memory functioning. In fact, the patient's neuropsychological studies demonstrate such deficits. This is an excellent example of how brain imaging technology can interface with neuropsychological test findings to establish the most accurate and specific assessment of behavioral and cognitive changes in a patient with TBI.

The integration of different imaging technologies is only in its infancy. Scientists have yet to fully explore interrelationships among different neurodiagnostic procedures. The greatest potential of these tools may lie in assessing the neuropsychological functions *during* neurophysiologic procedures. The tools that appear most valuable at this time are fMRI, MEG, quantitative EEG, PET, and SPECT. This direction will lead to a multidimensional and increasingly comprehensive approach to the functioning of the brain, bridging the gap between psychology and biology.

Summary

The neuropsychology student may believe that the level of technology is so sophisticated that behavioral techniques add little to the overall information about a human being. This is true to some extent, particularly in the area of diagnosis. The presence of tumors, stroke, and hydrocephalus is most easily, efficiently, and accurately discerned by modern imaging techniques. However, some diagnoses are so subtle and diffuse that only comprehensive neuropsychological tests can identify them. Although the neuropsychologist's role in diagnosis has shrunk, behavioral techniques still play a major role in diagnosing early stages of dementia or attention deficit disorder. Furthermore, sophisticated medical examination procedures cannot provide a functional assessment of an individual, and certainly not an understanding of the patient's quality of life or perception thereof. A functional assessment is most effectively conducted by neuropsychologists using behavioral tools.

Moreover, remember that most of the outlined procedures provide a static picture of the brain, and that neuropsychological dysfunction may extend considerably beyond the pathology that modern imaging techniques uncover. No doubt the alphabet soup of new imaging technologies has become a powerful tool in the study of brain–behavior relationships. But will this new technology fulfill what the phrenologists were unable to do, that is, create a precise functional map of the brain? Probably not. Many constraints hinder the use of functional imaging in studying the human brain. For example, ultimately, the image rendered is not a direct representation of the mechanism involved in the mental activity, but some correlate. Furthermore, functional imaging captures brief moments, most suitable for analyzing a neuroimage or process involved in sensorimotor operations or a specific neuropsychological task. But it is doubtful that imaging technology will ever be able to assess a thought or investigate personality.

One of the most exciting advances in the imaging of the living brain is the collaboration among different disciplines, including biomedical engineers, psychiatrists, neurologists, neurosurgeons, and neuropsychologists, to define and differentiate between the normal and the malfunctioning brain. We turn next to the developing brain and its often complex behavioral sequelae.

Critical Thinking Questions

- What are the differences among electrical, magnetic, and metabolic technologies in imaging?
- Why is co-registration, that is, the use of multiple assessments using different technologies, an important advancement in neuropsychology?
- Which medical technology to examine your brain would you volunteer for? Why?
- Will neuropsychology be outdated by the increased use of sophisticated brain imaging technology? Why or why not?

Key Terms

Golgi, Camillo	Computed transaxial tomography (CT)	Wada technique	Positron emission tomography (PET)
Nissl, Franz		Electroencephalography (EEG)	
Myelin staining	Hypodensity		Magnetic resonance imaging (MRI)
Horseradish peroxidase (HRP)	Hyperdensity	Electrocorticography (ECoG)	
Röntgen, Wilhelm Conrad	Enhanced CT	Evoked potential (EP)	Magnetoencephalography (MEG)
X-ray	Angiography	Single-photon emission computed tomography (SPECT)	Lumbar puncture
Air encephalogram, or pneumoencephalogram	Femorocerebral angiography		Neurologic examination
	Digital subtraction angiography		Neuropsychological evaluation

Web Connections

http://www.med.harvard.edu/AANLIB/home.html
The Whole Brain Atlas—Harvard University site that provides neuroimaging primer and overview of brain anatomy and physiology, including images of CT, MRI, PET, MPEG movies, and SPECT. This site can be used as a general reference for exploring the latest in brain imaging.

http://www.bic.mni.mcgill.ca
Brain Web: Simulated Brain Database—Contains simulated brain MRI data based on two anatomic models. Full 3-D volumes have been simulated using a variety of slice thicknesses. Data are available for viewing in three orthogonal views.

Chapter 3

NEUROPSYCHOLOGICAL ASSESSMENT AND DIAGNOSIS

The teacher is faced with the eternal dilemma, whether to present the clear, simple, but inaccurate fact, or the complex, confusing, presumptive truth.
—*Karl Menninger*

Keep in Mind

- What do clinical neuropsychologists do?
- How is clinical neuropsychology distinguishable from clinical psychology or from neurology?
- What makes a neuropsychological test reliable and valid?
- What different roles do neuropsychologists play?
- What individual differences influence neuropsychological test interpretation?
- How can a neuropsychologist improve a patient's quality of life?

Overview

Jeanne was a passenger on a motorcycle with her husband when at an intersection a car ran a stop sign and hit them. Although her husband received only minor injuries, Jeanne was thrown about 5 feet. Luckily, she was wearing a helmet. However, Jeanne thinks she must have been knocked out, because she does not remember anything until the ambulance arrived. Emergency department personnel attended to her knee injury. She also had a terrible headache. Magnetic resonance imaging (MRI) did not detect any contusions or lesions. The hospital released Jeanne that day and told her to see her general practitioner if she had any more problems.

Jeanne recovered for a week at home, and then went back to her job as a medical records clerk. She also returned to school to enroll in coursework for a nursing degree. First, she noticed that she often forgot a client's seven-digit medical record number between the time she looked at it and went next door to get the chart. Her grades also started slipping. Before the accident, she was earning As and Bs; but on her first biology test a month after the accident, she received a D. She also continued to have headaches, which she had not had before. Four months after her injury, after several visits to her general practitioner and a neurologist, neither of whom could find anything medically wrong with her, her practitioner referred her for a neuropsychological evaluation. The request was to evaluate Jeanne to determine whether she had suffered a brain injury as a result of her accident or if her symptoms might be a psychosomatic reaction, that is, related to increased stress in dealing with the accident and the aftermath.

What can neuropsychology offer Jeanne? Many people who have head injuries or suffer whiplash injuries in car accidents, sports injuries, or falls may have a brief lapse of consciousness. They may feel temporarily confused or disoriented. They may or may not go to a doctor or to the hospital, and if they do, they are usually released after a brief observation. Computed transaxial tomography (CT) or MRI results are quite likely to be negative for any small or microscopic contusions or lesions. Only after going home and trying to resume the normal tasks of working or going to school may someone such as Jeanne feel unable to concentrate or often forget things. The person may have other odd symptoms that he or she does not understand, such as becoming more easily frustrated or just not feeling "herself." If these problems do not resolve and the person is persistent, or the physician perceptive, then the physician should make a referral for neuropsychological testing.

General Considerations in Neuropsychological Testing

This chapter describes the most frequently used assessment techniques in neuropsychology and outlines the scientific and theoretical principles of neuropsychological measurement. We stress that clinical neuropsychologists use a number of different methods to evaluate and treat individuals with brain dysfunction. Simply put, neuropsychologists are foremost clinical psychologists who have specialized in neuropsychological conceptualizations and methods. For neuropsychologists to understand the individual, they must view psychology as the expression of neuropsychology. From this perspective, neuropsychology is a broad field, and the neuropsychologist's roles span

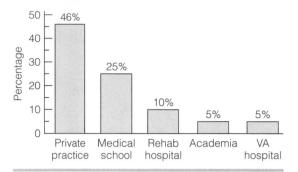

Figure 3.1 Distribution of neuropsychology practice, based on a survey of more than 2000 members of the National Academy of Neuropsychology. (Reproduced from Gordon, A., & Zillmer, E. A. [1997]. Integrating the MMPI and neuropsychology: A survey of NAN membership. *Archives of Clinical Neuropsychology, 4*, 325–326, by permission of Elsevier.)

the range from evaluation to rehabilitation to research. This provides flexibility for employment in diverse settings. Figure 3.1 outlines representative employment settings of clinical neuropsychologists. Almost half of all clinical neuropsychologists work in private practice, 24% in medical schools, 11% in rehabilitation hospitals, 5% in university settings, and 5% in Veterans Affairs (VA) medical centers. Other employment settings for clinical neuropsychologists include community mental health centers/clinics, school systems, military settings, and prisons/correctional facilities. Across all settings, the "average" clinical neuropsychologist devotes 63% of his or her professional time to neuropsychology, has approximately 12 years of experience in practicing neuropsychology, is 45 years of age, and is predominantly male (73%) (Gordon & Zillmer, 1997).

In private practice, the role of the neuropsychologist is perhaps the most varied and flexible, but also the most ambiguous, because the amount of time devoted to neuropsychology depends on the type of patient population. Thus, neuropsychologists in private practice may provide neuropsychological evaluation and diagnosis, as well as psychotherapy, family therapy, biofeedback, and other forms of traditional psychological services. Most often, clinical neuropsychologists in private practice are generalists; that is, they have grounding in clinical psychology with expertise in clinical neuropsychology. Some private practitioners have teaching or clinical appointments in universities or medical schools and participate to some degree in teaching and research.

In medical schools and hospitals, and in VA medical centers, clinical neuropsychologists most frequently work in psychiatry and rehabilitation departments and, to a lesser extent, in neurology or neurosurgery departments.

The role of the neuropsychologist in the medical arena is typically neuropsychological diagnosis, evaluation, and intervention. The major difference compared with the private practice setting is the degree to which neuropsychologists participate in research. Particularly in medical schools, research plays an important role, and neuropsychologists are often important participants in multidisciplinary research. In rehabilitation hospitals, neuropsychologists are essential in interventions for and remediation of disabilities related to brain impairment. In the academic setting, neuropsychologists predominantly teach undergraduate students in psychology and graduate students in clinical psychology. Academic neuropsychologists typically run active research programs. Clinical service delivery may play a minor role. Neuropsychologists in university settings may treat patients in an integrated university neuropsychology clinic, or they may participate in a small private practice. Common to all employment settings is the emphasis on clinical diagnosis and evaluation, research, and rehabilitation and intervention. Figure 3.2 outlines the typical patient populations that clinical neuropsychologists serve. A combined total of more than 70% of the patients who neuropsychologists treat are rehabilitation, psychiatry, or neurology patients. To a lesser degree, neuropsychologists treat patients referred with learning disabilities, forensic issues, dementia, general medical conditions, and seizure disorders.

WHY TESTING?

In the past, the interest in clinical neuropsychology, specifically in assessment, reflected a perceived need to expand the clinical understanding of behavior to include

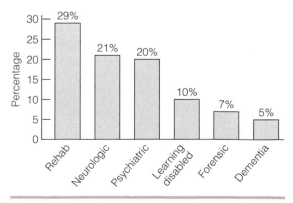

Figure 3.2 Types of patients treated by neuropsychologists. (Reproduced from Gordon, A., & Zillmer, E. A. [1997]. Integrating the MMPI and neuropsychology: A survey of NAN membership. *Archives of Clinical Neuropsychology, 4*, 325–326, by permission of Elsevier.)

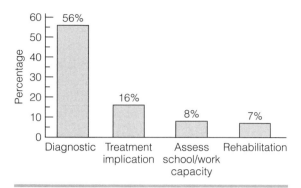

Figure 3.3 Overview of the neuropsychologist's role in assessment. (Reproduced from Gordon, A., & Zillmer, E. A. [1997]. Integrating the MMPI and neuropsychology: A survey of NAN membership. *Archives of Clinical Neuropsychology, 4,* 325–326, by permission of Elsevier.)

effects on human functioning caused by brain dysfunction. As a result, evaluation of brain functioning through the development of neuropsychological testing has been a major contribution to psychology. Clinical neuropsychologists, however, have often been—not undeservedly—pigeonholed as "brain damage testers" or reductionistic "lesion detectors." But this notion is outdated. Clinical neuropsychology is a quickly evolving field in which the neuropsychologist can play several roles. One of those roles traditionally has been conducting psychological evaluations of brain–behavior relationships. Understand that neuropsychologists gain expertise in neuropsychological assessment and diagnosis over years of study and clinical practice, which they usually pursue at predoctoral and postdoctoral levels. The purposes of administering psychological assessment instruments are to identify a patient's cognitive and behavioral strengths and weaknesses, to assist in the differential diagnosis of mental disorders, and to aid in treatment and discharge planning. Figure 3.3 reviews the neuropsychologist's role in assessment and diagnosis by summarizing the general purposes of neuropsychological assessments.

A majority (>50%) of all neuropsychological evaluations are diagnostic in purpose. In essence, the question to understand is whether there are indications of a decline in cognitive abilities and whether they suggest a specific diagnosis or neuropathologic condition. In many cases that involve obvious pathology (such as brain tumor and stroke), neuropsychological evaluations are a precursor or are complementary to more in-depth neurologic or neuroimaging procedures that can establish the exact medical or neurologic diagnosis. In other cases (such as learning disabilities, attention deficit disorder, dementia, or minor

head injury), the medical diagnosis is much more obscure and cannot be verified precisely by medical imaging techniques. Neuropsychological evaluations play a major role in assessing such conditions, because the diagnosis often rests largely on behavioral symptoms. In some medical conditions (such as epilepsy, multiple sclerosis, and AIDS), neuropsychological assessments have only minor diagnostic value, but they are used for documenting the extent of cognitive strengths and weaknesses, to outline effective treatment strategies and appropriate placements for school or vocational settings. Thus, many neuropsychological evaluations are conducted with more descriptive purposes in mind. As a result, the neuropsychologist's role has evolved from that of a strict diagnostician to providing descriptions of cognitive functioning, current adaptation, and future prognosis.

RATIONALE OF THE NEUROPSYCHOLOGICAL EXAMINATION

You cannot determine whether a certain function of the brain is impaired unless you test that function. The **neuropsychological evaluation** is an objective, comprehensive assessment of a wide range of cognitive and behavioral areas of functioning, which the neuropsychologist typically integrates with intellectual and personality assessments and evaluates within the context of CT and MRI scans. When based on a thorough description of abilities and deficits, neuropsychological testing leads to recommendations for rehabilitation and treatment. In using such tests, clinical neuropsychologists are interested principally in identifying, quantifying, and describing changes in behavior that relate to the cognitive integrity of the brain. Serial assessments can demonstrate gradual improvement or deterioration in mental status over time, allow better differentiation of cognitive deficits, and assist in treatment and disposition planning (Lezak, Howieson, & Loring, 2004). Thus, the neuropsychologist may address issues of cerebral lesion lateralization, localization, and progress. Neuropsychological evaluations can provide useful information about the impact of a patient's limitation on his or her educational, social, or vocational adjustment. Because many patients with neurologic disorders, such as degenerative disease, cerebrovascular accidents, or multiple sclerosis, vary widely in the rate at which the illness progresses or improves, the most meaningful way to equate patients for severity of illness is to assess their behavior objectively, using neuropsychological procedures.

The neuropsychological evaluation has a number of advantages that many standard neurodiagnostic techniques do not share; for example, it is noninvasive and provides descriptive information about the patient. Specific tests used in neuropsychological assessment batteries may vary, although most assessments include objective measures of intelligence, academic achievement, language functioning, memory, new problem solving, abstract reasoning, constructional ability, motor speed, strength and coordination, and personality functioning (Zillmer & Greene, 2006).

You can conceptualize neuropsychological assessment as a method of examining the brain by studying its behavioral product. Because the subject matter of neuropsychological assessment is behavior, it relies on many of the same techniques and assumptions as traditional psychological assessment. As with other psychological assessments, neuropsychological evaluations involve the intensive study of behavior by means of standardized tests that provide relatively sensitive indices of brain–behavior relationships. Neuropsychological tests have been used on an empirical basis in various medical and psychiatric settings, are sensitive to the organic integrity of the cerebral hemispheres, and can often pinpoint specific neurologic or psychological deficits. Neuropsychological assessment has also become a useful tool for clinical service delivery and for research regarding the behavioral and cognitive aspects of medical disorders.

APPROPRIATE REFERRALS FOR NEUROPSYCHOLOGICAL EVALUATION

Because a neuropsychological workup may take from 30 minutes to 8 hours of professional time, health practitioners should request consultations with some discrimination for cost-effectiveness and utility. The interpretation and diagnosis of the patient's profile ultimately depends on the referral question, the neuropsychologist's test selection, and the process by which the neuropsychologist interprets the data. Referrals should specify exactly what questions or problems prompted the referral, what the referral source hopes to obtain from the consultation, and the purpose for which the referrer will use the information. The advanced student in neuropsychology often feels frustrated by the failure of medical professionals to give a clear referral question. Note, however, that generating appropriate referral questions, as well as questions from the patient about the goals of the evaluation, is the responsibility of the neuropsychologist. Thus, it is often necessary to educate the professional community about the purpose and goals of a neuropsychological evaluation. Having the patients themselves ask specific questions about the goals of the evaluation (e.g., whether they can go back to work) often makes the evaluation process more meaningful to patients, and typically motivates them to put forth a good effort.

In a medical setting, the neuropsychologist is most helpful to the treatment team as a neurobehavioral describer of functional strengths and weaknesses, as well as a provider of neurodiagnosis. As mentioned earlier, such disorders as mild head injuries, early stages of Alzheimer's dementia, or learning disabilities may show no symptoms beyond the cognitive dysfunction that formal neuropsychological testing assesses so well. Following is a listing of instances in which a neuropsychological consultation is generally useful:

- Differential neurologic diagnosis
- Acute versus static
- Focal versus diffuse
- Location of damage
- Establishment of a baseline for neuropsychological performance from which future evaluations can assess improvement or deterioration
- Descriptions of the effects of brain dysfunction on behavior
- Determinations of disability levels for compensation in personal injury litigation
- Evaluation of vocational potential
- Assessment of environmental needs after discharge from hospital (disposition planning)
- Development of remedial methods for rehabilitation of the individual brain-damaged patient
- Measurement of residual abilities during rehabilitation
- Patient management

Psychometric Issues in Neuropsychological Assessment

The success of psychological testing procedures to assess and select individuals to become officers and undertake special assignments in World War I was the impetus for some of the earliest recognition of psychology as a scientific field. Since then, the science of standardized clinical psychological testing has evolved to the point that there are now hundreds of psychological assessment instruments in use today. It is important for the neuropsychology student to understand the scientific principles of psychological measurement before examining neuropsychological assessment instruments in more detail.

Psychometrics, the science of measuring human traits or abilities, is concerned with the standardization of psychological and neuropsychological tests. A **standardized test** is a task or set of tasks administered under standard conditions and designed to assess some aspect of a person's knowledge or skill. Standardized psychological tests typically yield one or more objectively obtained quantitative scores, which permit systematic comparisons to be made among different groups of individuals regarding some psychological or cognitive concept. Most neuropsychologists agree that tests are rarely used alone and are not interpreted in a vacuum. Almost always, neuropsychological tests are only one of multiple components of information used to make important decisions about an individual. Neuropsychological assessment, therefore, depends on the complex interplay among the neuropsychologist, the patient, the context of the assessment, and the data from neuropsychological testing.

RELIABILITY

For any psychological test to be useful, it must be both reliable and valid. **Reliability** is the stability or dependability of a test score as reflected in its consistency on repeated measurement of the same individual. A reliable test should produce similar findings on each administration. If test scores show a great deal of variation when administered to the same individual on several occasions, the test scores are unreliable and there is concern about error. Interpretation of the scores becomes difficult. There are several different forms of reliability, including test-retest reliability, split-half reliability (the correlation between two halves of the test), or internal consistency (the degree to which items of a scale measure the same thing, also known as Cronbach's alpha). Thus, the concept of reliability is not as simple as it first appears, and test developers must present substantial detail when making claims of test reliability.

VALIDITY

The **validity** of a test is the meaningfulness of specific inferences made from the test scores; that is, does the test really measure what it was intended to measure? If a test is unreliable, it cannot be valid. For example, if you take the same language test on three different days and obtain three different scores, it is easy to conclude that there is no consistency and, therefore, the test cannot possibly be used to predict anything about your language abilities. A reliable test is not necessarily a valid one. Let us say a test was purported to measure how well you make organized

extemporaneous speeches. The test requires you to generate as many words as you can in 1 minute. On three different days you took the test, and on three days you got a similar score. The test has high reliability. But is it telling us about your ability to make impromptu speeches? Not necessarily. An analysis of the test's validity may show that it is primarily measuring your ability to search and retrieve words from memory. It may have little to do with your ability to put your thoughts together and come up with a good speech.

Although the concept of a test accomplishing its purpose is easy to grasp, applying this concept often results in confusion. Many tests that neuropsychologists use originally were designed for purposes or diagnostic groups other than those for which they are used now. Rather than discuss validity in overgeneralized terms, scrutinize an evaluation of a test's validity in relation to the specific purpose and the specific population it is used in. That is, never consider a test *generically* "valid" or "invalid." The question to ask is: "Is this test valid for this particular purpose?"

You can use several different strategies for determining validity. **Construct validity** focuses primarily on the test score as a measure of the abstract, psychological characteristic or construct of interest (such as memory, intelligence, impulsiveness, and so forth). Construct validity would be most important if you wanted a demonstration of the cognitive or functional abilities a test measures (e.g., visuospatial problem solving or perceptual-motor functioning).

Content validity pertains to the degree to which a sample of items or tasks makes conceptual sense or represents some defined psychological domain. Various items of the test should correspond to the behavior the test is designed to measure or predict, such as measuring how fast someone can tap a finger, to assess upper extremity motor speed. Finally, **criterion validity** demonstrates that scores relate systematically to one or more outcome criteria, either now (concurrent validity) or in the future (predictive validity). Criterion-related validity traditionally has been an area of prime concern in neuropsychology related to the correct classification of diagnostic groups including brain-impaired, psychiatric, and normal individuals. There is also the issue of whether the test is being used as a measure to describe current everyday functioning. Criterion-related predictive validity is important if a test is designed to predict decline or recovery of function or future behavior of any type (such as medication management or ability to drive a car).

FALSE POSITIVES AND BASE RATES

A **false positive** (also known as a type I error or false alarm) is a case in which a neuropsychological test erroneously indicates a pathologic condition—such as "brain damage"—in an individual who is actually "normal." In setting a cutoff score on neuropsychological tests, statisticians attend to the percentage of false alarms (or false positives), as well as to the percentages of successes and failures within the selected group. In most medical (life-threatening) situations, statisticians set the cutoff point low enough to exclude all but a few false alarms (such as on tests that detect the presence of cancer). When the selectio n ratio is not externally imposed, the cutting score on a test can be set at a point yielding the maximum differentiation between criterion groups. You do so, roughly, by comparing the distribution of test scores in the two criterion groups, including the relative seriousness of false alarms and acceptances.

The validity resulting from the use of a test depends not only on the selection ratio but also on the base rate of the test. **Base rate** is the frequency with which a pathologic condition is diagnosed in the population tested. For example, if 10% of a psychiatric population of a hospital has organic brain damage, then 10% is the base rate of brain damage in this population. Although introducing any valid test improves predictive or diagnostic accuracy, the improvement is greater when the base rates are closest to 50% (closest to chance). With extreme base rates found in rare pathologic conditions (e.g., <1%), an improvement with a neuropsychological test may be negligible. Under those conditions, the diagnostic use of a neuropsychological test is unjustifiable when you take into account the cost of its administration and scoring. When the seriousness of a condition makes its diagnosis urgent, as in Alzheimer's disease (AD), neuropsychologists may often use tests of moderate validity in early stages of sequential decisions. Table 3.1 demonstrates a simple decision strategy for neuropsychological procedures. A single test is administered, and the decision to reject or accept a diagnosis is made with four possible outcomes.

Table 3.1 *Decision Making in Neuropsychological Assessment*

Decision	Positive (presence of pathology)	Negative (absence of pathology)
CORRECT	Valid acceptance (hit)	Valid rejection (correct rejection)
INCORRECT	False positive (false alarm, type I error)	False negative (miss, type II error)

Table 3.2 *Types of Tests Most Commonly Used by Psychologists*

Type of Test	Characteristics Measured
Achievement	Profit from past experience
Aptitude	Profit from future training and educational experiences
Behavioral/adaptive	Basic adaptive behaviors (e.g., self-care, communication, socialization)
Intelligence	Ability to adapt to novel situations quickly
Neuropsychological	Brain–behavior relationships
Personality	Psychopathology and ability to adapt and cope with stress
Vocational	Success in a specific occupation or profession

Neuropsychological Tests

Table 3.2 reviews the most frequently used types of neuropsychological measures currently in practice. Different types of tests have different goals and applications. **Achievement tests** measure how well a subject has profited by learning and experience, compared with others. Typically, achievement is most influenced by past educational attainment. Achievement tests are not designed to measure the individual's future potential, which is typically measured by aptitude tests. **Behavioral-adaptive scales** examine what an individual usually and habitually does, not what he or she can do. Neuropsychologists most frequently use such scales in evaluating the daily skills of individuals who are quite impaired (such as the mentally retarded or the severely brain injured). **Intelligence tests** are complex composite measures of verbal and performance abilities that are related, in part, to achievement (factual knowledge) and to aptitude (e.g., problem solving). **Neuropsychological tests** traditionally have been defined as those measures that are sensitive indicators of brain damage. Today, scientists consider a measure to be a neuropsychological test if a change in brain function is systematically related to a change in test behavior. Most available neuropsychological tests, therefore, have a broader function (see later in this chapter for a more detailed description of these tests). Another area of psychological testing concerns the nonintellectual aspects of behavior. Tests designed for this purpose are commonly known as **personality tests**—most often, measures of such characteristics as emotional states, interpersonal relations, and motivation. Finally, **vocational inventories** assess opinions and attitudes that indicate the individual's interest in different fields of work or occupational settings.

Neuropsychologists generally recognize that there is considerable overlap among all types of psychological tests. For example, it is difficult to measure aptitude without measuring achievement, to measure vocational interest without measuring personality, or to measure intelligence without measuring neuropsychology. One way to deal with this overlap is to reduce the complexity to two basic neuropsychological constructs: "crystallized" and "fluid" functions. Psychologists consider **crystallized functions** to be most dependent on cultural factors and learning. In contrast, they believe **fluid functions** to be culture free and independent of learning. Problem-solving and abstract reasoning abilities are considered fluid, whereas spelling and factual knowledge are considered crystallized. Nevertheless, even this simple differentiation of psychological test properties is controversial. For example, much discussion concerns whether intelligence tests tap mostly crystallized or fluid forms of behavior. Actually, it is nearly impossible to measure all aspects of a complex skill or group of skills with a single test. As a result, neuropsychologists prefer to administer a number of different tests, known as a *test battery*, that address different areas of brain–behavior functioning. After all, testing behavior, whether vocational or adaptive, is mediated by brain function. Thus, neuropsychologists use the preceding tests to some degree to evaluate specific questions about an individual. The neuropsychological interview is also an important part of the neuropsychological evaluation. The benefits of talking to the patient include an understanding of the patient's symptom presentation; the patient's awareness of his or her symptoms; and a review of the patient's educational, marital, social, and developmental histories.

The best way to understand the purpose of the neuropsychological assessment is to examine the evaluation process. Because neuropsychological assessment batteries typically evaluate a wide range of behaviors, they are considered multidimensional in their approach to measuring higher cortical functions. Thus, the neuropsychological examination involves accurately evaluating multiple cognitive abilities (Table 3.3). The usual categories of the neuropsychological examination include the following functional areas, which are listed hierarchically; that is, higher cognitive functions depend to a large degree on intact lower functions, which are listed first:

Let us examine each of these areas in greater depth. For each neuropsychological domain, we present an example to elucidate the construct measured and the method used

to do so. In addition, we present examples of frequently used neuropsychological tests for each neuropsychological domain.

ORIENTATION (AROUSAL)

Brain impairment affects not only a person's intellect or muscle movement but all other aspects of performance as well, including his or her level of consciousness. Patients who are lethargic or tired all the time tend to perform poorly compared with patients who have good energy. Lethargy is sometimes a symptom of brain damage and sometimes a symptom of depression. It is the psychologist's job to determine which factors are at work in a given case.

Alertness is the most basic aspect of cognition. Patients who cannot demonstrate adequate arousal may have difficulty participating in a neuropsychological evaluation and are, perhaps, unlikely to benefit from rehabilitation or psychological intervention. **Orientation** describes a patient's basic awareness of himself or herself to the world around them. Specifically, in neuropsychology, orientation refers to an individual's knowledge of who he or she is (orientation to person), what the date is (orientation to time), and where he or she is (orientation to place). If a patient is fully oriented, the neuropsychologist will say that he or she is "oriented times three," meaning that those three areas of awareness are intact.

Neuropsychological Items (Orientation)

The neuropsychological assessment typically involves the common evaluation of orientation in the three spheres; for example, "What is your full name?" (both first and last names are required) "Where do you live?" (specific town or city is required), or "How old are you?" In addition, neuropsychologists may also ask additional questions that relate to an individual's ability to recall his or her specific whereabouts, the purpose of the hospitalization, and any part of his or her address: "What is the name of the place you are in now?" (a response indicating that the patient knows he or she is in a hospital is considered correct) and "What town or city are you in now?" (any response indicating adequate orientation to the hospital's location is scored). The following two examples are examples of the patient's orientation to well-known current facts involving famous individuals: "Who is President of the United States right now?" and "Who was president before him?"

Table 3.3 *Common Areas of Neuropsychological Assessment Grouped Hierarchically by Function*

Orientation
Arousal
Degree of confusion
Disorientation
Place
Person
Time
Awareness of change/time

Sensation/Perception
Recognition
Familiarity of stimuli
Relationship among features
Visual acuity
Auditory
Taste/smell
Tactile/proprioceptive
Internal/environmental
Awareness

Attention
Span
Selective attention
Shifting
Sustained attention
Vigilance
Neglect
Fatigue

Motor
Cerebral dominance
Initiation and perseveration
Manual dexterity

Graphomotor skills
Balance
Ambulation
Motor speed
Speech regulation
Motor strength

Visuospatial
Construction
Route finding
Spatial orientation
Facial recognition

Language Skills
Receptive speech (following directions, reading comprehension)
Expressive speech (verbal fluency, naming, writing, math)
Articulation (stuttering, stammering, articulation voice, fluency)
Speech production (articulation fluency, voice)
Syntax and grammar
Aphasias: Broca's, Wernicke's, conduction, fluent, transcortical, subcortical

Memory
Verbal
Visual
Immediate
Short term
Long term
Recognition
Encoding

Storage
Retrieval
Chunking
Declarative
Procedural

Abstract Reasoning/Conceptualization
Comprehension
Judgment
Calculations
Problem solving
Organizational abilities
Higher level reasoning
Sequencing

Emotional/Psychological Distress
Depression
Attitude toward rehabilitation
Motivation
Locus of control
Family relationships
Group interaction
One-to-one interaction
Behavioral impulsivity
Aggressive/confrontational

Activities of Daily Living
Toileting
Dressing
Bathing
Transferring
Continence
Feeding

Neuropsychological Tests (Orientation)

To measure orientation, neuropsychologists frequently use the Galveston Orientation and Amnesia Test (GOAT) (Levin, O'Donnell, & Grossman, 1979). This short mental status examination assesses the extent and duration of confusion and amnesia after traumatic brain injury. Like the Glasgow Coma Scale (GCS; see Chapter 13), it was designed for repeated measurements and can be used several times a day and repeated over days or week as necessary. The GOAT yields a score from 0 to 100, with a suggested cutoff score of 75 or better indicating relatively intact orientation and the capacity of the patient to undergo formal neuropsychological testing. Both the GCS and the GOAT are simple to administer; therefore, the treatment team often uses them. Because these scales quantify level of patient arousal, researchers have frequently used them in examining outcome of brain injuries that involve an alteration in consciousness.

SENSATION AND PERCEPTION

Sensation is the elementary process of a stimulus exciting a receptor and resulting in a detectable experience in any sensory modality; for example, "I hear something." **Perception** depends on intact sensation and is the process of "knowing"; for example, "I hear music, it is Pearl Jam." The perceptual process begins with arousal and orientation, sensation is the second stage, and perception the third. In assessing sensation and perception, the neuropsychologist is interested in quickly and grossly evaluating the patient's visual, auditory, and tactile functional levels. Screening for impaired sensation and perception yields important information by ruling out the contributions of dysfunctional visual or auditory sensation to test performance. In addition, discovering unilateral sensory deficits aids in diagnosis of lateralized brain injury. It is important to understand that neuropsychologists are interested in a more or less general assessment of a patient's sensory functioning. Specialists, including audiologists (hearing) or optometrist (visual), perform diagnostic evaluations.

Neuropsychological Items (Sensation and Perception)

Sample items of testing the sensory and perception domain may include assessing the intactness of the patient's left and right visual fields (see Chapter 8 for a description of visual field deficits). This is achieved by administering a visual field examination, common in a neurologic examination. For this procedure, the examiner must sit facing the patient, at a distance of approximately 3 to 4 feet, and ask, "I would like you to look straight at my nose. I am going to put my arms out like this, and I want you to tell me which finger I am moving. You can point to it if you like." The examiner extends the index finger of each hand in a vertical fashion with arms spread out at shoulder height and presents the stimuli by moving each finger slightly, waiting for the patient's response between trials. Discrimination of similar auditory, verbal stimuli may be tested by the examiner saying, "I am going to say two words, and I want you to tell me whether I am saying the same word twice or two different words," to assess auditory functioning:

house – house	(same)
people – peanut	(different)
bar – bar	(same)
first – thirst	(different)

To assess the patient's ability to sense or feel objects, the examiner may say, "I am going to place an object in one of your hands. I would like you to close your eyes, feel the object, and tell me what it is." This procedure measures stereognosis, recognition of objects by touch.

Neuropsychological Tests (Sensation and Perception)

Some neuropsychologists have standardized their procedures for examining sensory and perceptual functioning and developed scoring systems as well. For example, part of the well-known and often used Halstead–Reitan Neuropsychological Battery includes a sensory-perceptual examination that tests for finger agnosia, skin writing recognition, and sensory extinction in the tactile, auditory, and visual modalities (Reitan & Wolfson, 1993).

ATTENTION/CONCENTRATION

Attention is a critical requirement for learning. To remember, you first have to pay attention. Some patients are incapable of attending to their environment. Others may be able to attend to a learning task, but only for a limited amount of time. Still others may be able to attend to a task only if there are no distractions in the environment. Psychologists divide the concept of attention into separate categories such as sustained attention, paying attention to something over a prolonged period, and selective attention, paying attention to more than one thing at a time.

Neuropsychological Items (Attention/Concentration)

Tasks requiring mental control involve simple, overlearned information, but also require the person to maintain an adequate level of attention throughout the item. Errors in this area may indicate extreme fatigue or impairment in concentration skills. For example,

"Count from 1 to 20 as quickly as you can."
"Recite the days of the week backward beginning with Sunday."
"Say the alphabet *(A, B, C . . .)* all the way through."
"Count by threes, beginning with 1 and adding 3 to each number. For example, 1, 4, 7, and so on. (Stop when you reach 22.)"

Another form of attention in this cognitive skill area is attention span. Here, the examiner asks the patient to attend to various verbal stimuli, then repeat them. The stimuli become progressively more complex. In this manner, it is possible to evaluate a patient's span of attention for unfamiliar combinations of stimuli.

"I am going to say some numbers, and after I finish, I would like you to repeat them."

TRIAL 1	5	8	9	
TRIAL 2	9	2	7	5
TRIAL 3	7	1	6	3	2

"Now I am going to say some more numbers; but this time when I finish, I want you to say them backward. For example, if I say 3 – 6, you say 6 – 3."

TRIAL 1	5	8	
TRIAL 2	2	6	1

Sustained attention is the ability to concentrate over a period of time. For example, you can assess verbal attention with the following task: "Tap on the table when you hear me say the number 4":

| 2 | 3 | 5 | 4 | 7 | 4 | 6 | 4 | 4 | 2 |
| 1 | 8 | 1 | 7 | 8 | 4 | 5 | 4 | 2 | 3 |

Neuropsychological Tests (Attention/Concentration)

Standardized tests of attention include the Symbol Digit Modalities Test (SDMT) (Smith, 1982), which requires the respondent to fill in blank spaces with the number that is paired to the symbol above the blank space as quickly as possible for 90 seconds. The SDMT primarily assess complex scanning, visual tracking, and sustained attention. An interesting test of selective attention is the d2 Test of Attention (Brickenkamp & Zillmer, 1998). The d2 Test is a timed test of selective attention and is a standardized refinement of a visual cancelation test. It has been translated into four languages and is the most frequently used test of attention in Europe. In response to the discrimination of similar visual stimuli, the test measures processing speed, rule compliance, and quality of performance, allowing estimation of individual attention and concentration performance (Figure 3.4). The test was originally developed in 1962 in Germany and Switzerland as an assessment tool for driving efficiency. Subjects who fail the d2 task tend to have difficulty concentrating, including difficulty in warding off distractions.

MOTOR SKILLS

Neuropsychologists are interested in assessing a person's ability to demonstrate motor control in the upper and lower extremities. Simple motor skills require little coordination, whereas more complex items tap into higher motor processes. As items progress in difficulty, the patient must show more integration of cognitive skills to perform the task successfully. The following neuropsychological procedures measure varied aspects of a patient's motor functioning. The hierarchic nature of the item presentation can yield clues to the patient's limits in motor functioning.

Neuropsychological items (motor) that involve gross-motor movement assess one of the most basic cortically mediated motor responses such as a response to a single command; for example, "Raise your right hand," or "Move your left leg." You can evaluate motor speed from the patient's ability to "touch your thumb to your forefinger as quickly as you can," and fine-motor ability can be evaluated from the command, "Touch your thumb to each finger, one after the other." These previous items assess the ability to perform a particular response; the following items tap the patient's ability to perform and inhibit motor behavior: "If I clap once, you clap twice." (Clap hands one time.) "Now, I clap twice, you clap once." (Clap hands two times.) Neuropsychologists consider this a higher level cognitive process, because it requires the patient to shift between initiating and inhibiting behavior.

Neuropsychologists often examine graphomotor skills. The following items assess the ability to copy shapes with increasing degrees of difficulty. They involve the integration of visual perception (input) and a complex motor response (output). "Copy these designs. Take your time and do your best." The patient's drawings are scored related to the correct shape, size, symmetry, and integration (Figure 3.5).

Motor apraxia items assess the intactness of common motor sequences. In general, the term *apraxia* refers to an inability to perform purposeful sequences of motor behaviors. Although basic motor skills may be intact, the patient may be unable to perform even overlearned motor sequences. The form of apraxia assessed here is **motor apraxia** or **ideomotor apraxia**. Impairments in this area may stem from an inability to access a stored motor

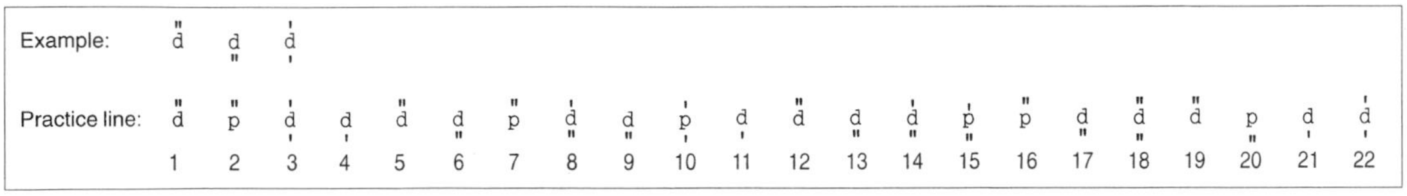

Figure 3.4 Practice line of d2 Test of Attention. The test items consist of the letters *d* and *p* with one to four dashes, arranged either individually or in pairs above and below the letter. The subject must scan across each line to identify and cross out each *d* with two dashes. In the manual, these items (correct hits) are called "relevant items." All other combinations of letters and lines are considered "irrelevant," because they should not be crossed out. The one-page d2 Test form provides sections for recording identifying data and test scores and provides a practice sample. On the reverse side is the standardized test, consisting of 14 lines, each with 47 characters, for a total of 658 items. The subject is allowed 20 seconds per line. (Reproduced from Brickenkamp, R., & Zillmer, E. A. [1998]. *d2 test of attention* [p. 7]. Göttingen, Germany: Hogrefe & Huber by permission.)

Example I

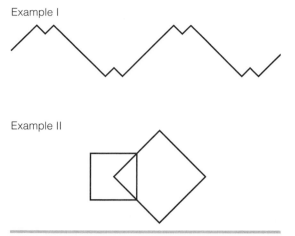

Example II

Figure 3.5 Visual integration examples. (Samples are from Zillmer, E. A., Chelder, M. J., & Efthimiou, J. [1995]. *Assessment of Impairment [AIM] Measure*. Philadelphia: Drexel University.)

sequence or an inability to relay that information to the motor association areas. An example to test this is, "Show me how you would make a telephone call from beginning to end."

Neuropsychological Tests (Motor)

Examples of standardized motor tests include a measure of grip strength and finger-tapping speed, both from the Halstead–Reitan Neuropsychological Battery. Grip strength simply measures the patient's ability to squeeze the dynamometer (Figure 3.6) as hard as he or she can. The Finger Oscillation or Finger Tapping Test requires the patient to tap as rapidly as possible with the index finger

on a small lever attached to a mechanical counter (see Figure 3.6).

VERBAL FUNCTIONS/LANGUAGE

Neuropsychologists screen for intactness of language. Initial items test the patient's ability to understand simple spoken language. More complicated areas of expressive language are then evaluated by assessing word repetition, naming, and word production.

Neuropsychological Items (Language)

Receptive speech evaluates the patient's ability to comprehend simple spoken commands such as "Wave hello," or a more difficult, three-step command: "Turn over the paper, hand me the pen, point to your mouth." Expressive speech focuses on vocabulary knowledge and recognition of concepts and objects; for example, "Please tell me what the word *happiness* means." Additional tests involve word and phrase repetition ("Repeat: 'No if's, and's, or but's'") and sentence generation ("Make up a sentence using the word *vacation*"). Deficits in verbal fluency and naming are also tested; for example, "Name all the animals that you can think of as quickly as you can." Visual naming can be evaluated by pointing to a picture and saying, "Tell me what this object is" (Figure 3.7).

You can evaluate writing by assessing the quality of writing at the word and sentence levels. You can also assess deficits in the motor component of writing (dysgraphia), simple reading (dyslexia), and spelling skills (spelling dyspraxia): "Please write down the name of this picture" (Figure 3.8).

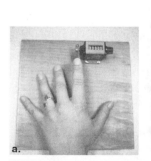 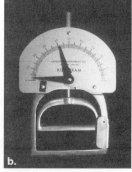

Figure 3.6 The Finger Tapping and Strength of Grip tests. (Courtesy Jeffrey T. Barth, University of Virginia, Charlottesville, VA.)

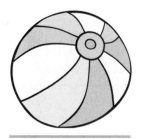

Figure 3.7 Naming example #1. (Reproduced from Zillmer, E. A., Chelder, M. J., & Efthimiou, J. [1995]. *Assessment of Impairment [AIM] Measure*. Philadelphia: Drexel University.)

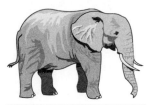

Figure 3.8 Naming example #2. (Reproduced from Zillmer, E. A., Chelder, M. J., & Efthimiou, J. [1995]. *Assessment of Impairment [AIM] Measure.* Philadelphia: Drexel University.)

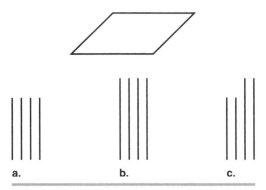

Figure 3.9 Visuospatial test item. (Reproduced from Zillmer, E. A., Chelder, M. J., & Efthimiou, J. [1995]. *Assessment of Impairment [AIM] Measure.* Philadelphia: Drexel University.)

Neuropsychological Tests (Language)

Many standardized neuropsychological tests assess verbal and language functioning. A simple but effective test of auditory comprehension (receptive language) is the Token Test (e.g., see Boller & Vignolo, 1966). Almost every non-aphasic person who has completed fourth grade should pass this test in its entirety. The test consists of a number of commands (such as "Touch the small yellow circle." or "Touch the green square and the blue circle.") that relate to plastic tokens, which come in different shapes, sizes, and colors. This test is sensitive to disrupted linguistic processes that are central to aphasic disability.

The Controlled Oral Word Association (COWA) test (Benton & Hamsher, 1989) assesses the subject's ability to use expressive speech. It measures verbal fluency by asking the subject to name as many words as possible that start with a specific letter. For example, within 60 seconds, an undergraduate or graduate student should be able to name 15 words that start with the letter *R*. In the COWA, examiners administer three word-naming trials using the letters *C, F,* and *L*. These letters were selected by English word frequency. That is, words beginning with *C* have a relatively high frequency; the second letter, *F,* a somewhat lower frequency; and the third letter, *L,* a still lower frequency. Word fluency is a sensitive indicator of general brain dysfunction and expressive language dysfunction.

VISUOSPATIAL ORGANIZATION

In the visuospatial domain, neuropsychologists assess various aspects of processing. They ask the patient to perform tasks of map skills, route finding, spatial integration and decoding, and facial recognition. The results of these neuropsychological tests can provide information about specific disorders of visuospatial organization.

Neuropsychological Items (Visuospatial)

Neuropsychologists can evaluate spatial orientation with simple directional skills and mazes, and then proceed through clock drawing and motor-free constructional tasks: "If this were a compass on a map and you were facing north, which direction would be behind you?" or "Draw the face of a clock, showing all the numbers, and set the hands to read 10 minutes after 11." Testers may evaluate visuospatial processing by asking, "Which of these sets of lines makes up this figure at the top: A, B, or C?" (Figure 3.9).

Facial recognition is the patient's ability to recognize a familiar face, as well as to compare similar faces and identify facial affect. For example, the examiner may ask, "Show me 'the happy face, the sad face, the angry face'" (Figure 3.10).

Visual sequencing also involves more integration and higher order processing. The person must comprehend the overall meaning of the activity, and then be able to correctly assemble the pictures to form the sequence of steps; for example, "This card has three pictures on it. If the pictures are put in the right order, they tell a story. Look carefully at the pictures, tell me the story, and point to the one you think comes first in the story. Now point to the one that would come second, and the picture that would finish the story" (Figure 3.11).

Neuropsychological Tests (Visual-Spatial)

The Bender Gestalt test consists of nine geometric designs, which the patient must reproduce exactly (Bender, 1938; Hutt, 1985). The "Bender," as it is often called, is a popular measure of visuospatial construction. It measures

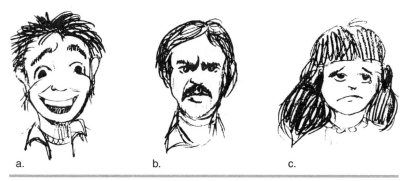

Figure 3.10 Test of facial recognition. (Reproduced from Zillmer, E. A., Chelder, M. J., & Efthimiou, J. [1995]. *Assessment of Impairment [AIM] Measure.* Philadelphia: Drexel University.)

a patient's ability to organize visuospatial material and has been shown to be sensitive to changes in neuropsychological status, particularly visual-graphic disabilities. Rey (1941) and Osterrieth (1944) devised another drawing test to investigate perceptual organization. The Rey–Osterrieth Complex Figure Test presents the subject with an intricate figure to reproduce. For both the Bender and the Rey–Osterrieth tests, scoring systems have been developed that evaluate specific copying errors.

MEMORY

You can look at memory in many ways. For example, as we noted earlier, to remember things, people must pay attention first. After paying attention, people must encode the information (do something meaningful with the information such as rehearsing it) to put it into more permanent storage. Once information is in storage, people must be able to retrieve the information as needed.

Neuropsychological Items (Memory)

Neuropsychologists assess general memory and new learning skills in a variety of modalities. There are immediate and delayed memory tasks in both verbal and visual formats. Performance on free recall and recognition tasks can help identify different aspects of memory function and dysfunction. Multiple trials of a list learning task can assess immediate verbal memory. For example, the examiner presents the patient with five words, repeated over four trials regardless of the patient's success on the item's initial trials: "I'm going to say a list of five words. Please try to remember them, and repeat them when I finish: *train, radio, apple, fork, chair.*"

You can assess delayed verbal memory by asking the patient, at a later point during the examination (such as 30 minutes), to say whether each word had been included in the list: "I am going to read a list of words. Tell me which of these words were in the earlier list I asked you to

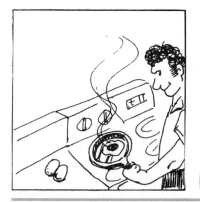
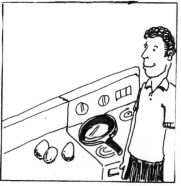
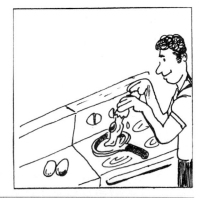

Figure 3.11 Example of picture arrangement. (Reproduced from Zillmer, E. A., Chelder, M. J., & Efthimiou, J. [1995]. *Assessment of Impairment [AIM] Measure.* Philadelphia: Drexel University.)

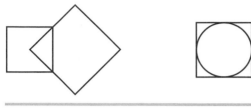

Figure 3.12 Example of design copy test.

recall several times: *clock,* ***apple,*** *book,* ***train,*** *table,* ***fork,*** *sandwich, truck,* ***radio, chair.***"

Delayed visual memory assesses the patient's ability to remember visual information the examiner presented earlier in the testing (an intermediate delay), as well as the ability to remember simple visual figures after a short delay. The examiner presents these items in a recognition format rather than a free recall format, so the patient chooses among similar stimuli, one of which is the correct figure. "Earlier I asked you to copy four designs. Which of these designs was it?" (Figure 3.12).

You can assess contextual or logical memory, immediate and delayed, by testing the patient's free recall ability. The examiner presents a short story to the patient, testing memory for information presented in a specific contextual structure. After an interference item, the examiner again asks the patient to tell the story. Slashes separate each unit of information in the following example.

I am going to read to you a short story. When I finish, I want you to tell me as much of the story as you can remember. Try to remember it in the same words as I have used: "Joseph / Green / left his house / and headed for the subway. / He was on his way / to the supermarket. / He purchased / wine, / steak, / and ice cream. / Later that day / he had dinner / with his boss / from the office." Now, tell me as much of the story as you can remember.

A completely verbatim response is not necessary, because neuropsychologists are mostly interested in whether the individual has formed a memory. For example, an acceptable substitution for /steak/ is "meat" or "beef."

Neuropsychological Tests (Memory)

To provide thorough coverage of the varieties of memory disabilities, researchers have developed batteries of memory tests. One of the memory assessment instruments most frequently used by neuropsychologists is the Wechsler Memory Scale (WMS; first introduced by Wechsler in 1945), which is now in its third revision (WMS-III). The WMS consist of seven subtests, which include personal and current information, orientation, mental control,

logical memory (which tests immediate recall of two verbal stories), digit span, visual reproduction (an immediate visual memory drawing task), and associate learning (which requires verbal retention). The WMS is sensitive to memory disorders and memory defects associated with aging.

JUDGMENT/PROBLEM SOLVING

A patient's ability to use abstract reasoning relates, in part, to his or her capacity to understand concepts. In determining a patient's ability to use abstract reasoning, the neuropsychologist examines the patient's ability to generalize from one situation to another. This skill is known as "transfer of learning." For example, if a rehabilitation patient can learn to transfer from the mat to the wheelchair with minimal assistance during physical therapy, one would normally expect the same patient to be able to generalize that skill from the physical therapy wing of the hospital to the nursing wing. Otherwise, the patient's learning is circumstantial.

Often, neuropsychologists are interested in evaluating insight specific to the patient's capacity to realize the implications of his or her disorder. At times a patient presents to a neuropsychologist, and says, "I'll be fine as soon as I get home," or "There is nothing wrong with me, I can drive a car." Initially, the neuropsychologist will measure his or her own evaluation against those by other team members. For example, if the patient has had a mild stroke and is hindered only by his or her own dislike of the hospital setting, it may be true that the patient will be "fine" on discharge. If the patient has experienced a moderate or more severe brain injury, the patient's communication may be evaluated as demonstrating lack of insight. One of the jobs of the neuropsychologist is to evaluate the insight that a patient has regarding the nature and the implications of his or her own disability.

Neuropsychological Items (Problem Solving)

You can evaluate higher order cognitive functioning and abstract thinking skills by asking the patient to interpret proverbs, solve everyday problems, or perform mental arithmetic. For example, you can assess abstract reasoning by asking a patient to interpret a common proverb, scoring responses based on degree of abstraction. Proverb interpretations are a traditional feature of the neuropsychological examination, assessing the ability to reason beyond the concrete level. For example, "What does this saying mean: 'You can't judge a book by its cover?'" An abstract answer may be, "Don't judge a person by their looks"; a

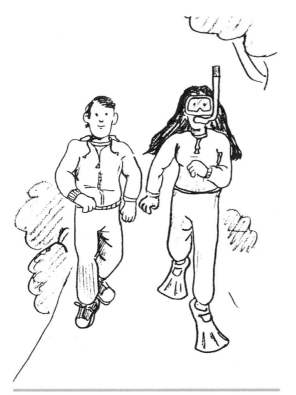

Figure 3.13 Example of a visual absurdity. (Reproduced from Zillmer, E. A., Chelder, M. J., & Efthimiou, J. [1995]. *Assessment of Impairment [AIM] Measure.* Philadelphia: Drexel University.)

concrete answer may be, "You don't know what is inside the book just by looking at its cover."

A common way to assess concept formation is to use a similarities/differences paradigm or analogies. The following items involve the abstract categorization of objects and concepts. They assess whether the patient can determine the appropriate abstract links between the objects and discriminate form and function: "How are an eagle and a robin alike?" or "Please complete this sentence: 'Banana is a fruit, cat is an animal. Father is a man, mother is a . . .'"

Problem-solving tasks tap the patient's ability to formulate solutions to a common, everyday situation. Responses can often demonstrate impulsivity and poor social judgment, as well as decreased functional independence or a need for supervision. "What should you do if you can't keep an appointment?" Sometimes tests present absurdities to evaluate reasoning skills, attention to abstract details, and the ability to formulate an abstract verbal response: "What is strange about this sentence: 'When the cook discovered that he had burned the meat, he put it in the refrigerator to fix it'?" or "What is funny or strange about this picture?" (Figure 3.13).

Neuropsychological Tests (Problem Solving)

Neuropsychologists have been creative in developing assessment procedures that evaluate executive abilities, and literally dozens of tests measure this neuropsychological domain. Only a few are mentioned here. The Trail Making Test B, part of the Halstead–Reitan Neuropsychological Battery, requires the participant to draw lines to connect consecutively numbered and lettered circles by alternating the two sequences (1 to *A, A* to 2, 2 to *B,* and so on). This timed task necessitates complex visual scanning, motor speed, mental flexibility, and attention.

The Wisconsin Card Sorting Test (WCST) (Berg, 1948; Heaton, Chelune, Talley, Kay, & Curtis, 1993) is widely used to study "abstract behavior" and "shifting sets." The examiner gives the subject a pack of 64 cards on which are printed 1 to 4 symbols—triangle, star, cross, or circle, in red, green, yellow, or blue. No two cards are identical. The patient's task is to place them one by one under four stimulus cards according to a principle that the patient must deduce from the pattern of the examiner's responses to the patient's placement of the cards. For example, if the principle is color, the correct placement of a red card is under one red triangle, regardless of the number of symbols. Thus, the subject simply starts placing cards and the examiner tells him or her whether the placement is correct. After 10 cards have been placed correctly in a row, the examiner shifts the principle, indicating the shift only to the patient by the changed patterns of "right" and "wrong" statements. A poor performance on this test often suggests that the patient has trouble organizing his or her own behavior or has difficulty applying one set of rules to different situations. The WCST is a sensitive neuropsychological measure, particularly for injuries to the frontal lobes.

Culbertson and Zillmer (2005) designed the Tower of London–Drexel University (TOL^{dx}) as a neuropsychological measure of executive planning and problem solving based on the original Tower of London (Shallice, 1982). The TOL^{dx} measures executive planning that involves the ability to conceptualize change, respond objectively, generate and select alternatives, and sustain attention (Lezak et al., 2004). The frontal lobes, in systematic interaction with other cortical and subcortical structures, support executive planning. The TOL^{dx} test materials include two identical tower structures (Figure 3.14), one for the subject and one for the examiner to use. Each structure consists of three pegs of descending lengths and three colored beads that the patient can place on the pegs in different configurations or patterns. The examiner asks the subject to move the beads of his or her tower structure to match

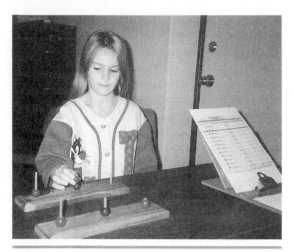

Figure 3.14   Administration of the Tower of London–Drexel University test, which evaluates frontal lobe functioning, that is, anticipatory-, pre-planning, and goal-oriented planning. (Courtesy Eric Zillmer.)

bead configurations that the examiner presents. In solving the bead patterns, the subject must adhere to two strictly enforced problem-solving rules: Only move one bead at a time, and do not place more beads than fit on each peg. The examiner records number of moves, rule violations, and time the subject uses in solving the bead patterns. Interpreting the subject's performance involves an analysis of both quantitative and qualitative variables. Empirical studies (Culbertson & Zillmer, 2005) show that the TOL^{dx} is sensitive to a complex set of cognitive processes, including planning computations, working memory, mental flexibility, attention allocation, and response inhibition.

Symptom Validity Testing in Forensic Neuropsychology

Unlike traditional therapy clients, the potential monetary compensation associated with personal injury or insurance claims may motivate patients tested to exaggerate or distort their symptoms. For example, individuals suffering from neuropsychological dysfunction as a result of trauma frequently report problems in attention and memory. Therefore, neuropsychologists learn to assess for a client's response bias. Psychologists have had a long and rich history of evaluating deception (e.g., polygraph procedures, assessing feigning of somatic symptoms). Through the use of their expertise in psychometrics and test theory, neuropsychologists have generated assessment procedures to measure symptom validity.

Although symptom validity tests are commonly referred to as malingering tests, **malingering** is just one possible

cause of invalid or biased performance. Test bias on the part of the client may range from outright malingering and conscious distortion of test performance to subtler, nonoptimal approaches to his or her performance, such as exaggeration. Thus, the neuropsychologist must also be expert in evaluating the test-taking approach and motivation of each individual. In some instances, these biased test-taking approaches actually stem from the patient's neurologic symptoms. For example, patients with right parieto-occipital stroke often have limited insight into their condition.

According to the *Diagnostic and Statistical Manual of Mental Disorders,* Fourth Edition (DSM-IV) (American Psychiatric Association, 1994, p. 683), malingering is "the intentional production of false or grossly exaggerated physical or psychological symptoms, motivated by external incentives such as avoiding military duty, avoiding work, obtaining financial compensation, evading criminal prosecution, or obtaining drugs." Thus, it has become a standard procedure for neuropsychologists to perform an assessment of malingering when performing independent neuropsychological evaluations (Zillmer, 2004; Zillmer & Greene, 2006), for example, using the Test of Memory Malingering (TOMM) (Tombaugh, 1996, 2003).

NEUROPSYCHOLOGICAL DIAGNOSIS

With the advent of modern medical diagnostic procedures (see Chapter 2), including single-photon emission computed tomography (SPECT), MRI, CT, positron emission tomography (PET), angiography, and evoked potential, using behavior-based assessments to diagnose organic-functional causative factors has become less essential. It has become less important for neuropsychologists and psychologists to act in the capacity of "lesion detectors" and more important to document the precise effects of brain dysfunction on behavior for purposes of remediation and treatment (Zillmer & Perry, 1996). Nevertheless, clinical neuropsychologists continue to figure prominently in uncovering the behavioral syndromes that correspond to impaired brain regions and neuronal circuits and may play an important role in diagnosing neuropathologic conditions (e.g., see Goldman-Rakic & Friedman, 1991).

Medical teams still ask clinical neuropsychologists to aid in diagnosis, not merely confirming what might appear on PET or MRI images, but adding behavioral and descriptive information about a patient's cognitive strengths and weaknesses. If a neurologist wants to know whether a patient has had a left hemisphere stroke, a CT scan or an MRI can show this. Neuropsychological testing would be redundant and not as precise as sophisticated imaging equipment for exactly locating the lesion within the brain. Imaging technology, however, does not provide information about how brain damage may affect behavior. Clinical neuropsychologists provide invaluable and unique diagnostic information in areas where behavioral information provides an important piece of the diagnostic puzzle. Those areas include the diagnoses of mild head injury, attention-deficit/hyperactivity disorder, learning disability, or AD. Currently available imaging techniques are not sufficient to diagnose AD. Brain biopsy after death is the only certain method. Thus, Alzheimer's dementia is a diagnosis largely determined by behavioral methods. Through careful observation and history taking with the patient and family, the neuropsychologist documents the extent and probable progression of the behavioral deterioration. Then, through repeated evaluations spread out over time, the neuropsychologist charts the severity and course of the neuropsychological impairments. If the team can rule out all other medical causes of dementia, then the person can be diagnosed as having "possible" or "probable" AD. In fact, the diagnosis of most dementia subtypes requires close collaboration between neurologists and neuropsychologists (see Chapter 14).

Mild-to-moderate head injuries also present diagnostic issues that neuropsychology can help clarify. With many head injuries, particularly of the mild variety (such as concussion), it is not immediately evident whether the person has actually sustained a brain injury. In many cases, the diagnostic aim of the neuropsychological evaluation is to determine the presence and severity of brain injury. The diagnosis is made, not to answer the outdated question, "Is this patient 'organic'?" but to answer the question, "Does this neuropsychological profile fit with what is known about the neuropsychological pattern of impairment after closed head injury?" CT and MRI may not show microscopic shearing, tearing, stretching, and bruising of axons. Even if they did, you could not predict clear behavioral symptoms from looking at radiologic or imaging data. As in AD, behavioral testing largely determines the diagnosis and severity of brain damage after closed head injury. Thus, neuropsychologists play an important role in determining patterns of neuropsychological dysfunction characteristic with a variety of central nervous system disorders. In addition, and to address the entire diagnostic picture, many neuropsychologists conduct comprehensive examinations of emotion and personality, to understand how the patient is adapting. For example, they not uncommonly diagnose depression or significant deficits in stress tolerance in patients who have experienced a head injury. The neuropsychologist's diagnostic skills as a psychologist helps differentiate between the impact of emotional/personality problems and brain dysfunction.

Neuropsychological diagnosis remains an important component of the neuropsychologist's role. However, diagnosis usually is not the only question of interest when a patient seeks neuropsychological testing. The next section discusses certain other issues that practicing neuropsychologists address.

DESCRIBING FUNCTION, ADAPTATION, AND PROGNOSIS

Describing behavioral functioning—that is, a patient's cognitive strengths and weaknesses—puts the "psychology" into neuropsychology. Psychology is the science of behavior; neuropsychology is the science of brain–behavior functioning. Although neuropsychology combines neurologic and psychological foci, the neurologic goal of detecting and classifying lesions dominated clinical neuropsychology through the 1970s. Since then, emphasis has shifted to a more behavioral focus, assessment of the human person, ranging from assessing cognitive abilities to evaluating quality-of-life indicators. In this approach, the goal as a clinical neuropsychologist is to describe brain–behavior functioning in such a manner as to accurately depict the current and future adaptive capabilities of the individual. Such information is important in evaluating the rehabilitation needs of a patient to facilitate adaptive functioning and prognosis, or in assessing the degree and type of assistance needed in the home and work environments. This chapter addresses these important issues in neuropsychological description, its similarities to and differences from generic psychological description, how it seeks to describe current adaptation in the real world, and how neuropsychologists use it to predict the course of recovery or decline of an individual.

Interpreting Neuropsychological Assessment Data

By now it should be obvious that the neuropsychological examination is a complex undertaking. Not only are no two patients alike, but how neuropsychologists administer the tests and which tests they select often differ. In addition, many procedures we have reviewed measure more than one functional domain, making it difficult to interpret the neuropsychological construct and cause underlying an impaired performance. This section presents an overview of interpretative guidelines for the neuropsychologist.

We provide quantitative and qualitative dimensions of neuropsychological performance, as well as case studies; elucidate neuropsychological diagnosis; and detail evaluation. Although this depends on the specific referral question, the clinical neuropsychologist is primarily interested in generating **interpretive hypotheses** about the patient and in answering specific questions about the test data, including the following:

Is there any cerebral impairment?
Evidence of behavioral deficits?
Behavioral changes caused by lesion?
How severe is the injury?
Is the injury medically significant?
Does the injury impair the person's ability to function in his or her daily activities?
Is the lesion progressive or static?
Is the lesion diffuse or lateralized, or are there multiple lesions?
Is the impairment anterior or posterior? Can it be localized?
What is the most likely pathologic process? What is the prognosis?
What are the individual's cognitive/behavioral strengths and weaknesses, and how do they relate to daily living skills, treatment, and rehabilitation?
Do the neuropsychological deficits influence the patient's quality of life?
What is the patient's reaction to the injury and/or impairment?

APPROACHES TO NEUROPSYCHOLOGICAL INTERPRETATION

Clinicians disagree somewhat in their approach to neuropsychological interpretation. These differences center on both practical and theoretical test issues and have become a source of debate. In making determinations regarding the evolution of a specific assessment and interpretation approach, practical and theoretical issues are often intertwined. A typical example is test selection and time needed for completing the neuropsychological examination. Neuropsychologists usually broaden information regarding a patient by administering a wider range of tests (such as memory, motor, learning, and language); they deepen information by administering a number of tests examining varying aspects of the same cognitive domain (such as selective attention or sustained attention). They must balance these theoretical considerations against the practical reality of examination length. Many patients cannot tolerate long testing sessions because of

fatigue effects. Given the current climate in which managed health care reduces specialized services to patients, most clinicians are also concerned about cost-effectiveness in time spent on evaluating the patient.

The approaches presented here include the major strategies of neuropsychological assessment and interpretation from which numerous variations have developed. We discuss the pros and cons of each approach in regard to both theoretical and practical issues.

Standard Battery Approach

Halstead (1947) and Reitan (1966) pioneered the use of a **standard battery approach** of tests for identifying brain damage. First, Halstead and Reitan identified tests that were sensitive to the integrity of cortical functioning. Then they sought to incorporate the evaluation of all the major cognitive, sensory, motor, and perceptual skills that a neuropsychological examination should reflect. The purpose of the Halstead–Reitan Neuropsychological Battery was to allow the development of various principles for inferring psychological deficit as applied to results obtained on individual subjects (Reitan & Wolfson, 1993). In this approach, the clinician gives the same tests to all patients, regardless of his or her impression of an individual patient or the referral question. Typically, a technician administers the neuropsychological procedures, rather than a doctoral-level psychologist, because the tests are administered according to standardized rules of procedure, without variations. Using technicians allows more testing for the same cost, because the more expensive time of a doctoral-level neuropsychologist is not needed.

This standard battery approach has several advantages. First, it can ensure that all subjects are evaluated for all basic neuropsychological abilities. This makes it unlikely that the diagnosis could overlook a condition of importance. Second, the neuropsychologist can use the data to identify objective patterns of scores that he or she can consider in diagnosing various neuropathologic conditions. Patterns within the data can help in diagnosing the probability of certain causes of brain dysfunction. Knowledge of causes can be useful in providing the patient, physician, or treatment team with tentative diagnoses, as well as in predicting the course of a disorder. Finally, the standard battery approach lends itself to the teaching of neuropsychological assessment and interpretation, because the beginning neuropsychology student need not make decisions about test selection, and the interpretation is objective and data driven. Finally, because the test instructions, test selection, and test interpretation are all standardized, this approach is particularly useful for empirical studies and facilitates comparison across different research projects.

There are also drawbacks to the test battery approach. The time involved in testing any patient can be considerable. Problems such as fatigue or loss of motivation may develop. The time involved forces the use of a testing technician to ensure a reasonable cost and reasonable use of the neuropsychologist's time. As a result, the neuropsychologist may have little contact with the patient outside of the interview and, thus, loses the opportunity to make a qualitative analysis of the patient's behavior. Obtaining qualitative impressions of the patient's appearance and behavior often is important, however. For example, we once observed a neuropsychologist who used the standard battery approach make an interesting misdiagnosis. This particular neuropsychologist strictly favored the neuropsychological battery approach and therefore typically did not interview his patients. He claimed that the subjective presentation of the case would "contaminate" his ability to make an objective interpretation. During a neuropsychological examination of a patient, the neuropsychologist's psychometrician indicated on her data summary sheet that the patient's performance on the Finger Tapping test was zero. The neuropsychologist proceeded to interpret this score as "severe, right-sided, upper extremity motor slowing with possible corresponding left hemisphere cortical dysfunction." But visual inspection of the patient would have made it obvious that the patient was not suffering from motor slowing and "brain damage"—instead, his right arm was amputated! The issue of using psychometricians to administer the neuropsychological tests remains controversial in contemporary neuropsychology.

The original choice of tests to include in the battery heavily influences standard batteries. The theoretical beliefs of the person doing the choosing often bias the choice. A poorly chosen test battery, no matter how many times it is given, will continue to yield unsatisfactory results. In different situations, alternate areas of assessment may be more effective in providing information. However, because the user of a standard battery gives no additional tests, he or she would never discover this. For example, the Halstead–Reitan Neuropsychological Battery does not include a memory test.

You can see a common problem of interpreting the empirical approach in composite tests that require the examinee to have a number of cognitive skills. For example, the Hooper Visual Organization Test (Hooper, 1983) requires the subject to name or write more or less readily recognizable cut-up objects. The Hooper consists of 30 stimuli. The maximum score is 30, and a score below 20

typically indicates "organic brain pathology." Because examiners think the measure primarily measures perceptual integration, a function often associated with right hemisphere function, they often interpret low scores as perceptual fragmentation most likely related to dysfunction of the right hemisphere. However, left hemisphere stroke patients often make low scores on this test, not related to impaired perceptual functioning, but related to the patient's impairment in naming objects. Thus, critiques of the battery approach often suggest that understanding why a patient failed a task is as valuable as that the person failed (Luria, 1966). Such information, they argue, often can be more useful than test scores in making intervention and diagnostic decisions. Furthermore, opponents of the empirical approach argue that complex behavior cannot and should not be reduced to a single number or test score. For example, the Hooper demands include comprehending the instruction; visually scanning the stimulus figure; mentally rotating the cut-up parts of the object to form a whole; and recognizing, naming, and articulating the object, either in writing or orally. Thus, this seemingly simple task actually requires the person to integrate a number of neuropsychological processes to generate a correct response.

The standard battery method also fails to recognize that altering a test procedure is sometimes valuable in determining a specific deficit. A standard battery may not be appropriate for all patients, especially when there are peripheral deficits, such as injury to the limbs, a serious visual loss, or spinal cord injury. Such patients' inability to complete a given test may reflect a peripheral motor or visual problem, rather than a dysfunction of the central nervous system. Consequently, data from such a patient on a standard battery may be useless for diagnosis, evaluation, and intervention. Finally, interpreting even a standard battery requires considerable skill, knowledge, and experience. Nevertheless, as standard rules and norms develop, standard batteries are somewhat easier to interpret and to teach.

Although the criticisms of the battery approach are valid, many psychologists remain faithful to administering a "core battery." Approximately 55% of neuropsychologists favor a flexible, modified battery approach, suggesting that the type of patient treated and the nature of the referral question play important roles in test selection.

Process Approach

The **process approach** to neuropsychological testing, often called the *hypothesis approach,* rests on the idea that the neuropsychologist should adapt each examination to the individual patient. Rather than using a standard battery of tests, the neuropsychologist selects the tests and procedures for each examination, using hypotheses he or she has made from impressions of the patient and from information available about the patient. As a result, each examination may vary considerably from patient to patient for length and test selection. The clinician may use standard tests, or may alter and adapt tests as he or she tries to form an opinion on the nature of the deficits (Christensen, 1979; Lezak et al., 2004). Altering tests to discover the patient's strategies is a popular method within the process approach to neuropsychological assessment (e.g., see Milberg, Hebben, & Kaplan, 1986). Many conclusions reached in the examination follow the clinician's qualitative interpretations of the test results and the patient's behavior. The clinician also grounds the conclusions on his or her experience and knowledge of the clinical literature. The principal developers of the process approach are Alexander Luria and Edith Kaplan.

The process approach has several advantages. First, it acknowledges the individual nature of the patient's deficits and seeks to adapt the examination to this individuality. Under the proper condition, such a technique can yield more precise measurements of a subject's skill on a given ability than just the patient's score on a given test. Second, the examination can concentrate on those areas the neuropsychologist sees as most important for the patient. It can ignore areas not important for the patient's prognosis. Because the time for any examination is limited, this enables the clinician to more thoroughly investigate significant areas.

Perhaps most important, the flexible/process approach emphasizes in what manner a patient fails or succeeds in a specific cognitive task. For example, a patient is unable to answer the question, "What is the capital of the United States?" Does this relate to the patient not understanding the question (speech comprehension), does it indicate an inability to answer verbally (expressive aphasia), or does the patient not know the answer (poor factual knowledge)? The standard battery approach does not allow a deviation from the standard instructions of the test, because deviating would invalidate the results. If the patient is unable to answer the question, the process approach allows for further investigation. For example, the examiner can show the patient a multiple-choice card with the answer and several wrong alternatives. If the patient points to the correct answer, "Washington, D.C.," the neuropsychologist would interpret this response as meaning that the patient knows this factual knowledge but cannot express this information either verbally or in writing.

Thus, the process approach lets the clinician concentrate on tasks related to the most important deficits that the patient exhibits.

The process approach also has several disadvantages. Because the content of the examination emphasizes areas that the clinician believes are important, the examination may selectively confirm the clinician's opinion. Because the clinician may never test areas that he or she sees as irrelevant, no one may realize that a deficit has been missed. Because the test's focus is just on the patient and his or her expected problems, the data may be biased toward confirming the original hypothesis. Thus, many neuropsychologists believe this more subjective approach relies willy-nilly on clinical experience, hunches, colleagues' anecdotes, intuition, common sense, folklore, and introspection (Meehl, 1973).

Using tests not standardized for a clinical population, or tests that have been adapted, also presents potentially serious problems. The interpretation of a test that has not been adequately standardized is always questionable. The clinician's subjective impression of what a score should mean for a given patient may be quite wrong. A test that appears to measure one thing in a normal population may measure something entirely different in a brain-injured population. In each of these situations, the accuracy of the individual clinician's judgment becomes the accuracy of the test. Thus, in the process approach, the opinion of the clinician is as good as his or her reputation. Currently, no measures of such accuracy exist, but probably this varies considerably among clinicians.

The use of different examinations and procedures for each patient precludes the experimental validation of individual tests in applied clinical settings. It also precludes evaluation of the process as a whole, because conclusions do not come from test scores, but from the clinician's judgments. Clinicians may, in such a situation, continue using an ineffective test because it appears to work. The process approach, therefore, does not lend itself to large-scale research, but often relies on case studies.

Structuring an examination on an individual basis may mean that it assesses only some of the basic functions mediated by the brain. Rehabilitation and prognosis depend on the state of the brain as a whole; the lack of information on the entire brain can impede an intervention program or invalidate a prognosis. In practice, it is not unusual to see patients with secondary deficits that appear unrelated to their primary referral problem and to the impression that the patient gives. For example, it is not unusual for a patient with a major stroke to have had smaller, secondary disorders of cerebral circulation. The deficits might have existed before the patient's current

Table 3.4	*Summary and Comparison of Approaches to Neuropsychological Interpretation*

Standard Battery Approach	Process Approach
Same tests or "core battery" given to all	Examination administered by a neuropsychologist
Tests administered according to standardized rules	Tests not administered in a standard way
Interpretation based on standardized norms	Conclusions based on clinical experience
Advantages	
Comprehensive evaluation of abilities	Acknowledges the individuality of patient
Objective interpretation based on normative data	Examination focuses on most important deficits
Facilitates teaching because of standard rules/norms	Emphasizes how a task is failed or solved
Useful for empirical studies	Useful for clinical case studies
Disadvantages	
Time demanding and labor intensive	Test procedure may be biased by clinician
Tests only as good as standardization	Opinion of the clinician is subjective
Relatively inflexible approach to testing	Difficult to teach, because it requires experience
Scores may not reflect a single cognitive process	Does not lend itself to large-scale research

problem arose. Whatever the source of the deficits, the clinician must identify and consider them in making any recommendations for a client. Finally, the flexible/process approach is more difficult to teach to students, because few "rules" and "procedures" exist. Test selection, adaptation, and interpretation depend largely on extensive clinical experience. This approach is also time-consuming, because the neuropsychologist, rather than a technician, must perform the evaluation. Table 3.4 reviews the advantages and disadvantages of the standard battery and process approaches.

Paul Meehl, a preeminent psychodiagnostician and former president of the American Psychological Association, addressed the complex decision-making process involved in psychological assessment. In 1957, he wrote the now-classic essay entitled "When Shall We Use Our Heads Instead of the Formula?" (1973). With this question he examined the rationale for when to use more empirical (psychometric) compared with more clinical approaches (qualitative) to psychological assessment, interpretation, and diagnosis. By the term *formula,* Meehl implied the scientific, empirical, and data-driven approach to psychology, consistent with those neuropsychologists who favor the fixed battery approach. By "using our heads," in contrast, Meehl was referring to the more clinical, commonsense, approaches typically used by the process approach in neuropsychology. Meehl suggested that the two answers to his question—"Always" and "Never"—were equally unacceptable. He also proposed that it would be silly to answer, "We use both methods; they go hand in hand." If the formula and your head invariably yield the

same predictions about an individual, you should use the less costly method, because the more costly one is not adding anything. If the methods *do not* always yield the same prediction—and most empirical studies show that they do not—then the psychologists cannot use both, because they cannot predict in opposite ways for the same patient.

This discussion remains a central theme in any type of psychological assessment, although the empirical approach has been increasingly refined since Meehl wrote his famous paper. Empirical and theoretic considerations suggest that the field of neuropsychology would be well advised to continue to concentrate efforts on improving actuarial techniques, rather than to focus on calibrating each clinician for each of many different diagnostic problems. In the meantime, neuropsychologists continue to make descriptions, interpretations, and predictions about human behavior. How should neuropsychologists be making interpretive decisions? Should they use the process approach, or should they follow the empirical, psychometric approach? Mostly, neuropsychologists will use their heads, because researchers have not developed adequate empirical batteries for every type of neuropsychological problem. In those cases in which there are good empirical approaches to neuropsychological problems (as in estimating intelligence), they should use an empirical approach. What if there is a case in which the formula disagrees with the clinical opinion of the process approach? Which approach should neuropsychologists use then? Meehl, a staunch scientist, suggested that in such a situation, they should use their heads very, very seldom—

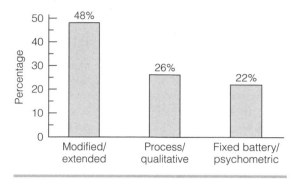

Figure 3.15 Approaches to neuropsychological test interpretation. (Reproduced from Gordon, A., & Zillmer, E. A. [1997]. Integrating the MMPI and neuropsychology: A survey of NAN membership. *Archives of Clinical Neuropsychology, 4,* 325–326, by permission of Elsevier.)

except, of course, if the issue is as clear as a broken leg or amputated arm.

Considerable controversy has raged about the preceding approaches to performing and interpreting a neuropsychological evaluation. Although there are certainly schools of thought about this, almost 50% of neuropsychologists report using parts of both approaches (Figure 3.15). That is, a majority of neuropsychologists use a modified battery approach, in which they choose specific tests to answer a referral question. They may interpret some tests in an empirical fashion and other test behavior in a more qualitative way. Approximately 25% report that they strictly adhere to a standard/fixed battery approach or a process/qualitative approach.

We caution the neuropsychology student that diagnostic and treatment decisions warrant integrating data drawn from a number of sources, including neuropsychological measures, pertinent neuromedical findings, and the patient's developmental and medical histories. Neuropsychologists typically do not render diagnostic decisions based on a single neuropsychological measure. Obviously, site, nature, and severity of the injury/disease process, premorbid personality, and a host of other moderating variables affect neuropsychological test performance. Interpreting the neuropsychological data requires a thorough understanding of neuropsychological principles, developmental findings, and psychopathology.

Interpretation of the neuropsychological protocol can then proceed through several levels of analysis, including the following:

- Overall level of impairment
- Pattern of impairment

- Lateralizing and localizing signs
- Qualitative observations

Once interpretation proceeds through these levels, the neuropsychologist can then evaluate test data to determine consistency with a patient's known medical conditions and presenting diagnoses, as well as to predict functional abilities and limitations.

ASSESSING LEVEL OF PERFORMANCE

Use of Norms in Neuropsychology

The use of norms in neuropsychology entails comparing an individual's test scores and available **normative data.** This approach provides the neuropsychologist with information regarding an individual's ability in comparison with others. This method compares the patient's score on a test to an expected score, or norm. The method determines the expected test score from the performance of a normative sample of patients and control subjects. Such norms may take into account such factors as age, sex, education, and intelligence. Many neuropsychological tests have a **cutoff score.** A patient scoring worse than the cutoff score is labeled as impaired; a patient scoring better is labeled as within normal limits.

The selection of any specific cutoff point relates to factors of test **specificity** and test **sensitivity.** When seeking to identify people whose cognitive abilities are abnormal (e.g., brain damage), neuropsychologists prefer a sensitive test. In such cases, they set the cutoff score so that as few errors as possible arise in classifying a disease entity. However, sensitive tests that rely on measuring impaired cognitive functioning may also include false-positive errors, for example, erroneously identifying psychiatric patients as brain damaged. Such a test is of little value to the neuropsychologist, who wants to delineate the precise nature of a patient's deficits. Rather, the clinician needs tests that examine specific aspects of neuropsychological functions; that is, tests that have high specificity. Such tests may assess more general areas of cognitive functioning, including sustained attention or immediate memory. But they may miss patients who have impairments outside of those specific areas of cognitive functions, which results in false-negative errors. Of course, tests that have high sensitivity and high specificity are most useful in neuropsychology. In reality, there is always a tradeoff between aspects of how specific a procedure is versus its usefulness as a sensitive test. Thus, neuropsychologists often set cutoff scores at an intermediate point at which the chances of misclassifying either impaired performance or normal performance are about equal.

Statistical Approaches

When administering a battery of tests, it is important to be able to compare performance on tests that measure widely different skills. As you gain enough experience with a set of tests, this skill often becomes automatic. However, the easiest way to accomplish this task is to use standardized scores rather than raw scores. A raw score is a score that is presented in terms of the original test units. It is simply the number of items passed or points earned. A standard score, in contrast, is a derived score that uses as its unit the standard deviation of the population on which the developers standardized the test. Thus, a standard score is a deviation score. A standard deviation relates to the variability or scatter of test scores. This pattern is known as a *distribution* of test scores. The normal probability distribution (also known as the *bell-shaped curve*) represents the frequency with which many human characteristics are dispersed over the population. For example, intelligence and spatial reasoning ability are distributed in a manner that closely resembles the bell-shaped curve.

In the **normal distribution,** 68.2% of all cases fall between ±1 standard deviation (SD) from the mean, 95.4% of the cases fall between ±2 SD from the mean, and 99.7% of the cases fall within ±3 SD from the mean. The normal distribution is the basis for the scoring system on many standardized tests. For example, on the Scholastic Aptitude Test (SAT), the developers set the mean at 500 and the standard deviation at 100. Hence, SAT scores reflect how many SDs above or below the mean a student scored. For example, a score of 700 means that you scored 2 SDs above the mean, exceeding approximately 97% of the population on which the test is normed. Thus, test scores that place examinees in the normal distribution can always be converted to percentile scores, which are often easier to interpret. A percentile score indicates the percentage of people who score below the score you obtained. For example, if you score at the 60th percentile, 60% of the people who take the test scored below you, and the remaining 40% scored above you. Tables are available that permit transformation from any SD placement in a normal distribution to a percentile score.

Neuropsychologists use a variety of standard scores. They determine standard scores by a mathematical formula that can convert raw scores from tests to a standard scale. For example, Table 3.5 lists commonly used standardized scores in clinical neuropsychology.

Once you know the test score frequency of a neuropsychological measure, you can easily compute a standard score. For example, determine the standard score (SS) by first subtracting the mean score from a normative group

Table 3.5 *Examples of Different Standardized Scores*

Name of Standardized Score	Mean	Standard Deviation	Tests Used
Z-score	0	1	None
Sten score	5	1	16 personality factors
Scaled score	10	3	Wechsler subtests
T-score	50	10	Minnesota Multiphasic Personality Inventory, many norms
Standard score (SS)	100	15	Wechsler Intelligent Quotient scores

for a test from the person's actual score. Divide the result by the SD of the scores in the normative sample. Multiply this result by 15 (the SD), and add 100 (the mean) to this answer. The formula for standard score is as follows:

$$SS = 100 + \frac{(\text{Score obtained minus average normative score})}{\text{Standard deviation (normative sample)}} \times 15.0$$

The standardized score approach to neuropsychological assessment has several advantages. First, all scores are roughly comparable. Second, you can make adjustments for such factors as age and education. You do this by determining normative means and SDs for different age or educational levels. You can then include the normative scores corresponding to a given person's age or education. Of course, not all neuropsychological measures result in normal test distributions. Some distributions skew in one direction or another. Some neuropsychological tests, particularly those that the process approach favors, are relatively "easy." That is, most "intact" individuals would have few problems passing the test. For example, "On a plain piece of paper, draw a clock with all the numbers and the hands of the clock positioned at 10 minutes after 11." Most individuals would pass this task, but patients with disturbances in visuospatial perception or planning ability may "fail." Thus, the resulting test score distribution is dichotomous (pass/fail) and does not present a normal distribution. It is inappropriate to calculate standard scores from such a test distribution. A great pitfall of the statistical approach to neuropsychological interpretation is that developers have transformed to standard scores many tests that are not normally distributed, thus providing inexact estimations of performance.

Neuropsychology in Action 3.1

Case Example: The Neuropsychology of Lyme Disease

by Eric A. Zillmer

David was an active, 66-year-old, right hand–dominant, married man who had completed 11th grade before joining the U.S. Armed Forces. Before retiring, David was employed as a medical technician in a psychiatric hospital. His wife, a nurse, was his supervisor. In August 1992, David began experiencing periods of blurred vision, headaches, nausea and "feeling ill all over, as if I was coming down with the flu." The family doctor suspected a heart problem because David had a history of mild hypertension and angina beginning in 1987, but a 24-hour electrocardiogram (EKG) monitor showed no heart malfunction. Over the next month, David experienced five similar episodes. Then, in September 1992, he awoke with numbness and weakness on the right side, as well as slurred speech, and was subsequently hospitalized. Initial neurologic findings indicated that David was awake and alert with dysarthria and right hemiparesis. The examiner noted periods of paralysis, with the comment that the patient felt "locked in" when these occurred. Physicians at the hospital diagnosed him as having had a transient ischemic attack (TIA; see Chapter 12). After a 10-day course of treatment, the patient was sent home. Hospital records noted that he was "fully recovered" at this point.

MRI of the brain suggested prominence of the ventricular system and subarachnoid spaces consistent with moderate atrophy. The report also noted mild white matter changes on the periventricular region. CT and MRI films of the coronal (Figure 3.16) planes showed a subacute cerebellar infarct (stroke). CT scans

of the head, without intravenous contrast infusion, confirmed the atrophy and previously visualized infarct in the left cerebellum. Repeat CT scan of the head without contrast 3 weeks later showed an additional new small infarction in the left thalamus (see Figure 3.16). Intracranial and neck angiogram sequences revealed no stenosis of the right or left carotid artery bifurcations. Taken together, radiologic data suggested moderate atrophy, postacute left cerebellar infarct, a small left thalamic infarct, and minimal thickening of the common, internal, and external carotid arteries. The radiologic studies did not indicate the presence of intracranial hemorrhage or any significant stenosis or plaque in the right or left carotid system. Electroencephalogram showed no definite focal or epileptogenic features.

David continued to have episodes of nausea and blurred vision, and in October 1992, he was again hospitalized with right hemiparesis, dizziness, and slurred speech. Initial diagnosis was that he had suffered another TIA. He was experiencing projectile vomiting and had episodes of high fever and brief periods when he could move only one eye. He also had behavioral digressions during which he would not recognize anyone and would pull out his IV tubes and exhibit other strange behaviors until he had to be restrained to the bed. The medical staff was mystified as to the causes of David's symptoms.

A few weeks into David's treatment, the Centers for Disease Control and Prevention (CDC) notified the hospital that David had tested positive for Lyme disease. Puzzled by

the cause of David's symptoms, his family doctor previously had taken a blood serology before the second hospitalization and forwarded samples to the CDC. David was given a course of treatment appropriate for

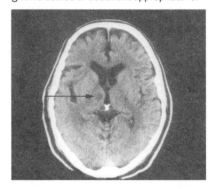

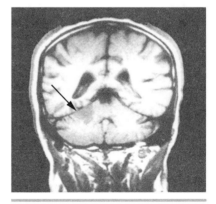

Figure 3.16 Horizontal computed axial tomography scan (top) showing infarction in left thalamus. Coronal magnetic resonance image (bottom) demonstrating subacute cerebellar infarct, as well as moderate atrophy. (Courtesy Eric Zillmer.)

DEFICIT MEASUREMENT

Deficit measurement, as an approach, is standardized and group oriented. It is useful for understanding general conditions and disease states. By comparing a person with "the norm," you can determine statistically probable deficits. By examining a battery of tests, you can examine an individual's pattern of strengths and weaknesses. You

can compare these with known, general profiles. But clinicians are also concerned with the uniqueness and dynamic qualities of each individual. The adaptive approach to neuropsychology mirrors developments in other areas of psychology. To paraphrase Howard Gardner, the Harvard psychologist, neuropsychologists should not be asking, "How smart is this person?" but "How is this person smart?" In clinical neuropsychology, the focus is not only

both stroke and Lyme disease. As a result, David's strange symptoms abated and have not returned, though the hemiparesis and dysarthria remain. The hospital physician did not agree that Lyme disease was responsible for David's symptoms. David was discharged to a rehabilitation hospital for continued care, where he was referred for neuropsychological testing to evaluate his cognitive status and his ability to participate in speech and physical therapies. Table 3.6 reviews the results of the neuropsychological battery.

David exhibited generalized deficits, with impaired performance across cognitive areas. His performance on the neuropsychological tests indicated impaired attentional capacity, motor slowness, weakness in the nondominant upper extremity (the patient was unable to use his dominant hand), impaired fine-motor ability, left auditory suppressions, impaired visuoconstructional ability, deficient spatial memory, and poor executive functioning. David's memory performance demonstrated slightly impaired verbal recall, moderately impaired visual recall, and moderately to severely impaired delayed recall for both verbal and visual material. His intellectual performance, as measured by the Wechsler Adult Intelligence Scale, Third Edition (WAIS-III), was in the Low Average range. David's IQ scores indicated slightly higher verbal than performance ability, again partially because of his right hemiplegia, but also because of impaired perception of visual material, especially visual details. The visual impairment was further documented by his borderline performance on the Hooper Visual Organization Test. On the Wisconsin Card Sorting Task, David failed to complete any categories and used the maximum possible number of trials to complete the test. Results of clinical

personality testing (Minnesota Multiphasic Personality Inventory [MMPI]) did not indicate significant psychopathology or psychological dysfunction. However, factors reflected in the protocol did suggest susceptibility to developing psychological problems including denial, somatic concern, and tension. Individuals with similar profiles are often mildly dysphoric, pessimistic about the future, and difficult to engage in psychological therapies because of their defensiveness and lack of insight.

The neuropsychological evaluation did not shed any light on whether Lyme disease was the "culprit" for David's medical problems (for a more detailed description of the clinical, radiologic, and neuropsychological manifestations of Lyme disease, see Bundick, Zillmer, Ives, & Beadle-Lindsay, 1995). David's case analysis demonstrates that psychological and neuropsychological assessment may serve to aid in the more definitive diagnosis and improved intervention/rehabilitation of patients exhibiting complex symptoms.

Table 3.6 *Neuropsychological Profile of Patient with Lyme Disease*

Age, years	66
Sex	Male
Education, years	11
Occupation	Retired medical technician
Intellectual functioning (WAIS-III)	
Verbal IQ	91 (31)
Performance IQ	84 (28)
Full Scale IQ	87 (27)
Abstract reasoning, cognitive efficiency, mental flexibility	
TMT A (seconds)	109 (26)
TMT B (seconds)	255 (35)
Wisconsin Card Sort (in perseveration errors)	65 (34)
Memory: WMS-R	
Logical Memory I	19 (36)
Logical Memory II	5 (11)
Motor speed and coordination	
Finger Oscillation DH	Not attempted
Finger Oscillation NDH	31 (29)
Grooved Pegboard (seconds) DH	Not attempted
Grooved Pegboard (seconds) NDH	154 (34)

Note: WAIS-III = Wechsler Adult Intelligence Scale, Third Edition; IQ = intelligence quotient; TMT = Trail Making Test; WMS-R = Wechsler Memory Scale–Revised; DH = dominant hand; NDH = nondominant hand.

T-scores in parentheses from Heaton, Grant, and Matthews (1991).

on the level of deficits and strengths to describe functioning; for example, "How adapted (normal) is this person?" but also, "How does this person adapt to his or her condition?" Neuropsychologists should question what is lost in terms of understanding the brain if they do not consider the range and extent of individual adaptations to injury, tumor, and disease.

Differential Score Approach

The deficit measurement approach compares a patient's score on two tests. One test is theoretically highly sensitive to brain damage (e.g., a new problem-solving task); the second is theoretically insensitive to brain dysfunction (e.g., a measure of factual language). The insensitive test is supposed to reflect the individual's ability before any brain injury occurred, whereas the sensitive test reflects the effects of brain damage. If the sensitive test score is significantly worse, the neuropsychologist assumes the difference is caused by a brain injury. In general, you combine two test scores to get a single score measuring their difference. You may accomplish this by simply subtracting or dividing one score by the other. Then analyze this single score by treating it as described in earlier in the Assessing Level of Performance section.

Pattern Analysis

A modification of the differential score approach is **pattern analysis,** which examines the relationships among the scores in a test battery. It seeks to recognize patterns consistent with specific injuries and particular neurologic processes and has value in identifying mild disorders that cause relatively little disturbance in level of performance. For example, in early stages of Alzheimer's dementia, neuropsychologists would expect a deficit in memory functioning compared with performance on verbal tests, which may be relatively normal. If you plot all the neuropsychological data on a standardized norm worksheet, a profile of cognitive skills may emerge. You can then observe the interrelationships among these differing cognitive skills areas. A basic method of pattern analysis involves observing strengths and weaknesses in the highest and lowest scores. You can evaluate cognitive strengths and weaknesses relative to the normative group by observing which scores fall above, below, or within the average range. You can also determine strengths and weaknesses relative to the individual's specific profile. Again, high and low scores are highlighted, but without regard for where they fall relative to the normative sample. Finally, you can integrate information about cognitive strengths and weaknesses with therapeutic suggestions to family and the treatment team to improve the patient's recovery.

The differential score method and pattern analysis have the advantage of recognizing that each individual starts at a different level of performance. Thus, it avoids error of misclassifying all people with low ability as "brain injured." However, this approach has several potential sources of error. First, a sensitive test may fail to reflect the impairment present. Currently, no test is sensitive to all forms of brain dysfunction. Second, the brain injury may lower a score on an insensitive test. Because all abilities depend on the brain, brain damage can affect all abilities. No test is fully insensitive to brain injury. Finally, relatively little is known about specific patterns of deficits that correlate with specific neurologic disorders, or how to set any cutoff points to identify those conditions.

LATERALIZING SIGNS

The two cerebral hemispheres control the contralateral sides of the body for most sensory and motor behaviors. If one side of the body performs significantly worse than the other, the opposite hemisphere may have been injured. Lateralizing signs are specific test results or behaviors that suggest right or left cerebral hemisphere dysfunction. This approach resembles the differential score approach in that one side of the body serves as the control for the other. Generally, you subtract the scores from the two sides of the body to obtain a single difference score. You then treat this score as described in the level-of-performance approach. This approach may yield inaccurate conclusions, however, when an injury involves both hemispheres, or when an injury to the spinal cord is involved, because such injuries may also cause lateralized motor or sensory deficits or impair performance bilaterally.

PATHOGNOMONIC SIGNS (QUALITATIVE OBSERVATIONS)

Examining **pathognomonic signs** is a method that clinical neurologists commonly use. In the medical model, the clinical examination often assumes that specific, distinctive characteristics of a disease or pathologic condition can be detected. These signs or symptoms are often labeled *pathognomonic* (derived from Greek meaning "fit to give judgment"), because often a specific diagnosis can be made from them. The medical model is a causal model in which specific signs stem either from a specific medical condition or from the disease itself. Thus, a standard medical examination is often a series of medical tests for pathognomonic signs. Once a disease has been diagnosed, it can be treated. This model has served the field of medicine rather well. For example, the model attempts to fit (pigeonhole) the available information from the medical examination into often rigid and inflexible diagnostic criteria. Also, if the signs from the medical examination do not precisely fit, or are contradictory, and if some symptoms are transient, the model does not work well, because no substantive diagnosis can be established; thus, no treatment can be offered.

Pathognomonic signs occur rarely in normal individuals. In clinical neurology, this includes such signs as an eye that will not move from side to side. In neuropsychology, examples of pathognomonic signs include the rotation of a drawing or the failure to draw the left half of a figure. You can count the number of pathognomonic signs within a given test to get a summary number. You can treat this number as a level-of-performance score. In other cases, the simple presence of a particular pathognomonic sign is taken as an indication of brain damage.

See Neuropsychology in Action 3.1 for a case example related to the neuropsychological interpretation and diagnosis.

Summary

The neuropsychological evaluation is a method of examining the brain by studying its behavioral product. As with other psychological assessments, neuropsychological evaluations involve the comprehensive study of behavior by means of standardized tests that are sensitive to brain–behavior relationships. In effect, the neuropsychological examination offers an understanding of the relationship between the structure and the function of the nervous system. Thus, the goal of the clinical neuropsychological examination is to be able to evaluate the full range of basic abilities represented in the brain. In practice, the neuropsychological assessment is multidimensional (concerned with evaluating many different aspects of neurofunctioning from basic to complex), reliable (stable across different situations and time), and valid (meaningful).

The neuropsychologist's role in evaluation has evolved from a diagnostic emphasis to one in which current neuropsychological functioning is described and the individual's adaptation to the unique demands of his or her environment is evaluated. The focus is on performance in the testing setting, as well as on a task analysis of the cognitive requirements of home and work. Neuropsychological testing profiles can aid in identifying general categories of neurologic disease and conditions. The purpose of the neuropsychological evaluation examines the individual's strengths and weaknesses, ability to deal with stress, adaptation, and overall social and occupational functioning. It is in this latter, more descriptive role that neuropsychologists have made their most recent advances.

Critical Thinking Questions

- Why are the concepts of reliability and validity so important in psychological and neuropsychological assessment?
- What kinds of questions and tests do neuropsychologists use in a neuropsychological evaluation?
- How are neuropsychology assessment procedures the same? How are they different?
- What sort of recommendations and treatments can neuropsychologists give to brain-impaired people that will be useful in their daily lives?
- How do the major two approaches (process and battery) to interpreting neuropsychological data differ?

Key Terms

Neuropsychological evaluation	Base rate	Orientation	Normative data
Psychometrics	Achievement tests	Sensation	Cutoff score
Standardized test	Behavioral-adaptive scales	Perception	Specificity
Reliability	Intelligence tests	Motor apraxia	Sensitivity
Validity	Neuropsychological tests	Ideomotor apraxia	Normal distribution
Construct validity	Personality tests	Malingering	Deficit measurement
Content validity	Vocational inventories	Interpretive hypotheses	Pattern analysis
Criterion validity	Crystallized functions	Standard battery approach	Pathognomonic signs
False positive	Fluid functions	Process approach	

Web Connections

http://ericae.net
ERIC Clearinghouse on Assessment and Evaluation—Extensive site on psychological and educational testing and assessment; includes test locator, frequently asked questions, search engine for ERIC, and many other links.

http://www.unl.edu/buros
Buros Institute of Mental Measurement—Home page of the *Buros Mental Measurements Yearbook,* tests in print, test reviews, and test locators.

http://www.mindtools.com/page12.html
Psychometric Testing—Interactive page that lets you discover your learning style; provides "IQ test," Myers–Briggs Personality Test(R), and other measures.

http://www.toldx.com
More information on the Tower of London test.

http://www.sportsci.org/resource/stats/index.html
A New View of Statistics—This site features a web-based book about the ins and outs of statistical procedures using simple sports analogies and common everyday problems. Within this site you can find concrete examples of simple statistical terms and validity and reliability procedures on interpretation discussed in this chapter.

Part Two

THE FUNCTIONING BRAIN

Chapter 4

CELLS OF THOUGHT

Immense numbers of individual units, the neurons, completely independent, simply in contact with each other, make up the nervous system.

—Santiago Cajal

An invitation is offered to cross a bridge as vast as the infinite space surrounding us and as small as the width of a neuron's membrane. This is a journey into unknown territory, a voyage into the mind. To know the mind is to know the universe.

—Fred Alan Wolf

Neurons and Glial Cells
Communication within a Neuron: The Neural Impulse
Communication among Neurons
Regeneration of Neurons

Neuropsychology in Action

4.1 Short-Circuiting Neurons: Multiple Sclerosis
4.2 Neuronal Firing: Clinical Examples
4.3 What Can We Learn from Songbirds?
4.4 Stem Cell Research: Science and Ethics

Keep in Mind

▨ How does the unicellular neuron differ from a one-celled creature?

▨ What are the purposes of different cell types in the central nervous system?

▨ How do neurons communicate?

▨ Are damaged neurons able to regenerate?

Overview

Cells are the building blocks of all living organisms. Evolutionarily old, one-celled creatures such as the amoeba show elementary responses to sensation and have decision-making capabilities. In their universe of a droplet of water, amoebas can move about, locate food, and engulf it. They can differentiate light from dark and warmth from cold. This unicellular organism uses complex electrochemical processes, but has no nervous system and no brain. Moving up the evolutionary ladder, increased complexity of behavior corresponds with a more specialized nervous system, which is essential for speeded communication. The "jelly-fish," for example, has a rudimentary nervous system, which allows coordinated movement, but still has no brain.

The human central nervous system (CNS) contains billions of interconnected cells. Of the two main types of cells, neurons alone account for about 100 billion cells, and estimates suggest that glial cells outnumber neurons by 10 to 1. Considering there are approximately 6 billion people on earth, the number of cells in one human brain is more like the number of stars in the sky. The CNS is not connected in a simple, linear fashion, but in a densely packed tangle of interconnected networks. If 1 neuron connected only to 100 others, the emerging network would be staggering in its size and complexity. However, evidence suggests that the number of connections actually ranges from 1000 to 100,000, averaging about 10,000 per neuron (Beatty, 1995; Hubel, 1988). Cells of the CNS are specialized and interact with each other in a unique manner. Their processing systems require a great deal of energy and consume the most oxygen and glucose of any bodily system.

This chapter focuses on the essential building blocks of thought and behavior: neurons and glial cells. Neurons and glia are classes of cells that contain subtypes based on their structure and function. Neurons are considered the most important cells, and the basic electrical-chemical processes of neuronal communication have been well described by scientists. Although glial cells traditionally have been described as having a supporting function for neurons, science now suggests that glial cells may have a larger role to play in thought and learning. The neuron can be studied as a universe unto itself, but neuropsychology is also focused on the effect of behavior related to neuronal disruption. Clinical problems such as multiple sclerosis (MS) and spinal cord injury are the direct result of disease or injury at the neuronal level. The ability of the neuron to repair itself is intriguing because of the enormous implications for treatment.

Neurons and Glial Cells

The neuron differs from other cells in that it is specialized for information processing. To some degree all functions that sustain life, as well as those that make us human, are coordinated and depend on the communication of neurons. Neurons are anatomically independent; they come very close to each other but do not touch. The nervous system thus consists of separate units rather than one continuous structure.

The neuron has often been studied by scientists with the idea that by studying the fundamental parts, a better understanding of the whole can be achieved. This reductionistic view attempts to investigate complex phenomena by dividing them into more easily understood components. Reductionists may describe their work as mapping the brain. Everything, they argue, exists at a particular location (Churchland, 1993). The neuron hypothesis is in accord with this viewpoint suggesting that (1) all neural function is reflected in behavior, and (2) all behavior has an underlying neural correlate (Pincus & Tucker, 1985). Reductionists argue that the healthy mature brain produces the mind's range of functions and experiences, which are perfectly correlated to precise biological phenomena. In other words, the reductionist viewpoint argues that every human experience can be reduced to a physical phenomenon. Although reductionism is considered outdated and oversimplified because it is not possible to correlate behavior with individual neurons, some neuropsychologists study the relation of behavior to assemblies of neurons and interconnected neural networks.

The structure of neurons is similar to that of other body cells in that they have a cell body that contains a nucleus, genes, cytoplasm, mitochondria, and other organelles necessary to conduct protein synthesis and energy production. However, neurons are quite different from other body cells in several ways. For example:

1. They possess *specialized extensions,* **dendrites** and **axons,** which allow for communication. Dendrites are treelike or feathery extensions that branch from the neuron into the immediate neighborhood of the cell body. The axon extends from the cell body to transmit information.
2. They possess *specialized structures,* particularly **terminal buttons,** which produce neurochemicals.
3. Neurons communicate through an *electrochemical process.*

The structure of neurons allows them to communicate with each other in an interesting way. Most body cells communicate with each other or the outside world through energy exchange and intercellular transport, using the cellular membrane. Neurons, however, communicate with each other by *axonal firing,* which allows electrochemical transmission across the **synapse,** the tiny gap between two neurons. The process of such communication releases chemical **neurotransmitters,** permitting highly sophisticated combinations of reactions that influence downstream neuronal behavior.

Neurons also have properties of formation and regeneration that differ from those of other body cells. In general, no new neurons form after birth (Cowan, 1990). In fact, during certain periods of development, massive **pruning** occurs as important neural connections form in response to learning and maturation. Excess neurons, which may

cause distracting associations, die off. An important question for brain science is to what extent neurons can regenerate once damaged. Neurons in the periphery can regenerate; for example, if surgeons reattach an amputated finger, the finger may regain some mobility. Neurons in the spinal cord and brain do not heal spontaneously. This is most evident in the complete severing of neurons in the spinal cord, which leads to paralysis. Recent findings, however, suggest that some regrowth may be possible. Research on reactivating damaged neurons is ongoing, so perhaps some day scientists will be able to reverse spinal cord damage (Naugle, Cullum, & Bigler, 1998). Later in this section (see Regeneration of Neurons) we examine the question of neurogenesis, regeneration, and attempts to regain function after injury.

STRUCTURE AND FUNCTION OF THE NEURON

Neurons vary in shape and size, but have four common features (Figure 4.1):

1. A cell body with a nucleus
2. Dendrites
3. An axon
4. Terminal synaptic buttons

Neurons are specialized to exchange information, specifically the reception, conduction, and transmission of electrochemical signals.

Cell Body

The functioning and survival of the neuron depend on the integrity of the cell body that controls and maintains the neuronal structure. Because these cell bodies are gray, the term **gray matter** is used to describe areas of the brain that are dense in cell bodies, such as the cortex. The cell soma contains mitochondria, amino acids, and DNA, and it has the same properties of other cells in the body. Protein synthesis cannot occur in the axon, so all axonal proteins come from the cell body.

Dendrites

Neurons generally receive chemical transmissions from one another through dendrites, feathery extensions that branch from the neuron into the immediate neighborhood of the cell body. There are often thousands of dendrites per neuron, and they differ in relation to the different functions of the neurons. The profuse branching of dendrites allows them to receive communication from a large number of axonal terminals across the synapse. The shapes of dendritic "trees" are often among the most characteristic morphologic

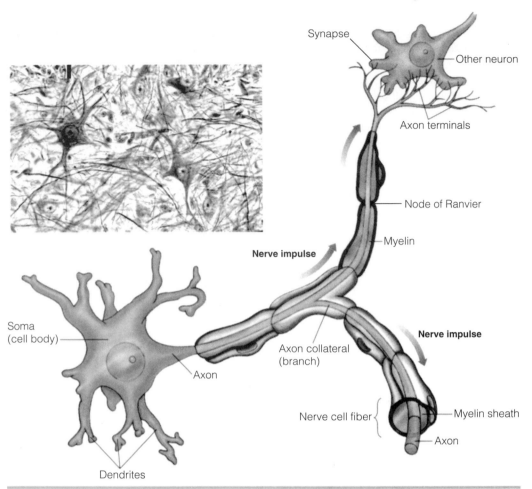

Synapse

Other neuron

Axon terminals

Node of Ranvier

Myelin

Nerve impulse

Nerve impulse

Soma
(cell body)

Axon collateral
(branch)

Axon

Nerve cell fiber

Myelin sheath

Axon

Dendrites

Figure 4.1   An example of a neuron, or nerve cell, showing several of its important features. The right foreground shows a nerve cell fiber in cross section, and the upper left inset gives a more realistic picture of the shape of neurons. The nerve impulse usually travels from the dendrites and soma to the branching ends of the axon. The neuron shown here is a motor neuron. Motor neurons originate in the brain or spinal cord and send their axons to the muscles or glands of the body. (From Martini, F. H., Timmons, M. J., and McKinley, M. P. Human Anatomy. 3rd ed. Prentice Hall, 2000. Reprinted by permission of Pearson Education, Upper Saddle River, NJ.)

features of a neuron (Figure 4.2). For example, dendrites of **Purkinje cells** (see Figure 4.2*a*), which are found in all areas of the cerebellar cortex, are characteristically spread out in one plane and have thousands of **dendritic spines.** Many dendrites are covered with spines, or small knobs, that form the synaptic connection with communicating neurons. Dendrites are tiny, only visible under an electron microscope, and are usually shorter than the axon, but they can have up to thousands of synapses or contacts with other neurons. Neuroscientists estimate that the total possible connectivity among neurons in the human brain is approximately 10^{15}, or 10,000,000,000,000,000—more numerous than the known stars in the universe (Beatty, 1995;

Williams & Herrup, 1988). Dendrites comprise most of the receptive surface of a neuron.

A x o n

The axon extends away from the cell body. Its primary function is to transmit electrochemical information from the cell body to the synapse through microtubules along its length. Axons are anywhere from less than 1 millimeter (mm) in length to 1 meter (m) or more. Large motor neurons have long axons, some of them reaching from the lower end of the spinal cord to the foot muscles. Other neurons, including those that coordinate activity within a specific region of the CNS, have short axons. Unipolar axons proceed from

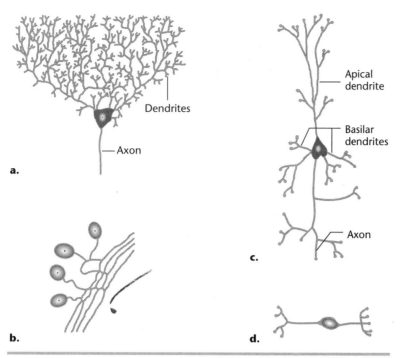

Figure 4.2 Neurons of various shapes: (a) Purkinje cell; (b) sensory neurons; (c) pyramidal cell; (d) bipolar cell. (From Kalat, J. W. [2007]. *Biological psychology* [9th ed., p. 34, Figure 2.9]. Belmont, CA: Thomson Wadsworth.)

one region in the CNS to another without branching. In bipolar or multipolar axons, the branching is elaborate.

Many axons are surrounded with a **myelin sheath** that increases the speed of axonal transmission (Beatty, 1995). This is especially important in longer neurons. Myelin is lipoprotein that wraps around the axon like the layers of an onion, giving neurons their characteristic **white matter** appearance. The sheath begins at the first segment of the axon, where the nerve impulse or **action potential** begins. The myelin serves as an electric insulator that increases conduction velocity. The myelin sheath is formed

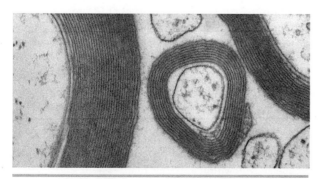

Figure 4.3 Cross section of a myelinated axon. (© Dennis Kunkel Microscopy, Inc.)

by **glial** cells, termed *oligodendrocytes,* in the CNS and by **Schwann cells** in the peripheral nervous system (PNS). The layers of the myelin wrap around the axon like layers of onion skin (Figure 4.3). Gaps called the **nodes of Ranvier** interrupt it at regular intervals (see Figure 4.1). The projections of the surface membrane of each of those cells fan out and coil around the axon of neurons to form myelin sheaths. Because the nerve impulse jumps from node to node, the length of the myelin segment is of considerable importance. The longest axonal fibers, which can have a conduction velocity of up to 100 m/sec, may have myelin segments longer than 1 mm.

Myelination begins soon after birth and continues for many years. The development of the myelin sheath corresponds to behavior. Babies are unable to control their bladder and bowel functions: This is caused by insufficient myelination of neurons; therefore, children cannot be toilet trained before about age 2 or 3. In adults, a breakdown of the myelin sheath is a consequence of MS (Neuropsychology in Action 4.1).

The speed of neuronal conduction is important in the adaptation of all species to potentially dangerous events in the environment. Given that, in some cases, the built-in conduction speed is not fast enough, the nervous system has evolved to process important sensory data at levels

Neuropsychology in Action 4.1

Short-Circuiting Neurons: Multiple Sclerosis

by Eric A. Zillmer

The destruction of the myelin sheath around the axon can result in significant and often striking behavioral changes, including blindness and paralysis. Such conditions are called *demyelinating disorders,* of which multiple sclerosis (MS) is the best known. MS is the most common neurologic illness in the United States, affecting 50 of every 100,000 young adults. Symptoms are most often first noticed between the ages of 20 and 40. Because MS is more frequent in certain geographic locations than in others (polar latitudes), an environmental agent may be implicated in the cause of the disease, perhaps one related to a demyelinating slow virus or an autoimmune process (Ebers & Sadovnick, 1993).

Although the contracting factor of MS remains an enigma, the course of the disease is known; it is related to the localized loss of myelin in the white matter of the brain and subsequent neuronal death. The loss of myelin initially results in "scrambled" electrical impulses, thus neuronal information slows or never reaches its target. The symptoms vary according to where the hardened patches, known as *sclerotic plaques,* lie in the brain and spinal cord, but most manifest visually (sudden unilateral blindness), in the brainstem and cerebellum (wide-based gait, intention tremors), and in the spinal cord (spastic gait, loss of position sense, and paraplegia). Relapses are usually acute and persist for several weeks. Postmortem studies of MS patients have revealed hundreds of lesions smaller than 1.5 cm (Adams & Victor, 1993). Furthermore, there is little potential for regrowth of myelin.

There is no known effective treatment or cure for MS. The prognosis is a gradual deterioration of the patient's condition over many years. Death can result if the demyelination affects vital centers of the brain.

closer to their origin. The knee reflex is an example. The sensory information that you are about to fall is sent to your spinal cord, which relays it directly back with "instructions" to extend your knee. This occurs without any higher cognitive processing. If the same sensory information traveled to the brain, the relay would take too long to process, which could result in a fall. Another example is the reflex arc in response to pain, such as a burn. The sensation is relayed to your spinal cord, which gives the appropriate response: "Withdraw finger!" The information also reaches your brain, of course, although somewhat later; it is then processed at that higher level: "Did I burn my finger?"

In large animals, such as dinosaurs, to compensate for the relatively long distances sensory and motor neurons have to travel, large dinosaurs had a small additional brain at the level of the pelvis. Presumably, the brain integrated many sensory and motor functions at this level so the dinosaur could respond adaptively to the environment.

Terminal Buttons

Near the end of the axon are branches with slightly enlarged ends called *axonal terminals* or terminal buttons. The site of interneuronal contact, where neurochemical information transmits from one neuron to another, is called a synapse (see later in this section for a detailed discussion of synapses). The terminal button is the presynaptic portion of the synapse, the place where electrical nerve impulses cause the release of a neurotransmitter. This chemical in turn affects another neuron or muscle in either an excitatory or an inhibitory manner. Signals that travel along the axon are electrical, and the transfer of neurotransmitters across synapses, from one neuron to another, is chemical. Researchers can therefore study and analyze the brain through electrical means—for example, using the electroencephalograph, evoked potential, or electrical stimulation—or through biochemical or metabolic techniques such as positron emission tomography.

Neuron Classification and Terminology

Neurologists commonly classify neurons either by morphology (shape) or by function. The three principal classes of neurons are defined by the number of processes emanating from their cell bodies. Most are **multipolar neurons,** with more than two processes, or extensions from the cell body (see Figures 4.2*a, c*). One of these is the axon, and the others are dendrites extending from various parts of the cell body. **Bipolar neurons** have two processes (see Figure 4.2*d*). **Monopolar neurons** have a single or unipolar process, and do not have dendrites originating directly from the cell body or soma (see Figure 4.2*b*). Neurons with short axons are called **interneurons;** they integrate neural activity within a specific brain region.

In classifying neurons by their function, **motor neurons** make muscles contract and change the activity of

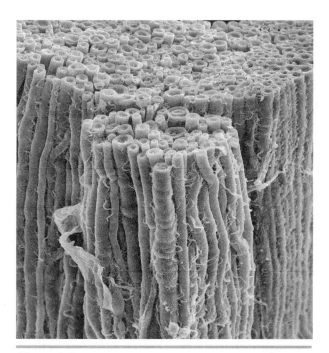

Figure 4.4 Bundles of myelinated neurons make up tracts, pathways, or fibers in the central nervous system and nerves in the peripheral nervous system. (© SPL/Photo Researchers, Inc.)

glands; **sensory neurons** respond directly to changes in light, touch, temperature, odor, and so on. The majority of neurons are interneurons, or "between" neurons, because they receive input from and send output to other neurons.

Neurons are organized in collective structures; that is, behavior arises from the firing of many neurons, not a single neuron. These bundles—large collections of neurons—are known as **tracts, pathways,** or **fibers** in the CNS and **nerves** in the PNS (Figure 4.4). The three major types of fibers all primarily consist of myelinated axons that appear as white matter:

1. **Intracerebral** (or *association*) **fibers** connect regions within one hemisphere.
2. **Intercerebral** (or *commissural*) **fibers** connect structures in the two hemispheres.
3. **Projection fibers** connect subcortical structures to the cortex and vice versa.

Anatomists often discuss pathways by the direction of the projection and the systems they connect (England & Wakely, 1991). For example, the corticostriatal pathway is where fibers connect cortical areas to the striatum. Likewise, the hypothalamocerebellar tract projects from the hypothalamus to the cerebellum.

Aggregations of cell bodies—predominantly dendrites and terminal buttons—are grayish; their actual color in the living state is pink. As noted earlier, gray matter is typically found on the surface of the cerebral cortex, in the center of the spinal cord, and on large subcortical nuclei (e.g., in the thalamus). In the CNS, clusters of gray cell bodies are called **nuclei** (singular, *nucleus*), a term often used to designate a group of nerve cells in direct relation to the fibers of a particular nerve. In the PNS, clusters of gray cell bodies are called **ganglia** (singular, *ganglion*). The presence of nuclei in the brain is important to neuropsychologists because nuclei often signal strategic clusters of neuronal cell bodies. Vital integration of neuronal information may be occurring at a specific neuroanatomic location. Some functional roles have been attributed to certain nuclei. The precise role of any one nucleus is, however, difficult to delineate, because the dendrites and axons may extend for a considerable distance outside of the boundary of the nucleus. In addition, some nuclei consist of different neurons with different neurotransmitters from other neurons, which increases the complexity. In some cases, it may be more useful to conceptualize function according to neuronal regions or networks rather than by nuclei. Nevertheless, mapping and identifying specific nuclei in the brain continues to occupy brain scientists.

GLIAL CELLS

Glial cells (also known as neuroglia or glia) outnumber neurons by a factor of 10, but because of their small size (1/10 that of a neuron), they make up about 50% of the volume of the nervous system, with neurons comprising the other half. The term *glia* (derived from Greek *gliok,* meaning "nerve glue") comes from an old notion that glial cells offer purely structural support to neurons. This is just part of the story; glia have more functions. Glial cells are often described as "servants" to neurons. They help support neurons by physically and chemically buffering them from each other, and they supply nutrients and oxygen to neurons to support their very high metabolic rate, because neurons cannot store their own nutrients. Some glial cells act as housekeepers, metabolizing and removing the carcasses of neurons destroyed by injury or disease, and as discussed earlier, certain glial cells form the protective myelin sheath around axons. There is new evidence, however, that some glial cells (i.e., astrocytes) may function more like "parents" than "servants" in directing and regulating neuronal behavior.

Glial cells are found throughout the CNS and PNS. The three main types of glial cells in the CNS are oligodendrocytes, **microglia,** and **astrocytes.** The primary

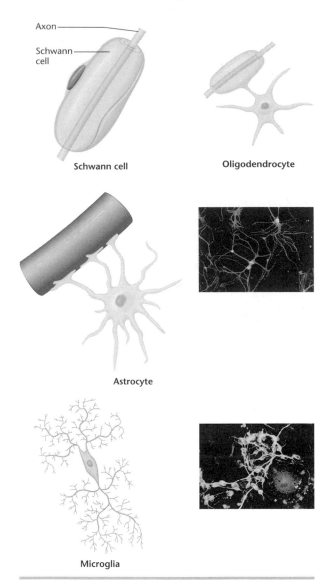

Axon

Schwann cell

Schwann cell

Oligodendrocyte

Astrocyte

Microglia

Figure 4.5   Glia cells of the central and peripheral nervous systems. Glia cells are of special interest to neurologists and neurosurgeons because they are the site of the principal tumors of the brain and spinal cord. (From Kalat, J. W. [2007]. *Biological psychology* [9th ed., p. 35, Figure 2.10]. Belmont, CA: Thomson Wadsworth. Photos: © Nancy Kedersha/UCLA/SPL/Photo Researchers.)

As mentioned earlier, oligodendrocytes in the CNS and Schwann cells in the PNS are myelin-forming glia cells that envelope axons and neurons. These cells perform a vital function in wrapping the nerve cell with a lipid layer of myelin and increasing the speed with which a neuron conducts its impulse along an axon. Schwann cells myelinate only a single segment of one cell, whereas oligodendrocytes may myelinate several segments of the same axon or several different axons.

Microglia are small cells within the CNS that undergo rapid proliferation in response to tissue destruction, migrating toward the site of injured or dead cells, where they act as scavengers and metabolize tissue debris.

Astrocytes are fibrous, star-shaped cells (derived from Latin *astra,* meaning "star") with many small "feet" or processes that interpose themselves between neuronal cell bodies, dendrites, and the vasculature providing structural support. The "servant," or housekeeping, functions of astrocytes are well known. These functions include: (1) "border patrol" of the brain via the **blood–brain barrier** to protect neurons from potential pathogens transported by the blood, (2) maintenance of local ionic and pH balance between groups of neurons, and (3) delivery of energy to neurons in the form of glucose and other metabolic substances.

The border patrol via the blood–brain barrier is accomplished because blood vessels in the CNS have a lining of tightly joined endothelial cells, which the "feet" of the tightly joined astrocytes hold in place (Figure 4.6). This wrapping of blood vessels keeps large molecules out and permits only restricted transfer of soluble material between blood and brain. The blood–brain barrier allows water, gases, and small lipid-soluble substances to pass across. Certain substances (some drugs, for example) are totally barred from the brain, and other substances require an active transport system across the blood–brain barrier.

Astrocytes help regulate the local intercellular ionic and pH balance. The receptor sites on the cellular membranes respond to ions such as calcium (Guthrie et al., 1999), and they restore the ion balance by removing excess ions after neuronal firing. Astrocytes also clear neurotransmitters released through synaptic firing and clean up intercellular metabolic waste.

Astrocytes also supply glucose to neurons through the blood–brain barrier. The "feet" of astrocytes, attached to capillaries and blood vessels throughout the brain, act as a suction system, drawing glucose up from the bloodstream via astrocytes and into neurons. Before being passed on, glucose is partially metabolized by astrocytes into a form usable by neurons.

corresponding cell in the PNS is the Schwann cell (Figure 4.5).

Of tumors that invade the brain, the most prevalent arise from glial cells and are termed **gliomas.** Unfortunately, gliomas are often relatively fast-growing tumors. Astrocytes respond to brain injury by swelling or proliferating to fill a damaged space. With injury, astrocytes can also degenerate and form scar tissue.

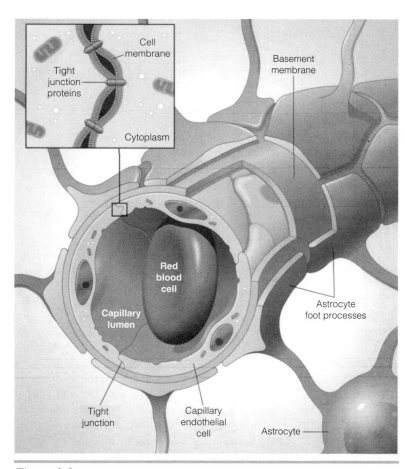

Figure 4.6 Blood–brain barrier. (Courtesy Jim Perkins and Netter Images.)

The most interesting role of astrocytes, however, may be their "parent" role. It recently has been suggested that astrocytes may play an important role in regulating and coordinating neuronal firing (see review by Nedergaard, Ransom, & Goldman, 2003). Astrocytes may act locally to help define not only structural but communication pathways among neurons. That is, according to this conceptualization, astrocytes are not just the support crew and the nurturers but the parental directors. Examples of this are seen in the ways that astrocytes can communicate among themselves and also affect neurons. They can, for example, release captured neurotransmitters and affect the synchronization of neurons. Astrocytes can also communicate among themselves through neuron-independent signaling. Whereas neurons communicate through a combination of electrical impulse and chemical transmission, astrocytes rely on chemical signaling only. Their receptor sites respond to ions and specific neurotransmitters. Whereas the response time of electrical signaling in neurons is lightning fast, chemical responding through glial cells may take 15 seconds or longer (Fields & Stevens-Graham, 2002). Because astrocytes can detect the ionic character of the intercellular space, particularly the synaptic space between neurons, they are in a position to modify the strength of connections between neurons and synchronize neuronal firing. For example, in animal models, it has been demonstrated that the synaptic connections between neurons can be strengthened through stimulation by adjacent astrocytes (see review by Nedergaard, Ransom, & Goldman, 2003). Therefore, astrocytes appear to have a bigger role in learning and memory than previously thought (Fields & Stevens-Graham, 2002). Also, astrocytes participate in the formation of new neuronal synapses and help to specify the connections they make (Pfrieger & Barres, 1997). Finally, radial glial cells, a type of astrocyte, appear to aid in directing nervous system development (Lemke, 2001).

In summary, the role of astrocytes is emerging from one that was believed to be purely structural, to one of a servant role, to one that has an integrative and possibly directing role in the functioning of the nervous system. Interestingly, mammals have a greater percentage of glial cells in relation to neurons than creatures lower on the evolutionary scale. It is also interesting that Einstein's brain, although having no greater density of neurons than other people, had a higher percentage of glial cells in areas of the brain related to higher cognition (Paterniti, 2000). This group of findings is leading brain scientists to pursue the study of glial cells to determine the manner in which they interact with and influence neurons.

Communication within a Neuron: The Neural Impulse

The message that travels along the axon from the cell body to the terminal buttons is electrical, but the neuron does not carry it down the axon the way an electrical wire conducts electricity. Rather, chemical alterations in the membrane of the axon result in exchanges of various ions between the axon and the fluid that surrounds it, producing an electrical current. This electrical signaling is the foundation of neuronal communication.

RESTING MEMBRANE POTENTIAL

As with all living cells, a cell membrane protects the neuron from other matter. Neurons show a **resting potential** or **membrane potential** when they are inactive; that is, they show a slight electrical imbalance between the inner and outer surfaces of the membrane caused by the separation of electrically charged ions. Neural communication requires the passage of **ions** through tiny channels in the axon wall. Ions are atoms or molecules that have acquired an electrical charge by gaining or losing one or more electrons. Four ions are important: sodium (NA^+), potassium (K^+), calcium (Ca^{++}), and chloride (Cl^-). Electrophysiologic equipment makes it possible to measure the electrical potentials (transmembrane potential) of axons. The inside of the axon is electrically negative with respect to the outside of the neuron; thus, an electrical potential difference exists between the interior and exterior of the axon that is synonymous with the membrane potential. In the giant axon of the squid, this difference is approximately –70 millivolts (mV). An electrical imbalance can occur because the membrane of the axon is semipermeable to allow the flow of chemicals across the axonal membrane (Figure 4.7). Some molecules, including oxygen and water, flow through the membrane constantly, and other chemicals, such as potassium, chloride, and sodium, cross through

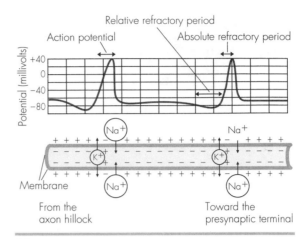

Figure 4.7   During the resting state of the membrane, the unequal distributions of sodium (Na^+) and potassium ions (K^+) between the inside and the outside of the neuron produced a difference in voltage. (From Kalat, J. W. [1998]. *Biological psychology* [6th ed., p. 41, Figure 4.18]. Pacific Grove, CA: Brooks/Cole.)

gates that control the rate of passage. When the neuron is not firing and the membrane is at rest, the sodium ions (Na^+) are trapped outside of the neuron. The imbalance in an electrical charge maintains the cell in a state of tension, ready to fire rapidly in response to a stimulus.

The positively charged sodium ions are located in greater concentrations outside the neuron, even though the electrostatic field (negative charges inside the membrane) tends to attract them inside. The biological transport system that exchanges three sodium ions for every two potassium ions across the membrane of the axon is called the **sodium–potassium pump.** Many individual protein molecules in the membrane pump sodium out of the axon. This active transport system exchanges three sodium ions for every two potassium ions that push in, and it consumes considerable energy—up to 40% of the neuron's metabolic resources. The concentration of potassium reflects an equilibrium of competing processes. The pump actively moves potassium into the neuron, expending energy in the process. Concurrently, potassium ions flow passively from an area of greater concentration to an area of lesser concentration by the force of diffusion.

ACTION POTENTIAL

To generate a nerve impulse, a cell membrane must first depolarize. Depolarization begins when a sodium channel across the membrane briefly opens and sodium ions pass through it into the cell, reducing voltage. Depolarization occurs only when the membrane achieves a threshold of at least 35 mV reduction of polarization toward zero. When this occurs, the membrane suddenly opens its sodium gates, permitting a rapid, massive, explosive flow of ions. When sodium enters the cell in this fashion, the neuron fires with an action potential. Subthreshold stimulation does not result in an action potential, but any stimulation beyond the threshold does. Thus, neurons fire in an all-or-none fashion. The force of the action potential does not depend on the intensity of the stimulus initiating it, and a neuron cannot send stronger action potentials down its axons. In fact, neurons fire more or less continuously, and the timing and sequences of impulses and pauses determine the message. Figure 4.8 illustrates the varying stages of an electrical potential across a neuron

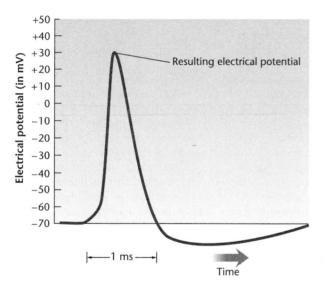

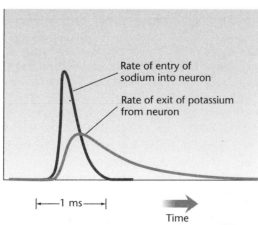

Figure 4.8 Action potential. (From Kalat, J. W. [2007]. *Biological psychology* [9th ed., p. 43, Figure 2.16]. Belmont, CA: Thomson Wadsworth.)

membrane during electrical stimulation. The nerve impulse spreads down the axon as the voltage-controlled sodium channels open sequentially, like falling dominoes.

Neurons may be in different states of preparedness for firing. Some may be just a few millivolts below the critical voltage level, requiring little additional excitation to reach firing threshold. Others may need to overcome a larger voltage difference between the inside and the outside of the axon to generate an action potential. Once a neuron has fired, there is an associated recovery period when the neuron resists re-excitation and is incapable of firing. This **refractory period** lasts 1 or more milliseconds, during which the membrane cannot produce another action potential in response to stimulation of any intensity.

Neurons communicate through synapses. Chemical messages between neurons are carried by neurotransmitters and have one of two effects on the receiving neuron: excitation or inhibition. The inhibitory and excitatory properties of neurons on behavior are of special interest to neuropsychologists. The ability to sit quietly and read this book requires many functions, both excitatory and inhibitory. It is common for patients with generalized brain trauma to have difficulties sitting still, concentrating, and reading for a prolonged period (Golden, Zillmer, & Spiers, 1992). Such problems are related to that many of the neuronal collections in the CNS, particularly those of the frontal lobe, serve to inhibit rather than excite behavior. This is of clinical importance because losing inhibitory neurons to trauma or disease may result in impulsivity and inappropriate behavior known as **disinhibition.**

It is the firing rate, not the magnitude of electrical activity of the neuron, that can change—that is, increase. For example, if inhibitory fiber collections increase their rate of firing, inhibition increases and behavior correspondingly decreases. This is why many traumas to the brain often cause both a loss of function, such as the inability to initiate behaviors, and disinhibition, which may include impulsiveness, hypersexuality, and inappropriate expression of emotions such as crying or silliness.

Communication among the cells of the brain is the basis of all behavior. Our previous discussion centered on how the individual neuron works. We now discuss how neurons communicate with each other. The anatomic location of this communication is known as the *synapse.* The synapse is the gap between the terminal button and the receptors of the next neuron.

The language of human neural communication is chemical. In fact, almost all mammalian synapses are chemical in nature, although researchers have found electrically transmitting synapses in invertebrates and lower vertebrates. The chemical messengers are called *neurotransmitters.* In simple

---

Neuropsychology in Action 4.2

Neuronal Firing: Clinical Examples

by Eric A. Zillmer

The influence of neuronal firing on behavior is easily seen in a variety of related clinical phenomena.

Seizures

Seizures, which are unusual electrical events in the brain, have a wide range of causes, including trauma, tumors, and epilepsy. **Seizures** result from massive waves of synchronized nerve cell activation that may involve the entire brain. You can thus conceptualize them as "electrical storms." Seizures may have dramatic behavioral manifestations, including uncontrolled muscle contractions, changes in perception, and alterations in mood and consciousness.

Drugs

Certain drugs and poisons specifically alter the flow of sodium and potassium through the membrane. Most drugs act at the level of the synapse, but several substances directly influence the firing rate of the axon, changing the person's perception or mood and, in some cases, causing death. For example, scorpion and black widow venoms overexcite the nervous system by keeping sodium channels open and closing potassium channels, causing prolonged depolarization that renders the neuron helpless to convey information. As a result, life-sustaining behavior may cease (e.g., breathing may stop), or there may be a lack of disinhibition (such as a continuous involuntary flexing of a

muscle or tic). Novocain, a topical anesthetic used by dentists, attaches itself to the sodium gates of the neuronal membrane and prevents sodium ions from entering. Consequently, the action potential is blocked and sensory nerve messages, including pain, cannot reach the brain because the neurons that typically convey this message cannot fire.

Chloroform decreases brain activity by promoting the flow of potassium ions out of the neuron. This reduces the number of sodium ions that spontaneously pass through the cell membrane and hyperpolarizes the neuronal membrane, which reduces the responsiveness of the nervous system. Tetrodotoxin (TTX), a poison found in the Japanese blowfish, directly blocks voltage-gated sodium channels. Lithium, a simple salt extracted from rock, is the most effective treatment for bipolar disorder (manic-depressive illness), which is characterized by severe mood swings (Freedman, Kaplan, & Sadock, 1978). Lithium stabilizes mood most effectively during the manic stage. Its overall effect on brain activity is not clearly understood, but lithium is chemically similar to sodium and may partly take its place crossing the membrane.

Electroconvulsive Therapy

Early in the twentieth century, a physician named Ladislaus von Meduna noted that psychotic patients who had epilepsy improved in mood immediately after each

epileptic attack. Reasoning that the electrical storm of neural activity in the brain somehow improved mental activity, Meduna applied a large amount of electricity to the skull of depressed patients, causing the collective firing of neurons—a seizure. **Electroconvulsive therapy (ECT)** sometimes improves severe forms of depression within a few days. Although researchers do not clearly understand the mechanism, currently, clinicians use ECT when it is important to intervene quickly to prevent a patient from acting on suicidal thoughts.

Death

When is a human considered dead? When the heart stops beating? Or when the lungs stop breathing? Because the brain is the *Zentralorgan* (German meaning "central organ") that coordinates the beating of the heart and the breathing of the lungs, the clinical moment of death is precisely when the firing of the brain ceases. Thus, in most states, once an unconscious patient has been admitted to a hospital, the staff monitors brain electrical potential data with an **electroencephalograph.** As long as there is brain activity, the patient is considered alive. Interestingly, even after a brain has stopped generating action potentials, the brain mass itself can hold its own electrical charge for a short time. This can be measured by placing a dead brain slice on an apparatus that is sensitive to small electrical charges.

---

terms, a chemical message transfers across the synapse from one neuron to another, where it influences the neuron or neurons to fire or not to fire. In reality, this particular exchange is extremely complex, involving many different molecules. The process is so intricate that a neuroscientist can easily dedicate an entire career to the study of one neurotransmitter exchange. But human brains, and minds, are affected not only by internally produced chemical messengers but also by externally originating chemicals that find their way to the synapse. Such chemicals are known as

psychoactive drugs, and they include caffeine, cocaine, nicotine, and alcohol, among many others.

Chemical transmission is very much at the center of human behavior and emotions. In fact, many of the most fascinating discoveries about the brain concern the chemical nature of neuronal transmission. For example, researchers have established that the large numbers of individual nerve cells or units in the nervous system are related to each other through synapses in a more or less continuous fashion, creating a *network* (Neuropsychology in Action 4.2).

Communication among Neurons

STRUCTURE OF SYNAPSES

The presynaptic neuron delivers an action potential down its axon until it loses its myelin sheath and divides into many branches called *buttons,* or **synaptic knobs.** These buttons swell at the end to increase the area of contact with the postsynaptic neuron. The buttons themselves do not touch the postsynaptic cell, which is covered with myelin and surrounded by glia cells. Between the two neurons lies a small space known as the *synaptic cleft* or *synaptic gap.* This space is so tiny (about 200–300 Å) that it is observable only through an electron microscope.

Terminal buttons harbor oval structures called **synaptic vesicles,** which contain neurotransmitters. These vesicles are unique cellular structures that typically cluster close to the presynaptic membrane. Neurotransmitters are synthesized until they are delivered to the **receptor sites** on the postsynaptic neuron. There are numerous neurotransmitter

molecules, each shaped differently and with its own key fit to a specific receptor. This mechanism determines how the synaptic endings evoke excitation or inhibition in the postsynaptic neuron. Researchers have identified two major types of receptor sites (Beatty, 1995): the symmetric synapse, which appears to be involved in inhibitory functions, and the asymmetric synapse, which plays a role in excitatory processes. The anatomic location of the terminal button in relation to the postsynaptic membrane can vary. It may be on the dendrite, the soma, or the axon of the postsynaptic neuron.

SYNAPTIC TRANSMISSION

The synapse includes the presynaptic membrane, the synaptic cleft, and the postsynaptic membrane. When the neural impulse from the presynaptic neuron reaches the button, the vesicles release a specific amount of a neurotransmitter (typically 1000–10,000 molecules) into the synaptic cleft (Figure 4.9).

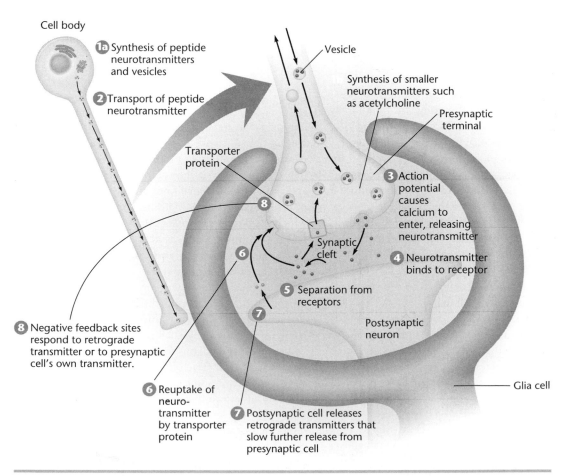

Figure 4.9 Events in synaptic transmission. (From Kalat, J. W. [2007]. *Biological psychology* [9th ed., p. 59, Figure 3.8]. Belmont, CA: Thomson Wadsworth.)

Several scenarios are possible after the release of a neurotransmitter. The molecules may not fit a specific receptor site and, therefore, do not bind to the cell membrane. In this case, the neurotransmitter has no effect on a receiving neuron, and no communication takes place. Or, neurotransmitters may be released in areas with no immediate postsynaptic receptors. In this case, the transmitter may diffuse over a wider area, affecting neurons far from the point of release. If the released neurotransmitter keys into the receptor site, it will bind to the cell membrane. Depending on the type of neurotransmitter, it will affect the ultimate firing or inhibition of the postsynaptic cell in one of two ways. Some neurotransmitters activate the postsynaptic receptors, which triggers an alteration in the ionic permeability of the cell membrane. Transmitters affecting the postsynaptic cell in this matter are considered to be rapid transmitters, because the onset of ionic action in the postsynaptic cell is fast, in the order of milliseconds. Other neurotransmitters (e.g., serotonin) activate the postsynaptic receptor to transmit a chemical message through the cell membrane. The messenger, in turn, triggers a *second messenger* (intracellular molecule) that initiates a cascade of reactions within the postsynaptic cell. This intracellular activity produces a number of cellular changes, including an alteration in the ionic permeability of the postsynaptic membrane. Second-messenger transmission is considered to be slow with regard to onset of postsynaptic activity; that is, onset can range from hundreds of milliseconds to seconds (Schwartz & Kandel, 1991; Preston, O'Neal, & Talaga, 1997). The ionic changes initiated by the two forms of neurotransmitter actions are similar. If the alteration in the permeability of the cell results in increased levels of Na^+ and Cl^- moving into the postsynaptic cell and smaller amounts of K^+ moving out, the postsynaptic cell depolarizes. This depolarization, known as an **excitatory postsynaptic potential (EPSP),** increases the probability that the postsynaptic cell will reach its threshold. An EPSP makes it more likely that the membrane threshold will reach an action potential and that the postsynaptic neuron will fire.

During an inhibitory exchange, the presence of a neurotransmitter increases the permeability of the postsynaptic membrane, particularly to K^+. This results in an ionic current that hyperpolarizes the postsynaptic neuron. Thus, greater depolarization than normal is required to reach an action potential. This depolarization, called **inhibitory postsynaptic potential (IPSP),** becomes less probable. Next, the synaptic vesicle either dissipates or is reabsorbed by the presynaptic membrane, which allows the recycling of neurotransmitters and completes the cycle. This summation of EPSPs and IPSPs, analogous to

Table 4.1	*Neurotransmitters*
Biogenic amines	Acetylcholine (ACh)
	Serotonin (5-HT)
Catecholamines	Dopamine (DA)
	Norepinephrine (NE) (noradrenalin)
	Epinephrine (EPI) (adrenalin)
Amino acids	Gamma-aminobutyric acid (GABA)
	Glycine
	Glutamate
	Aspartate
Peptides	Vasopressin
	Oxytocin
	Thyrotropin-releasing hormone (TRH)
	Corticotropin-releasing factor
	Substance P
	Tachykinins
	Cholecystokinin

yes/no messages, is the main principle of neural communication. The nervous system is exceedingly complex, because one single neuron may have many synaptic terminals on it that could influence the action potential of thousands of other neurons.

NEUROTRANSMITTERS

Neurotransmitters permit the exchange of information among neurons and between neurons and other cells. Neurotransmitter types (Table 4.1) are classified according to molecular size. For example, the biogenic amines and amino acids are small-molecule messengers, consisting of fewer than 10 carbon atoms, and the neuropeptides, which are larger molecules. Although smaller molecule neurotransmitters, such as **acetylcholine (ACh), serotonin,** and the **catecholamines,** have traditionally received the most scientific study, neuropeptides are more numerous in the brain, with more than 40 different neuropeptides currently identified (Kalat, 1998).

Just as each neurotransmitter has a specific shape, comparable with a key, each receptor site also has a specific structure analogous to a lock. Thus, a specific neurotransmitter will attach itself only to a receptor with an appropriate fit. In some cases, a variety of neurotransmitters can adhere to a single type of receptor molecule: Many different keys may fit the same lock. At times, different neurotransmitters may compete for the same receptor molecule. For example, even though neurotransmitter A might have adhered to receptor Z at one time, in competition with neurotransmitter B, A may fail to activate because B fits better. This scenario may occur thousands of times even at the individual level of one neuron. Chemical transmission allows tremendous flexibility and refinement.

Distribution of Neurotransmitters

Many distinct neurotransmitter pathways define the brain chemically and anatomically. The tracing of neuronal pathways along neurotransmitter systems has been at the center of the neurosciences since the development of modern staining methods. Investigations show that neurotransmitters are both localized to specific regions and widely dispersed in the brain. The pathways of the catecholamine transmitters such as **dopamine** (DA) and norepinephrine are relatively specific in their targeting of brain regions, whereas other transmitters (e.g., glutamate) are widely distributed throughout the brain.

Acetylcholine—In the early 1900s, ACh (or choline) was the first neurotransmitter to be identified; researchers discovered that it stimulates the parasympathetic nervous system. It plays a prominent role in the PNS, influencing motor control, and in autonomic nervous system functioning. ACh also is a predominant neurotransmitter at the neuromuscular junction, stimulating muscular contraction. In the CNS and brain, ACh affects a wide behavioral repertoire. One of its most important functions might be to influence alertness, attention, and memory.

ACh has a simple chemical structure, but its method of action is complicated and is yet to be fully understood. One component necessary for synthesizing ACh is choline, which is supplied by foods such as liver, kidneys, egg yolks, seeds, and many vegetables and legumes. It is synthesized in the liver and recycled in the brain. Choline easily crosses the blood–brain barrier. There is evidence that shows an influx of choline in the brain after eating and an outflow when plasma choline levels are lower, that is, between meals (see Feldman, Meyer, & Quenzer, 1997). Like other neurotransmitters, ACh binds to a variety of postsynaptic receptor subtypes. The two main subtypes of ACh are **muscarinic choline** and **nicotinic choline,** named after the bitter botanical alkaloids that stimulate the receptors (muscarine from the fly agaric mushroom, *Amanita muscaria,* and nicotine from tobacco, *Nicotiana tabacum*). The implication is that the action of ACh may differ from one receptor subtype to another. Nicotinic receptor binding creates an excitatory response, whereas muscarinic responses may be either excitatory or inhibitory. Therefore, in the PNS, for example, glands and muscles may be either excited or inhibited, depending on the subtype of ACh receptor. Certain drugs act on nicotinic receptors, and others are specific to muscarinic receptors.

As in the PNS, distribution of ACh is widespread in the brain, where it has many possible behavioral functions. First, cholinergic (ACh) neurons in the **striatum,** a collection of brain structures named after their striped or striated appearance, influence motor system functioning. Degeneration of striatal neurons is associated with Huntington's disease.

Second, ACh functions in arousal and in the sleep/wake cycle. The **reticular activating system** is a network of neurons that arises from the brainstem and projects throughout the cortex. One of its primary functions is to regulate brain activation. For example, Sitaram, Moore, and Gillin (1978) report that an ACh antagonist such as scopolamine extends the normal interval (about 45 minutes) between rapid eye movement (REM) sleep. Although many neurotransmitter systems are involved in the sleep cycle, ACh appears to play a role in activating the cortex. Increased levels of ACh in the brainstem and **basal forebrain** are associated with increased cortical arousal and wakefulness. Researchers can elicit REM sleep, which is characterized by increased cortical activity, by activating muscarinic ACh receptors.

Third, a major cholinergic system thought to influence attention, memory, and learning emerges from the basal forebrain and projects throughout the cortex and to structures important for consolidating memory, such as the **hippocampus.** An important cholinergic nucleus in the basal forebrain is the **nucleus basalis of Meynert** (named after its discoverer). Its degeneration as a factor in Alzheimer's disease became evident when researchers found that patients with this disorder had measurably lower than normal levels of ACh in their brains. Alzheimer's disease is associated with severe memory dysfunction, and this observation led researchers to wonder whether ACh plays a role in memory functioning. Scopolamine, a drug that blocks ACh at muscarinic receptor sites, causes deficits in encoding and consolidation into long-term memory (see Polster, 1993). Surgical patients given scopolamine often have amnesia for the events before surgery. These findings led to the development of drugs that serve as ACh agonists binding to the same receptors as ACh and increasing ACh levels for use in clinical trials with patients with Alzheimer's disease. However, this intervention was largely disappointing, perhaps in part because Alzheimer's disease involves much more than one neurotransmitter system. It is also possible that ACh has a less direct influence on memory, and instead functions to maintain a higher level of cortical alertness and attention that may be a necessary precursor to adequate memory functioning.

Serotonin—Serotonin is widely distributed throughout the brain, but the serotonin system originates in a small area of the brainstem called the **nuclei of the raphe.** The raphe nuclei consist of a collection of neurons throughout the midline of the brainstem. The serotonin pathways of the raphe nuclei branch out toward the cerebellum. Those pathways in the medulla oblongata project toward the spinal cord, and axons of the cells in the rostral group of the nuclei branch out to the forebrain. Ascending fibers of serotonergic neurons project to the limbic system, a major collection of subcortical structures involved in the modulations of mood and emotion. Destroying the raphe nuclei leads to insomnia, and serotonin plays a major role in the sleep/wake cycle. Low levels of serotonin are also associated with severe depression. Several studies have demonstrated that depressed individuals are more likely to commit suicide if they have unusually low levels of serotonin being produced and released in the brain (Roy, De Jong, & Linnoila, 1989; Träskmann, Asberg, Bertilsson, & Sjöstrand, 1981). Alterations in serotonin also accompany violent and aggressive behavior in animals (Brown & Linnoila, 1990) and in humans (Elliott, 1992).

Norepinephrine—**Norepinephrine** (NE) forms predominantly among neurons and their nuclei in a brainstem site named the **locus ceruleus** (the "blue place"), located below the wall of the fourth ventricle. NE pathways innervate many areas in the forebrain, the cerebellum, and the spinal cord. Its functions are complex and widespread. Research suggests that NE is important in regulating mood, hormones (via the hypothalamus), cerebral blood flow, and motor behavior. Similar to DA, NE plays a role in arousal and attentional regulation (specifically, the focusing of attention), as well as other cognitive operations such as memory and speed of information processing. NE is implicated in clinical disorders involving depression, anxiety, and inattention (Stahl, 2000). Researchers have also found that stressful situations can increase the production and release of NE in the hypothalamus in rats (Cenci, Kalen, Mandel, & Bjoerklund, 1992).

Dopamine—DA is an important neurotransmitter that has been implicated in a number of clinical disorders. Three relatively distinct brain dopaminergic pathways are implicated in neuropsychological functioning (Figure 4.10). The first pathway, the mesolimbic pathway, projects from the ventral tegmental area of the brainstem to the nucleus accumbens (basal ganglia), other limbic areas of the brain, and prefrontal cortex. This pathway is associated with the experience of pleasurable sensations, including euphoria

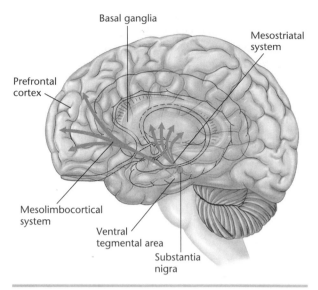

Figure 4.10 Dopamine pathways. (From Kalat, J. W. [2007]. *Biological psychology* [9th ed., p. 479, Figure 15.20]. Belmont, CA: Thomson Wadsworth.)

with the abuse of certain drugs, and the positive symptoms (e.g., hallucinations and delusions) of schizophrenia. Most antipsychotic drugs that target the positive symptoms of schizophrenia operate to block DA receptors. The second pathway, the mesocortical DA pathway, also originates in the ventral tegmental regions of the brainstem, but transverses to the frontal cortex and limbic regions. This pathway has been implicated in the pathogenesis of the negative symptoms of schizophrenia and the mediation of a number of cognitive functions (verbal fluency, serial learning, attention regulation, and regulation of behavior based on social cues) (Stahl, 2000). The third DA pathway, mesostriatal, projects from the **substantia nigra** of the brainstem to the caudate nucleus and putamen of the basal ganglia. This pathway is involved in the regulation of voluntary motor functions and initiation of behavior in response to environmental stimuli (Feifel, 1999). Decreased DA activity in the pathway is associated with motor symptoms such as rigidity, loss or slowing of movement, and tremors. In contrast, excessive DA in the system appears to prompt motor tics, chorea, and other motor behavior disruptions. Two subcortical disorders implicated in the overactivity and underactivity of the nigrostriatal pathways are, respectively, Parkinson's and Huntington's diseases.

Amino Acids—**Amino acids** are the building blocks of protein and are present in every cell in the body. In the brain,

---

Neuropsychology in Action 4.3

What Can We Learn from Songbirds?

by Mary V. Spiers

Can the adult brain form new neurons? The common wisdom has been that at birth the brain has all the neurons it will ever possess. In fact, the brain goes through a necessary process of pruning neurons as learning strengthens certain neural associations and others become unnecessary. There is evidence in some species of songbirds, however, that new brain cells form in conjunction with seasonal changes in mating songs. Researchers Ball and Hulse (1998) have reviewed this literature and report intriguing findings. Male canaries and sparrows, some of the most studied songbirds, have complex mating songs that show seasonal variation, being most prominent in spring. Neurobiologists have precisely mapped the vocal system of these songbirds and have found a consistent structure–function relation between specific nuclei and singing behavior.

For example, the high vocal center (HVC) is responsible for vocal production, and the robust nucleus of the archistriatum (RA) aids in coordinating respiration with singing. Within this circuit of nuclei are neurorecep-tors that are specific for sex hormones, such as androgens and estrogens. Receptors for these steroid sex hormones are not present in the vocal control circuitry of birds that are not songbirds. The complexity of song production differs in male and female songbirds, with males singing more songs and more complex songs. Researchers think this greater production in males serves as a mating function, to attract females and establish territory. This sex difference in singing behavior corresponds to structural differences in the vocal control systems of males and females. Specifically, in male songbirds, the HVC and RA are larger and contain more hormonal receptor nuclei. These differences aroused the curiosity of researchers. Male song production is seasonal, so might there be seasonal changes in the brains of males?

In fact, there were. In male canaries, the HVC had increased in size by nearly 100% in the spring compared with the fall! The RA had increased by a factor of about 75% (Nottebohm, 1981). The next question was, "What was causing this increase?" Was the size or volume of existing neurons changing? For example, might new dendritic connections form during this time? Or were new neurons developing? Evidence showed that the nuclei that control singing increase in volume when the blood levels of testosterone rise. New staining techniques involving a traceable radioactive tag of newly forming cells indicated that new neurons formed in the ventricles of canaries and migrated to the vocal control system, specifically the HVC and RA (Goldman & Nottebohm, 1983). This was an astonishing finding. Further evidence indicates that adults of other species also generate new neurons, and that this co-occurs with learning. Such research has exciting implications for the study of human language. Will the findings of neurogenesis in adult canaries generalize to human language or other types of learning? And if new neurons can be formed, what is the implication for rehabilitation from brain injury and for lifetime adult learning programs?

---

amino acids are involved in the basic neuronal transmission that depends on rapid communication among neurons. Of the more than 20 amino acids, the most common are **gamma-aminobutyric acid (GABA),** which has strong inhibitory properties, and **glutamate,** an excitatory neurotransmitter. In fact, GABA is so common in the CNS that researchers believe one third of all synapses are receptive to it. Glutamate also occurs in high concentration throughout the nervous system and is the major excitatory neurotransmitter. The most prominent GABAergic projection system consists of the inhibitory Purkinje cells that extend into the deep portions of the cerebellar nuclei. Some of the major projecting systems of the basal ganglia that are also inhibitory are the striatum, globus pallidus, and substantia nigra. The inability of patients with Huntington's disease to control their own motor behavior perhaps relates to the loss of inhibitory GABAergic neurons in the basal ganglia.

Peptides—Peptides are short chains of amino acids; scientists have identified more than 60 peptides. High levels of peptides are present in the hypothalamus and the amygdala, and to a much lesser extent, in the cortex, the thalamus, and the cerebellum. Naturally produced peptides with opiate properties are called **endorphins.** Endorphins have received much scientific attention for their analgesic effects and their possible role in a pain-inhibiting neuronal system. Psychologists have always been interested in new procedures to alter the perception of pain, and research suggests that acupuncture and electrical stimulation of the brainstem arouse the pain-inhibiting endorphin system. The nervous system has specific receptor sites that bind the drug morphine and related opiate compounds. The presence of opiate receptors suggests that the brain itself can create opiate neurotransmitters, perhaps to produce a natural high after prolonged physical stress or in the event of a catastrophic injury. Endorphins that

Neuropsychology in Action 4.4

Stem Cell Research: Science and Ethics

by Meghan L. Butryn, Danielle Kerns, and Heather W. Murray

As scientific inquiry has evolved, so too have ethical dilemmas. Nowhere is this illustrated more prominently than in the area of stem cell research. Stem cells are undifferentiated cells; they do not yet have either an identified or specialized function. They eventually differentiate into the building blocks of tissues and organs. Another unique characteristic of stem cells that distinguishes them is their ability to proliferate or replicate themselves for long periods.

Stem cells used for research typically are either embryonic or adult stem cells (Committee on the Biological and Biomedical Applications of Stem Cell Research, 2002, p. 13). Embryos usually come as a donated by-product of in vitro fertilization (National Institutes of Health, 2002). Embryonic stem cells can be stimulated to differentiate into specific cell types such as heart muscle

cells, blood cells, or nerve cells. Stimulation includes changing "the chemical composition of the culture medium," altering "the surface of the culture dish," or modifying "the cells by inserting specific genes" (National Institutes of Health, 2002). The goal of such procedures is the future ability to produce, on demand, specialized cells that can be used as a treatment for certain diseases where there is degeneration or destruction of cells.

Adult stem cells have been located in "bone marrow, peripheral blood, brain, spinal cord, dental pulp, blood vessels, skeletal muscle, epithelia of the skin and digestive system, cornea, retina, liver, and pancreas" (Department of Health and Human Services, 2001). It was not until the 1990s that scientists discovered that the brain contains stem cells. These stem cells

are able to generate the brain's major cell types: astrocytes and oligodendrocytes, which are nonneuronal glial cells, and neurons. Stem cells in adults have been identified in the subventricular zone of the telencephalon (Alvarez-Buylla & Garcia-Verdugo, 2002) and in the dentate gyrus of the hippocampus (Gould & Gross, 2002; Song et al., 2002); these cells were demonstrated to differentiate into any type of nervous tissue cell (Alvarez-Buylla & Lois, 1995; Gage, 2000; Weiss et al., 1996).

The pluripotency, or plasticity, of embryonic cells has been one of the touted advantages of embryonic stem cells compared with adult stem cells. However, recent research supports that at least some adult stem cells may also demonstrate this pluripotency, with the possibility that further research will uncover other adult stem cells

---

originate in the brainstem may interfere with pain impulses via their action on the spinal cord.

Regeneration of Neurons

To what extent a patient recovers from an injury to the PNS or CNS pathways depends largely on the regenerative capacity of the damaged neurons. The capacity for regeneration in the PNS is actually quite good; useful function can often be restored with surgical nerve repair. Surgeons have reattached fingers and even complete limbs, and much sensory and motor function has been restored (Neuropsychology in Action 4.3).

The regeneration of neurons in the CNS is more complex. Once damaged, neurons do not heal spontaneously after the developmental period. Generally speaking, humans are born with as many neurons as they will ever have, although new research has suggested that adult humans do generate new neurons from some **stem cells** in various parts of the brain. This fact is related, in part, to the structure of the CNS, which is infinitely more complicated than that of the PNS. As a result, the CNS has

little of the spontaneous cellular regeneration required to reconnect a damaged axon to its normal target. Most often, the projections of such neurons, as well as the targets of other neurons, are lost. Later chapters discuss why the brain can compensate when neurons are lost and also how neuronal plasticity and the reconfiguration of functional systems are important to the developing brain. Recently, a flurry of research activity has focused on establishing procedures that facilitate neuronal growth through stem cell research (Neuropsychology in Action 4.4) or by attempting to coax injured neurons into regrowing.

Injuries and diseases that result in neuronal loss or degeneration are a major health concern and can significantly affect the quality of life in individuals with CNS disorders. For example, more than 100,000 people in the United States have paraplegia or quadriplegia, a disabling condition that results from severed neurons in the spinal cord. Head injuries—in which axonal shearing, a form of stretching caused by physical forces, is common—affect about 3 million people. Stroke, which is neuronal cell death due to insufficient oxygen, affects about 2 million people; degenerative conditions such as Alzheimer's, Parkinson's, and Huntington's diseases burden millions more. It is thus important for

that are multipotent. A second key difference is related to the ease of growth in cultures, with embryonic stem cells being more easily grown. Researchers are attempting to determine why embryonic stem cells proliferate for a year or more in the laboratory without differentiating, whereas most adult stem cells appear to have a more limited capacity for doing so (Carpenter, Mattson, & Rao, 2003). Finally, the ability to use an individual's own adult stem cells eliminates the risk for rejection by the immune system.

If scientists can direct the differentiation of stem cells into specific cell types, they may be able to treat many diseases and injuries. Patients who have conditions in which destruction of cells occurs within a defined area, such as stroke or spinal cord injury, may be candidates for transplantation. Patients with diffuse conditions such as Alzheimer's disease, where neurochemical destruction of many types of cells occurs, may be more difficult to treat with stem cell transplantation because many different types of neurons would need to be replaced in many different locations (Armstrong, Watts, Svendsen, Dunnett, & Rosser, 2000).

Similarly, replacement of entire circuits, which would likely be necessary to treat conditions such as Huntington's disease, may prove to be more difficult. Cell-specific conditions, such as **amyotrophic lateral sclerosis (ALS)** and Parkinson's disease, where destruction is limited to certain tracts of cells, and demyelinating conditions, such as MS, are also considered candidates for advanced research in stem cell transplantation. Other conditions that eventually might be treated with stem cell transplantation include Purkinje cell degeneration and vision and hearing loss.

ALS, also known as Lou Gehrig's disease, is a progressive disease that degenerates cholinergic motor neurons in the brain and spinal cord. As the disease progresses, patients with ALS eventually become paralyzed and, on average, die 5 years after onset. In a study conducted by Kerr and colleagues (2003), rats were exposed to the Sindbis virus, which destroys motor neurons and causes paralysis in a way that mimics ALS. These researchers selected embryonic stem cells that were barely differentiated and that had two molecular markers of motor cells and

injected them into the spinal cords of these rats. Three months after transplantation, treated rats had regained movement in their hind limbs, including the ability to walk, whereas untreated rats remained paralyzed. The transplanted stem cells migrated throughout the spinal cord and further developed molecular markers of motor neurons.

In addition to typical ethical issues of research, stem cell research involves procedures that are controversial, particularly regarding use of embryonic stem cells. The heart of the stem cell research debate is based on the definition of life. There is a push to develop less controversial alternative treatments to replace embryonic stem cell transplantation. But the lack of plasticity of adult stem cells in comparison with embryonic stem cells leads some researchers to suggest that advancements in stem cell research will come largely from further investigation of embryonic stem cells. Limiting research with embryonic cells, it is believed, will only slow the progression of learning about the development of increased plasticity of adult stem cells (Civin, 2002).

---

neuropsychologists to understand the life cycle of a neuron and what happens when it becomes damaged or diseased.

Some immediate recovery of function can be observed after traumatic or vascular lesions to the CNS. A lesion is any pathologic or traumatic discontinuity of tissue resulting in the loss of neurons. Interestingly, recovery is related to a reduction of swelling in surrounding brain or spinal cord tissue, not to a spontaneous healing of neurons. A process called *collateral sprouting*, which occurs in nearby intact neurons, may also facilitate functional reorganization (Figure 4.11). Researchers have made great advances in stimulating the growth responses with which the CNS

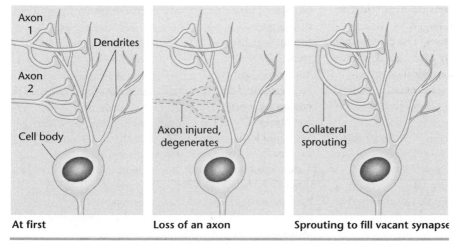

At first   **Loss of an axon**   **Sprouting to fill vacant synapse**

Figure 4.11 Example of collateral sprouting. (From Kalat, J. W. [2007]. *Biological psychology* [9th ed., p. 141, Figure 5.16]. Belmont, CA: Thomson Wadsworth.)

typically reacts to trauma, replacing tissue lost to injury or disease with neuronal transplants and developing assessment, prosthesis, and cognitive rehabilitation techniques for disrupted functional systems. One major finding by

neuropsychologists has been that an active training rehabilitation program facilitates recovery of function. It is within this area of assessment and intervention that clinical neuropsychologists have made some of their greatest advances.

Summary

This chapter discusses the structure and function of the important "cells of thought." Each of these classes of cells contain subtypes that are specialized for different types of information processing. Although scientists know most about the electrochemical processes of neurons, the chemical processes of glial cells are gaining more attention for their role in cognitive functioning. At its most fundamental level, all human behavior originates from the basic processes mediated by the structural interconnections and the chemical influences of neurons and glial cells with each other. Clinical disorders of neurons include diseases or conditions that physically damage the neuron or disrupt communication. In this chapter, we discuss multiple sclerosis and introduce disorders that will be examined in more depth in later chapters, such as epilepsy and spinal cord injury. Research related to the mechanisms of structural neuronal repair as well as a better understanding of the chemical interplay of these cells is helping to inform treatment.

Critical Thinking Questions

- Will it be possible one day to "map" the circuits of the human brain?
- Actor Christopher Reeve suffered a severe spinal cord injury and died without fulfilling his pledge to walk again. What is the outlook for other people with paralysis caused by spinal cord injury?
- Is it possible for a drug to be effective if it does not activate a naturally occurring brain chemical receptor?
- What scientific and ethical questions will need to be resolved for research into neuronal repair and neurogenesis to be successful?

Key Terms

Dendrites	Interneurons	Sodium–potassium pump	Striatum
Axon	Motor neurons	Refractory period	Reticular activating system
Terminal buttons	Sensory neurons	Disinhibition	Basal forebrain
Synapse	Tracts	Seizures	Hippocampus
Neurotransmitter	Pathways	Electroconvulsive therapy (ECT)	Nucleus basalis of Meynert
Pruning	Fibers	Electroencephalograph	Nuclei of the raphe
Gray matter	Nerves	Synaptic knobs	Norepinephrine
Purkinje cells	Intracerebral fibers	Synaptic vesicles	Locus ceruleus
Dendritic spines	Intercerebral fibers	Receptor sites	Substantia nigra
Myelin sheath	Projection fibers	Excitatory postsynaptic potential	Amino acids
White matter	Nuclei	(EPSP)	Gamma-aminobutyric acid
Action potential	Ganglia	Inhibitory postsynaptic potential	(GABA)
Glia	Microglia	(IPSP)	Glutamate
Oligodendrocytes	Astrocytes	Acetylcholine (ACh)	Peptides
Schwann cells	Gliomas	Serotonin	Endorphins
Nodes of Ranvier	Blood–brain barrier	Catecholamines	Stem cells
Multipolar neurons	Resting potential	Dopamine	Amyotrophic lateral sclerosis
Bipolar neurons	Membrane potential	Muscarinic choline	(ALS)
Monopolar neurons	Ions	Nicotinic choline	

Web Connections

http://psych.hanover.edu/Krantz/neurotut.html
Basic Neural Processes Tutorials
A good tutorial on the basics of neural processing. Includes a glossary of terms and quizzes on the structure of the neuron and the brain.

http://www.neuroguide.com
Neurosciences on the Internet
A searchable page that provides links to sites in neuroscience.

Chapter 5

FUNCTIONAL NEUROANATOMY

Anatomy is for physiology what geography is for the historian: It describes the scene of action.

—*Jean Fernel*

The Brain—is wider than the sky—
For—put them side by side—
The one the other will contain
With ease—and You—beside—

—*Emily Dickinson*

Keep in Mind

▪ What are the stages and processes of anatomic development?

▪ How are the subsystems of the brain organized?

▪ How does the brain protect and nourish itself?

▪ Does brain structure follow brain function?

▪ What are the major divisions of the brain?

Overview

Neuroanatomy is best understood within a conceptual framework of structure–function relationships. In neuropsychology, a primary goal is to understand the psychological functions and systems of the brain. Rather than memorizing structures for structure's sake, a more meaningful picture emerges from knowing how the subdivisions of the brain are related, and what roles they play in initiating and regulating behavior. Neuroanatomy and neuroscience texts present slightly different variations of organization within the major subdivisions of the brain. Some authors focus on morphology as the organizing scheme, some on physiology, and some on embryonic and fetal development. Despite the daunting array of structures, the basic logic of neuroanatomy is straightforward. The organization presented in this chapter shows the relationships between the often-confusing terms and groupings. This goal is accomplished by using the foundation of the developing brain within the context of evolution, which provides a useful picture of functioning from basic to more complex behaviors.

This chapter discusses individual structures and terminology, shows their location in the brain, and gives a brief overview of function. The material covered here is not a detailed review of the content often covered in courses on neuroscience or sensory motor systems, but rather constitutes an illustrated account of the functional anatomy of the major components of the nervous system. With the foundation of the gross anatomy and functioning this chapter presents, you can appreciate the normal and abnormal phenomena associated with brain dysfunction. The structures are the important topographical features on which the various processing systems of the brain depend. This chapter is a stepping-stone for subsequent chapters related to functional systems and, indeed, for the entire book. We develop these structures further as we examine functional brain systems and neuropsychological disorders.

To set the stage for our discussion of the functional neuroanatomy of the brain, we discuss the prenatal and postnatal development of the human brain. The gestation of the brain is a significant developmental period when you consider that the rate of neuronal development is estimated at 250,000 neurons *per minute,* for a total, at birth, in excess of 100 billion (Cowan, 1979; Papalia & Olds, 1995). Despite this astonishing rate of early brain development, the process is both orderly and systematic. That is, the brain develops in accordance with genetically predetermined templates or "blueprints" that guide the unfolding of structure and function. The developmental process does not stop and wait for better conditions such as optimal maternal health and nutrition, nor does it reverse direction to repeat developmental stages that are compromised by insults engendered by trauma, drugs, or environmental toxins. Accordingly, it is not surprising that negative events during gestation account for a significant number of childhood neurologic disorders.

The first section presents an overview of the anatomic development of the brain, followed by a presentation of the major components of the nervous system. We also introduce the necessary terminology for a common orientation to the geographical locations of structures. Next, we present structural features that protect and sustain the brain. Finally, we discuss principal divisions of the brain, from lower, evolutionarily older structures to higher order structures.

Anatomic and Functional Development of the Brain

Beginning as a hollow tube, the brain develops steadily through temporally distinct stages to its final anatomic and functional state of well-delineated cellular layers and regions. The development of the **central nervous system (CNS)** is orderly and systematic, generally unfolding from head (cephalic) to tail (caudal), from near (proximal) to far (distal), and from inferior (subcortical) to dorsal (cortical). The earliest stage, **neurogenesis,** involves the proliferation of neurons of the neural tube and the migration of these cells to predetermined locations. This stage is primarily genetically determined, although environmental influences can have an impact on this process. Subsequent stages include the growth of axons and dendrites, formation of synaptic junctures, myelination of axons, and synaptic reorganization involving strengthening or loss of synaptic connections. The latter stages complete much of their maturation during postnatal development. In general, prenatal development is primarily concerned with the formation of the CNS, whereas postnatal development involves the increasing emergence of functionality.

NEUROGENESIS AND CELLULAR MIGRATION

Both the CNS and **peripheral nervous system (PNS)** develop from the outer ectoderm layer of the fertilized egg at approximately 18 days after conception. Ectodermal tissue (neural plate) rises, then subsequently folds and fuses at approximately the fourth week to form the **neural tube** (Figure 5.1). The cavity of the neural tube gives rise to the ventricular system of the CNS, and the cells lining the wall of the neural tube, termed **precursor or progenitor cells,** create the neurons and **glial cells** (astrocytes, **oligodendrocytes,** and **microglia**) of the brain (Martin & Jessell, 1991). Developing cells do not proliferate at the same rate along the expanding neural tube. The timing and location of these cells are genetically predetermined and relate to their final placement and function in the mature brain. Once the proliferation of a specified group of neurons is complete, the **migratory process** commences and the cells move outward toward their genetically determined destination in temporally different waves. As the cells reach their destination, they begin to develop the characteristics of the cell types that are intrinsic to that particular brain region (Kolb & Fantie, 1997). The process of increasing regional specialization of cells is referred to as **differentiation.** The migrating cells do not differentiate at the same

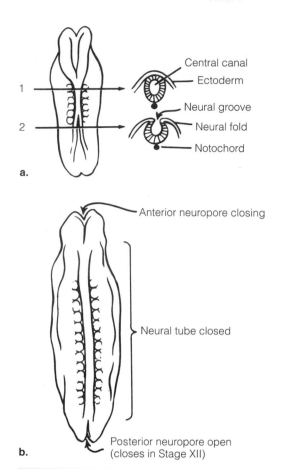

a.

b.

Figure 5.1   Formation and closure of the neural tube. (a) Start of neurulation, two cross-sectional views. (b) Late stage of neurulation, showing the anterior and posterior closing. (From Lemire, R. J., Loeser, J. D., Leech, R. W., & Alvord, E. C. [1975]. *Normal and abnormal development of the human nervous system.* Philadelphia: Lippincott Williams & Wilkins, by permission.)

rate; for example, the cells destined for the hippocampus differentiate at a faster rate than the cells of the cortex (Monk, Webb, & Nelson, 2001).

The open ends of the neural tube close at approximately the 26th day of gestation, with the anterior end subsequently creating the brain, and the posterior end forming the spinal cord. The process of forming and closing the neural tube is called **neurulation.** Failure of the neural tube to close during development can cause a number of developmental disorders. For example, neuroscientists believe that **spina bifida,** a congenital developmental disorder characterized by an opening in the spinal cord, results from a disruption of the proliferation rate of neural cells or from the failure of these cells to differentiate properly in the neural tube. In contrast, when the anterior end of the tube fails to close, the brain fails to develop anatomically, producing a condition termed **anencephaly.** In this condition, the brain is a vascular mass and the infant does not survive.

The development of the cortex, **corticogenesis,** begins in the sixth to seventh embryonic week. The rapidly proliferating cells along the wall of the neural tube migrate outward at different predetermined times. The neurons migrate in sheets (laminae) along nonneuronal (glial) fibers that span the cortical wall. Ultimately, these neuronal sheets constitute the six laminated layers of the cortex and the subcortical nuclei. The inner layer forms first, followed by the development of the outer layers of the cortex. Each successive generation of migrating cells passes through the previously developed neuronal cells. Thus, the cortex develops from inside out, with migration beginning earlier for the more anterior and lateral areas of the cortex (Rakic & Lombroso, 1998). By the 18th week of gestation, virtually all cortical neurons have reached their designated locations and cell proliferation ceases. The exceptions are the cells of the hippocampus and cerebellum that continue to proliferate after birth (Anderson, Anderson, Northam, Jacobs, & Catroppa, 2001). After migration, many of the glia cells transform into astrocytes, whereas others merely disappear (Monk et al., 2001).

Disruption in the migratory process can result in significant and extensive malformations of the developing brain. For instance, abnormalities of cell migration can produce developmental anomalies of the corpus callosum and other subcortical structures. Similarly, disruption of cell migration during the first trimester of development is associated with malformations of the cerebral cortex. An example is the condition of **agyria,** or **lissencephaly,** a disorder that occurs during the 11th to 13th weeks of gestation and involves the underdevelopment of the cortical gyri (Hynd, Morgan, & Vaughn, 1997). Severe neurologic problems accompany this condition, such as severe mental retardation, motor retardation, seizures, and reduced muscle tone. Most infants with agyria do not survive beyond 2 years of age.

AXON AND DENDRITE DEVELOPMENT

As the neurons migrate along the glial fibers, **axons** begin to form rapidly and travel to other neurons of the brain, allowing for cortical–cortical, cortical–subcortical, and interhemispheric communication. The intercommunications afforded by axonal connections are crucial to the integrative functioning of the brain. As the migrating neuronal cells reach their designated positions, **dendrites**

begin to sprout in a process called **arborization.** Subsequently, little extensions called **dendritic spines** begin to extend out from the dendrites. The dendrites and dendritic spines create synapses for gathering information to transmit to the neuron. Dendritic growth begins prenatally and proceeds slowly, with the majority of arborization and spine growth actually occurring postnatally. The most intensive period of dendritic growth occurs from birth to approximately 18 months of age.

The development of the dendrites and dendritic spines is highly sensitive to the effects of environmental stimulation. This sensitivity fosters the growth and differentiation of the brain; yet, it increases its vulnerability to damage. An example of this vulnerability is the discovery, for certain groups of mentally retarded children, of abnormalities of the dendritic spines that are not attributable to genetic factors. In these cases, neuroscientists suspect some form of environmental insult as having produced the anomaly.

SYNAPTOGENESIS

Paralleling the growth of the axons and dendrites of the brain is the formation of synapses, that is, **synaptogenesis.** Synaptogenesis begins during the second trimester as neuronal migration approaches completion. Thus, at the 28th gestational week, synaptic density is low in all cortical regions, particularly the **prefrontal cortex.** Whereas the occipital lobe begins developing before birth and rapidly achieves near adult-level synaptic density between ages 2 and 4, the more slowly developing prefrontal cortex does not reach adult levels until late adolescence or adulthood. Likewise, the synaptic development of the motor speech cortex (Broca's area) follows a slow trajectory paralleling that of the prefrontal cortex (Huttenlocher & Dabholkar, 1997). Regional increases in synaptic density accompany the emergence of function. For example, a rapid increase in synaptic density of the frontal lobes during the latter part of the first year of life correlates with the emergence of rudimentary executive functions.

MYELINATION

As cellular migration nears completion, oligodendrocytes begin to encircle the axons, providing a protective white insular sheath called **myelin** (see discussion in Chapter 4). The process of myelination begins in the spinal cord, proceeds through the subcortical regions, and finally completes the cortical circuitry. The cortical regions myelinate at different times, beginning in the posterior regions of the brain and moving in an anterior direction, with the parietal and frontal lobes completing the process last. The myelination of the latter two regions begins after birth, and in the case of the frontal regions, continues into adolescence and adulthood. The significant increase in brain weight in the postnatal years is primarily a function of the brain's increased myelination. Furthermore, the myelination of regional circuitry generally correlates with the emergence of function. Thus, similar to synaptic density, myelination is a "marker" of increasing functional maturity of brain circuitry. For example, myelination of the optic nerve begins at birth and is completed by the third month, consistent with the emergence of vision.

PRUNING

During the early months of neurodevelopment, the neurons and synaptic processes of the brain are initially overproduced. Researchers believe that the synaptic connectivity of the neurons is not completely genetically preprogrammed, and many of the initial connections may be random, unnecessary, or poor. Subsequent development eliminates, or **prunes,** large numbers of neurons, with the process often beginning at the sites of the dendritic spines. Pruning does not appear to be random, but rather to be a purposeful sculpting of the brain; that is, synaptic connections that are strengthened through sensory input and motor activity are spared. In contrast, pruning eliminates weakly reinforced or redundant connections, thus promoting neural efficiency. Economy in structure and function appears to be an overarching principle of evolutionary development. This process is exemplified by the development of speech and language specific to one's culture. At birth, the infant is sensitive to the range of sounds that are evident in all languages. However, the reinforcement of speech sounds unique to one's culture results in the loss of sensitivity to sounds *not* evident in the language. Neuroscientists speculate that neurons and synaptic processes representing the understimulated sounds are pruned. Functionally, this pruning potentially accounts for the greater difficulty encountered in learning a second language at an older age as opposed to at an earlier age.

Pruning is primarily a postnatal process, eliminating 40% of the cortical neurons of the brain during childhood. The remaining neurons are eliminated during adolescence, and possibly into early adulthood. The observed reduction in cortical gray matter during adolescence is believed related to synaptic pruning (Gogtay, Giedd, Lusk, Hayashi, Greenstein, Vaituzis, et al., 2004). Pruning of brain regions proceeds at different times and rates. Thus,

reduction of the synapses in the **visual cortex** begins at 1 year of age and is completed by age 12, whereas pruning of the prefrontal region proceeds from 5 to 16 years of age (Pfefferbaum, Mathalon, Sullivan, Rawles, Zipursky, & Lim, 1994).

REGIONAL DEVELOPMENT

As noted earlier, the anterior, cranial end of the neural tube expands to form the brain, and the posterior end evolves to form the spinal cord. Before neurulation is complete, three vesicles (dilations or expansions) develop at the anterior end. These vesicles subsequently form the **forebrain (prosencephalon), midbrain (mesencephalon),** and **hindbrain (rhombencephalon).** In the fifth week of development, the forebrain and hindbrain each subdivide, whereas the third vesicle, the midbrain, maintains its regional structure. The division of the prosencephalon results in the formation of the **telencephalon** and **diencephalon.** The rhombencephalon subdivides to form the **metencephalon** and **myelencephalon.** These regions, in turn, give rise to the cortical and subcortical structures of the brain. The five subdivisions, in combination with the ventricular system and spinal cord, constitute the seven major divisions of the CNS. Figure 5.2 presents the regional development of the brain.

LOBULAR AND CONVOLUTIONAL DEVELOPMENT

As the cerebral cortex moves forward in development, it first expands anteriorly to form the frontal lobes, then dorsally to form the parietal lobes, and finally, posteriorly and inferiorly to form the temporal and occipital lobes. The posterior and inferior expansion pushes the cortex into a C-shape. As a result, this C form also shapes many of the underlying structures, including the lateral ventricles, the head of the caudate of the basal ganglia, the hippocampus and fornix, and the cingulate and parahippocampal gyri (Martin & Jessell, 1991).

In the initial stages of prenatal development, the brain surface is smooth, lacking both **gyri** and **sulci.** The gyri and sulci patterns of the cortex form after neuronal migration, and they reflect the processes of neuronal specialization, dendritic arborization, synaptic formation, and pruning.

The major sulci dividing the cerebral lobes appear first, whereas the gyri within the individual lobes emerge later. At approximately 14 weeks gestation, the longitudinal fissure dividing the two cerebral hemispheres and the **Sylvian (lateral) fissure** demarcating the border of the parietal and frontal lobes are visible. Gyrification continues in

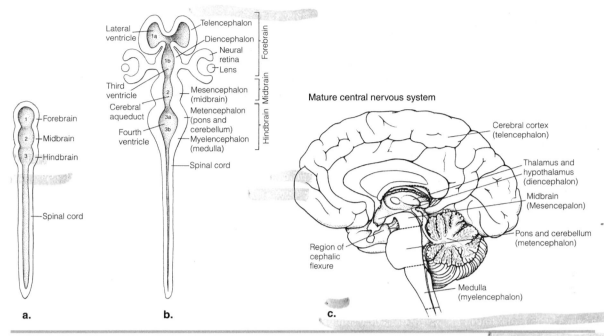

Figure 5.2 Regional development of the brain. (a) Three-vesicle stage of the neural tube in early development of the brain and spinal cord. (b) Five-vesicle stage of the brain and spinal cord at a later stage of development. (c) The regions of the mature central nervous system (spinal cord not shown). (From Martin, J. H., & Jessell, T. M. [1991]. Development as a guide to the regional anatomy of the brain. In E. R. Kandel, J. H. Schwartz, & T. M. Jessell [Eds.], *Principles of neural science* [5th ed., pp. 298–299, Figures 21-2a.b and 21-3c]. New York: Elsevier Science, by permission of the McGraw-Hill Companies.)

an orderly and symmetric fashion through gestation, and by birth, the gyral patterns of the adult are present (Hynd & Hiemenz, 1997). Table 5.1 details this progression.

The formation of the gyri signals that intracortical connections are established. Although the gyri and sulci pat-

terns of each person differ slightly, unusual or extreme alterations suggest deviations in cortical connections and potential cognitive and behavioral deficits (Hynd & Hiemenz, 1997). For example, an insult to the brain (such as intrauterine infection) during the fifth and sixth month of gestation can produce **polymicrogyria,** a condition characterized by the development of small, densely packed gyri. This anomaly is associated with learning disabilities, mental retardation, and epilepsy (Hynd et al., 1997).

VENTRICULAR AND SPINAL CORD DEVELOPMENT

As the CNS matures, the cavities within the cerebral vesicles of the neural tube subsequently form the ventricular system and the central canal of the spinal cord. The cavities of cerebral vesicles differentiate into (1) the two lateral ventricles, formerly called the first and second ventricles of the forebrain; (2) the narrow cerebral aqueduct, or aqueduct of Sylvius, of the midbrain; and (3) the fourth ventricle of the hindbrain (Martin & Jessell, 1991). The transformation of the ventricles into their characteristic C-shape begins at approximately 3 months. **Cerebrospinal fluid (CSF)** is produced in the ventricles,

Table 5.1 *Embryonic Development of the Cortical Gyri in Humans*

Gestational Age (weeks)	Gyrus
16–19	Gyrus rectus, insula, cingulate
20–23	Parahippocampal, superior temporal
24–27	Prerolandic and postrolandic, middle temporal, superior and middle frontal, occipital
28–31	Inferior and transverse temporal, medial and lateral orbital, angular, supramarginal
32–35	Paracentral
36–39	Anterior and posterior orbital

Source: Adapted from Benes, F. M. (1997). Corticolimbic circuitry and the development of psychopathology during childhood and adolescence. In N. A. Krasnegor, G. R. Lyon, & P. S. Goldman-Rakic (Eds.), *Development of the prefrontal cortex: Evolution, neurobiology, and behavior* (pp. 211–240). Baltimore: Paul H. Brookes, by permission.

cushions the brain and spinal cord within the skull and **vertebral column,** and removes waste products from the brain.

The spinal cord does not divide; rather, it segments during development. These units correspond to the cervical, thoracic, lumbar, sacral, and coccygeal levels of the mature spinal cord. Throughout early prenatal development, the spinal cord grows at the same rate as the vertebral column and occupies the entire length of the vertebral canal (space within the vertebral column). Later in development, the growth of the vertebral column exceeds that of the spinal cord. At birth, the caudal end of the spinal cord extends only to the lumbar vertebra (Martin, 1996).

POSTNATAL DEVELOPMENT

During the last 3 months of prenatal life and the first 2 years of postnatal development, the brain changes rapidly. At birth, a baby's brain is one-fourth the weight of its final adult weight of approximately 1300 to 1500 grams (Majovski, 1997). By age 2, the brain has achieved three fourths of its eventual adult weight and the cortical surface area of the hemispheres has doubled. During this rapid growth period, significant synaptic and dendritic interconnections form, and pruning and myelination are occurring. Other maturational processes are also evident during this period, including increases in neurotransmitters and related biochemical agents and changes in electroencephalographic wave patterns.

Positron emission tomography (PET) studies of infants are providing insights into the early postnatal development of the brain. Glucose is a primary energy source of the brain, and the rate at which glucose is used (metabolized) in various brain regions provides a measure of the activation of these regions. PET imaging can capture the glucose metabolism of brain structures. Moreover, the pattern of glucose metabolism of brain regions correlates with the behavioral, neurophysiologic, and neuroanatomic maturation of the brain (Chugani, Muller, & Chugani, 1996). In the newborn (5 weeks), four brain regions show the highest rate of glucose utilization. These areas include the sensorimotor cortex, thalamus, brainstem, and cerebellum. In contrast, glucose utilization is generally at low levels in other regions of the cortex and basal ganglia. This pattern of regional utilization indicates that the phylogenetically older brain structures (primarily subcortical) are rapidly developing, consistent with the reflexive and limited behavioral repertoire of the newborn. Cortical functions are at a rudimentary level and are limited to the primary sensory and motor areas. As the infant begins to demonstrate more coordinated visuomotor movements during the second to third month, increases in glucose metabolism are evident in the parietal, temporal, primary visual cortical regions, basal ganglia, and cerebellum. Primitive neural reflexes become less prominent as subcortical and cortical regions integrate. Between 6 and 8 months, the frontal and association cortices increase in activation. This increase correlates with the emergence of more advanced cognitive behaviors. For example, by the eighth month, the infant is able to perform the delayed response task, a rudimentary measure of working memory (see Chapter 9). Continued changes in regional metabolism and associated behavioral maturation are evident through childhood.

Total brain volume does not significantly increase after 5 years of age. This stability of total brain volume belies the progressive and regressive growth of white and gray matter; that is, white matter volume increases are offset by decreases in gray matter volume. White matter increases are evident throughout childhood into adulthood, although the growth varies across and within different brain regions. Cortical and subcortical gray matter initially increases, with peak volumes being achieved at different temporal points. For example, the peak in gray matter volume for the parietal lobes is between 10 and 11 years of age, the temporal lobes by 16 years of age, and the frontal lobes by 11 to 12 years of age (Casey, Giedd, & Thomas, 2000; Giedd, 2004). Progressive loss of gray matter occurs after these peaks. This loss of gray matter volume reflects the developmental processes of pruning and cell death of neurons and glial cells. Among the last maturing cortical regions, as evidenced in achievement of adult gray-to-white matter volumes, is the dorsolateral prefrontal cortex. The relatively late maturation of the dorsolateral prefrontal cortex is consistent with the protracted development of higher order or "executive" cognitive, emotional, and social processes and functions. The increase in white matter significantly enhances the speed of neural transmission, whereas the reduction in gray matter represents a form of neural "streamlining" to support complex and efficient processing. Developmentally, the maturation of gray and white matter parallels the emergences of ever increasing cognitive, affective, and social behaviors. That is, brain regions associated with primary sensory and motor functions mature first, followed by regions supportive of higher order integrative (e.g., association brain areas) and executive functions (Gogtay et al., 2004).

This discussion of the anatomic development of the brain completes our first step. We now examine the organization and function of the nervous system.

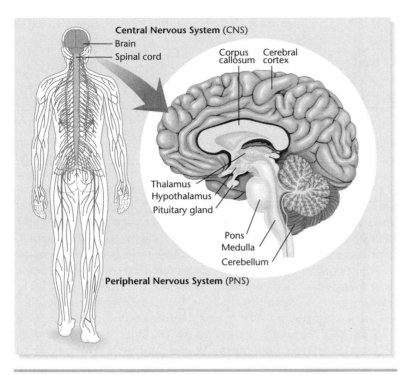

Figure 5.3 Human nervous system. (From Kalat, J. W. [2007]. *Biological psychology* [9th ed., p. 82, Figure 4.1]. Belmont, CA: Thomson Wadsworth.)

Organization of the Nervous System

The nervous system is customarily divided into two parts: the PNS and the CNS (Figure 5.3 and Table 5.2). This division stems from the different properties and functions of neurons and systems within the two systems. Chapter 4 discusses neuronal differences, specifically the special properties of neurons within the CNS; this chapter discusses functional differences. The PNS includes all the portions of the nervous system outside the CNS. The PNS consists of the **somatic nervous system (SNS),** which interacts with the external environment, and the **autonomic nervous system (ANS),** which participates in regulating the body's internal environment. The ANS has two divisions: the **sympathetic** and **parasympathetic nervous systems.** The PNS and the CNS are in constant communication with each other.

The CNS includes the **brain** and **spinal cord.** It communicates with the PNS by exchanging sensory and motor information via the spinal nerves and cranial nerves. You can imagine the spinal cord as a cable carry-ing bundles of spinal nerves from the body up to higher processing areas in the brain. It serves as the CNS conduit of the majority of sensory and motor information to and from the body. The **cranial nerves** also carry very specific sensory and motor information directly to the brain, bypassing the spinal cord.

Table 5.2	*Principal Divisions of the Nervous System*

1. Central nervous system (CNS)
   Brain
   Spinal cord

2. Peripheral nervous system (PNS)
   Somatic nervous system
      Cranial nerves
      Spinal nerves

   Autonomic nervous system (ANS)
      Sympathetic
      Parasympathetic

Peripheral Nervous System

In principle, all components of the PNS inform the CNS about events in the environment and transmit commands from the CNS to the body. The somatic nervous system consists of **afferent nerves** or sensory nerves that convey messages from the sense organs to the CNS (incoming) and **efferent nerves** that carry motor signals from the CNS to muscles (outgoing). Most nerves of the somatic nervous system project at regular intervals to the spinal cord via the spinal nerves, except for 12 pairs of cranial nerves, which synapse directly with the brain.

The function of the ANS is the neural control of internal organs (e.g., heart and intestines). The ANS consists of both peripheral and central parts and includes a sympathetic division that is involved in activities that expend bodily energy. This expenditure most often occurs in response to, or anticipation of, a stressful event. A simplified summary of the role of sympathetic activation is that it prepares the body for action based on the "fight-or-flight" principle. Sympathetic activity mobilizes the energy necessary for psychological arousal. It includes an increase in blood flow, blood pressure, heart rate, and sweating, and a decrease in digestion and sexual arousal.

The parasympathetic division of the ANS acts to conserve energy and is typically associated with relaxation. It increases the body's supply of stored energy and facilitates digestion and gastric and intestinal motility. Most autonomic organs receive both sympathetic and parasympathetic input and are influenced by the relative level of sympathetic and parasympathetic activity. For many bodily functions, the sympathetic and parasympathetic divisions act in opposite directions. You can think of the two branches of the ANS as balancing each other, like two sides of a scale. People generally consider the functions of the ANS automatic, not under voluntary control. The view that the response of the ANS to stress is not under voluntary control provided the basis for the development of the lie detector test. However, biofeedback, meditation, hypnosis, and other forms of stress management have shown that these functions are not as "automatic" as once thought, although some controversy has focused on the degree to which humans can control them (Zillmer & Wickramaserkera, 1987).

Although it is useful to divide the nervous system as outlined above, real functional anatomic circuits and systems pay little heed to these boundaries. For example, many nerve cells described as part of the PNS have their cells of origin or terminal branches actually situated in the CNS. Consider the divisions within the nervous system as somewhat flexible; they follow the organizational need to separate complex phenomena into discrete and less complex units.

Central Nervous System

The brain and spinal cord form a continuous communication system of the CNS. The CNS has several unique features. First, as discussed earlier, CNS neurons have some properties that differ from PNS neurons in that, for example, they do not show similar properties of regeneration. Second, you can recognize the importance of the CNS by the extra protection the body provides it. Structurally, it is located within the bony cavities of the skull and spine. Coverings called the **meninges** protect it, and it is surrounded by and floats in the protective CSF. The CNS, and especially the brain, is the most well-nourished area of the body, being supplied with an intricate system of arteries designed with "backup" systems. The body gives it priority in receiving nutrients and oxygen, and at the same time, gives it more protection, through the blood–brain barrier, from potentially harmful substances circulating in the body.

BRAIN

Anatomically, the brain is continuous with the spinal cord, from which it emerges. From an exterior view, the brain appears to be one organ with a left and a right hemisphere. It actually consists of several divisions with many identifiable structures.

How the brain is organized into subsystems that ultimately result in human behavior is a challenging question, one on which the rest of this text focuses. Consider that the brain occupies a relatively small space of about 1000 to 1500 cm^3, roughly the size of a cantaloupe. Within this space functions an incredible array of different types of cells. There is also an almost infinite number of possible connections that make up exceedingly complex networks. From this complexity a sense of order and organization emerges that supports basic life, behavior, and consciousness. The human brain represents the most advanced stage of this integration.

Anatomic Terms of Relationship

Because the brain is a three-dimensional structure, neuropsychologists use a number of terms that describe specific parts, planes, and directions. Unfortunately, the terminology is complex and not entirely standardized. This is related, in part, to the fact that we still use nomenclature proposed in Latin or Greek more than a century ago. In some instances, anatomists disagree about the boundaries of a specific brain structure; thus, several terms may describe overlapping brain regions. Early anatomists used names to describe structures simply because they reminded them of something else. For example, the outer part of the brain was named *cortex,* meaning "bark," because it is a thin mantle or covering for the brain. Thus, whenever we use the original meaning of the names of brain structures to help the reader form association about the nomenclature, we also provide precise anatomic terms to clear up any resulting confusion. Additionally, these precise anatomic terms will enable the reader to accurately communicate about the geography and topology of the brain.

Descriptions usually divide the brain into one of the three main planes (using the *x-*, *y-*, and *z-*axes). Table 5.3 lists terms that describe the planes and orientation of brain anatomy.

SPINAL CORD

Overview

■ *Gross anatomic features:* spinal nerves, internal organization of the spinal cord (gray and white matter)

■ *Function:* relays information to and from the brain, responsible for simple reflexive behavior

Structure

The spinal cord is continuous with the brain and extends downward along the back for about 46 cm. Like the brain, it is protected by bone, meninges, and CSF. The spinal cord is physically housed in the spinal column, which consists of alternating bony vertebrae and intervertebral disks made up of cartilage that absorb mechanical shocks sustained to the spinal column. The spinal cord itself is considerably smaller than the vertebral canal and the meninges. Fat, CSF, and veins combine to protect against contact with bony surroundings.

The spinal nerves consist of both sensory and motor neurons. At each of the 30 levels of the spinal cord, a pair of incoming (afferent) dorsal root fibers signals incoming sensory information and a pair of outgoing (efferent) ventral root fibers controls motor nerves and muscles (Figure 5.4). These nerves conduct information related to both the somatic and autonomic nervous systems in the periphery. In the spinal cord, white matter (myelinated axons) makes up the outside of the cord, whereas gray matter (cell bodies) is located on the interior. Each area of the spinal cord corresponds to a specific body location and controls sensation

Table 5.3	*Planes of the Brain and Directions of Orientation to the Central Nervous System*

Planes bisecting the brain:

Horizontal plane—plane (*x*-axis) that shows the brain as seen from above or parallel to the ground.

Coronal plane—plane (*y*-axis) that shows the brain as seen from the front (frontal section). Typically, this plane is viewed from behind to provide consistency for right and left directions of the brain and the picture.

Sagittal plane—plane (*z*-axis) that shows the brain as seen from the side or perpendicular to the ground, bisecting the brain into right and left halves (derived from Latin *sagitta,* meaning "arrow").

Directional terms: Most often, directions in the human nervous system are related to the orientation of the spinal cord.

Anterior: toward the front or front end

Posterior: toward the back or tail

Inferior: toward the bottom, or below

Superior: toward the top or above

Medial: toward the middle/midline, away from the side

Lateral: toward the side, away from the midline

Rostral: toward the head

Caudal: toward the rear away from the head

Proximal: near the trunk or center, close to the origin of attachment

Distal: away from the center, toward the periphery, away from the origin of attachment

Dorsal: toward the back; the top of the brain is dorsal in humans

Ventral: toward the belly; the bottom of the brain is ventral in humans

Ipsilateral: on the same side

Contralateral: on the opposite side

and movement of the associated body area: skin, muscle, and internal organs. There are 1 coccyx, 5 sacral (S), 5 lumbar (L), 12 thoracic (T), and 8 cervical (C) spinal cord levels. The spinal nerves form ringlike innervations around the trunk of the body at each level of the spinal cord. The innervations of the limbs are extensions of the body rings. For example, the nerves to the arms and hands are extensions of C-6, C-7, and C-8 innervations from the trunk.

Function

The spinal cord relays somatosensory information from the trunk and limbs to the brain. The cord also relays simple motor messages from the brain to the trunk and limbs.

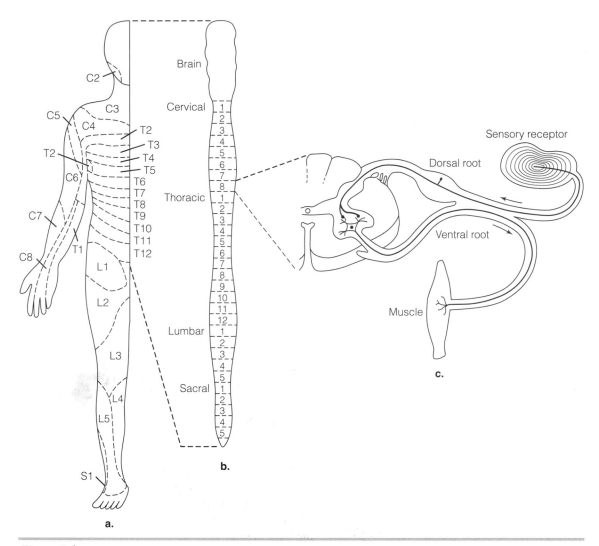

Figure 5.4   Spinal nerves and areas of body innervation. (a) The body segments of spinal innervation are segmented in rings around the body. (b) The divisions of the 30 segments of the spinal cord. (c) Cross section through a segment of the spinal cord showing sensory input through the dorsal root and motor output through the ventral root. (Adapted from Kolb, B., & Wishaw, I. Q. [1996]. *Fundamentals of human neuropsychology* [4th ed., p. 46, Figure 3.3]. New York: W. H. Freeman and Company, by permission of Worth Publishers.)

It does some integration of information that involves basic reflexive behavior. Spinal cord lesions can result in motor and sensory impairment. Although neuropsychologist often place greater emphasis in their evaluations on whether sensory or motor impairments relate to brain lesions, similar symptoms may also reflect spinal cord or even peripheral nerve damage. A thorough neurologic evaluation in combination with a comprehensive neuropsychological evaluation often clarifies the location of the dysfunction. Spinal cord injuries frequently occur with brain injury caused by whiplash, which may go unnoticed until after the trauma of paralysis has been stabilized.

Gross Anatomy: Protection and Sustenance of the Brain

The body affords extra protection and sustenance to the CNS because of its special status. The structural and physiologic protections extend to the spinal cord and the brain, although the focus is on the brain. Structurally, bone provides a type of "armor" to surround both the brain and spinal cord. In most cases, the skull holds the brain snugly and physically protects it from injury. However, as in closed head injury (see Chapter 13), the gelatinous brain may accelerate and scrape against the bony projections of the skull. It is important to understand the skull–brain relationship to understand how the brain may be vulnerable to skull-related damage. Under the hard protection of bone, protective membranes called *meninges* form a flexible structural but semipermeable protective pad that completely surrounds the brain and spinal cord. The covering of the meninges forms another layer of protection. However, certain types of tumors called **meningiomas** may form here and impact on the brain. The CSF circulates around and throughout the CNS via the **ventricular system,** which provides not only an additional structural fluid cushion but also physiologic protection through its immunologic functions and its ability to act as a "waste disposal" system. The unique **vascular system** of the brain not only supplies nutrients to the energy-demanding brain but also adds a layer of protection through the blood–brain barrier. The blood–brain barrier (see discussion in Chapter 4) is formed by tightly formed endothelial cells in the walls of the capillaries of the brain, held in place by astrocytes that prevent the passage of certain substances into the brain.

SKULL

Overview

■ *Gross anatomic features:* fused connection of bony plates covering the brain

■ *Function:* protection of the brain

Structure

The skull consists of the frontal bone (in some individuals, the frontal bone develops in two parts), two parietal bones, two temporal bones, the occipital bone, and the sphenoid bone (Figure 5.5). The cerebral lobes derive their names from the cranial plates of the skull, whose corresponding outline they generally follow. This has led to an imprecise nomenclature of the cortex because the external aspects of the skull are easily differentiated, unlike those of the cortical lobes. The skull provides grooves for blood vessels in the roof (calvaria) of the cranium, conspicuous ridges in the base of the skull, known as **fossae,** that hold the brain in place, and more or less symmetric orifices or **foramina** in the base of the skull that provide passage for nerves and blood vessels. The largest of these orifices is the **foramen magnum,** which provides a large median opening in the occipital bone for the spinal cord to pass through to the brainstem.

In the newborn, the skull is a relatively large part of its body, accommodating the disproportionally large brain.

At birth, the brain is approximately 25% of its adult size, weighing about 500 grams, but will reach about 75% of its mature size by its first year of maturation. Facilitating this rapid development of the brain, the bony plates that comprise the skull are not fused as they are in later years, but are separated by membranous, soft tissue. In the newborn, the membranous gaps are largest at the corners of the parietal bone. These soft openings are labeled **fontanelles** ("small fountains") and may fluctuate with changes in intracranial pressure. The largest of these openings is the anterior fontanelle, located at the top of the head between the frontal and parietal bones. It does not fully close until 2 years after birth.

Function

The skull completely encases the brain, protecting it from external influences. Although normally the shell of the skull is an asset, in some instances, it can actually be a liability. The fact that the skull is rigid can become life threatening when the internal pressure of a swelling, injured brain cannot be released. Because the skull is not smooth on the interior, but rather consists of bony projections designed to hold the brain in place, injury to the areas around the bony projections of the frontal and temporal lobes is common with whiplash and other head injuries, which cause the gelatinous brain to reverberate in the skull. The skull varies in thickness; particularly, the areas around the temporal and sphenoid bones are relatively thin and are easily fractured by a blow to the side of the head. Fractures to the base of the skull can lead to serious damage of the brain related to shearing of the cranial nerves, leakage of the CSF from the nose, and bleeding from the auditory canal.

MENINGES

Overview

■ *Gross anatomic features:* dura mater, arachnoid membrane, pia mater

■ *Function:* protective covering of the CNS, location of venous drainage and CSF absorption

Structure

The brain and spinal cord are the only human structures completely enclosed in protective bone. In addition, they are covered by the meninges, a set of thin membranes that hold the brain and spinal cord in place and act as a protective buffer. The meninges of the CNS consist of three meningeal membranes and completely surround the brain and the spinal cord. Inner to outer they can be remembered

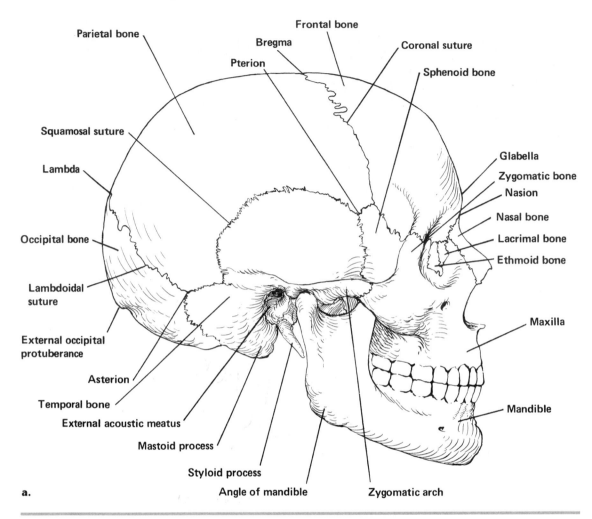

Frontal bone
Parietal bone
Bregma
Pterion
Coronal suture
Sphenoid bone
Squamosal suture
Glabella
Zygomatic bone
Nasion
Lambda
Nasal bone
Lacrimal bone
Occipital bone
Ethmoid bone
Lambdoidal suture
Maxilla
External occipital protuberance
Asterion
Temporal bone
Mandible
External acoustic meatus
Mastoid process
Styloid process
Angle of mandible
Zygomatic arch

a.

Figure 5.5 Lateral (a) and basal (b) views of the skull. (From Chusid, J. G. [1982]. *Correlative neuroanatomy & functional neurology* [p. 256, Figure 19.3; p. 257, Figure 19.4]. New York: Appleton & Lange, by permission of the McGraw-Hill Companies.)

with the mnemonic PAD: pia mater, arachnoid membrane, and dura mater (or simply dura) (Figure 5.6). The thin **pia mater** (derived from Latin meaning "pious mother") directly adheres to the surface of the CNS, following its contours closely. The **arachnoid membrane** (spider web–like membrane) overlies the **subarachnoid space,** which contains CSF. The **dura mater** (derived from Latin meaning "tough mother") is a dense, inelastic, double-layered membrane that adheres to the inner surface of the skull. The meningeal veins are in the outer portion of the dura. The space between the two dural layers is the **epidural space.** The space between the dura and the arachnoid is the **subdural space.** Cerebral veins crossing the subdural space have little supporting structure

and, therefore, are most vulnerable to injury and bleeding as a result of trauma (e.g., **subdural hematoma**).

Function

The meninges provide a protective covering by encasing the brain and spinal cord. They have no function in cognitive activity, but are of importance to neuropsychologists because of clinical complications during injury. For example, a head trauma frequently tears large blood vessels in the subarachnoid space. In addition, the meninges are susceptible to inflammation, usually by bacterial infection, resulting in **meningitis.** Meningitis can be caused by both bacteria and viral infection. The disease is dangerous because it can progress quickly, within 24 hours,

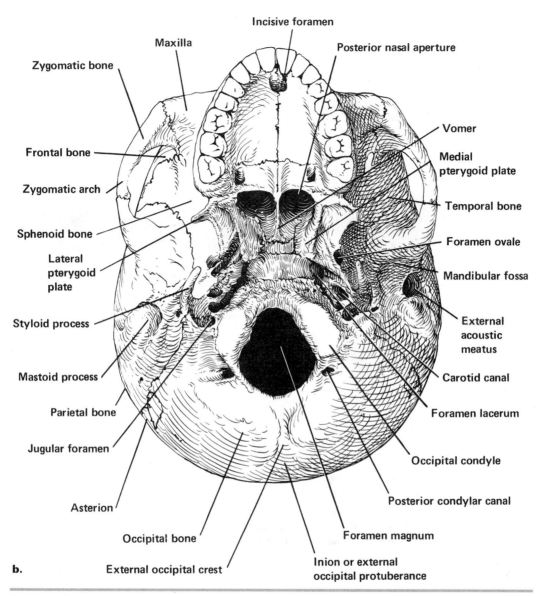

Zygomatic bone

Maxilla

Incisive foramen

Posterior nasal aperture

Frontal bone

Zygomatic arch

Sphenoid bone

Lateral pterygoid plate

Styloid process

Mastoid process

Parietal bone

Jugular foramen

Asterion

Occipital bone

External occipital crest

Inion or external occipital protuberance

Foramen magnum

Posterior condylar canal

Occipital condyle

Foramen lacerum

Carotid canal

External acoustic meatus

Mandibular fossa

Foramen ovale

Temporal bone

Medial pterygoid plate

Vomer

b.

Figure 5.5 *(continued)*

from a respiratory illness with fever, headache, and a stiff neck to changes in consciousness, including stupor, coma, and death.

VENTRICULAR SYSTEM

Overview

- *Gross anatomic features:* lateral (first and second), third, and fourth ventricles; choroid plexus; cerebral aqueduct; arachnoid granulations

- *Function:* intracranial pressure, CSF production and circulation

Structure

Within the brain are four interconnected, fluid-filled cavities known as the **ventricles** (Figure 5.7). There are two lateral ventricles, one in each hemisphere, the third ventricle, and the fourth ventricle. The lateral ventricles are the largest and are seen easily in many types of brain imaging, because they occupy what appears to be a large hollow in each hemisphere. They are connected by a small opening, the **interventricular foramen** or **foramen of Monro,** to the third ventricle, which is situated between the two lateral ventricles at the level of the thalamus and the hypothalamus. The third ventricle has a single opening that leads downward through a narrow channel known as the

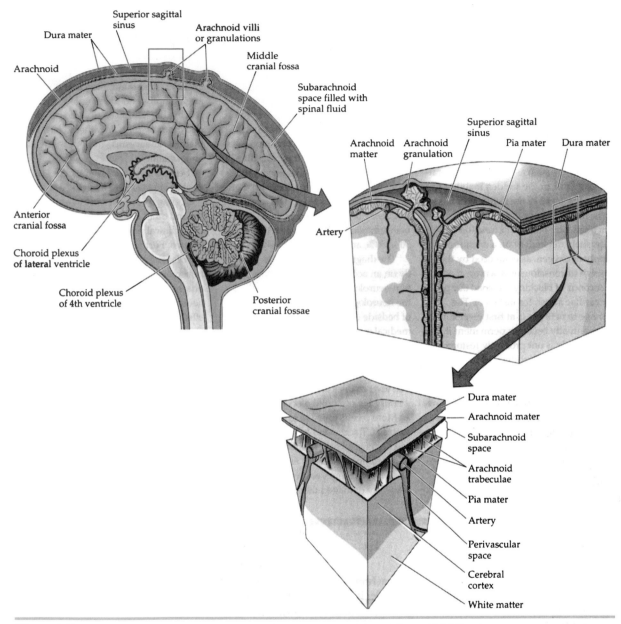

Figure 5.6 The meninges. (top left) Midsagittal view of the three layers of the meninges. (right) Panels are enlarged to show the details of the meninges. (From Purves, D., Augustine, G. J., Fitzpatrick, D., Katz, L. C., LaMantia, A., McNamara, J. O., & William, S. M. [Eds.]. [2001]. *Neuroscience* [2nd ed., p. 34, Figure 1.18]. Sunderland, MA: Sinauer Associates, by permission.)

cerebral aqueduct (or **aqueduct of Sylvius**), connecting it to the fourth ventricle. The cerebral aqueduct passes through the midbrain and expands into the fourth ventricle, which lies in the brainstem, just beneath, and anterior to, the cerebellum. Early anatomists such as Leonardo da Vinci were fascinated by the ventricles, which were believed to contain the spirit (Figure 5.8).

Within these ventricles the **choroid plexus** tissue secretes CSF, which flows from the upper to the lower ventricles. The choroid plexus is a highly vascularized network of small blood vessels that protrude into the ventricles from the lining of the pia mater. It continually produces CSF. The CSF circulates through the ventricles and around the spinal cord and brain. In humans, approximately 450 ml

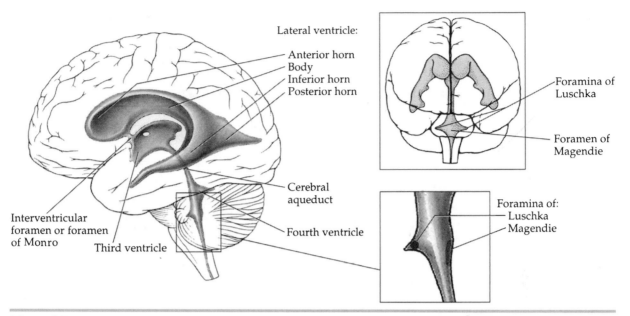

Figure 5.7 Ventricular system (lateral view, left panel). (right) Panels show the locations of the foramina of Luschka and Magendie in the fourth ventricle viewed from the ventral (top) and lateral surfaces (bottom). (From J. H. Martin, *Neuroanatomy: Text and Atlas,* 2nd ed., 1996, p. 19, Figure 1.10. Reproduced by permission of the McGraw-Hill Companies.)

CSF (somewhat more than a 12-ounce soft drink can) is produced every day, mostly by the choroid plexus in the lateral ventricles. Then, after flowing through the interventricular foramen of Monro, CSF volume is increased by fluid produced in the third ventricle.

The fourth ventricle has three openings in its membranous roof, the **foramen of Magendie** and two lateral **foramina of Luschka,** that allow the CSF to flow outside the brain and recirculate. The cycle is completed via the continuous reabsorption of CSF from the subarachnoid space between the arachnoid and the pia mater. From the expansions of the subarachnoid space called **cisterns,** most of the CSF moves upward along pressure gradients to a large sinus called the **superior sagittal sinus** and is reabsorbed into the blood system into larger blood-filled spaces. Within the subarachnoid space are also small pockets of veins, termed **arachnoid villi** or **granulations** (see Figure 5.6). These cauliflower-like projections serve as pathways for the CSF to be absorbed and re-enter the venous circulation. The fluid recirculates every 6 to 7 hours.

The ventricular system not only boasts some of the most exotic terms of the brain but is also important to any study of brain anatomy. The reason for this is that the brain shapes the ventricular system; thus, any changes in the anatomy of the brain can distort the ventricular system. The location of the fourth ventricle, for example, near the cerebellum, is important for neuroradiology.

When neuroradiologists view two-dimensional pictures of the brain, locating any of the four ventricles helps precisely locate the brain image, because the structure of the surrounding brain defines the ventricles. If brain tissue is distorted, ventricle size and shape are usually distorted.

Function

The ventricles and the CSF are involved in two principal processes. First, CSF protects the brain and the spinal cord by acting as a buffer. The ventricles of the brain, the central canal of the spinal cord, and the subarachnoid spaces all contain CSF with a normal intracranial pressure of 0 to 15 torr (1 torr = pressure necessary to support a column of mercury 1 mm high). The CSF thus floats the CNS like a buoy and protects the brain by acting as a liquid buffer or cushion to absorb internal and external forces. This is easily appreciated in patients who had some of their CSF drained as part of the now outdated X-ray diagnostic procedure known as *pneumoencephalography* (see Chapter 2). These patients experienced severe headaches and stabbing pain with any head movement because of injected air and less support to the brain.

The second function of CSF is in disposing of waste products from the brain, which are thus absorbed via cisterns into the venous vascular system. Chapter 1 notes that medieval scientists attributed significant mental and spiritual processes to the presence of CSF within the ventricular

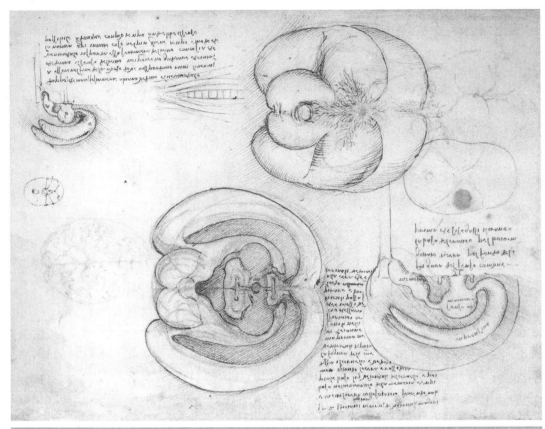

Figure 5.8 Although many of Leonardo da Vinci's (1452–1519) early brain anatomy drawings were inaccurate, he later became a keen observer of neuroanatomy. For this drawing, which presented an anatomic breakthrough, he poured melted wax into the ventricles of an ox, then cut away the brain tissues to determine the true shape of the ventricles. (The Royal Collection © 2007, Her Majesty Queen Elizabeth II.)

chambers of the brain. This theory became known as the ventricular localization hypothesis and later formed the basis for the cell doctrine. On gross dissection of the brain, the lateral ventricles are the most striking features; thus, this theory, although wrong, persisted robustly.

The ventricles have no direct role in cognitive function. However, abnormal intracranial ventricular pressure (>15 torr) may lead to general cognitive deficits. A sequence of events can occur in which the ventricles become enlarged with fluid, occupying greater space than usual. This results in brain swelling and an increase in intracranial pressure. The squeezing or displacing of brain tissue, in turn, leads to changes in behavior and cognition. This expansion of the ventricles accompanied by increased intracranial pressure results in a medical condition called **hydrocephalus,** which may be caused by an imbalance in the rate of CSF production or absorption, or by blockage (such as by a tumor) of the circulation. The skull itself

may actually swell. If hydrocephalus occurs in childhood before the cranial bones have closed, the skull may enlarge to enormous size (Figure 5.9). Acute hydrocephalus can be life threatening. Because the fused plates of the skull cannot accommodate the additional space, untreated hydrocephalus among adults and older children results in chronic dilation of the ventricles and a thinning of the cortex. A variant of hydrocephalus in adulthood, particularly the elderly, is **normal-pressure hydrocephalus (NPH),** characterized by the presence of normal levels of intracranial CSF. The term may actually be a misnomer insofar as research (Vanneste, 2000) suggests that there appears to be an initial stage of increased CSF pressure with a subsequent enlargement of the ventricles. As the ventricles expand, the CSF pressure returns to upper normal to normal levels. However, there may be further transient episodes of increased intraventricular pressure. It is believed that the mechanism of action that produces the

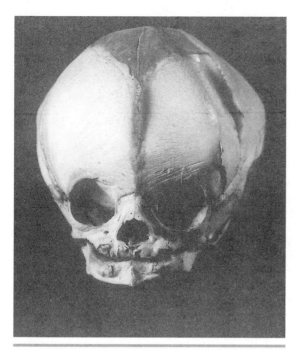

Figure 5.9 Skull of a child with severe hydrocephalus. Note the enlarged fontanelle. (Mütter Museum, College of Physicians of Philadelphia.)

expansion of the ventricles is a reduction in CSF absorption at the arachnoid villi (see Figure 5.6), resulting in an abnormal increase in intracranial CSF pressure. However, the validity of this mechanism of action has been challenged, and alternative mechanisms have been proposed (Vanneste, 2000). Events that often precede the development of NPH include subarachnoid hemorrhage, meningitis, and head injury, although the cause in other cases is frequently unknown. Regardless of the originating cause, a triad of progressive neuropsychological signs alerts the clinician to possible NPH (Verrees & Selman, 2004). Walking difficulties and postural imbalance is usually the first sign of the disorder. Later, dementia and urinary incontinence develop. With treatment, particularly early treatment, these symptoms can be reversed or reduced.

Because the subarachnoid space extends down toward a small central channel that runs the length of the spinal cord, it is possible to collect a small sample of CSF at the level of the lower back by tapping into the subarachnoid cisterns of the lower lumbar vertebrae. This can be done without damaging the integrity of the spinal cord using an invasive diagnostic procedure known as a lumbar puncture or "spinal tap" (see Chapter 2). The CSF sample can then be examined under the microscope for the abnormal presence of blood, infection, or cancerous cells.

VASCULAR SYSTEM

Overview

- *Gross anatomic features:* arteries (Table 5.4), veins, circle of Willis
- *Function:*
  Arteries: nourishment: supply of oxygen, nutrients
  Veins: carrying away of waste products

To function properly, the brain must receive adequate oxygen and many nutrients (such as glucose) from the blood vessels. If a blood vessel is obstructed or bursts, the brain cells supplied by that vessel cannot function properly and begin to die. When brain cells do not function, neither do the parts of the body controlled by those neurons or other related parts of the brain to which the damaged neurons project (targets). Becoming familiar with the blood supply of the brain can make important vascular disorders such as stroke more understandable.

Arteries That Supply the Brain

All major cerebral arteries and the meninges are supplied by four large arteries to the brain. They are the right and left **internal carotid arteries,** as well as the two **vertebral arteries** (Figure 5.10 and Table 5.4). These vessels originate directly or indirectly from branches of the **aortic arch,** which arises from the left ventricle of the heart. The internal carotid arteries supply the anterior portions of the brain, and the vertebral arteries supply the posterior portion.

The two vertebral arteries join together at the level of the brainstem to form the **basilar artery.** The basilar artery divides into the left and right **posterior cerebral arteries.** This vertebrobasilar system provides approximately 20% of the total cerebral blood circulation mostly to the posterior portions of the brain, and a corresponding 20% of all **cerebrovascular accidents (CVAs),** or strokes, are restricted to this territory.

Circle of Willis

The cross-brain connections from both the internal carotid and basilar systems form a remarkable vascular structure near the base of the brain, the **circle of Willis** (Figure 5.11), named after its discoverer, English anatomist and physician Thomas Willis (1621–1675). The circle is formed by the anterior cerebral branches of the internal carotid artery and its connections, the anterior communicating artery, the posterior communicating artery, and the posterior cerebral branches of the basilar artery. The circle of Willis is the most important intracranial

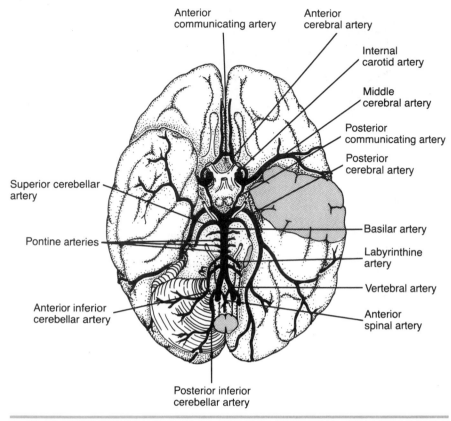

Figure 5.10   Major arteries to the brain. The cerebral arteries are seen from the base of the brain. The left half of the cerebellum and the tip of the left temporal lobe have been removed. (From Burt, A. M. [1993]. *Textbook of neuroanatomy* [p. 179, Figure 9.8]. Philadelphia: W.B. Saunders.)

collateral blood supply, and it allows a certain degree of redundancy among blood vessels and blood supply to the various areas of the brain.

CEREBRAL ARTERIES

The internal carotid artery on each side of the body divides into the **anterior cerebral artery** (which supplies the anterior paramedian cerebral hemisphere) and the larger **middle cerebral artery** (which supplies the lateral hemisphere and most of the basal ganglia). Figure 5.12 shows the areas of the brain served by each of the three cerebral arteries. The left and right anterior cerebral arteries are connected by the **anterior communicating artery.** The **posterior communicating arteries** arise from the internal carotid arteries and connect the middle and posterior cerebral arteries. The major cerebral arteries have multiple cortical branches (these branches are not discussed in

detail here). Disrupting blood supply to any of the cerebral arteries or its branches may cause relative uniform and characteristic symptoms related to each brain area served by the artery. Of the major arteries that supply the brain, blockage of the carotid arteries most often results in a stroke affecting the middle cerebral artery. The anterior cerebral artery is not as commonly involved in stroke because the anterior communicating artery can supply blood.

In the normally functioning brain, there is little arterial crossover from one hemisphere of the brain to the other, or between anterior and posterior arteries. In the event of a stroke to a major artery, other intact blood vessels can take over for injured blood vessels. For example, if the basilar artery is occluded, shutting off blood supply to the posterior communicating artery, the internal carotid arteries may provide blood to posterior circulation via the posterior communicating artery. However, there is

Table 5.4 *Arteries to the Brain*

Artery	Origin	Distribution
Basilar	Junction of right and left vertebral arteries	Brainstem, internal ear, cerebellum, posterior cerebrum
Carotid, common	Brachiocephalic (right), aorta (left)	Internal and external carotid
Carotid, external	Common carotid artery	Neck, face, skull
Carotid, internal	Common carotid artery	Middle ear, brain, choroid plexus of lateral ventricles
Cerebellar, inferior anterior	Basilar artery	Lower anterior cerebellum, inner ear
Cerebellar, inferior posterior	Vertebral artery	Lower part of cerebellum, medulla, choroid plexus of fourth ventricle
Cerebellar, superior	Basilar artery	Upper part of cerebellum, midbrain, pineal body, choroid plexus of third ventricle
Cerebral, anterior	Internal carotid artery	Orbital, frontal, and parietal cortex, corpus callosum, diencephalon, corpus striatum, internal capsule, choroids plexus of lateral ventricles
Cerebral, middle	Internal carotid artery	Orbital, frontal, parietal and temporal cortex, corpus striatum, internal capsule
Cerebral, posterior	Basilar artery	Occipital and temporal lobes, basal ganglia, choroid plexus of lateral ventricles, thalamus, midbrain
Ophthalmic	Internal carotid artery	Eye, orbit, facial structures
Spinal, anterior	Vertebral artery	Spinal cord
Spinal, posterior	Vertebral artery	Spinal cord
Vertebral	Subclavian artery, which arises from brachiocephalic (right), aorta (left)	Neck muscles, vertebrae, spinal cord, cerebellum, cortex

much individual variation in the circle of Willis; parts of the system may actually be missing in some people (e.g., in 15% of normal brains, the posterior cerebral artery is a direct extension of the posterior communicating artery).

VENOUS SYSTEM

The veins are located in the outer portion of the dura and pass blood through vessels back to the heart. Venous drainage starts with the superficial cerebral veins, which originate in the brain substance within the pia mater and empty into the superior sagittal and transverse sinuses, the deep veins of the brain, and the straight sinus, which connects to the internal jugular vein. As noted earlier in the discussion of the ventricular system, the subarachnoid space contains pockets of veins called *arachnoid granulations* that serve as pathways for the subarachnoid CSF to be absorbed and re-enter the venous circulation. Arachnoid granulations first appear in childhood, around age 7, and increase in size and number during adulthood. Unlike the arterial blood supply, the venous system of the brain does not have a right and left system. Thus, there is free circulation within the venous system, which may facilitate the spread of infectious agents from one hemisphere to the other. Chapter 12 gives a detailed description of vascular disorders.

Principal Divisions of the Brain

The brain can be subdivided into three major divisions based on the development of the human embryo (see earlier). As the embryo's neural tube closes, it begins to differentiate into three bulges. The topmost becomes the *forebrain (prosencephalon),* the middle is the *midbrain (mesencephalon),* and the third is the *hindbrain (rhombencephalon).* The remainder of the neural tube develops into

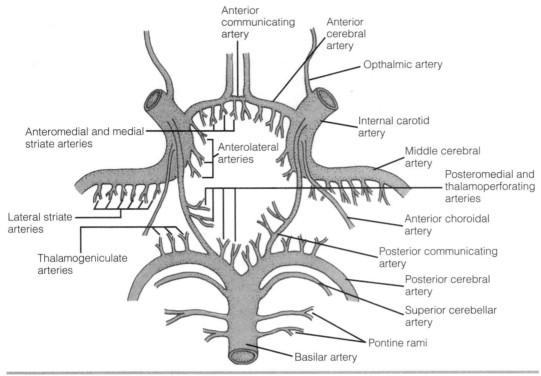

Anterior communicating artery

Anterior cerebral artery

Opthalmic artery

Internal carotid artery

Middle cerebral artery

Posteromedial and thalamoperforating arteries

Anterior choroidal artery

Posterior communicating artery

Posterior cerebral artery

Superior cerebellar artery

Pontine rami

Basilar artery

Anteromedial and medial striate arteries

Anterolateral arteries

Lateral striate arteries

Thalamogeniculate arteries

Figure 5.11   Circle of Willis. (From Banich, M. T., Neuropsychology: The Neural Basis of Mental Function, p. 13, Figure 1.7. Copyright © 1997 by Houghton Mifflin. Adapted with permission.)

the spinal cord. The three major subdivisions of the brain further differentiate into five subdivisions: (1) telencephalon, (2) diencephalon, (3) mesencephalon, (4) metencephalon, and (5) myelencephalon. This framework organizes the study of the primary structures evident in the adult. Table 5.5 and Figure 5.13 depict the relationships among the principal anatomic divisions, subdivisions, and major structures of the brain.

Traditionally, neuropsychologists focus on the brain areas of complex processing within the telencephalon, primarily the **cerebrum.** In fact, the major structures of the telencephalon, including the cerebrum, basal ganglia, and **basal forebrain,** comprise about 85% of the brain's weight (Burt, 1993). Therefore, although this is only one subdivision of the brain, it covers much area and is of great importance in understanding higher cognitive abilities. Consequently, a common manner of dividing the brain is to differentiate between the telencephalon and the brainstem. The brainstem includes all the subdivisions below the telencephalon (diencephalon, mesencephalon, metencephalon, and myelencephalon), except for the cerebellum, and mediates many primary regulatory processes of the body. We begin by discussing the major

structures of the brainstem and cerebellum, and then move to the telencephalon.

Brainstem and Cerebellum

The brainstem and the cerebellum, in terms of evolution, form the most primitive area of the brain. The **cerebellum,** which looks like a "little brain," connects to the dorsal aspect of the brainstem. Figure 5.14 shows the brainstem and cerebellum in relation to the entire brain.

The **brainstem** extends from the spinal cord and comprises about 4.4% of the total weight of the adult brain; the cerebellum makes up about 10.5% (Burt, 1993). The four parts of the brainstem include the **medulla oblongata** (myelencephalon), the **pons** (metencephalon), the structures of the midbrain (tectum and tegmentum), and the structures of the diencephalon (thalamus and hypothalamus). Although the brainstem and cerebellum account for relatively smaller areas of the brain and function more primitively than the telencephalon, these areas consist of a number of different structures relevant to understanding the basics of brain functioning. We first discuss the structures

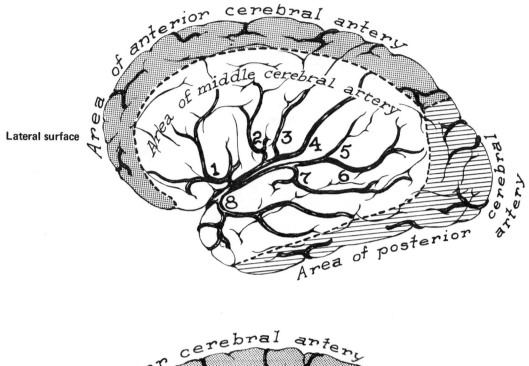

Lateral surface

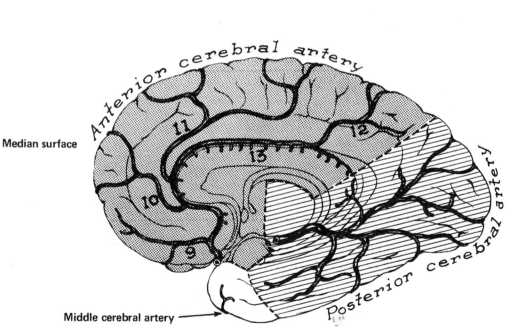

Median surface

Middle cerebral artery →

1. Orbitofrontal artery.
2. Prerolandic artery.
3. Rolandic artery.
4. Anterior parietal artery.
5. Posterior parietal artery.
6. Angular artery.
7. Posterior temporal artery.

8. Anterior temporal artery.
9. Orbital artery.
10. Frontopolar artery.
11. Callosomarginal artery.
12. Posterior internal frontal artery.
13. Pericallosal artery.

Figure 5.12 Blood supply to the cortex. Major arteries and areas of cortical profusion. (a) A lateral view shows the middle cerebral artery and its branches. (b) The course of the anterior and posterior cerebral arteries in midsagittal view. (From J.G. Chusid, Correlative Neuroanatomy & Functional Neurology, NY: Appleton & Lange, 1982, p. 50, Figure 1-54. Reproduced by permission of the McGraw-Hill Companies.)

Table 5.5   *Principal Anatomic Divisions of the Brain*

Major Division	Subdivisions	Structures	Cavity
Forebrain (prosencephalon)	Telencephalon (endbrain)	Cerebral cortex Basal ganglia Basal forebrain Hippocampal complex Corpus callosum	Lateral ventricles
	Diencephalon (between brain)	Epithalamus Thalamus Hypothalamus	Third ventricle
Midbrain (mesencephalon)	Mesencephalon (midbrain)	Tectum Tegmentum	Cerebral aqueduct
Hindbrain (rhombencephalon)	Metencephalon	Pons Cerebellum	Fourth ventricle
	Myelencephalon	Medulla oblongata	

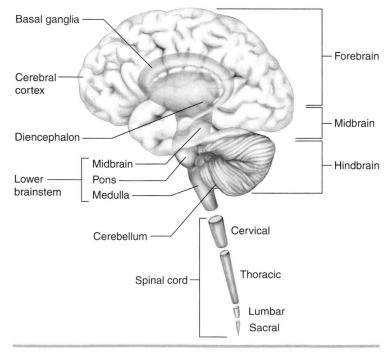

Figure 5.13   The three divisions of the brain. (From Banich, M. T.,
Neuropsychology: The Neural Basis of Mental Function, p. 13, Figure 1.7.
Copyright © 1997 by Houghton Mifflin. Adapted with permission.)

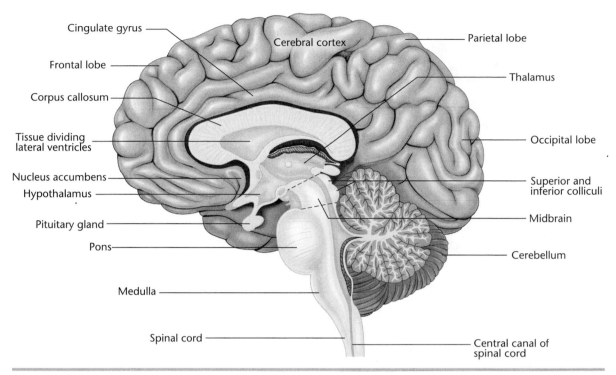

Figure 5.14 Human brain in midline and brainstem. (From Kalat, J. W. [2007]. *Biological psychology* [9th ed., Figure 4.10]. Belmont, CA: Thomson Wadsworth.)

of the lower brainstem (medulla, pons, and midbrain), then the upper brainstem (diencephalon), and finish by considering the cerebellum.

LOWER BRAINSTEM

Overview

■ *Gross anatomic features:*
Hindbrain: medulla oblongata (myelencephalon), pons (metencephalon)
Midbrain: tectum and tegmentum
Cranial nerves
Reticular activating system

■ *Function:* relay information to and from the brain; responsible for simple reflexive behavior

Structure

The lower brainstem resembles a road system of neural interconnections. In it, large tracts ferry information between telencephalon and spinal cord and between cerebellum and brainstem. It also contains smaller groups of nerves such as the cranial nerves, specialized nuclei, and the network of the **reticular activating system (RAS).** The medulla oblongata, pons, and midbrain structures are old structures, from an evolutionary perspective. Interestingly, they are relatively uniform in shape and organization over the range from evolutionarily less complex species such as fish to more complex humans (Figure 5.15). However, the size of the pons appears to increase in proportion to the degree of neocortical organization across species (Burt, 1993). The medulla is immediately superior to the spinal cord and forms an intermediary zone between the elementary neuronal configuration of the spinal column and the complex neural organization of the brain. It contains myelinated tracts that carry motor and sensory information between the brain and spinal cord, where the tracts **decussate,** switching transmission of information from one side of the body to the contralateral side of the brain. From this point upward, the left side of the brain controls the right side of the body and vice versa. The pons ("bridge") resembles two bulbs immediately superior and anterior to the medulla and inferior to the midbrain. The cerebellum connects to its posterior aspect, and information from the cerebellum funnels through the pons by way of large tracts termed **cerebellar peduncles** (see Figure 5.22 in Cerebellum section).

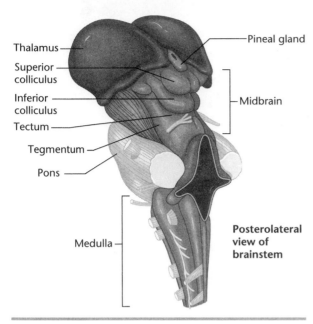

Thalamus
Superior colliculus
Inferior colliculus
Tectum
Tegmentum
Pons
Medulla

Pineal gland
Midbrain

Posterolateral view of brainstem

Figure 5.15 Brainstem structures. (From Kalat, J. W. [2007]. *Biological psychology* [9th ed., p. 88, Figure 4.8]. Belmont, CA: Thomson Wadsworth.)

The midbrain lies between the cerebrum and the pons and is the smallest portion of the brainstem. It merges anteriorly with the hypothalamus and thalamus. Although its beginning and end are not well outlined, it can be divided into the **tectum** ("roof") and the **tegmentum** ("covering"). Within the roof of the tectum are four small elevations, a pair of **inferior colliculi,** and above these, a pair of **superior colliculi.** The tegmentum surrounds the tiny cerebral aqueduct, which connects the third and fourth ventricles. The lower brainstem contains many important nuclear groups, including the cranial nerves and important pathways connecting the spinal cord and cerebellum with the telencephalon. The major motor and sensory tracts to and from the cerebral hemispheres all pass through the lower brainstem. The lower brainstem also contains a network of neurons known as the RAS, or reticular formation (the cranial nerves and the RAS are discussed separately later in this section).

Function

The lower brainstem serves several functions in addition to conducting information from spinal cord to brain. This complex system with many different nuclei and ascending and descending connections plays a crucial role in reflexive functions necessary for life, as well as in arousal level, auditory processing, visually guided movements, and the control of movement. The medulla mediates vital functions such as respiration, blood pressure and heart rate, and basic muscle tone. Damage to this area can interrupt motor and sensory pathways and threaten life itself. The pons serves as a major juncture for information passing between the structures of the spinal cord, brain, cerebellum, and some of the cranial nerves. It also plays a role in balance, vision, and auditory processing.

Together with the midbrain, structures of the lower brainstem play an important role in orientating to visual and auditory information. The superior colliculi contain important reflex centers for visual information and contain some retinal fibers via the optic tracts and the visual cortex. The inferior colliculi serve as an important relay center for the auditory pathway. Interestingly, compared with humans, bats have proportionally enlarged inferior colliculi. This is related to their sonar-like system, which allows them to receive echoes, and thus determine structures in space. Tracts originating in the colliculi connect to established motor nerve cells and influence the movement of the neck and head in response to visual and auditory information.

Cranial Nerves: Structure and Function

Overview

■ *Gross anatomic features:* located within the brainstem

■ *Function:* conduit of specific motor and sensory information

The lower brainstem is also the site of origin of 10 of the 12 cranial nerves. These nerves, which are directly connected to the brain, carry information to muscles or sensory information back to the brain. The cranial nerves were originally numbered by Galen, and each one also has a name associated with it. Cranial nerves I through IV arise from nuclei in the midbrain and forebrain, and nerves V through XII originate from the medulla and pons in the hindbrain (Figure 5.16).

The cranial nerves integrate sensory information and motor output. Table 5.6 lists the individual cranial nerves and their functions. These nerves are very old from an evolutionary point of view. Some aspects of facial emotional expressions are also organized at this level, suggesting that our basic facial expressions are ancient and consistent across all human cultures. Because cranial nerves have more or less specific sensory or motor responsibilities, neurologists often test them during a clinical examination. For example, difficulties with eye tracking or numbness on one side of the face are clear symptoms of dysfunction with a cranial nerve.

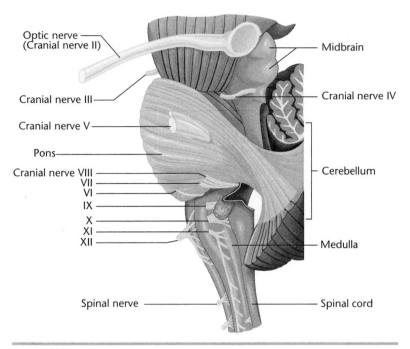

Figure 5.16 The 12 cranial nerves. (From Kalat, J. W. [2007]. *Biological psychology* [9th ed., p. 89, Figure 4.9]. Belmont, CA: Thomson Wadsworth.)

Reticular Formation Overview

- *Gross anatomic features:* a neural network located within the lower brainstem transversing between the medullae to the midbrain

- *Function:* nonspecific arousal and activation, sleep and wakefulness

Structure—The reticular formation is, evolutionarily, one of the oldest systems in the nervous system (Figure 5.17). The brains of primitive vertebrates are almost exclusively made

Table 5.6 *Cranial Nerves*

Number	Name	Function
I	Olfactory	Sensory: smell
II	Optic	Sensory: vision
III	Oculomotor	Sensory: eye muscle; motor: eye movement, pupil constrictions
IV	Trochlear	Sensory: eye muscle; motor: eye movement
V	Trigeminal	Sensory: skin of face, nose and mouth; motor: chewing and swallowing
VI	Abducens	Sensory: sensation from eye muscles; motor: eye movement
VII	Facial	Sensory: taste; motor: facial expression, crying
VIII	Statoacoustic	Sensory: hearing, equilibrium
IX	Glossopharyngeal	Sensory: taste; motor: swallowing
X	Vagus	Sensory: taste, sensation from neck; motor: control of larynx, parasympathetic nerves to heart and viscera
XI	Accessory	Motor: movements of shoulder and head
XII	Hypoglossal	Sensory: tongue; motor: movement of tongue

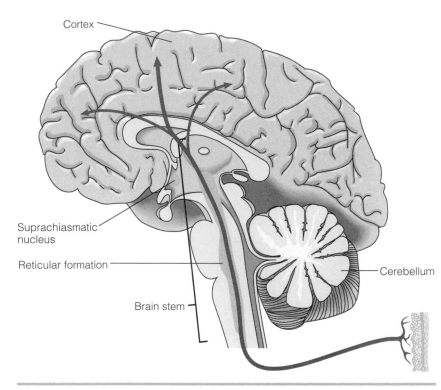

Figure 5.17   Reticular formation. (From Goldstein, E. B. [1994]. *Psychology* [p. 188, Figure 5.8]. Pacific Grove, CA: Brooks/Cole.)

up of a reticular or "netlike" formation. Humans retained the reticular formation over the course of evolution, as the more organized parts of the nervous system appeared. The formation has a diffuse arrangement of both ascending and descending neurons that form a system of networks (hence "reticular"). The network interacts with all major neural tracks of the brain. The reticular formation is not a singular set of nuclei, but rather consists of many clusters of nerve cells (Lezak, Howieson, & Loring, 2004).

Function—The reticular system is the starting point for the brain's vital activity. Life-sustaining nuclei and widespread connections here lead to the cerebral cortex. The reticular formation plays a role in nonspecific arousal, cortical activation and tone, and regulating sleep and wakefulness. Because of the system's role in arousal, it is often called the reticular activating system (RAS), which may be stimulated by outside, environmental events or by internal events. The reticular system forms the basis of Unit 1 in Luria's conception of the brain (Units 2 and 3 reside in the cerebral hemispheres; see Chapter 1). Defects in the reticular system can lead to a variety of problems. The major deficit, seen in many neurologic disorders, is a change in the level of consciousness, ranging from sleepiness to coma. The role of the RAS in sleep and wakefulness is discussed in Chapter 16.

As mentioned in the earlier discussion of the medulla, the medullary levels of the reticular formation contain important respiratory and cardiovascular centers. Injury to these areas can result in death due to impaired respiratory rate, heart rate, and blood pressure. Thus, low-level RAS injuries (or high-level spinal cord injuries; e.g., C-1, C-2, and C-3) may result in respiratory deficits. One such example is that of actor Christopher Reeves, who fractured his neck at the C-2 level while horse jumping. Not only was he paralyzed after the accident, he also required an artificial respirator because part of his brainstem, and specifically the reticular formation, was injured.

In addition to the task of arousal, the RAS is also responsible for selective attention. The system must decide what information to let pass on its way to the cortex and what information to filter. This is an important function because there is generally too much competing information at any one point in time for the brain to analyze it all. Thus, a further deficit or injury to this structure is one of filtering. Such a deficit can be related to RAS injuries that occur at or near birth. In these cases, the ability of the brain to filter information is either increased or decreased to an abnormal level. In the case of decreased filtering, the child is stimulus bound, easily distractible, and more pliable in low-stimulus sensory environments. In the case of increased filtering skills, the child shows symptoms of sensory deprivation. This can result in a complete withdrawal from the external world, similar to the deficit seen in some autistic children.

In general, the brainstem, and the RAS in particular, plays a major and vital role in regulating wakefulness and in mediating and filtering ascending and descending sensory and motor information. As such, the brainstem constitutes the starting point of the brain's analysis of information. Disruption of the brainstem, specifically of the RAS, affects the level of arousal, orientation, and general awareness of one's surroundings. Neuropsychologists are interested in the often profound symptoms associated with dysfunction of these areas. Neuropsychologists can systematically assess general arousal when it is important to monitor the progress of people who are recovering from RAS injuries. Individuals with acute brainstem injuries may be placed in inpatient medical care, because such patients may be in a stupor or coma, and thus dependent on external life support.

UPPER BRAINSTEM: DIENCEPHALON

The diencephalon (also known as the *interbrain* or "between brain") is located at the head of the brainstem connecting the cortex with lower structures of the brain. The diencephalon is part of the larger forebrain, and its evolution has paralleled that of the cortex. The diencephalon consists of two prominent brain structures, the **thalamus** and the **hypothalamus,** which contain many nuclei that are of interest to neuropsychologists because of their functions in regulating behavior. Phylogenetically, the thalamus consists of ancient nuclei that may have originally reacted reflexively to pleasant and unpleasant environmental stimuli before the cerebral cortex evolved. The hypothalamus, part of the limbic system, is considered instrumental in controlling the autonomic system. This system regulates emotional responses and other functions such as thirst, appetite, digestion, sleep, temperature of the body, sexual drive, heart rate, and smooth muscles of the internal organs.

Hypothalamus
Overview

■ *Gross anatomic features:* structure of the hypothalamus, hypothalamic nuclei, major fiber systems, third ventricle

■ *Function:* activates, controls, and integrates the peripheral autonomic mechanisms, endocrine activity, and somatic functions, including body temperature, food intake, and development of secondary sexual characteristics

Structure—The hypothalamus is the portion of the diencephalon that forms the floor and part of the lateral wall of the third ventricle. Anatomically, it is defined by the optic chiasm rostrally and the mamillary bodies caudally. The boundaries of the hypothalamus are easily described, but it does not form a well-circumscribed region and extends into surrounding parts. The hypothalamus itself is small by weight (pea size, about 4 grams in adults), but contains a grouping of small and complex nuclei located at the junction of the midbrain and the thalamus (close to the roof of the mouth). Within the hypothalamus lie at least a dozen identifiable cell clusters named the *hypothalamic nuclei* (Figure 5.18). The exact number depends on how the clusters are organized, but is similar in most vertebrates, suggesting that little has changed over time and across species. Originally thought of as "a trifling part of the human brain," the hypothalamic nuclei have become known over the past half century as an important collection of nuclei, "the brain within the brain." The hypothalamus plays an important role in regulating, activating, and integrating peripheral autonomic processes, endocrine activity, and somatic functions.

In general, the hypothalamus has three longitudinal zones: lateral, medial, and periventricular. The medial aspects of the hypothalamus have rich connections with the thalamus. The lateral nuclei have efferent and afferent connections to and from regions outside the hypothalamus, including brainstem fiber systems and preoptic and olfactory areas. In addition, the hypothalamus is an interaction center for several neurotransmitter substances. The hypothalamus, therefore, is a complex diencephalic structure in terms of its communicating neurotransmitters and dendritic and axonal interconnectedness.

Function—The hypothalamus is interconnected to the adjacent "master gland" of the brain, the pituitary (also known as *hypophysis*). The hypothalamus regulates the endocrine activity of the pituitary, both directly and indirectly (Kupfermann, 1991). The direct route involves the transport of hormones via axons from hypothalamic neurons extending downward to the posterior region of the pituitary. These axonal bundles constitute, in part, the **pituitary stalk.** Stimulation of these cells results in the release of the hormones by the pituitary directly into the bloodstream. The direct route controls the release of the *antidiuretic hormones* and *oxytocin,* which are actually produced by the hypothalamus, but are stored in the pituitary gland. The antidiuretic hormones are involved in homeostatic regulation, and oxytocin influences uterine contractions at birth and lactation. The indirect track

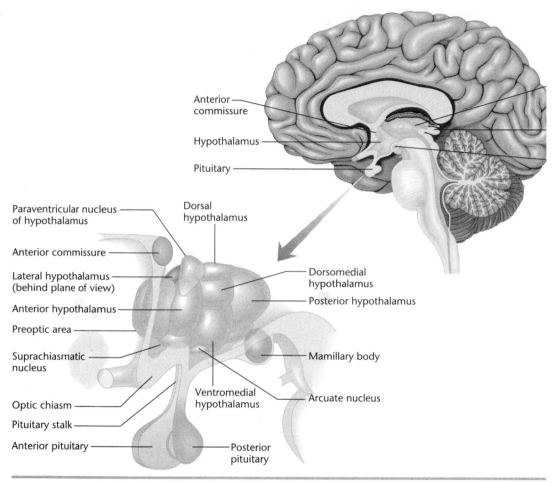

Anterior commissure

Hypothalamus

Pituitary

Paraventricular nucleus of hypothalamus

Dorsal hypothalamus

Anterior commissure

Lateral hypothalamus (behind plane of view)

Dorsomedial hypothalamus

Anterior hypothalamus

Posterior hypothalamus

Preoptic area

Suprachiasmatic nucleus

Mamillary body

Optic chiasm

Ventromedial hypothalamus

Arcuate nucleus

Pituitary stalk

Anterior pituitary

Posterior pituitary

Figure 5.18   Hypothalamus and pituitary. (From Kalat, J. W. [2007]. *Biological psychology* [9th ed., p. 300, Figure 10.5]. Belmont, CA: Thomson Wadsworth.)

involves the transport of releasing and inhibitory hormones via the vascular-capillary system interconnecting the hypothalamus and the anterior region of the pituitary. These regulating hormones signal the pituitary to release (or inhibit) a variety of hormones into the bloodstream. These hormones, in turn, regulate endocrine glands and body organs throughout the body. For example, the corticotropin-releasing hormone signals the release of **adrenocorticotropic hormone (ACTH)** in response to stress and pain. ACTH, in turn, stimulates the release of cortisol and other hormones by the adrenal cortex as part of the body's autonomic response to stress.

Thus, the hypothalamus, through its interactions with the pituitary and other brain structures and systems, is essential for body homeostasis, physical growth, sexual di-morphism, reproductive activities, and response to stress. The regulation of body temperature, food intake, and development of secondary sex characteristics are also important functions of the hypothalamus. Furthermore, the hypothalamus plays a role in digestion, sexual arousal, and circulation. It also influences thirst, hunger, and circadian rhythms (Victor & Ropper, 2001).

Many pathologic processes can influence the function of the hypothalamus. Of these, tumors are the most frequent, including hypothalamic tumors and the more frequent tumors of the pituitary (see Chapter 12). Disturbances of the medial aspects of the hypothalamus (the ventromedial nucleus) may lead to severe behavioral disorders, because these nuclei have important connections with the frontal cortex and the amygdaloid complex.

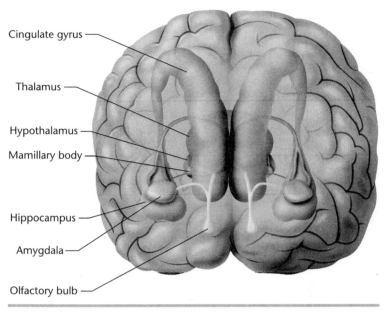

Cingulate gyrus

Thalamus

Hypothalamus

Mamillary body

Hippocampus

Amygdala

Olfactory bulb

Figure 5.19 The thalamus. (From Kalat, J. W. [2007]. *Biological psychology* [9th ed., p. 91, Figure 4.12]. Belmont, CA: Thomson Wadsworth.)

Thalamus

Overview

- *Gross anatomic features:* structure of the thalamus, its nuclei, and thalamocortical connections
- *Function:* complex relay station, handling major sensory and motor inputs to and from the ipsilateral cerebral hemisphere

Structure—The thalamus consists of two symmetric large nuclei embedded in the cerebral white matter toward the base of the cerebral hemispheres superior to the hypothalamus (derived from Greek *hypo,* meaning "beneath"). Each cerebral hemisphere contains half of the thalamus (Figure 5.19). Each half is a relatively large (about 4 cm in length), ovoid, gray mass that sits partially within the hollow made by the internal capsule and helps form the lateral walls of the third ventricle. The word *thalamus* means "bridal chamber," a name that reflects the deep, hidden, and secure location of the thalamus within the two hemispheres. On dissection of the brain, the relatively well-defined thalamus is easily visible because of its grayish color, signaling the presence of many nerve endings.

Cortical and thalamic functions are significantly interrelated. The thalamic nuclei consist primarily of gray matter and are connected extensively with most other parts of

the CNS. For example, many pathways that carry information from the brainstem to the cortex relay their information through the thalamic nuclei before reaching the cortex. Thus, the thalamus plays a central role in processing most information that reaches the cortex. The thalamic nuclei are relatively well-defined geographic areas that can be divided into groups, based on their geographic location within the thalamus and their specific function. Some major nuclei of the thalamus are the pulvinar nucleus (PN), ventral posterolateral (VPL), ventral posteromedial (VPM), medial geniculate (MG), lateral geniculate (LG), ventral lateral (VL), and dorsal medial (DM).

In addition to receiving ascending input, all thalamic nuclei receive descending input from the cerebral hemispheres, principally from the cortical regions to which they project. As such, the thalamus plays a key role in providing a complex "relay station" for all sensory systems, except for olfaction, that project to the cerebral hemispheres. The thalamus and the hypothalamus together make up an important part of the activities of the limbic system (see later in this chapter for a more detailed description). Figure 5.20 shows the relation of the thalamus and hypothalamus to other brain structures.

Function—As the gateway to the cortex, the thalamus serves as the major pathway for primary sensory and motor impulses to and from the cerebral hemispheres. The one exception is olfactory sensory information (cranial nerve I),

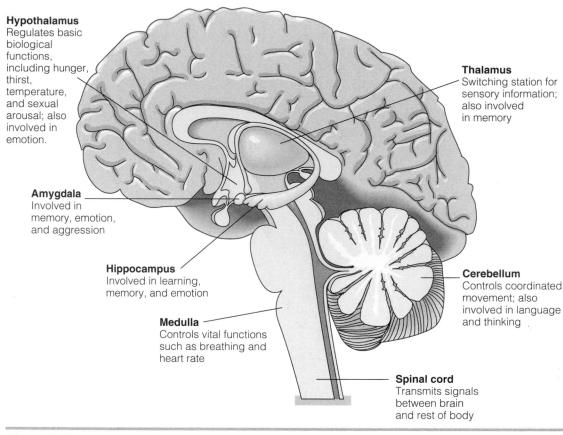

Hypothalamus
Regulates basic biological functions, including hunger, thirst, temperature, and sexual arousal; also involved in emotion.

Thalamus
Switching station for sensory information; also involved in memory

Amygdala
Involved in memory, emotion, and aggression

Hippocampus
Involved in learning, memory, and emotion

Cerebellum
Controls coordinated movement; also involved in language and thinking

Medulla
Controls vital functions such as breathing and heart rate

Spinal cord
Transmits signals between brain and rest of body

Figure 5.20 Subcortical structures of the brain. (From Goldstein, E. B. [1994]. *Psychology* [p. 89, Figure 3.8d]. Pacific Grove, CA: Brooks/Cole.)

which bypasses the thalamus and progresses directly from olfactory receptors to olfactory bulbs to the cerebral cortex. Other neuronal fibers that do not pass through the thalamus are those that are involved in arousal.

The thalamus is analogous to the concept of a large, busy, commuter train station. It makes preliminary classifications, integrates information, and "sends" it on to the cortex for further processing. Specifically, each half of the thalamus sends information to, and receives information from, the cerebral hemisphere on the same (ipsilateral) side of the brain. In this fashion, the descending projections serve as a two-way system between each cortical region and the corresponding thalamic nuclei.

The nuclei of the thalamus can be divided into two groups by their structure, connections, and function. The first group includes *nonspecific nuclei,* which are located primarily toward the median portion of the thalamus. These nuclei project widely to other brain structures, including other thalamic areas, and to the cortex, particularly its frontal regions. They receive input from the spinal

cord and the reticular formation and appear to play a role in monitoring the overall excitability of neurons in the cortex and the thalamus.

The second group of thalamic nuclei is referred to as *specific nuclei,* which are involved in sensory and motor processing (Figure 5.21). Specific nuclei project to restricted regions of the cortex. For example, specific sensory nuclei include the *VPL* and *VPM* (not shown) nuclei, which receive input from somatosensory relay neurons and project directly to the primary and secondary somatosensory cortex. The *LG body* receives input from the optic tract and projects to the primary visual area in the occipital cortex. The *MG body* receives input from the auditory relay nuclei and projects to the primary auditory cortex in the temporal lobe. Specific nuclei of the thalamus that are involved in controlling motor activity include the *VL* and *ventral intermedial* (*VI;* not shown) nuclei, which receive input from the cerebellum. The lateral portion of the *ventral anterior (VA)* nucleus receives ascending fiber tracts from the basal ganglia, which are

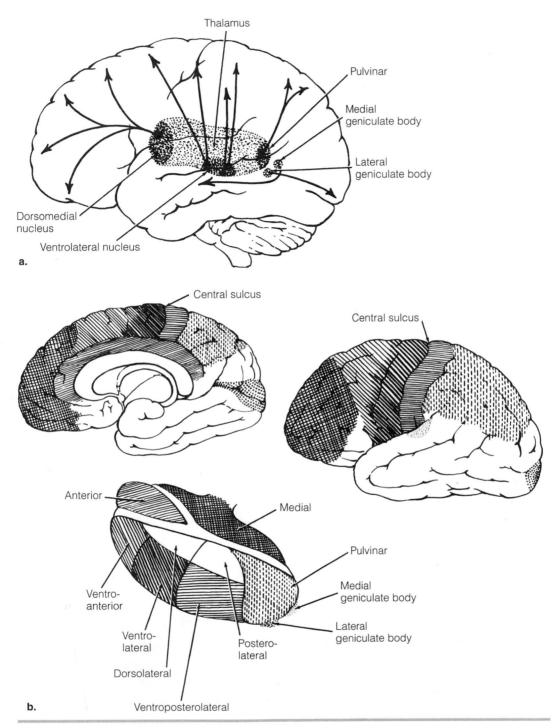

Figure 5.21 Thalamocortical radiations. (a) Principal thalamocortical projections. (b) Relation of cortical areas to thalamic nuclei. (a: From J. G. Chusid, Correlative Neuroanatomy & Functional Neurology, NY: Appleton & Lange, 1982, p. 19, Figure 1.10 and p. 20, Figure 1.21. Reproduced by permission of the McGraw-Hill Companies; b: reproduced with permission from original drawings by Frank H. Netter, MD; first appeared in Ciba Clinical Symposia. Copyright ©1950, Ciba Pharmaceutical Co.)

involved in regulating motor behavior. All three thalamic nuclei (VL, VI, and VA) project to the precentral motor areas of the cortex. Finally, the *DM* nucleus has many connections to the limbic system, which regulates emotional activity. In addition, the DM nucleus is one of the thalamic nuclei involved in memory. This list of thalamic nuclei provides only an overview of the neuropsychological function, because the connections of the thalamus are extremely complicated and an understanding of them all lies beyond the scope of this text.

Lesions, particularly vascular accidents, and to some extent tumors, have been most often associated with the thalamic syndrome, marked deficits in gross areas of sensory or motor function. For example, lesions of the left thalamus have been implicated with depressed scores on cognitive-verbal tasks (Vilkki & Laitinen, 1974; Zillmer, Fowler, Waechtler, Harris, & Khan, 1992). Lesions of the right thalamus have been associated with defects in spatial ability (Bundick, Zillmer, Ives, & Beadle-Linsay, 1995; Jurko & Andy, 1973), facial recognition (Vilkki & Laitinen, 1974), and the perception of music (Roeser & Daly, 1974). Consequently, many sequelae of thalamic injury are those you might expect from the interruption of essential relay elements in pathways to and from the

cerebral hemispheres. In some thalamic lesions, the symptoms are short lived, indicating that alternative pathways are quickly formed.

CEREBELLUM

Overview

- *Gross anatomic features:* cerebellar cortex, cerebellar white matter, and glia
- *Function:* coordination of movements, posture, antigravity movements, balance, and gait

Structure

The cerebellum (derived from Latin meaning "little brain"), surprisingly, contains nearly 50% of the neurons of the brain, even though it makes up only 10% of its weight. On visual inspection, the cerebellum is a spectacular brain structure because of its clearly defined morphology and symmetry (Figure 5.22). The cerebellar cortex is heavily infolded, and the numerous parallel sulci give it a layered appearance. The cerebellum also has several deep fissures dividing each cerebellar hemisphere into separate lobes. Its histologic structure, however, is relatively

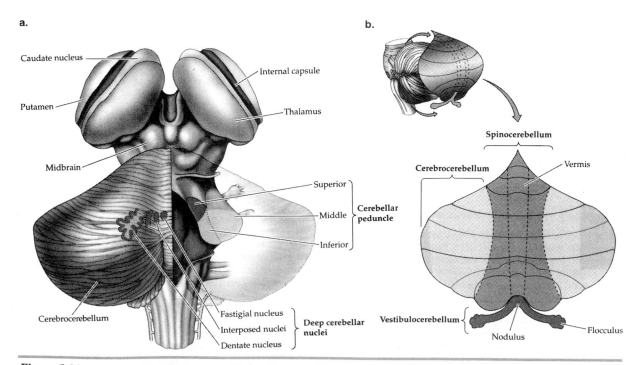

a.

Caudate nucleus
Putamen
Midbrain
Cerebrocerebellum
Internal capsule
Thalamus
Superior ⎫
Middle ⎬ Cerebellar peduncle
Inferior ⎭
Fastigial nucleus ⎫
Interposed nuclei ⎬ Deep cerebellar nuclei
Dentate nucleus ⎭

b.

Spinocerebellum
Cerebrocerebellum
Vermis
Vestibulocerebellum ⎨
Nodulus
Flocculus

Figure 5.22 Structure of the cerebellum. (a) Dorsal view of the left cerebellar hemisphere with the right hemisphere removed to reveal the cerebellar peduncles. (b) Flattened view of the cerebellar surface showing the three major subdivisions and vermis. (From Purves, D., Augustine, G. J., Fitzpatrick, D., Katz, L. C., LaMantia, A., McNamara, J. O., & William, S. M. [Eds.]. [2001]. *Neuroscience* [2nd ed., p. 410, Figure 19.1]. Sunderland, MA: Sinauer Associates, by permission.)

simple compared with that of the cortex. The neurons appear to be organized in repeating patterns. The cerebellum is located posteriorly and superiorly to the pons and medulla, just inferior to the posterior portion of the cerebral hemispheres. The cerebellum is attached to the brainstem at the level of the pons ("bridge") via the cerebellar peduncles and consists of two large oval hemispheres connected by a single median portion, termed the **vermis** (derived from Latin meaning "worm").

Function

The cerebellum is phylogenetically old and may have been the first brain structure to specialize in coordinating motor and sensory information. Observing patients with cerebellar disease makes clear the importance of this center for coordinating movement and postural adjustments. The cerebellum is heavily involved in basic processes necessary for general motor behavior, as well as in coordinating movements. The oldest areas of the cerebellum are concerned with keeping the body oriented in space motorically. The cerebellum also helps control muscles keeping the body upright despite the pull of gravity and monitors background muscle tone involved in voluntary movement.

Lesions of the cerebellum, depending on location, may cause a variety of disorders, including deterioration of coordinated movement, irregular and jerky movements, intention tremor when attempting to complete a voluntary task, static tremor when resting, impairment of alternating movements, impairment in balance, disturbances of gait, and uncontrolled nystagmic movements of the eyes. Evidence exists that people born without a cerebellum can function completely normally, because other brain structures have adapted to take over its functions. Neuropsychologists often erroneously ignore the cerebellum because no obvious cognitive properties have been associated with lesions of the cerebellum. However, it now appears that the cerebellum stores memories for simple learned motor responses and is involved in attentional shifting, as well as other cognitive functions (Diamond, 2000).

Telencephalon

The telencephalon, or endbrain, consists of the two cerebral hemispheres connected by a massive bundle of fibers, the corpus callosum. The outer layer of the cortex consists primarily of cell bodies (gray matter) and affects thinking, memory, and voluntary behavior, as well as the regulation of motor behavior. Within each hemisphere is a lateral ventricle and a collection of several large nuclei known as the basal ganglia, which contain the cell bodies of motor control neurons. The basal forebrain is also recognized as a prominent division of the subcortical (below the cortex) aspect of the cerebrum. This area, surrounding the inferior tip of the frontal horn, is strongly interconnected with limbic structures, and some researchers (e.g., Crosson, 1992) consider it part of the limbic system.

BASAL GANGLIA

The **basal ganglia,** also called the **basal nuclei,** are a collection of deep nuclei of the telencephalon (basal means "lowest level"; Figure 5.23) The basal ganglia communicate with motor regions in the cortex via the thalamus. With their complex interconnections and efferent outputs and afferent inputs, the basal ganglia participate in the control of higher order movement, particularly in starting or initiating movement.

Overview

■ *Gross anatomic features:* structures of the caudate nucleus, putamen, globus pallidus, substantia nigra, and subthalamic nuclei

■ *Function:* important as relay stations in motor behavior (e.g., the striato-pallido-thalamic loop), coordinating stereotyped postural and reflexive motor activity, and supporting higher order cognitive functions

Structure

Embedded deep within the cortex lies a group of symmetric subcortical gray matter structures known collectively as the *basal ganglia.* They partially surround the thalamus and are themselves enclosed by the cerebral cortex and cerebral white matter. They have sensory projections to the cerebral hemispheres, interconnections between parts of the cortex, and outflow from the cerebral cortex to other nervous system structures. Neuropsychologists most often conceptualize the basal ganglia within the context of the motor system and, thus, typically exclude the amygdala (located at the tail of the caudate nucleus) and a large part of the thalamus. However, the substantia nigra and the **subthalamic nucleus** have important motor functions and are usually included as part of the basal ganglia.

The two major structures of the basal ganglia are the **caudate nucleus** and the **putamen,** with the adjacent medial and lateral **globus pallidus.** In general, these structures

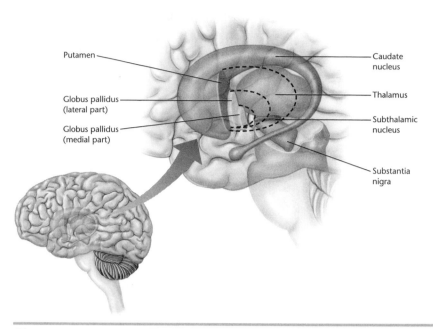

Figure 5.23   Basal ganglia within the cortex. (From Kalat, J. W. [2007]. *Biological psychology* [9th ed., p. 251, Figure 8.16]. Belmont, CA: Thomson Wadsworth.)

connect with the cortex, via the thalamus, the reticular formation, and the midbrain, but to a lesser degree with the spinal cord. The caudate nucleus connects to the putamen via the anterior limb of the internal capsule. This conglomeration is so difficult to identify as separate structures that it is usually referred to as the **striatum** because of its striped or striated appearance.

The precise circuitry of the basal nuclei is not fully understood, but researchers think they act as a relay station between the cerebral cortex via the thalamus. The major output from the basal ganglia targets the thalamus.

One major pathway between different structures comprising the basal ganglia is the *striato-pallido-thalamic loop*. This communication loop greatly interests neuropsychologists because it provides a mechanism for processing and integrating information from different regions of the brain before cortical processing. The input side of the basal ganglia, the striatum, receives information (descending connections) from separate sources, including the motor system, sensory and higher integrative areas of the cortex, the language centers of Broca's and Wernicke's areas, the thalamic nuclei, and the substantia nigra. The striatum, in turn, projects to the globus pallidus, which directly projects to the motor areas of the thalamus. The **substantia nigra** plays an important role in basal ganglia function via the dopaminergic *nigrostriatal system*. Its links

to the globus pallidus, and the thalamus can influence motor behavior, which is organized by the cortex.

Function

Researchers think the primary activity of the basal ganglia regulates voluntary movements, specifically related to planning and initiating motor behavior. The basal ganglia, together with the red nucleus and substantia nigra of the midbrain and the cerebellum, form what has clinically been termed the **extrapyramidal motor system,** which is responsible for stereotyped postural and reflexive motor activity. The system also acts to keep individual muscles ready to respond. The other major motor system, the **pyramidal system,** originates in the cerebral cortex.

Two general theories of the role of the basal ganglia have been advanced. One suggests that the basal ganglia are mostly integrative in nature and receive input from visual centers, from the balance centers of the brain, and from the muscles and joints of the body. An alternative hypothesis assigns less importance to the basal nuclei, suggesting they are, more or less, a relay station with few integrative properties (Noback & Demarest, 1975). The basal ganglia may also play a role in language, specifically motor planning and programming for speech, and perhaps even functions associated with attention and alerting before a motor response. Increasingly, research suggests that the basal ganglia, via their interconnections with the frontal lobes, participate in the generation, inhibition, and execution of higher order behaviors (Lichter & Cummings, 2001). For instance, damage to the caudate nucleus of the basal ganglia can impair cognitive or mental flexibility, a finding also evident with prefrontal damage.

Most understanding regarding the function of basal ganglia is gained from knowledge of movement disorders associated with basal ganglia dysfunction. Such abnormalities, which also include disorders of the cerebellum, have been labeled *extrapyramidal* and are characterized by atypical movements and changes in muscle tone. In contrast, *pyramidal* symptoms involve upper motor neuron disorders of the cortex and are more often associated with a loss of voluntary movement, including paralysis. Two relatively common basal ganglia disorders are Parkinson's disease and Huntington's disease (see Chapter 15).

Extrapyramidal symptoms also have been observed in schizophrenics who are treated with antipsychotic drugs. Those drugs, including Thorazine (chlorpromazine), Stelazine (trifluoperazine), and Haldol (haloperidol), block dopamine transmission. Although this reduces psychotic behavior and hallucinations, it has the side effect of Parkinson-like symptoms, including writhing movements of the mouth, face, and tongue. This neurologic presentation in schizophrenics who develop such symptoms is known as **tardive dyskinesia** and is irreversible. In general, the overall connections and functions of the basal ganglia are not fully understood, although the principal function of this formation is associated with motor behavior, specifically organizing ease and flow of movement.

LIMBIC SYSTEM

The anatomic term *limbic* (derived from the Latin word *limbus,* meaning "border") was first coined by Paul Broca (Schiller, 1982). Broca noticed that a ring of cortical tissue forms a border around the brainstem and medial aspects of the brain. Broca thought *"le grand lobe limbique"* was primarily involved with olfaction, because of its interconnections with the evolutionarily older **rhinencephalon,** or "smell brain." In 1937, James Papez suggested the presence of a more precise circuit or "limbic system," which he proposed was significantly involved in mediating emotional behavior. Indeed, proposing that a set of brain structures might be primarily involved in processing emotions was a bold statement at the time. Since then, however, the limbic system has received much attention for its major role in the expression of emotions, as well as in olfaction, learning, and memory.

Overview

- *Gross anatomic features:* structures of the amygdala, hippocampus, parahippocampal gyrus, cingulate gyrus, fornix, septum, and olfactory bulbs
- *Function:* the limbic system is closely involved in the expression of emotional behavior and the integration of olfactory information with visceral and somatic information

Structure

Broca defined the limbic lobe to include those structures on the medial and basal surfaces of the cerebral hemispheres. Because the limbic lobe is most developed in mammals, it is also known as the mammalian brain. In fact, in some primitive animals, such as the crocodile, the entire forebrain is limbic brain (the limbic cortex is part of the forebrain that developed first in evolution). The primary structures of the lobe include the medial cortex surrounding the corpus callosum, termed the **cingulate gyrus** (see Figure 5.14), and the medial cortex of the temporal lobes, or the **parahippocampal gyrus,** and the **hippocampal formation** (*hippocampus, dentate gyrus,* and *subiculum;* see Figure 9.2). The structures of the **limbic system** are often debated, but usually also include the **fornix,** some brainstem areas, particularly the **mammillary bodies** of the hypothalamus, specific basal forebrain structures, including the **amygdala** ("almond" because of its shape), and the **septum** (Figure 5.24). Several anatomic circuits have been described that include limbic system structures. The most likely role of the **basolateral circuit,** which centers around the amygdala, is in emotional processing. The **Papez circuit,** which centers around the hippocampus, is perhaps the most well-known loop. We further discuss these functional systems in Chapter 9.

Function

The limbic system is a most complex but important set of brain structures that has fascinated anatomists, neurologists, and neuroscientists for more than 50 years. The limbic system is a bit misnamed because there is no one-to-one structure–function relationship, as is evident in many sensory systems that are discussed in Chapter 7. The role of the limbic system in emotions and memory has generated a great deal of interest in neuropsychology. Extensive research has been conducted on several components of the highly interconnected limbic system. However, because of the interconnectivity of the system, it is often difficult to discern structure–function relationships. For example, the amygdala and hippocampus have specific

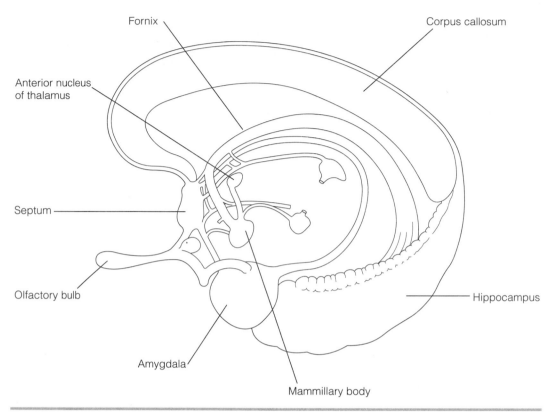

Fornix

Corpus callosum

Anterior nucleus of thalamus

Septum

Olfactory bulb

Hippocampus

Amygdala

Mammillary body

Figure 5.24 Limbic system with cortical area removed. (From Heller, K. W. [1996]. *Understanding physical, sensory, and health impairments* [p. 54, Figure 4.9]. Pacific Grove, CA: Brooks/Cole.)

connections with other brain structures and also have been studied as separate entities. The activities of the limbic system in memory consolidation, emotional behavior, and olfactory processing are topics on which we further elaborate in Chapters 7 and 9.

The limbic system is closely related to the hypothalamus, which researchers have singled out as the main brain structure for integrating and organizing autonomic processes related to the emotional expression of behavior. In humans, limbic system dysfunction has been associated with a variety of abnormalities, including emotional and behavioral problems (Glaser & Pincus, 1969) and sexual dysfunction (Rosenblum, 1974).

The hippocampal formation has been specifically associated with memory acquisition (Douglas & Pribram, 1966; Penfield & Milner, 1958; Scoville & Milner, 1957). The primary defect, seen after bilateral injury of the hippocampus, involves difficulty in learning new information. Such patients find themselves unable to retain newly learned information, although immediate and old memories remain relatively intact (Luria, 1971; Milner, 1968).

These effects on memory functioning are less profound when only one hippocampal gyrus is affected (McLardy, 1970). Lesions of the left hippocampal gyrus may cause problems with verbal memory (Russell & Espir, 1961), whereas lesions of the right hippocampal gyrus may cause greater impairment in spatial memory, including maze learning (Corkin, 1965).

The amygdala has ascending and descending connections with the cerebral hemispheres, the thalamus, the hippocampus, and even the spinal cord. The amygdala plays a specific role in fear conditioning and in impacting the strength of stored memory (LeDoux, 1994). The amygdala is discussed in greater detail in Chapter 9.

Numerous psychological disorders are characterized by emotional disturbances, and the limbic system has been implicated in many of them. Extreme violence in patients who exhibit rage attacks and frequent aggressive behavior can follow damage to the amygdala and its connections. In fact, removal of the amygdala (amygdalotomy) has been performed on extremely violent and aggressive patients in an attempt to stem rage reactions. Balasubramanian and

Ranamurthi (1970) have reported 100 cases of bilateral destruction of the amygdala in patients with behavior disorders.

Another clinical disorder associated with memory function of the limbic system is **Wernicke-Korsakoff's syndrome.** This is typically observed in severe alcoholics who show multiple nutritional deficiencies because they have essentially replaced solid food with alcohol. Such patients may develop a confusional state over time, as well as severe motor and new learning difficulties. This syndrome is related to vitamin B_1 (thiamine) deficiency.

Despite the limbic system's popularity among researchers, the complexity of the system's connections, internally as well as to other areas outside of the system, and the disagreement as to what brain structures should be included in the limbic system, it still puzzles modern neuropsychologists. In fact, some scientists suggest that neuropsychology needs to move away from the concept of the larger "system" of the limbic structures and should define them in more precise individual terms.

CORPUS CALLOSUM

Overview

- *Gross anatomic features:* a large set of myelinated axons connecting the right and left cerebral hemispheres

- *Function:* information exchange between the two hemispheres

Structure

The most prominent bundle of axons in the brain is a collection of intercerebral fibers known as the **corpus callosum,** an arched mass composed almost exclusively of myelinated axon bundles or white matter. The corpus callosum lies in the depths of the space between the two hemispheres called the **longitudinal fissure** and lies immediately inferior to the **cingulum,** a major intracerebral fiber within the cingulate gyrus (Figure 5.25).

Function

In the normal brain, information that enters one hemisphere crosses to the opposite side almost instantaneously (about 7–13 milliseconds). This happens via the corpus callosum, but also through smaller intercerebral fibers, the **anterior commissure** and **hippocampal commissure.** Because of the corpus callosum, both hemispheres share information, even though initially only one hemisphere may have received the information. The corpus callosum enables most communication and exchange of information between left and right hemispheres (Springer & Deutsch, 1993; Sperry, 1958).

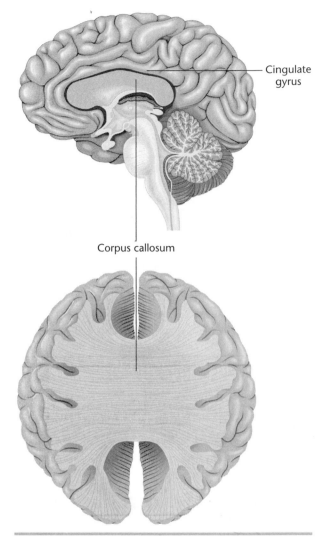

Figure 5.25 Corpus callosum. (From Kalat, J. W. [2007]. *Biological psychology* [9th ed., p. 418, Figure 14.2]. Belmont, CA: Thomson Wadsworth.)

An interesting problem for the brain arises if the corpus callosum is severed. This is intriguing to neuropsychologists, because now information presented to only one side of the body (or brain) is not shared with the other hemisphere. In very young children, cutting the corpus callosum has little apparent effect, because the brain develops alternative pathways to help compensate for the loss. In the adult brain, however, neural pathways have already developed. If the corpus callosum is severed surgically, which is sometimes done as a medical procedure to arrest the spread of seizures between hemispheres, the processing of some sensory information is confined to only one hemisphere. The study of such individuals, also known as *split-brain patients,* has helped provide extensive and interesting data on the independent functioning of the two cerebral hemispheres (Gazzaniga, 1966; Geschwind, 1965; Zaidel & Sperry, 1973). Researchers have learned from such cases that each hemisphere can function and process information in isolation. The idea that the brain might be composed of two independently functioning brain halves, perhaps even having two personalities or separate minds, is a question we explore in our later discussion of consciousness (see Chapter 16).

Summary

This chapter reviews the development, major structures, and functions of the brain. This anatomy lesson is important for a variety of reasons. It is important to understand the functional aspects of the brain as they relate to brain anatomy. Knowledge of brain structures, in and of itself, is not very useful to neuropsychologists. This is most interestingly demonstrated when students with little neuropsychological knowledge dissect a brain. They proceed in a most rapid manner with the dissection, naming each structure they are able to detect as they go along. Once finished, they are typically perplexed with the mess they have made and how little they have learned. They often ask, "Where has the brain gone?" Novices look at the brain as an anatomic object; neuropsychologists examine it as a functioning organ of interconnected systems.

This chapter serves as an overview of the basic neuroanatomic structures and functions of the CNS. However, it is typically the more integrated behaviors that interest neuropsychologists. Therefore, it is necessary to move from discussions of groupings of structures based on ontogeny to the idea of *pluripotentiality* of structures within functional systems. This concept, first introduced in Chapter 1, often transverses groupings based on migration of structures during brain development. It is to the systemic organization of regions of the cerebral hemispheres in support of behavior, particularly those involving higher order mental functions that we now turn.

Critical Thinking Questions

- Why is an understanding of the stages and processes of brain development important to the neuropsychologist?
- If a child was born without the telencephalon region of the brain, would the child be able to orient to visual and auditory stimuli, perform reflexive movements, and sit up? Explain why or why not.
- To what extent can behavioral functions be localized to specific brain structures?
- What level of brain mapping is most useful to the neuropsychologist?

Key Terms

Central nervous system (CNS)	Agyria or lissencephaly	Metencephalon	Spinal cord
Neurogenesis	Axons	Myelencephalon	Cranial nerves
Peripheral nervous system (PNS)	Dendrites	Gyrus (gyri)	Afferent nerves
Neural tube	Arborization	Sulcus (sulci)	Efferent nerves
Precursor or progenitor cells	Dendritic spines	Sylvian (lateral) fissure	Meninges
Glial cells	Synaptogenesis	Polymicrogyria	Horizontal plane
Oligodendrocytes	Prefrontal cortex	Cerebrospinal fluid (CSF)	Coronal plane
Microglia	Myelin	Vertebral column	Sagittal plane
Migratory process	Pruning	Somatic nervous system (SNS)	Anterior
Differentiation process	Visual cortex	Autonomic nervous system (ANS)	Posterior
Neurulation	Forebrain (prosencephalon)	Sympathetic nervous system	Inferior
Spina bifida	Midbrain (mesencephalon)	Parasympathetic nervous system	Superior
Anencephaly	Hindbrain (rhombencephalon)		Medial
Corticogenesis	Telencephalon	Brain	Lateral
	Diencephalon		Rostral

Caudal
Proximal
Distal
Dorsal
Ventral
Ipsilateral
Contralateral
Meningiomas
Ventricular system
Vascular system
Fossae
Foramina
Foramen magnum
Fontanelle
Pia mater
Arachnoid membrane
Subarachnoid space
Dura mater
Epidural space
Subdural space
Subdural hematoma
Meningitis
Ventricles
Interventricular foramen or
    foramen of Monro

Cerebral aqueduct or aqueduct
    of Sylvius
Choroid plexus
Foramen of Magendie
Foramina of Luschka
Cisterns
Superior sagittal sinus
Arachnoid villi or granulations
Hydrocephalus
Normal-pressure hydrocephalus
    (NPH)
Internal carotid arteries
Vertebral arteries
Aortic arch
Basilar artery
Posterior cerebral arteries
Cerebrovascular accident (CVA)
Circle of Willis
Anterior cerebral artery
Middle cerebral artery
Anterior communicating artery
Posterior communicating
    arteries
Cerebrum
Basal forebrain

Cerebellum
Brainstem
Medulla oblongata
Pons
Reticular activating system
    (RAS)
Decussate
Cerebellar peduncles
Tectum
Tegmentum
Inferior colliculi
Superior colliculi
Thalamus
Hypothalamus
Pituitary stalk
Adrenocorticotropic hormone
    (ACTH)
Vermis
Basal ganglia
Basal nuclei
Subthalamic nucleus
Caudate nucleus
Putamen
Globus pallidus
Striatum

Substantia nigra
Extrapyramidal motor system
Pyramidal motor system
Tardive dyskinesia
Rhinencephalon
Cingulate gyrus
Parahippocampal gyrus
Hippocampal formation
Limbic system
Fornix
Mammillary bodies
Amygdala
Septum
Basolateral circuit
Papez circuit
Wernicke-Korsakoff's
    syndrome
Corpus callosum
Longitudinal fissure
Cingulum
Anterior commissure
Hippocampal commissure

Web Connections

http://www.meddean.luc.edu/lumen/MedEd/GrossAnatomy/h_n/cn/cn1/mainframe.htm
The Cranial Nerves
This site provides excellent discussion of the cranial nerves.

http://www.neuropat.dote.hu
Neuroanatomy
This page features links to a number of resources in neuroanatomy.

Chapter 6

CEREBRAL SPECIALIZATION

Men are from Mars, and Women are from Venus.

—*John Gray*

The Cerebral Hemispheres
Hemispheric Anatomic and Functional Differences
Sex Differences and Hemispheric Specialization

Neuropsychology in Action

6.1 The Evolution of the Brain: A Focus on Brain Size
6.2 A Land Where Girls Rule in Math

Overview

This chapter focuses on the cerebral cortex with regard to structure, function, lateralization, and sex differences. Our discussion of the cortex provides a foundation for subsequent chapters that explore the functional systems of the brain that support complex behavior such as language, memory, and emotions. The cortical regions of the brain can be defined in a number of ways, although the most frequently used nomenclature involves the divisions of the cortex into four lobes (occipital, temporal, parietal, and frontal). Although there is greater correspondence between region and primary sensory functions of the posterior regions of the brain, higher order cognitive, emotional, and social functions are not specifically localized to a particular lobe. Rather, multiple pathways and regions underpin functions, particularly those that involve complex behavior.

The human brain is composed of two hemispheres that interact in the support of behavior. The hemispheres differ regarding structure and function, with certain human attributes being lateralized to either the left or right hemisphere. However, the lateralization of a function to one hemisphere does not mean that the other hemisphere is uninvolved in the support of the function. For example, speech and language are generally lateralized to the left hemisphere in most people (both right- and left-handed individuals), but the right hemisphere is also intimately involved in speech and language functions.

It is generally recognized that each person's brain is different from the brain of every other person. Putative cognitive and behavioral differences of male and female individuals have led to neuropsychological investigations to determine whether structural and functional differences exist between the brains of the two sexes. Significant attention has focused on the role of sex hormones in the organization and activation of the brain. You will soon realize that the relation of sex hormones to behavior is complex and not fully understood.

 ## The Cerebral Hemispheres

Overview

◾ *Gross anatomic features:* structures of the frontal, parietal, occipital, and temporal lobes

◾ *Function:* higher cognitive functioning, cerebral specialization, and cortical localization

The cerebral hemispheres represent the most recently evolved brain structure in humans, although they are approximately 1 to 3 million years old (see Neuropsychology

in Action 6.1). The complexity of the interhemispheric and intrahemispheric connections reflects this degree of evolution, which allows humans to use such abstract concepts as symbols, language, and art.

STRUCTURE

The largest part of the brain consists of the cerebrum, or the right and left **cerebral hemispheres.** The two hemispheres form a half globe with a flat basal surface. The hemispheres are separated by a deep midline cleft, the longitudinal fissure, and are connected via the corpus

Neuropsychology in Action 6.1

The Evolution of the Brain: A Focus on Brain Size

by Eric A. Zillmer

To understand the functioning brain, place it within the context of evolution. Two to three million years ago, humans living in East Africa were making stone tools, perhaps building simple dwellings. Their brains would, in the course of a spectacular evolution, eventually enlarge to the size and complexity of today. Humans could not possibly perform the numerous and complex behaviors that they do without brain mechanisms that have evolved over hundreds of thousands of years. Evolutionary psychology offers a coherent theory that may begin to explain the strategic differences and similarities in the structures and functions of the brain.

Central to the concept of evolution was Charles Darwin's (1809–1882) text *On the Origin of Species* (1859). His historic 1835 trip to the Galápagos Islands laid the foundation of his theory of biological evolution, even though he stayed for only 5 weeks. Darwin suggested that the mechanism for explaining how species evolve from existing forms is a process based on natural selection. He identified the process of natural selection as the mechanism underlying the evolution of all organisms. He reasoned that some individuals were better able to survive and reproduce than others, and that the characteristics that made these species more successful could then be transmitted to the next generation. Perhaps the most significant legacy of evolution is a powerful brain that has evolved to a degree allowing humans to learn from experiences.

Basic human psychological mechanisms related to brain processes are likely to be species specific. For example, most or all humans share certain psychological processes, including fear of darkness; characteristic emotions such as anger, love, and humor; weapon making; sexual attraction; and probably hundreds more (Wright, 1994). People often call these processes human nature, but they must be related to brain processes. One reason most humans share many psychological mechanisms relates to that natural selection tends to impose relative uniformity in complex adaptive designs, such as the brain. Thus, central to any theory on brain evolution is that certain aspects of the CNS remain stable, whereas others must adapt over time. This is most readily apparent at the level of human physiology and anatomy: All people have two arms, a heart, and a brain; that is, they do not vary in possessing basic physiologic mechanisms. According to evolutionary psychology, however, the brain must contain a large number of specialized psychological mechanisms; each designed to solve a different or related adaptive problem. Thus, individuals also differ, and fundamental individual differences must be central to any comprehensive brain theory.

One way that the human brain differs, compared with other species, is its size, particularly the size of the neocortex. For example, a general principle of neural organization indicates that the size and complexity of a structure is related to its functional importance of the structure. The brain, through the meninges, is firmly attached to the skull. Anthropologists measure the internal volume of skulls, which is easily preserved over time, to estimate the weight of the brain. Using this technique, researchers estimated the brains of our earliest ancestors, dated approximately 5 million years ago, to be relatively small, about 400 cm^3 (Changeux & Chavaillon, 1995). Anthropologic evidence suggests that approximately 3 million years ago the anatomic organization of the CNS and its associated functions evolved at a spectacular rate. Although the human brain was always relatively large in proportion to the body, and presented a modern organization, the relative size of the brain rapidly increased in size. About 1 million years ago, the occipital lobes began to develop, followed by the frontal, parietal, and temporal lobes. This new biological foundation enabled increased memory capacity, more frequent and specific spoken communication (language), a more elaborate social life, and a more extensive exploration of the environment. Humans no longer depended on gathering rocks, carcasses, and vegetables, but became proficient in animal capture. This evolution in the structural complexity and performance of the brain corresponded directly with the formation and development of diverse cultures.

Neanderthals are thought to have inhabited Europe and the Middle East as early as 100,000 years ago. It is not clear exactly how similar they were to us, but they certainly had an elaborate tool-using culture that included ritual burial (Changeux & Chavaillon, 1995). About 100,000 years ago, the growth in brain size started to level off, probably related to the fact that the female pelvis, and the size of the skull that can fit through it, had not kept pace with the evolution of the brain. This has made for a remarkable state of affairs as it relates to brain development in humans. At birth, the

callosum. The surface of each hemisphere folds in on itself in many places, creating grooves along the surface referred to as sulci (singular, sulcus). Very deep grooves are termed **fissures.** The irregularly shaped ridges between sulci are known as gyri (singular, gyrus). No two brains are exactly identical in the size or the shape of their gyri, although the general gyral pattern is consistent enough to locate major landmarks. The morphology of the brain's gyri can be thought of as somewhat related to the idea of a face, where the features such as the nose, eyes, and mouth are generally localizable but vary in shape according to the person. Perhaps, more like a fingerprint, each

brain is approximately 1/4 its eventual size, compared with the rest of the body, which is 1/20 its eventual size. Then, over the next 20 years of a human's life, the brain matures at an amazing rate, developing billions of connections and supporting cells. At age 16, it reaches a level of behavioral control and conscious realm (maturity) that the owner of the brain is allowed to drive himself or herself around in an automobile. At age 18, the brain is allowed to render an opinion, a vote, affecting other brains (through culture and society).

The basic brain structures are similar for all mammals, although brain size may vary considerably among different species. One of the many fascinating aspects of how humans have evolved as a species is related to this extreme and unprecedented growth of the human brain, the cerebral cortex, and specifically the prefrontal cortex, which Luria named the "organ of civilization." To many students, the size of an organism's brain may seem intuitively related to the intellectual properties of a species. Certainly, if you compare animals with humans, there is a relation between brain size and intelligence. Aristotle commented on that humans had proportionally the largest brains of all animals.

Consider, for example, that gorillas, although physically larger than humans, only have about one fourth of the brain size. In humans, the average adult brain size is about 1300 cubic centimeters (cm^3) and weighs about 1500 grams. But a blue whale's brain weighs 6000 grams, and an African elephant's brain 5700 grams. If, however, brain size is held constant as it relates to body size, humans compare very well. The brain of a whale accounts for only 1/10,000 of its body weight, the elephant's brain 1/600, and the human brain 1/40. Thus, if the range of brain size with body size is held constant, the human brain is 21,000 times larger and the neocortex is 142,000 times larger than that of the shrew, a very

small, mouselike mammal. This means that if a shrew were the size of a human, its brain would weigh only 46 grams. The body/brain weight formula, however, does not work well with all small animals. For example, the ferret's brain makes up 1/12 of its body weight. In fact, the best ratio appears to be between an organism's body surface (not body weight) and brain size. Certainly, it is logical to assume that the surface of the body, through which the organism has contact with the environment, is more directly related to brain function than is the total weight in bones and blood. When body surface is taken into consideration, the human comes in first among all vertebrates, with the chimpanzee and the dolphin following second and third (Changeux & Chavaillon, 1995).

Large brains are not necessarily more efficient or effective; in fact, absolute brain weight has no significance in itself. It may require a larger brain more time to process information than a smaller one. There are even differences in brain size among humans. Big people tend to have larger brains than smaller people. This does not imply that men, who are, on average, taller and heavier than women, are smarter. After correcting for body size, men and women have brains of approximately equal size.

The size of a brain has been an object of debate and controversy for many centuries. Broca, for one, argued that the size of the brains of human races had to account for something (1861). He proposed that "in general, the brain is larger in mature adults than in the elderly, in men than in women, in eminent men than in men of mediocre talent, in superior races than in inferior races . . . . There is a remarkable relationship between the development of intelligence and the volume of the brain" (1861, pp. 188, 304). As evidence, Broca offered findings that 51 unskilled workers had an average brain weight of 1365 grams, compared with the

brain weight of 24 skilled workers, which was an average of 1420 grams. Any student of statistics knows that this finding may not be statistically significant, given the large variation of brain weights in humans and, presumably, in Broca's sample as well. Furthermore, it is entirely possible that the unskilled workers were malnourished and, therefore, were smaller in stature than the skilled workers. In any case, Broca's data have not been confirmed by more recent studies, suggesting that his findings were due to chance. Nevertheless, Broca went to great lengths to "prove" his theory. One has to wonder what Gall himself must have thought of this—his brain measured "only" 1100 grams.

The measurement (or mismeasurement) of human intellectual properties according to brain size has been described by the evolutionary biologist Stephen J. Gould in *The Mismeasure of Man* (1981), in which he presented a fascinating historical account of phrenology and other pseudoscientific explanations of the size of the human brain and its relation to intelligence. What Broca and others did not realize was that body size, as well as many other factors, relates to the complexity of the brain and the nervous systems of humans and other species. In fact, the complexity of the brain depends on many dimensions in addition to brain size, including connectivity, cell density, cell morphology, neurotransmitter complements, and perhaps the most important variable, the rate and duration of neuronal sprouting. Among humans, no brain size–intelligence relation exists.

The brain of Albert Einstein, the Nobel Prize–winning physicist, underwent autopsy after his death on April 18, 1955. Gall and Broca would have been surprised to learn that the Princeton professor's brain was basically normal in appearance and of average size, although there were structural differences in the parietal lobe.

person has his or her own "brain print." So much variation is evident between the brains of people that researchers conducting imaging and histologic analyses must compensate for interindividual variability by standardizing and transforming formulas, rather than by comparing brains directly (Mai, Assheuer, & Paxinos, 1997). Figure 6.1 presents general gyral and sulcal features.

The surface of the cerebral hemispheres is covered by gray matter. As described in Chapter 4, the gray areas of the central nervous system (CNS) consist mainly of cell bodies of neurons that serve as the brain's functional units. Underlying the cortex is white matter that links structures within the cerebral hemispheres and the CNS as a whole. The size, shape, and distribution of the cells and fibers vary

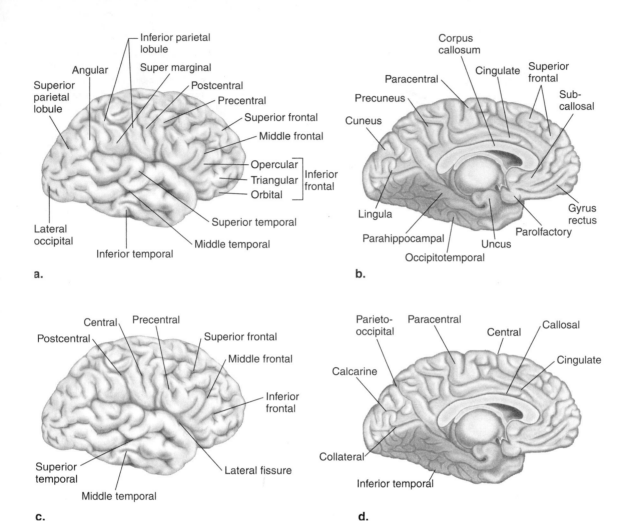

Figure 6.1   Major gyri and sulci of the cerebral hemispheres. (a) Lateral and (b) medial views of gyri; (c) lateral and (d) medial views of sulci. (Adapted from Kolb, B., & Wishaw, I. Q. [1996]. *Fundamentals of human neuropsychology* [4th ed., p. 51, Figure 3.5]. New York: W. H. Freeman and Company, by permission of Worth Publishers.)

from place to place within the cerebral cortex. In principle, there are many connections within the cortex itself, both horizontal and vertical, as well as to subcortical areas.

The **frontal, parietal, temporal,** and **occipital lobes** (Figure 6.2) are the four major divisions of each hemisphere. The frontal and parietal lobes are separated from the temporal lobe by the **lateral fissure.** The frontal and parietal lobes are separated by the **central sulcus.** The parietal and occipital lobes are separated by the parietal–occipital fissure and its imaginary extension across the lateral surface of the hemisphere to the **occipital notch.** The division and naming of the cortex into four lobes is quite arbitrary and is related to the names of the cranial plates that provide protective covering just superior to the lobes.

Another way of referring to the topography of the brain is related to the architectural arrangement of neurons in different regions throughout the brain. Brodmann (1909) divided the cortical surface according to these differences and showed that the anatomic organization of the cortex is similar in all mammals. He divided the brain into 52 sections, which are now referred to as **Brodmann's areas** (Figure 6.3). Correspondence between architectural regions and functional regions is, however, not precise. In fact, Brodmann's cytoarchitectural scheme is now considered questionable. For example, in humans, the cerebral cortex is much more developed than Brodmann's map suggests. In particular, the Brodmann system did not do justice to the degree of complexity of the brain's interhemispheric and intrahemispheric connections. Nevertheless, it is still

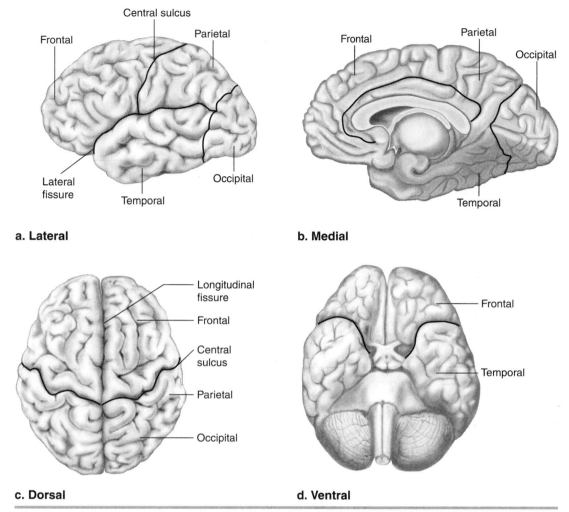

Figure 6.2 Lobes of the cerebral cortex. Four views of the frontal, temporal, occipital, and parietal lobes of the brain. (Adapted from Kolb, B., & Wishaw, I. Q. [1996]. *Fundamentals of human neuropsychology* [4th ed., p. 52, Figure 3.6]. New York: W. H. Freeman and Company, by permission of Worth Publishers.)

used widely for referring to particular parts of the cortex and is certainly more sophisticated than gross descriptions of the cerebral lobes. The publication of Brodmann's famous map of the human cortex in 1909 was instrumental in clarifying the confusion that existed until then. Using Brodmann's system, for example, Broca's area is called area 44.

FUNCTION

Because the cerebral hemispheres are responsible for the "higher mental functions" of humans, it is not surprising that neuropsychologists have shown particular interest in these structures. In essence, the cerebral cortex is what makes us uniquely human. The cerebral cortex organizes higher cognitive functions related to the following operations: (1) analyzing input, or processing of elementary sensory information such as touch, sound, or vision; (2) sorting, organizing, integrating, synthesizing, storing, or otherwise using the information; and (3) directing output through motor processing, which can range from activities such as walking to speaking.

The greatest one-to-one correspondences between structure and function within the cortex are in the areas of primary sensory input and primary motor output. For example, the **somatosensory cortex,** which occupies the anterior aspect of the parietal lobes, is responsible for receiving primary tactile sensation from the body, and the

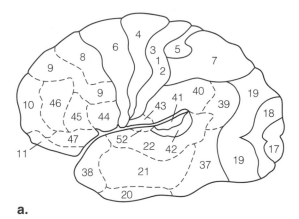

a.

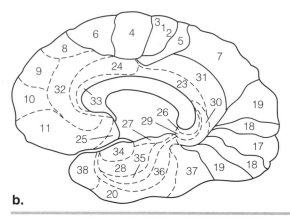

b.

Figure 6.3 Brodmann's map of the human cortex. This map is based on hypothesized cytoarchitectural differences between brain areas. Dashed lines refer to less distinct borders. (a) Lateral view; (b) midsagittal view. (Adapted from Kolb, B., & Wishaw, I. Q. [1996]. *Fundamentals of human neuropsychology* [4th ed., p. 55, Figure 3.3]. New York: W. H. Freeman and Company, by permission of Worth Publishers.)

primary motor cortex of the frontal lobe is concerned with initiating, activating, and performing motor activity. As a general rule, within the cortex, sensory processing occurs in the posterior aspects (the temporal, parietal, and occipital lobes), whereas motor processing is controlled primarily by the anterior aspects (frontal lobes).

The four lobes of the brain are associated with varied and identifiable functions in the primary sensory and association cortical areas. For example, in addition to the primary somatosensory and motor cortexes, elementary visual processing is associated with the occipital lobe, whereas the temporal lobes are concerned with receiving and interpreting auditory information. The interconnections of the auditory (temporal), somatosensory (parietal), and visual (occipital) segments of the

lobes combine to form complex, highly integrated areas of the cortex called **association or polymodal areas.** When one cortical area is activated by a stimulus, other areas also respond. This is caused by the rapid activity along a large number of precisely organized, reciprocally acting association pathways, which ensures coordination of sensory input and motor activity, as well as regulation of higher cognitive functions. For example, occipital input via the occipito-temporal pathway (the "what" pathway) to the inferior temporal region is integrated to support the function of object recognition and perception, whereas occipital input to the posterior parietal lobe via the occipito-parietal pathway (the "where" pathway) is processed for the support of spatial perception. Pathways from the temporal and parietal lobes to the frontal motor regions serve to orchestrate the motor movements related to visual object and spatial perception. Some of these neuronal pathways are short (intracerebral fibers), linking neighboring areas within the gray area, and others are long bundles, passing through the white matter connecting different lobes (intercerebral fibers).

The frontal lobe contains the motor cortex and also houses the prefrontal cortex. This area is akin to a conductor or executive of the brain—organizing, controlling, and managing behavior, and making high-level decisions about socially appropriate behavior; that is, when to act and when not to act. The prefrontal cortex makes it possible to perceive, even anticipate, the consequences of your brain's behaviors. It is very much responsible for the many aspects of what makes you unique—your personality and your conscience. Obviously, for such a suprasystem to function, it must have many connections to practically every major cortical and subcortical region of the brain. It must constantly be informed about events, both inside and outside the body, and it must overlap with important motor areas to immediately express and change the environment through behavior. Although there is not a one-to-one correspondence between a specific region and functions of the prefrontal lobes, certain divisions appear to make relatively distinct contributions to complex behavior. These divisions include the dorsolateral, orbital, and medial (anterior cingulate) regions (Figure 6.4). The dorsolateral prefrontal lobe is associated with higher order or executive function, the orbital region is intimately involved with the modulation of emotional-social behavior, and the anterior cingulate is central to motivational behavior.

As can be seen, whereas sensory-perceptual and motor processing are more easily associated with certain lobes, higher mental functions such as executive functions,

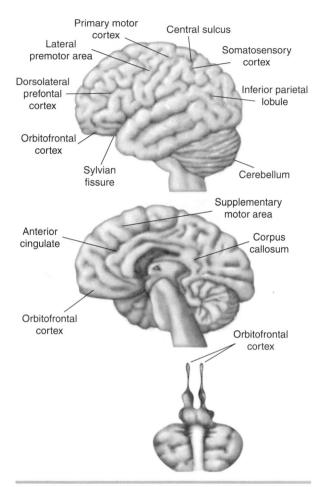

Figure 6.4 The prefrontal dorsolateral, orbital, and anterior cingulate regions in relation to other cortical brain areas. (top to bottom) Lateral (left hemisphere) and mesial views. (Adapted from John L. Bradshaw, 2001, Developmental Disorders of the Frontostriatal System, Philadelphia, PA: Psychology Press, p. 21, Figure 2.2. Reprinted by permission of Routledge/Taylor & Francis Group, LLC.)

language rule learning, memory, emotion, and social cognition rely on integrative functions and cross-sensory modalities. These functions do not wholly reside within the boundaries of a single lobe. For example, although encoding new information into memory is often associated with the temporal lobes, memory can best be conceptualized as a processing system spanning the limbic system structures, as well as aspects of the frontal, temporal, and parietal lobes. Likewise, reading is an exceptionally complex function that requires the systemic contributions of the occipital, temporal, parietal, and frontal regions, as well as subcortical regions such as the thalamus and basal ganglia. Aspects of higher mental processing such as memory, executive functioning, emotional processing, language, and consciousness are discussed as systems in subsequent chapters.

In general, damage to primary receptive areas produces identifiable deficits, whereas lesions in nonspecific or association areas of the cortex may produce a deficit far beyond the functional identity of that particular area, because the complex interconnections beneath that cortical region may also be damaged. For example, lesions of the somatosensory cortex may cause contralateral paralysis and loss of sensory reception. In contrast, lesions of the parietal-temporal-occipital association area often result in a more complex neuropsychological deficit, such as an inability to understand the numeric value of numerals even though the person is able to read them. Damage to the prefrontal area often produces deficits in concentration, ability to solve new problems, planning, and judgment.

ASYMMETRY, LATERALIZATION, AND DOMINANCE

Well-known differences in hemispheric functioning exist. This phenomenon has become so popularized, in fact, that many have taken to differentiating people according to the notion of being "right-brained" or "left-brained." Later in this chapter, we discuss the lateralization of hemispheric functions to determine whether this popular notion is, in fact, supported.

Much of what has been discovered about lateralization of function has come from the study of brains by one of four methods. In the first instance, destroying cortical tissue creates a situation similar to that which Broca encountered, whereby location of a function is inferred if damage to a particular area results in loss of that function. The second line of evidence has come from *split-brain patients* who have undergone the surgical separation of the corpus callosum, leaving the two hemispheres largely unable to communicate with each other. Third, epilepsy patients being considered for surgery typically submit to anesthesia of one cortical hemisphere at a time in a procedure called the **Wada test.** While one hemisphere is "unconscious," neurologists test the functional abilities of the opposite conscious hemisphere in isolation. Finally, neurosurgeons also electrically stimulate specific cortical areas to delineate boundaries of function before removing brain tissue. These methods have provided valuable converging evidence regarding general brain function and lateralization. However, all these methods seek to measure brain functioning in an "unnatural state." Can it be assumed from measuring the function of an isolated portion of the brain that functioning will remain the same within the context of whole-brain function? In addition, the patients being assessed typically have a brain disorder of some type. Dysfunctioning brains, particularly if the disorder has existed over a long period, may not behave the same way as intact brains. Now, through newer, noninvasive methods of brain imaging, such as positron emission tomography (PET), functional magnetic resonance imaging (fMRI), and single-photon emission computed tomography (SPECT), which show the dynamic workings of the brain (see Chapter 2), researchers can test normal subjects and pinpoint the centers of greatest brain activity for any one type of task. In addition, two innovative neuroimaging techniques, magnetic resonance spectroscopy (MRS) and diffusion tensor imaging (DTI), allow for even "finer" analysis of brain functioning. MRS provides visualization of the neurochemical activity of brain material, whereas the DTI maps the axonal connectivity of brain regions (Nordahl & Salo, 2004). These latter two techniques should further increase our understanding of hemispheric and regional brain functioning.

The term *hemispheric asymmetry* refers to the differentiation in morphology and physiology of the brain between the right and left hemispheres. The terms *lateralization* and *dominance* refer to the differences in functional specialization between the two hemispheres.

Probably the function most associated with laterality is speech. Paul Broca first determined that damage to the *frontal operculum* of the left hemisphere resulted in loss of speech (aphasia), whereas the right hemisphere appeared to play little or no role in language processing. Before Broca's seminal finding, it was widely believed that the two hemispheres were redundant in function. Broca's discovery led to the proposition that speech and language were properties of the left hemisphere. To say speech and language are lateralized to the left hemisphere denotes a functional dominance of the left hemisphere over the right hemisphere for language processing. Dominance does not mean that one hemisphere has complete or total responsibility for a function, but rather plays a primary or major role in the support of a function. For example, although there is significant empirical support for the lateralization of language to the left hemisphere (for most people), research has demonstrated that the right hemisphere is, in fact, able to perform a limited number of language functions such as understanding and processing of rudimentary linguistic contents. It is unable, however, to process complex linguistic information, and only rarely is able to communicate via speech. In addition, as discussed later, the right hemisphere plays a major and complementary role in regulating the nonverbal aspects of speech and language.

Because of the decussation of the sensory and motor tracks from the brain to the spinal cord, the right hemisphere shows greater involvement in the control of the left hand, whereas the left hemisphere is associated with modulation of the right hand. Broca (1861) proposed that a person's preferred handedness was opposite from the hemisphere specialized for language. Although the concept of preferred handedness appears simple to ascertain, there continues to be disagreement over the definition of the concept. For example, some researchers have defined preferred handedness based on the hand the individual uses to write, whereas others prefer to look to the hand the person uses across a number of activities to determine preference. The latter definition lends to representing handedness as a differential variable that ranges on a bipolar continuum, with one extreme indicating complete right-handedness and the other extreme complete left-handedness. The midpoint of the continuum would reflect mixed-handedness (ambidexterity). Finally, preferred handedness has been defined by the relative efficiency or speed of the hands. The latter definition shifts the emphasis from "preference" to "proficiency" of hand use.

Consistent with Broca's proposition, subsequent research demonstrates that the relation of preferred handedness to hemispheric lateralization is partially accurate when lateralization of right-handed individuals is considered. For example, an MRI study (Springer et al., 1999) of 100 healthy right-handed participants (48% female, 52% male) reported that 94% were left hemisphere dominant for language, whereas 6% showed bilateral, roughly symmetric language representation. None of the healthy participants were found to be right hemisphere dominant. In another study (Knecht, Dräger, Deppe, Bobe, Lohmann, Flöel, et al., 2000) of 188 healthy right-handed participants (59% female, 41% male), left language lateralization was identified in 92.5% of the participants, whereas 7.5% demonstrated right hemisphere lateralization.

Left-handed individuals are also likely to show left hemisphere lateralization for language, although to a lesser extent than right-handed individuals. Szaflarski et al. (2002) selected 50 healthy left-handed and ambidextrous participants for fMRI study. Predominately left hemisphere lateralization was found in 78% of the individuals, whereas 8% were predominantly right hemisphere lateralized, and 14% showed symmetric lateralization. In a larger study (Knecht, Dräger, Deppe, Bobe, Lohmann, Flöel, et al., 2000) with 326 healthy participants (198 females, 128 males), handedness was determined by the Edinburgh Inventory (Oldfield, 1971), a self-rating scale. This measure allows for a rating of handedness ranging from strong left-handedness to strong right-handedness. Seven groups were identified based on the Edinburgh Inventory. The determination of language laterality was made by having the participants perform word generation tasks while undergoing **Doppler ultrasonography (fTCD).** Overall results demonstrated a linear relation: the greater the right-handedness, the higher the incidence of left hemisphere language dominance, and vice versa. In extreme left-handers, the incidence of right hemisphere dominance was 27% compared with 4% for extreme right-handers with right hemisphere speech. The intermediate groups showed decreasing right hemisphere lateralization as the degree of right-handedness increased.

Initially, it was believed that "atypical" lateralization, particularly for right-handed people, was potentially an abnormal sign indicative of brain pathology or perturbations of brain organization. Support was drawn for this view from the finding that a significant number of individuals with brain abnormalities (e.g., epilepsy) demonstrated atypical lateralization. Yet, this assumption has been challenged by empirical findings demonstrating that a significant proportion of healthy individuals also show atypical language specialization without neuropsychological impairments (Hartlage & Gage, 1997). When there is a family history of left-handedness, the likelihood that left-handedness of offspring will be associated with brain pathology is significantly reduced.

In summary, empirical and clinical studies suggest that speech is generally lateralized to the left hemisphere for right-handed individuals (about 95%). Although the majority of left-handed individuals also show left hemisphere specialization for speech (about 70%), the incidence of bilateral or right hemisphere lateralization is greater in left-handed individuals.

Hemispheric Anatomic and Functional Differences

Although some structural differences between the hemispheres are known to correspond to functional differences in behavior, the relation between structure and function has not been fully determined. Table 6.1 outlines the differences in morphology between the two hemispheres. Figure 6.5 depicts some of the major hemispheric differences in structure.

Gross inspection of the two hemispheres of the brain reveals a number of differences. If you first look at the entire brain from the top down, it appears askew. This is because the right hemisphere often protrudes anteriorly from the frontal lobes, and the left hemisphere protrudes posteriorly from the parietal-occipital area. Turning the brain to the lateral surface of the cerebral hemispheres,

Table 6.1 *Anatomic and Physiologic Brain Asymmetries*

Morphology	Left Hemisphere	Right Hemisphere
Size	Greater density	Larger and heavier
Lobes	Parieto-occipital protuberance	Frontal protuberance
Frontal	Frontal operculum larger subcortical	Frontal operculum larger surface
Temporal	Larger planum temporale	Larger Heschl's gyrus (often 2)
Parietal		Larger area
Sylvian fissure	Longer and more horizontal slope	Steeper slope

the **Sylvian fissure** (which is normally the large fissure separating the frontal from the temporal and parietal lobes) is steeper in the right hemisphere than in the left. This results in a larger parietal and temporal area within the right hemisphere. It is reasonable to speculate that this allows higher level integration of visual, auditory, and proprioceptive information in the more spatially oriented right hemisphere. From an anterior view, the frontal operculum (Broca's area) of the right hemisphere has a larger surface area, whereas the surface area of the left hemisphere is more pronounced in the subcortical area. This may reflect differences in the language production abilities between the two hemispheres. If you remove the top half of the brain, allowing a view of the horizontal sectioning of the two hemispheres (see Figure 6.5), you can easily examine the area of the temporal lobes. Within the superior temporal lobes is **Heschl's gyrus,** and posterior to that is the **planum temporale.** The Heschl's gyrus (also known as the *primary auditory cortex*) of the right hemisphere is often larger than that of the left hemisphere, since it frequently consists of two gyri. In the left hemisphere, the planum temporale is larger than that of the right hemisphere. The structural differences here may account for the functional differences in auditory processing between the two hemispheres: Heschl's gyrus may have greater functional responsibility for the nonspeech aspects of language (pitch, tone, melody) and musical processing, whereas the planum temporale plays a larger role in speech comprehension. In addition to visible structural differences, there are also differences in neuronal architecture and neurochemistry, dependent on the side of the brain.

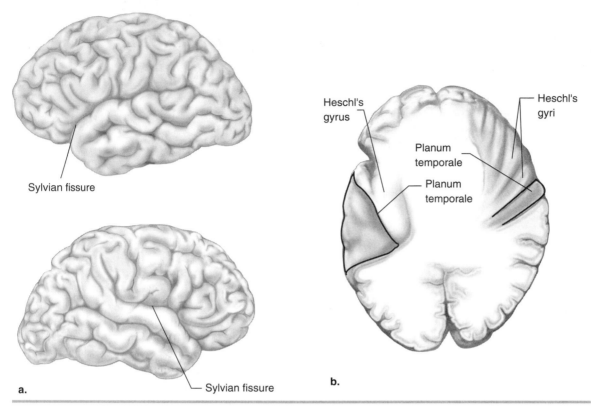

Figure 6.5   Brain hemisphere asymmetries. (a) The sylvian fissure on the right (bottom) has a steeper slope than on the left. (b) View cutting through the top portion of the brain at the level of the temporal lobes. (Adapted from Kolb, B., & Wishaw, I. Q. [1996]. *Fundamentals of human neuropsychology* [4th ed., p. 181, Figure 9.1]. New York: W. H. Freeman and Company, by permission of Worth Publishers.)

The gray and white matter composition of the two hemispheres provides clues to the type of processing associated with each hemisphere. The right hemisphere is heavier and contains more white matter than the left hemisphere. In contrast, the left hemisphere is composed of greater gray matter and more modality-specific sensory cortices. The composition of the left hemisphere suggests that it is more suited for single-modality and intraregion or within-region processing. A greater convergence of sensory regions is evident in the right hemisphere, signaling an increased representation of association regions. The increased association regions of the right hemisphere allows for multimodal and interregional processing (e.g., the association of the visual representation of an apple with its tactile representation). Because of these anatomic differences, it is hypothesized that the left hemisphere is better suited for processing information that is linear, sequential, rule-governed, or conforms to specific codes, such as language. In contrast, the right hemisphere appears more suited for holistic or

global processing of information; for example, determining the orientation of one's body in space (proprioceptive) or the spatial configuration and orientation of objects requires holistic or simultaneous processing of representative sensory input.

Empirical and theoretic efforts to associate hemispheric dominance to function have focused primarily on the content to be processed or the mental operation to be performed. Thus, differences in hemispheric dominance are generally associated with the type of content (e.g., verbal versus visuospatial), characteristics of the content (e.g., abstract versus concrete), or the mental functions recruited (e.g., analytic versus holistic operations). Based on a review of approximately 1000 studies of cerebral lateralization, Dean and Reynolds (1997) have summarized the functions and contents that are considered to show lateralization (Table 6.2). However, none of these characterizations of hemispheric dominance fully accounts for the functioning of the hemispheres. For example, Gazzaniga's (2000) research with

Table 6.2 *Lateralized Functions of the Left and Right Hemispheres*

Modes/Contents: Right Hemisphere	Modes/Contents: Left Hemisphere
Simultaneous	Sequential
Holistic	Temporal
Global	Local
Visual/Nonverbal	Verbal analytic
Spatial reasoning	Speech lateralization/verbal abilities
Depth perception	Calculation/arithmetic
Melodic perception	Abstract verbal thought
Tactile perception	Writing (composition)
Haptic perception	Complex motor functions
Nonverbal sound recognition	Body orientation
Motor integration	Vigilance
Visual constructive performance	Verbal paired-associates
Pattern recognition	Short-term verbal recall
Nonverbal memory	Abstract and concrete words
Face recognition	Verbal mediation
	Complex motor functions

split-brain individuals demonstrates that the processing of certain inputs (contents) shows greater association with one or the other hemisphere; yet, the hemispheres also differ in their processing orientation. The right hemisphere appears to show superiority to the left in "veridical processing" (accuracy of information representation), whereas the left tends to process information from an elaborative or explanatory perspective (interpretation and hypothesis generating), regardless of whether the content is verbal, facial, or abstract-figural.

There is a tendency to view the operations of the hemispheres as "either/or," rather than as overlapping or complementary operations. The involvement of the hemispheres in the processing of language exemplifies this mutual functioning. As discussed earlier, language is considered lateralized to the left hemisphere; however, neuroimaging studies (Vouloumanos, Kiehl, Werker, & Liddle, 2001) indicate that *both* hemispheres generally activate when language is processed, suggesting that complementary operations are necessary to support the comprehension and expression of language. Furthermore, individual differences in lateralization of functions are frequently encountered,

which argues against the rigid mapping of specific functions or processes to either the left or right hemisphere.

As you are aware, the brain is composed of two hemispheres that are interconnected by major pathways (e.g., corpus callosum). What factors would account for the lateralization of brain functions, and what are the advantages of hemispheric specialization? Although definitive answers to these questions are not evident, several related speculations have emerged. First, the efficiency and speed of processing would be improved if a hemisphere was specialized for processing. For example, speech involves the rapid sequencing of complex motor commands that may be better served by a single hemisphere, rather than by two hemispheres that are spatially and temporally separate. In essence, keeping functions "within house" would have an advantage over the "between-house" processing of two hemispheres. Of course, lateralization of a function poses a significant disadvantage when the designated hemisphere is damaged. The degree of loss would be greater after unilateral damage to the hemisphere supporting the function than if the function was represented asymmetrically. With asymmetric representation, the undamaged hemisphere continues to provide some degree of support of the function.

A second, although a variant of the previous proposal, relates to the differences in the manner and mode of processing of the left and right hemispheres. These differences could lead to competition or conflict if the two hemispheres shared equally in control of processing. Support for this view is provided by neuroimaging studies of chronic stutters that show the presence of bilateral hemispheric activation associated with speech. Training for the amelioration of stuttering appears to be associated with increased left dominance for speech (Fox et al., 1996).

Third, lateralization of one set of functions within a hemisphere frees the other hemisphere to specialize in a different set of functions. Gazzaniga (2000) notes that, as humans have evolved, the need for greater cortical space has increased. Lateralization of functions to separate hemispheres provides the needed cortical space and also reduces redundancy of cortical regions. The presence of the corpus callosum enables the lateralized brain functions to contribute to the entire cognitive system. The importance of adequate cortical space to support function is illustrated by the neuropsychological performance of young children who have undergone the removal of the left hemisphere (hemispherectomy). Some of these children are able to develop right hemisphere language. Yet, there appears to be a cost to the reorganization, as evidenced in the disruption of functions considered lateralized to the right hemisphere, namely, spatial processing. It has been hypothesized that the transfer of language to the right hemisphere "crowds out" certain spatial functions (Anderson, Northam, Hendy, & Wrennall, 2001).

NEUROPSYCHOLOGICAL AND BEHAVIORAL CEREBRAL DIFFERENCES

To understand the difference in styles between right and left hemisphere processing, consider how you would approach the following tasks: When asking for directions, do you prefer verbal instructions directing you to go three blocks to the first stop sign, then turn left and proceed three blocks, then take a right, and so on, or do you prefer a spatial map with directions marked on it? When you complete a puzzle, do you attempt to match individual features or concentrate on the overall gestalt? When learning or listening to music, are you more attuned to the rhythm or the melody? In math, are you more adept with mathematical calculations and algebra or with geometry? In each of these cases, the first preference corresponds to the verbal-sequential processing typically associated with the left hemisphere, and the second to right hemisphere spatial-holistic processing. The stereotype of "left-brained" or "right-brained" individuals has resulted from the oversimplified notion that one set of hemispheric skills will become dominant in a particular person. Perhaps you feel you use one style more than another. But in a normally functioning brain, all capabilities are used to some degree, although they may be developed to different degrees. Sometimes the contributions of various hemispheric abilities are not even noticed until their loss is made evident through brain damage or disease. When neuropsychologists discuss lateralization and dominance, the reference is to the division of labor for a particular skill in the brain, rather than the dominance of "brain traits" in any one person.

A number of behavioral differences are evident in the functioning of the two hemispheres. The correspondence between structural asymmetries and functional lateralization depends, in some measure, on the complexity of the behavior. The more simple primary sensory and motor functions show specific patterns of representation in each hemisphere. In general, except for smell and taste, sensory processing is funneled from the site of the sensory stimulation to the contralateral, or opposite, hemisphere. For example, the somatosensory strip of the parietal lobe of the left hemisphere processes objects placed in the right hand. The primary occipital cortices of the left and right hemispheres are involved in the processing of information in the right and left visual fields, respectively. These two senses are completely crossed, because the neural tracts project only to one hemisphere, opposite from the body site of stimulation. Audition is only partially crossed. The left hemisphere processes the majority of information presented to the right ear, whereas the right hemisphere processes a smaller portion of this auditory input. Olfactory information, which evolutionarily represents a more primitive sense, projects to the same (ipsilateral) hemisphere from each nostril; the right nostril is processed via the right olfactory bulb. Similarly, each hemisphere receives taste sensations from its respective side (ipsilateral) of the tongue. On the output side, the primary motor strip of the contralateral hemisphere controls primary motor processing. Thus, for instance, the motor strip of the left hemisphere controls motor movements of the right hand.

Higher order processing is, by definition, integrative in nature, involving multiple mental computations. Depending on the nature of the integration required, more or fewer brain areas are involved. Some may reside in the domain of a single hemisphere, and some may require both sides of the cortex. Although neuropsychologists recognize the integrative nature of higher order skills, some abilities demonstrate greater lateralization than others. As a general way of conceptualizing the differences between the hemispheres, the side that is dominant for verbal abilities (often the left) is usually more proficient in speech production and understanding. It is facile in manipulating the symbols of language, such as letters, words, and numbers. Both hemispheres are comparable in processing sound, with the left hemisphere (temporal region) responding selectively to meaningful language (Giraud & Price, 2001). Of interest, neuroimaging (PET) shows that communicative signing by congenitally and profoundly deaf individuals recruits similar left hemisphere regions (left inferior and middle frontal, and superior temporal gyrus) as individuals with normal hearing when processing language (Petitto et al., 2000).

The right hemisphere is more adept at processing the melodic, or prosodic, aspects of sound. Furthermore, the right hemisphere holds the advantage for visuospatial transformations, analysis of complex visual patterns, and emotional processing. Regarding emotional processing, the right hemisphere is thought to be more adept at reading emotions when expressed as gestures, tonal inflections, and facial expressions. When the right hemisphere is damaged, patients often speak in a monotone, fail to understand the emotional expressions of others, miss the gist of conversations, have problems expressing emotions nonverbally and verbally, and are limited in their understanding of humor and sarcasm (Beeman & Chiarello, 1998; Heilman, 2002; Meyers, 1999). Moreover, the right hemisphere, particularly the prefrontal cortex, exhibits preferential control of attentional functions such as arousal, sustained and selective attention, response inhibition, and self-monitoring. Although the left hemisphere is less involved in attentional functions, it does play a significant role in divided attention (Anderson, Jacobs, & Harvey, 2005).

Sex Differences and Hemispheric Specialization

Virtually every discipline of behavior has investigated the two sexes in an effort to identify and determine the origin and nature of putative behavioral and psychological differences. Neuropsychology and related professions have joined these efforts from the perspective of determining whether the sexes show brain-behavior differences. Although significant neuropsychological literature exists concerning sex differences, these empirical studies are inconsistent and often contradictory, precluding unequivocal conclusions. A number of morphologic (weight, volume, size, and composition) and functional differences have been identified through neuroimaging, electrophysiologic measures, and autopsy. Examples of structural and functional studies are presented in Tables 6.3 and 6.4, respectively. The most consistent findings relate to hemispheric differences, particularly in the morphology and activation of left temporal regions associated with language, as well as the anterior cingulate, corpus callosum, and gray/white matter ratios. However, not all studies have identified significant or similar differences (Sommer, Aleman, Bouma, & Kahn, 2004). For example, as presented in Table 6.3, Good et al. (2001) found that healthy male participants presented greater leftward asymmetry of the planum temporale than healthy female participants, whereas the opposite finding was evident in a study by Knaus, Bollich, Corey, Lemen, & Foundas (2004). Methodologic differences and weaknesses likely contribute to the inconsistencies in findings. The identification and control of moderating variables (age, handedness, hormonal levels, task type, method of administration, and so forth) and improved standardization of and advances in neuroimaging and related techniques should help determine whether, and under what circumstances, the brains of female and male individuals differ.

It has been proposed that men are more likely to show strongly lateralized speech functions, whereas women are more likely to demonstrate bilateral or right representation of speech. This came to light when researchers noticed that, after suffering a left hemisphere stroke, women were less likely to suffer the language impairment seen in men (see Levy & Heller, 1992). Support for this proposition is provided by an fMRI study (Shaywitz et al., 1995) of men and women while performing a rhyming task. Brain activation during the rhyming task was found to be more bilateral in women than men. Specifically, males demonstrated activation of the left lateralized inferior frontal gyrus, whereas females exhibited bilateral activation in this brain region. Similarly, a study (Saucier & Elias, 2001) of the relation of hand gestures to speech revealed that males made significantly more hand gestures with the right hand when speaking, yet when listening to conversation, demonstrated an increase in gesturing with the left hand. Females, in contrast, did not demonstrate asymmetries in gesturing during either speech or listening. These findings suggest that males are more functionally lateralized in speech than females. However, several subsequent investigations have challenged these findings. Frost and colleagues (1999) determined that males and females did not differ in their activation patterns in an fMRI study involving the performance of a language comprehension task. Similarly, Knecht and colleagues (2000a) presented a word fluency task to 188 healthy right-handed male and female participants while undergoing fTCD. The performance of the two groups did not differ in word fluency performance. Of importance, the distribution of language lateralization was equivalent for males and females. Finally, a recent study (Boles, 2005) of the relation of sex to performance on measures of lateralized cerebral functions demonstrates several significant differences, but these differences were small, accounting for less than 9% of shared variance (commonality of measurement). The investigator concludes that sex differences on measures of laterality are so small as to preclude the use of these measures for clinical prediction.

Empirical investigations reveal that females show superiority in language abilities, whereas males demonstrate greater proficiency in visuospatial skills (Gur et al., 1999; Voyer, Voyer, & Bryden, 1995). Before reviewing this issue, however, several caveats are in order. First, the superiority of the respective sexes with regard to verbal and visuospatial skills does not pertain to all forms of verbal or visuospatial tasks. Second, the differences in performance reflect group data and are not large in magnitude. In fact, there is substantial *overlap* in the performance of the two groups. Based on a recent review of studies of sex differences, Hyde (2005) concludes that the research indicates that the sexes are significantly more alike than different. Specifically, the differences between the sexes across multiple domains (cognitive, memory, motor, social, and personality) were, at

Table 6.3   *Comparisons of Female and Male Brain Structures*

Sex	Investigations		
Female	Smaller overall brain size (Kolb & Whishaw, 1996)	Leftward asymmetry of the planum temporale (Knaus et al., 2004)	Larger isthmus of the corpus callosum (Steinmetz et al., 1992)
	Higher percentage of overall gray matter; distribution of white matter and cerebrospinal fluid (CSF) symmetric for the hemispheres (Gur et al., 1999)	Greater density of neuronal material in the left planum temporale (Witelson, Glezer, & Kigar, 1995)	Larger corpus callosum (Dubb, Gur, Avants, & Gee, 2003; Steinmetz et al., 1995)
	Increased gray matter volume adjacent to the depths of both central sulci and in the left superior temporal sulci, right Heschl's gyrus and planum temporale, right inferior frontal and frontomarginal gyri, and cingulate gyrus (Good et al., 2001)	Larger volume of gray matter in the dorsolateral prefrontal cortex and superior temporal gyrus (Schlaepfer et al., 1995)	Larger splenium of the corpus callosum with increasing size with age (Dubb et al., 2003)
		Greater cingulate sulcus volume (Paus et al., 1996)	Increased volume of the hippocampus across childhood and adolescent development (Giedd, Castellanos, Rajapakse, Vaituzis, & Rapoport, 1997)
		Proportionally larger Broca and Wernicke areas (Harasty, Double, Halliday, Kril, & McRitchie, 1997)	
Male	Higher percentage of overall white matter and CSF; higher percentage of gray matter in left hemisphere, white matter symmetric, and greater percentage of CSF in the right hemisphere (Gur et al., 1999)	Symmetry of the planum temporale (Knaus et al., 2004)	Larger genu and decreasing genu size with age (Dubb et al., 2003)
	Increased leftward asymmetry in the Heschl's gyrus and planum temporale; greater gray matter volume, bilaterally in the mesial temporal lobes, entorhinal and perirhinal cortex, and anterior lobes of the cerebellum (Good et al., 2001)	Thicker cortex, higher neuronal density, and increased neurons in the left temporal lobe (Rabinowics, Dean, Petetot, & de Courten-Meyers, 1999)	Increased volume of the lateral ventricles and amygdala across childhood and adolescent development (Giedd et al., 1997)
		Greater hippocampal dendritic reduction in male rats with aging (Markham, McKian, Stroup, & Juraska, 2004)	Longer corpus callosum and decrease in width of the trunk and genu of corpus callosum with age (Suganthy et al., 2003)
		Greater paracingulate sulcus volume (Paus et al., 1996)	
		Greater asymmetry (L > R) of the anterior cingulate due to increased fissurization (Yücel et al., 2001)	

best, small in approximately 80% of the studies reviewed. Third, sex differences may relate more to differences in sociocultural expectations, socialization, and experiential history than to neurobiological factors.

Differences in cognitive performance favoring female individuals include verbal fluency and perceptual speed (Halpern, 1992; Kimura, 1999), delayed verbal memory and retrieval efficiency (Drake et al., 2000), mathematic computation (Eals & Silverman, 1994; James & Kimura, 1997), episodic olfactory memory (Öberg, Larsson, & Bäckman, 2002), and fine-motor dexterity (Agnew, Bolla-Wison, Kawas, & Bleecker, 1988). Females further excel in one form of spatial memory that involves the encoding and

retrieval of object location. However, the latter superiority has been related to the greater verbal facility of females, rather than to their spatial ability (Postma, Izendoorn, & De Haan, 1998). Conversely, males show an advantage with tasks that involve mental rotation and spatial perception (Burton, Henninger, & Hafetz, 2005; Siegel-Hinson & McKeever, 2002), mathematic aptitude, map reading, aiming at and tracking objects, geographic knowledge (Kolb & Whishaw, 1996), and three-dimensional maze performance (Grön et al., 2000; Kimura, 1999; Roberts & Bell, 2003). Voyer et al. (1995) performed a **meta-analysis** of 286 empirical studies that involved spatial abilities and sex differences. The findings of the analysis

Table 6.4 *Neuroimaging and Electrophysiologic Comparisons of Male and Female Brains*

Sex	Investigations		
Female	fMRI: Bilateral activation of the inferior frontal gyrus (rhyming task) (Shaywitz et al., 1995)	fMRI: Greater activation of the left ventral premotor cortex (hands mental rotation) (Seurinck, Vingerhoets, de Lange, & Achten, 2004)	EEG: Greater right parietal activation than left (two-dimensional mental rotation); greater right parietal activation than left (three-dimensional mental rotation) (Roberts & Bell, 2003)
	MRI: Bilateral activation of the superior and middle temporal gyri (linguistic listening) (Kansaku, Yamaura, & Kitazawa, 2000)	PET: Greater activation of the right inferior frontal gyrus and right precentral cortex (concrete naming/face orientation) (Grabowski, Damasio, Eichhorn, & Tranel, 2003)	PET: Enhanced activation of the left amygdala (emotional memory) (Cahill et al., 2001)
	fMRI: Greater activation of the left superior frontal gyrus and the right medial frontal gyrus, and right prefrontal cortex, right inferior and superior parietal lobe (mazes) (Grön, Wunderlich, Spitzer, Tomczak, & Riepe, 2000)	fMRI: Predominately left-sided activation (visual discrimination and construction tasks) (Georgopoulos et al., 2001)	PET: Symmetric dorsal premotor activation (tactile discrimination) (Sadato, Ibañez, Deiber, & Hallett, 2000)
			fMRI: Greater in the orbitofrontal lobe in response to both happy and sad, relative to neutral, faces (Amin, Constable, & Canli, 2005)
Male	fMRI: Activation of the left lateralized inferior frontal gyrus (rhyming task) (Shaywitz et al., 1995)	fMRI: Greater activation of the lingual gyrus (hands mental rotation) (Seurinck, et al., 2004)	EEG: Greater left parietal activation than right activation (two-dimensional mental rotation); greater right parietal activation than left (three-dimensional mental rotation) (Roberts & Bell, 2003)
	MRI: Left activation of the superior and middle temporal gyri (linguistic listening) (Kansaku et al., 2000)	PET: Greater activation of left inferotemporal regions and other left hemisphere regions (concrete naming/face orientation) (Grabowski et al., 2003)	PET: Enhanced activation of the right amygdala (emotional memory) (Cahill et al., 2001)
	fMRI: Greater activation of the left parahippocampal gyrus and left hippocampus proper and right hippocampal gyrus and left posterior cingulate (mazes) (Grön et al., 2000)	fMRI: Primarily right hemisphere activation (visual discrimination and construction tasks) (Georgopoulos et al., 2001)	fMRI: Greater activation in bilateral parietal to fearful, relative to neutral, faces (Amin et al., 2005)
		fTCD: Comparable hemispheric activation to females (word fluency task) (Knecht, Deppe, Dräger, Bobe, Lohmann, Flöel, et al., 2000)	fMRI: Comparable hemispheric activation to males (language comprehension task) (Frost et al., 1999)

Note: fMRI = functional magnetic resonance imaging; PET = positron emission tomography; fTCD = Doppler-ultrasonography; EEG = electroencephalography.

were as follows: males showed significantly greater proficiency relative to the performance of females with tasks that involve **mental rotation** (ability to mentally rotate two- or three-dimensional figures quickly and accurately) and **spatial perception** (ability to determine spatial relations despite the presence of distracting information). Further analysis demonstrated that sex differences generally did not emerge until after 13 years of age, and the magnitude of sex differences in mental rotation and spatial perception increased with age. Of significance, sex differences were evident on only certain measures of mental rotation and spatial perception, suggesting that (1) spatial

ability is not a unitary concept, but rather represents a group of relatively distinct component skills; and (2) males do not demonstrate an advantage across all tasks that involve spatial abilities.

A number of studies have endeavored to determine whether men and women recruit different brain circuitry during spatial processing (Voyer et al., 1995). Illustrating this research is a neuroimaging (fMRI) study by Grön and colleagues (2000) that determined a significant overlap in the neural circuitry activated while performing mazes, with exclusive activation in the left parahippocampal gyrus and left hippocampus proper for males, and in the left superior frontal gyrus and the right medial frontal gyrus for females. In addition, males showed greater activation of the right hippocampal gyrus and left posterior cingulate, as compared to females who demonstrated increased activity of the right prefrontal cortex, right inferior and superior parietal lobe. Finally, males were more proficient than females in solving the mazes. While males and females appear to use different neural circuitry during maze performance, this does not rule out the possibility that other factors (for example, experiential history with spatial activities) may account for the greater facility of males in maze performance.

A variety of explanations for the sex differences in spatial processing, particularly mental rotation, have been proposed. One explanation, consistent with our discussion, relates the male advantage in spatial processing to the greater specialization of this function to the right hemisphere. A second proposal is that men have more experience in spatial processing by virtue of socialization and role expectations. In a relatively recent lateralized tachistoscopic study (Siegal-Hinson & McKeever, 2002), males were found to be more right hemisphere specialized (left visual field superiority) and to have greater previous spatial activity experience than females. The magnitude of right hemisphere specialization correlated significantly and positively with mental rotation ability. Further analysis determined that sex differences in spatial ability were primarily related to right hemisphere specialization, and experiences with spatial activity were of only secondary importance. Thus, experience with spatial activities was not supported as a primary determinant of the difference in performance of the sexes. However, other lateralized tachistoscopic studies have not identified male-related visual field superiority in spatial processing (Siegal-Hinson & McKeever, 2002), highlighting the current contradictions in this area of study.

Women have been found to work more carefully than men when performing mental rotation tasks, suggesting that time may be a factor influencing overall performance (Voyer, 1997). Yet, when females and males were presented a mental rotation task without time constraints (Voyer, Rodgers, & McCormick, 2004), males once again showed an overall advantage in performance. Thus, behavioral style (careful, time-consuming approach) did not account for the difference in mental rotation performance. Spatial experiences and stylistic approach are but two of several factors that could account for sex differences in spatial performance. A multitude of social and cultural influences shape and maintain sex differences. Unfortunately, the ultimate impact of these sociocultural influences on sex are complex, often subtle, and not fully understood.

Adding to the complexity of determining whether sex differences exist in neuropsychological functioning is the realization that task variations can prompt the recruitment of different neural circuits. For example, mental rotation of two-dimensional figures appears to recruit more right parietal activation than left activation for females. The opposite pattern (left > right parietal activation) is evident for males. Yet, with three-dimensional figures, greater right parietal activation is evident for both males and females (Roberts & Bell, 2003). Further exemplifying the effects of task differences on level of performance and recruited neural processes is a recent fMRI study (Seurinck, Vingerhoets, de Lange, & Achten, 2004) that compares the performance of male and female healthy volunteers in the mental rotation of tasks that involve hands and tools. The neuroimaging findings of the participants with comparable levels of mental rotation performance demonstrated that both sexes activated a common neural substrate (superior parietal lobe, dorsolateral premotor cortex, and extrastriate occipital regions). However, activation differences were evident in the mental rotation of hands, with females showing greater involvement of the left ventral premotor cortex and males demonstrating greater activation of the lingual gyrus. These, as well as other studies, demonstrate the effects that task variations might have on neuropsychological performance both across and between the sexes. Moreover, task variations may contribute to the failure of investigators to replicate results and likely account for contradictory findings.

Although a number of studies report that females show greater facility with verbal skills, particularly verbal fluency, conflicting studies are also evident. Similar to the findings with spatial tasks, different verbal tasks may recruit different neural substrates for males and females. For example, men and women were asked to name concrete aspects of visually presented objects and perform a face orientation decision task while undergoing PET (Grabowski et al., 2003). Males showed greater activation of the left inferotemporal and other left hemisphere regions than females. In contrast, females demonstrated greater activation of the right inferior frontal gyrus and right precentral cortex, as compared to males who evidenced less activation or actual deactivation of these regions. These differences suggest that men and women use different strategies in processing similar contents.

Increasingly, empirical efforts to control variables that may account for differences in sex-related neuropsychological performance are evident, as illustrated in Georgopoulos and colleagues' (2001) study. Men and women were presented two visual tasks: one task required visual discrimination and another required visual object construction. The same visual stimuli were used for both tasks, thus reducing the likelihood that task differences accounted for performance. The visual discrimination task required the participants to judge whether pairs of square fragments were the same or different, whereas the visual object construction task required a determination of whether square fragments, when visually assembled and related, would make a "perfect square." Blood oxygen level–dependent (BOLD) fMRI did not show differences in left versus right hemispheric activation for the sexes when performing the visual discrimination task. However, the sexes did differ with respect to the visual object construction task, with females showing predominately left-sided activation, and males exhibiting both left and right hemisphere activation. The finding of increased right hemisphere activation was specific to the performance of men. The difference in performance between males and females could not be attributed to the features of the task employed, and thus reflected the cognitive operations recruited. That is, the two sexes appeared to utilize different cognitive strategies to solve the visual constructive tasks.

Sex differences have also been presented for emotionality. Wager, Phan, Liberzon, and Taylor (2003) conducted a meta-analysis of 65 neuroimaging studies related to sex, emotions, lateralization, and other relevant variables. These results indicate that the relationship between sex, brain activation, and emotional responses is much more complex than originally believed. Both sexes showed similar lateralized activation patterns for emotion, although men showed these patterns to a greater degree. Differences in neural activation by sex were most evident at the regional, rather than the hemispheric, level. At the regional level, the sexes recruited relatively distinct but overlapping areas, with some regions lateralized left and others right. When processing emotions, males activated the left inferior frontal cortex and posterior cortex, and females more reliably involved the midline limbic regions, including the **subcallosal anterior cingulate,** thalamus, midbrain, and cerebellum. Moreover, females showed left involvement in regions surrounding the amygdala **(sublenticular nuclei),** and males activated right-sided regions near the hippocampus. Based on these findings, Wager and colleagues speculate that males may be more biased toward processing the sensory aspects of emotional stimuli with regard to action, whereas females direct more attention to the subjective experience of emotion or, alternatively, show greater overt response to emotion. Finally, whether these regional and lateralized sex differences relate to actual or meaningful behavioral differences awaits further study.

The impact of sociocultural opportunities, resources, expectations, and attitudes regarding sex differences cannot be underestimated. For example, greater facility with mathematics has been attributed to males relative to females.

Although some have maintained that this greater facility is sex determined, Neuropsychology in Action 6.2 clearly challenges this supposition.

In summary, there are indications that females show an advantage in verbal abilities, while males tend to demonstrate superiority in visuospatial ability, particularly related to mental rotation tasks. However, these differences are not uniformly supported, and sex differences may be a consequence of sociocultural rather than neurobiological influences, or the interaction of these factors. Finally, differences in emotional processing are evident for males and females that do not conform to a simple left or right hemispheric specialization.

SEXUAL HORMONES

Because of the pervasive effects of sex hormones on development and functioning, investigations have sought to determine whether hormonal influences relate to sex differences in neuropsychological functioning. Much of this focus has been on the reproductive hormones (androgen and ovarian). An **androgen hormone** refers to any steroid hormone with a "masculinizing" effect. Up to 95% of androgens are produced by the testes. The principal functions of the androgen hormones include the masculinization of the fetus, production of sperm, and development of secondary sexual characteristics. The ovarian hormones (estrogens and progestins) are primarily secreted by the ovaries. These hormones are responsible for the in utero "feminization" of the brain, regulation of the ovarian-reproductive cycle, secondary sexual characteristics, and menopause. Sex hormones are believed to have both an organizing and activating effect. The organization effect relates to the effects of early exposure to hormones during prenatal development, whereas the activation effect refers to the effects of hormones during later development; that is, prenatal exposure to hormones organizes the way behavior is activated by hormones later in development. The masculinization and feminization of the prenatal brain exemplifies the organizing effects of sex hormones, while the physical and psychological changes associated with puberty and menstruation illustrate the activating effects. Notably, male and female hormones are not restricted to either sex in that both sexes produce androgen and ovarian hormones. Sex differences are evident in the hormonal-induced organization of the brain and the ratio of male-to-female circulating hormones in the respective sexes.

Efforts to determine whether reproductive hormones account for visuospatial sex differences have involved studies of healthy individuals, individuals with developmental abnormalities affecting hormone levels, and those

Neuropsychology in Action 6.2

A Land Where Girls Rule in Math

by Vivienne Walt

During January 2005, Harvard President Larry Summer reignited the debate over whether males and females differ with regard to cognitive aptitude with his statement that men may have more "intrinsic aptitude" for high-level science than women. Although the neurosciences have revealed sex differences in brains for size, rate of development, and regions of activation when problem solving and processing, these findings neither clarify the interactive contributions of brain neurophysiology and social-environmental forces to aptitude nor account for differences in performance. Although greater facility in mathematics has been attributed to males, Vivienne Walt provides evidence that this difference may not be sex specific:

> This fishing village of 1,480 people is a bleak and lonely place, even in a country suspended at the top of the world. Set on the southwestern edge of Iceland, the volcanic landscape is whipped by the North Atlantic winds, which hush everything around them. A sculpture at the entrance to the village depicts a naked man facing a wall of seawater twice his height. There is no movie theater, and many residents never venture to the capital, a 50-minute drive away.

> But Sandgerdi might be the perfect place to raise girls who have mathematical talent. Government researchers two years ago tested almost every 15-year-old in Iceland for it and found that boys trailed far behind girls. That fact was unique among the 41 countries that participated in the standardized test for that age group designed by the Organization of Economic Cooperation and Development. But while Iceland's girls were alone in the world in their significant lead in math, their national advantage of 15 points was small compared

with the one they had over boys like Sandgerdi, where it was closer to 30.

The teachers of Sandgerdi's 254 students were only mildly surprised by the results. They say the gender gap is a story not of talent but motivation. Boys think of school as purgatory on the way to a future of finding riches at sea; for girls, it's their ticket out of town. Margret Ingporsdottir, and Hanna Maria Heidarsdottir, both 15, students at Sandgerdi's gleaming school—which has a science laboratory, a computer room and a well-stocked library—have no doubt that they are headed for university. "I think I will be a pharmacist," says Hdeidarsdottir. The teens sat in principal Gudjon Kristjansson's office last week, waiting for a ride to the nearby town of Kevlavik, where they were competing in West Iceland's yearly math contest, one of many throughout Iceland in which girls excel.

Meanwhile, by the harbor, Gisli Tor Hauksson, 14, already has big plans that don't require speeding his afternoons toiling over geometry. "I'll be a fisherman," he says, just like most of his ancestors. His father recently returned home from 60 days at sea off the cost of Norway. "He came back with 1.1 million krona," about $18,000, says Hauksson. As for school, he says, "it destroys the brain." He intends to quit at 16, the earliest age at which he can do so legally. "A boy sees his older brother who has been at sea for only two years and has a better car and a bigger house than the headmaster," says Kristjansson.

But the story of female achievement in Iceland doesn't necessarily have a happy ending. Educators have found that when girls leave rural enclaves to attend universities in the nation's cities, their science advantage generally shrinks. While 61% of

university students are women, they make up only one-third of Iceland's science students. By the time they enter the labor market, many are overtaken by men, who become doctors, engineers and computer technicians. Educators say they watch many bright girls suddenly recoil in the face of real, head-to-head competition with boys. In a math class at a Reykjavik school, Asgeir Gurdmundsson, 17, says that although girls were consistently brighter than boys at school, "they just seem to leave the technical jobs to us." Says Solrun Gensdottir, the director of education at the Ministry of Education, Science and Culture: "We have to find a way to stop girls from dropping out of sciences."

Teachers across the country have begun to experiment with ways to raise boys to the level of girls in elementary and secondary school education. Last year Sandgerdi's teachers segregated the 10th-grade mathematics classes after deciding that boys needed intensive instruction. "The girls are strong students, so both the teachers and the students liked it," says Kristjansson. But left alone, "some of the boys had such behavior problems that they spoiled it for the lot."

The high school in Kevlavik tried the same experiment in 2002 and '03, separating 16-to-20-year-olds by gender for two years. That time the boys slipped even further behind. "The boys said the girls were better anyway," says Kristian Asmundsson, who taught the 25 boys. "They didn't even try."

Vivienne Walt, "A Land Where Girls Rule in Math," Time, March 7, 2005, pp. 56–57. Reprinted by permission of Time, Inc.

with surgically induced or naturally occurring reductions in hormone levels (Erlanger, Kutner, & Jacobs, 1999). Studies of healthy subjects show a possible inverted U-shaped curve regarding the effects of androgens on spatial performance (Moffat & Hampson, 1996); that is, a positive correlation is evident between testosterone levels and spatial task performance for females, but a negative correlation exists for males. Thus, males with elevated levels of testosterone exhibit poorer spatial performance, whereas females with increased levels demonstrate enhanced spatial performance. Additional investigations with healthy participants indicate that average, not extreme, levels of testosterone relate to optimal spatial performance; that is, high levels of testosterone for males and low levels for females are each associated with reduced spatial performance (McCormick & Teillon, 2001). Similarly, transsexuals undergoing cross-sex hormonal treatment also demonstrate differences in spatial performance. Individuals moving from a male to female gender demonstrate decreased spatial performance when administered antiandrogens and estrogen, whereas those moving from a female to male gender demonstrate improved spatial performance when treated with testosterone supplements (van Goozen, 1994; van Goozen, Cohen-Kettenis, Gooren, Frijda, & Van de Poll, 1995). Overall, these findings suggest that *increased* levels of male androgens enhance the spatial performance of females, but have a "demasculinizing" effect on male spatial performance. Notably, however, male androgens are not the only hormones that effect spatial performance. For example, higher levels of estrogen are associated with poorer spatial performance (Jones, Braithwaite, & Healy, 2003). Young women regularly taking oral contraceptives have near postmenopausal levels of estradiol and also perform more poorly on some spatial tasks than women not taking oral contraceptives (Mohn, Spiers, & Sakamoto, 2005).

The circulating levels of both male and female hormones warrant consideration when sex differences are the subject of investigation. For example, one study (Drake et al., 2000) demonstrated that sex hormones may affect cognitive abilities in a differential manner. In this study, the estrogen, progesterone, androstenedione (natural hormone that is a direct precursor to testosterone), and testosterone circulating levels of healthy elderly women were compared with measures of neurocognitive functioning. The results showed that high levels of estrogen were associated with better delayed verbal memory and retrieval, whereas low levels were correlated with better immediate and delayed visual memory. Interestingly, testosterone levels were positively associated with verbal fluency, but levels of progesterone and androstenedione did not have any relationship to cognitive performance.

In addition, circulating levels of female hormones may interact with brain organization. For example, as discussed earlier, right-handers are largely considered left hemisphere dominant for speech; however, sex may influence bilateral expression of speech or other abilities. It may also be that other brain organizing factors, such as degree of left-handedness in the family, termed **familial sinistrality,** may interact with the sexual organization of the brain. It has been suggested that right-handed women

with left-handed relatives (that is, familial sinistrals [FS+] women) may have shifted brain organization away from the "female" preference for high reliance on verbal strategies and toward more male strategies (Annett, 1985, 2002). This has been supported in investigations of spatial performance on the Rey Complex Figure test (Rey, 1941, translated by Corwin & Bylsma, 1993), where familial sinistrality accounted for performance and strategy regardless of academic major, with FS+ women performing as well or better than men (D'Andrea & Spiers, 2005a, 2005b). These investigators also report that across a range of spatial, verbal, and speeded motor tasks, familial sinistrality interacted with the menstrual cycle such that FS+ women performed better on all tasks during menses when ovarian hormone levels were low, whereas women without the hypothesized shift (FS− women) performed better on all tasks close to ovulation when ovarian levels were high (D'Andrea & Spiers, 2005a)

These various findings highlight the complexity of the relation of sex hormones to the performance of the sexes. Increasingly, we are realizing that the variables that interact with sex hormones and gender are multiple and not fully understood. Illustrating this issue is a relatively recent investigation (van Goozen, Gooren, Slabbekoorn, Sanders, & Cohen-Kettenis, 2002) in which individuals undergoing transsexual hormonal treatment did not demonstrate the predicted shift in spatial performance. Previous studies have frequently used "mixed" transsexual groups composed of right- and left-handed transsexuals who were either homosexual or heterosexual. In van Goozen and colleagues' study, the spatial performance of only right-handed, homosexual transsexuals was contrasted with the performance of heterosexual participants. The transitioning transsexuals were treated with the appropriate sex hormone supplements and pretested and post-tested with a battery of spatial measures. Post-testing was undertaken 3 months after the sex hormone treatment. Results regarding levels of pretest and post-test spatial performance were as follows: heterosexual male control participants showed a higher level of performance than homosexual males transitioning to female gender, who, in turn, demonstrated greater proficiency than homosexual females transitioning to male gender. Heterosexual female control participants achieved significantly lower scores than the previous three groups. Pretesting to post-testing did not demonstrate a significant effect of sex hormone treatment on spatial performance. The authors speculate that the failure to find the predicted effect may have been due to the unique composition of the transsexual group. They note that previous investigations have suggested that homosexual transsexuals are biologically more similar to their desired sex, and their spatial performance tends to be similar to the opposite sex. Accordingly, their level of spatial performance would more closely approximate the opposite sex before sex hormone treatment; thus, the degree or magnitude of possible change in performance would be limited ("ceiling effect") after the introduction of sex hormones. Second, the authors report that left-handed individuals are more sensitive to neuroendocrinologic interventions, and the omission of this group may have accounted for the failure to find an activating effect of sex hormone treatment. Although replication and expansion of this study is warranted, it serves to capture the difficulty of disentangling the effects of sex hormones on gender performance.

Investigations of individuals with developmental disorders that affect reproductive hormones have identified similar relations between androgen levels and visuospatial performance. For example, individuals with **congenital adrenal hyperplasia** (CAH; an endocrine disorder of prenatal origin characterized by excessively high levels of androgen hormones) have been the subject of research. Hampson and colleagues (1998) compared the visuospatial performance of preadolescent girls with CAH to unaffected control participants and found that the visuospatial performance of the CAH group was significantly higher. In the same study, boys with CAH hyperplasia showed lower visuospatial proficiency relative to the performance of unaffected control boys. In a similar vein, individuals with **androgen insensitivity** (genetic males who produce androgens but whose androgen receptors are not responsive to the hormone) demonstrate lower performance relative to verbal intelligence when contrasted with male and female control participants (Imperato-McGinley, Pichardo, Gautier, Voyer, & Bryden, 1991). The measure of performance intelligence involved tasks requiring visual, visuospatial, and visuomotor abilities.

For verbal abilities, a number of studies demonstrate that women, during the high-estrogen phase of their menstrual cycle, demonstrate enhanced cognitive skills in color naming and color reading, mental flexibility, and paired-associate learning (see Erlanger et al., 1999 for review). A comparison (Phillips & Sherwin, 1992) of the cognitive performance of women before and after hysterectomies who received either an estrogen supplement or a placebo revealed that the women who maintained their presurgical estrogen levels demonstrated comparable memory recall (paragraph recall). In contrast, those in the postsurgery placebo group exhibited a significant decline in memory performance. A similar decrement in memory performance has been documented in women who have been administered estrogen-suppressing agents (Sherwin & Tulandi, 1996). Shaywitz and associates (1999) investigated the fMRI activation patterns of postmenopausal females when tested with tasks of verbal and nonverbal memory. One group was treated for 21 days with estrogen, and the second group received a placebo. The estrogen-treated group showed greater left hemisphere activation during encoding and increased activation in the right frontal superior frontal gyrus during retrieval. Increased activation of the inferior parietal lobe was evident during storage of verbal information, and deceased activation of the inferior parietal lobe was observed during the storage of nonverbal information. Interestingly, the two groups, despite their differences in regional activation, performed in a comparable manner on the measures of verbal and nonverbal memory. A number of studies (see Cameron's [2001] review) have failed to support the enhancing effects of hormone replacement therapy on cognitive performance. The mixed results suggest that certain hormone regimens may have an enhancing (although subtle) effect on specific cognitive and memory processes.

Cognitive concerns are frequently voiced by women going through menopause. When the ovaries stop producing estrogen, only estrone (a weaker sex hormone produced by the adrenal glands) remains. Initially, it was believed that the risk for stroke, heart disease, vascular dementia, and osteoporosis were associated with decreased estrogen production. Although estrogen augmentation has been associated with improved cognitive performance in menopausal women, particularly in the area of verbal memory, other studies have provided contradictory results. A meta-analysis of studies (Yaffe, Sawaya, Lieberburg, & Grady, 1998) suggests that improved cognitive performance is evident only in women receiving estrogen therapy who were recently menopausal. More disturbing have been recent large-scale studies (Nelson, Humphrey, Nygren, Teutsch, & Allan, 2002; Shumaker et al., 2003, 2004; Wassertheil-Smoller et al., 2003) demonstrating that estrogen therapy for postmenopausal females may *increase* the risk for stroke, thromboembolic events, breast cancer (with 5 or more years of use), and cholecystitis (inflammation of the gall bladder). An increased risk for dementia appears to be evident for women 65 years or older (Espeland et al., 2004). Related to the latter finding, a recent study (Erickson et al., 2005) of elderly women who were maintained on estrogen treatment for up to 10 years demonstrated spared gray matter in the frontal cortex and increased performance on measures of executive function. In contrast, elderly women who continued estrogen treatment beyond 10 years exhibited increased prefrontal deterioration and a greater rate of decline on the measures of executive function. Currently, the increases in physical and cognitive risk associated with prolonged estrogen therapy in postmenopausal women appear to over-ride the modest gains initially evident in cognitive functioning.

Overall, sex hormones appear to have an organizing and activating effect on brain development and functioning. Studies of varied gender groups show that sex hormones have either an enhancing or depressing effect on cognitive performance depending on such factors as the levels of circulating hormones, the specific sex hormone manipulated, type of task introduced, and age of the participants. Notably, similar neural substrates are often implicated in the cognitive processing of the sexes, and identified differences are often more of degree than type. In addition, differences in activated or recruited neural substrates do not necessarily translate into observable or meaningful differences in cognitive performance.

Summary

In this chapter, we examined the major structures and functions of the cortex, setting the stage for examining the systematic interaction of brain regions (cortical and subcortical) that support the complex behaviors that are presented in subsequent chapters. Hemispheric differences exist, but they are not consistent with the simple notion that people are either "right-brained" or "left-brained" in their behavior. Generally, the brain functions as a cohesive whole with interconnected pathways and regions performing both distinct and overlapping functions. However, certain functions, such as speech, tend to be lateralized to one hemisphere or the other. Lateralization does not imply that the other hemisphere is not providing a complementary function. For example, the left hemisphere is generally specialized for verbal speech, whereas the right hemisphere plays an equally important role in providing the prosodic aspects to speech.

Sex differences in the performance of neuropsychological tasks are evident, although the sexes overlap in their performance and the actual differences are small. Morphologic and functional brain differences have been identified; however, there is a lack of empirical consensus. Because of the organizing and activating influence of sex hormones, the relation of these hormones to neuropsychological performance has been the subject of considerable investigation. Androgens appear to have an enhancing effect on visuospatial performance, whereas the bolstering effect of estrogen on verbal performance has received less support. Certainly, the relation of sex hormones to neuropsychological performance is complex, and additional studies are warranted to identify the factors that mediate this relation.

Critical Thinking Questions

- How would you explain the functional differences between the right and left hemispheres?
- Are there adaptive reasons why the cerebral hemispheres would gravitate toward either a bilateral or asymmetric organization? Explain.
- What ecologic or evolutionary factors could account for the advantage of males in visuospatial abilities?

Key Terms

Cerebral hemispheres	Occipital notch	Dominance	Spatial perception
Fissures	Brodmann's areas	Doppler ultrasonography	Subcallosal anterior cingulate
Frontal lobes	Somatosensory cortex	(fTCD)	Sublenticular nuclei
Parietal lobes	Primary motor cortex	Sylvian fissure	Androgen hormone
Temporal lobes	Association or polymodal areas	Heschl's gyrus	Familial sinistrality
Occipital lobes	Wada test	Planum temporale	Congenital adrenal
Lateral fissure	Hemispheric asymmetry	Meta-analysis	hyperplasia
Central sulcus	Lateralization	Mental rotation	Androgen insensitivity

Web Connections

Neuroanatomy

http://www.med.harvard.edu/AANLIB/hms1.html

Chapter 7

SOMATOSENSORY, CHEMICAL, AND MOTOR SYSTEMS

[W]e naturally came into conflict both with the naive mechanistic ideas of localization, in which mental functions are consigned to rigidly demarcated areas of the brain, and with the idealistic concept that the higher mental processes stand quite apart from the biological functions of the brain or result from the indivisible activity of the "brain as a whole."

—*Alexander Luria*

Somatosensory Processing
Chemical Senses
Motor Systems

Neuropsychology in Action

7.1 Synesthesia: Melded Sensory Integration
7.2 Phantoms of Feeling
7.3 Tourette Syndrome: Too Much Behavior

Keep in Mind

■ How does the brain map incoming sensory information?

■ Is sensory information processed in the same manner by each system?

■ What happens when brain alteration causes malfunctions of ordinary experiences of perception?

Overview

A functional system is a circumscribed area of behavior that corresponds to a specific neuroanatomic pathway or network of pathways. Some systems are well defined and traceable, and others remain incompletely mapped. The sensory systems are among the most well delineated.

At times tracing systems through the brain may appear mechanistic, like the "leg bone connected to the thigh bone" routine. Scientists have gained their current understanding of the brain by identifying individual functions and attempting to map them to structure hierarchically, from lower to higher order functions. However, many structures participate in multiple functions. A complex internetworking of functions is evident in the progression from the sensory and motor systems to higher functional systems where the work involves anatomic networks that are sometimes widely dispersed throughout the brain.

The brain is a dynamic biological network, but a small lesion in a strategic location can have devastating effects on the system. It is therefore impossible to gain a thorough understanding of sensory and motor systems by studying only intact brains. Russian psychologist Alexander Luria, whose pioneering work made possible our understanding of functional brain systems, has argued that although higher mental functions may be disturbed by a lesion in any of the many different links of the system, they are disturbed differently by lesions in different links (Luria, 1966). Luria's research profited greatly from his keen observations of neurologic patients. He noticed that anatomically different lesions were possible within the same behavioral syndrome. He also noticed that a lesion in one area could affect a number of different behaviors.

The functional systems we focus on in this chapter may be broadly categorized as arising from sensory input and resulting in motor output. This chapter focuses on the somatosensory and motor systems, as well as the chemical senses of taste and smell. In the next chapter, we examine the visual and auditory systems. We concentrate on how each system operates at the level of central brain mechanisms. Most sensory systems are anatomically mapped to specific cortical areas devoted to primary sensory processing, which provide information that is then routed to secondary processing areas where it is "perceived" and meaning is attached. All sensory systems except smell follow a pathway through the thalamus, where they are directed to primary and secondary cortical processing areas (Figure 7.1). This chapter examines how each system functions at the level of the brain, and what can happen when behavior goes awry because of injury or disease. In general, we discuss disorders that illustrate a specific breakdown of a system rather than broad-based disorders. Also, the odd phenomenon of synesthesia is presented as an interesting possible evolutionary mutation (Neuropsychology in Action 7.1). (We discuss disorders that involve multiple systems in later chapters.)

Sensation is the body's window to the world. The range of what humans can detect is unique to our species and becomes the raw material of our perceptions and the stuff of our experiences. Information comes in fragments and requires the central processor of the brain to literally "make sense" of the outside environment. Sensation begins with the process of **transduction** (derived from the Latin *transducere,* meaning to "lead across"). An environmental stimulus activates a specific **receptor cell,** creating energy, which is transduced into an electrical stimulus that is then carried to neurons for the brain to process. (Receptor cells are not technically neurons, although they do synapse with

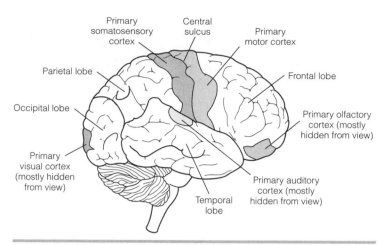

Figure 7.1   Primary sensory and motor cortexes. In general, primary sensory processing lies posterior to the central sulcus, and primary motor processing is anterior. The chemical senses of olfaction and taste are the exception. The primary gustatory cortex cannot be seen from this view. (Adapted from Banich, M. T. [1997]. *Neuropsychology: The neural bases of mental function* [p. 25, Figure 4.1]. Boston: Houghton Mifflin Company, by permission.)

neurons.) Sensory receptor cells throughout the body detect numerous stimuli, including sight, sound, pressure, pain, chemical irritation, smell, and taste, to name a few. We hear with our ears and see with our eyes, but if photoreceptor cells were on our hands, we would see with our fingers. Some sensory systems are complex. For example, taste uses multiple transduction processes to detect subtle differences of flavor. The visual system uses two primary types (rods and cones), and the auditory system uses a single basic mechanism.

> The hour is striking so close above me,
> so clear and sharp,
> that all my senses ring with it.
> I feel it now; there's a power in me
> to grasp and give shape to my world.
> I know that nothing has ever been real
> without my beholding it.
> All becoming has needed me.
> My looking ripens things
> and they come toward me, to meet and be met.
>
> —*Rainer Maria Rilke*

Agnosia, the inability to recognize the form and/or function of objects and people, occurs in every sensory domain. For example, **tactile agnosia,** also called **astereognosis,** is an inability to recognize objects by touch; for instance, failing to recognize a quarter or a pen held in the hand. Agnosia is possible in every sensory domain and can sometimes result in odd behavior. In his popular book of

neurologic tales, *The Man Who Mistook His Wife for a Hat* (1987), Oliver Sacks tells the story of a music professor who, coming upon his wife standing next to a coat rack, tried to lift her head instead of his hat. He no longer "knew" people or objects visually, but relied on distinctive voice characteristics and his other senses for identification.

Agnosia is not a single sensory phenomenon. It may strike any sensory domain, but the most commonly studied instances affect the somatosensory visual and auditory senses. Olfactory and taste agnosias have not been researched extensively. Agnosias, in general, are relatively rare, but they have received considerable attention in the neuropsychological literature, perhaps because they so strikingly alter consciousness.

Somatosensory Processing

The **somatosensory system** includes two types of sensory stimulation, external and internal. This system can monitor sensations such as cold and heat, whether the sensation comes from handling an ice cube or from a fever. Thus, the system processes external stimulation of touch (pressure, shape, texture, heat) in recognizing objects by feel and is also concerned with the position of the body in extrapersonal space, termed **proprioception.** Sensory dysfunctions that result in proprioceptive disorders of altered sense of bodily sensation or bodily position are of great interest to neuropsychology.

Neuropsychology in Action 7.1

Synesthesia: Melded Sensory Integration

by Mary Spiers

One of the more exotic and seemingly rare (reported by 1 in 500,000) alterations in sensory processing is the "cross-wiring" of senses called *synesthesia*. One woman reported that tasting lemon is like "points pressing against the face," and spearmint feels like "cool glass columns." The most reported form of synesthesia is *"audition colorée,"* or colored hearing, described vividly by the synesthete poet Arthur Rimbaud in his poem *"Les Voyelles"* ("The Vowels").

Probably the most completely described case of synesthesia was "S," reported by Luria in his book *The Mind of a Mnemonist* (1968). Every sound, including tones, words, music, voices, and other noises, summoned up a vivid visual image. One tone could be a "velvet cord with fibers jutting out on all sides," whereas another tone conjured up a strip, the color of "old tarnished silver." The sound of a voice could be "crumbly and yellow" or like a "flame with fibers." Seeing sounds could often be so attention grabbing that "S" could not follow the content of what people were saying to him unless they spoke very slowly.

The melding of sensory perceptions appears unique to each person, but the underlying neural processes may be quite similar. Neurologist Richard Cytowic (1993) has suggested that the source of synesthesia emanates from the most primitive reaches of the brain, specifically the limbic system. In his early studies, Cytowic used xenon inhalation to study the dynamic blood flow activity within the brain of synesthetes in mid *audition colorée*. Contrary to his initial expectations, neural activity in the cortex did not increase, but actually decreased an average of 18%. Surprisingly, it was the limbic system that "lit up." Cytowic

Vowels

A black, E white, I red, U green, O blue: vowels,
One day I will tell you latent birth.
A, black hairy corset of shining flies
Which buzz around cruel stench,

Gulfs of darkness; E whiteness of vapors and tents,
Lances of proud glaciers, white kings, quivering of flowers;
I, purples, spit blood, laughter of beautiful lips
In anger or penitent drunkenness;

U cycles, divine vibrations of green seas,
Peace of pastures scattered with animals, peace of the wrinkles
which alchemy prints on heavy studious brows;

O supreme Clarion full of strange stridor,
Silences crossed by worlds and angels:
O, the Omega, violet beam from HIS eyes!

—Arthur Rimbaud

hypothesizes that the neocortex "turns off" during synesthetic processing whereas a more ancient, fundamental processing system takes over. Finding limbic system involvement seems congruent in light of the way Luria's patient S describes his own experiences:

> S: I recognize a word not only by the images it evokes, but by a whole complex of feelings that image arouses. It's hard to express . . . . Usually I experience a word's taste and weight, and I don't have to make an effort to remember it— the word seems to recall itself. But it's difficult to describe. What I sense is something oily slipping through my hand . . . or I'm aware of a slight tickling in my left hand caused by a mass of tiny, lightweight points. When that happens I simply remember, without having to make the attempt. (Luria, 1968, p. 28)

Mood and memory are intimately linked through the limbic system. In the case of S, auditory and visual sensation also appear linked to this system. The final effect was effortless and seemingly unlimited memory capacity. A sound, once experienced, would always recall an image. S went on to use this strange gift as a professional performer of feats of memory, astounding audiences throughout Russia.

Many viewed synesthesia as an abnormal medical oddity. It is different from other "disorders" in that it is not an effect of acquired brain damage. This cross-wiring appears to be "hardwired" since birth. If, as Cytowic suggests, synesthesia is an evolutionarily more primitive form of processing sensory experience, there may be remnants of synesthesia in many of us. Do you ever feel blue?

The somatosensory system contains a conglomeration of receptor types and sensory information. Receptors on the skin are attuned to external sensations such as the pressure of a hand, a blast of wind, the pricking of a finger, the vibrational frequency of touch, the burn of a hot stove, and the itching of poison ivy. Somatosensory receptors are also spread internally throughout the body to monitor the stretching of the stomach during eating and digestion, the pain of muscle aches, and the spatial position of arms and legs, to name a few examples. The receptor types

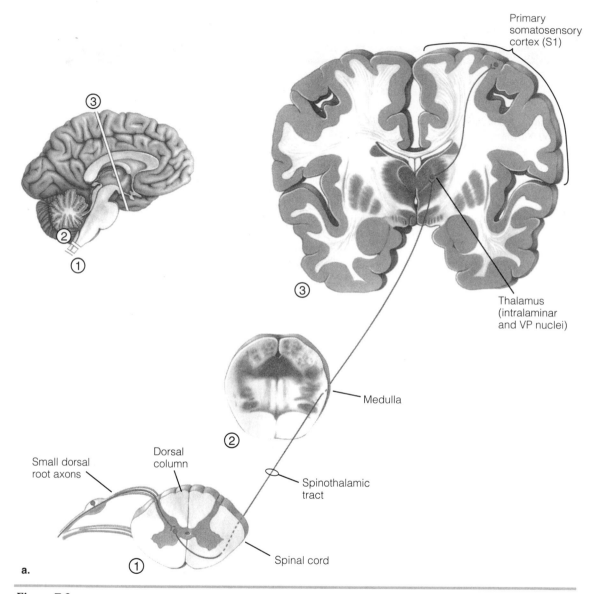

Primary somatosensory cortex (S1)

Thalamus (intralaminar and VP nuclei)

Medulla

Dorsal column

Small dorsal root axons

Spinothalamic tract

Spinal cord

a.

Figure 7.2 The two primary somatosensory pathways. (a) The ascending spinal-thalamic tract carries pain and temperature information. (b) The dorsal column medial lemniscal pathway carries touch and proprioceptive information. (Modified from Bear, M. F., Connors, B. W., & Paradiso, M. A. [1996]. *Neuroscience: Exploring the brain* [p. 327, Figure 12.15; p. 328, Figure 12.16]. Baltimore: Williams & Wilkins, by permission.)

and systems discussed in this section range over widely varying areas of function, from mechanical and chemical monitoring to damage and body position monitoring.

The somatosensory system begins at the level of receptors, of which five types are found on the skin and throughout the body. **Mechanical receptors** transduce energy from touch, vibration, and the stretching and bending of skin, muscle, internal organs, and blood vessels. A detailed discussion of subtypes is not necessary, but at least five different types of mechanical receptors exist. For ex-

ample, hair follicle receptors sense breezes or a brush of fern across the skin. They are essential to animals such as cats and mice in their whisker navigational system. **Chemoreceptors** respond to various chemicals on the surface of the skin and mucous membranes. They range from detecting level of stomach acidity to skin irritations. Smell and taste are special examples of chemoreception that we discuss separately. **Thermoreceptors** detect heat and cold. **Nociceptors** (derived from the Latin *nocere*, meaning "to hurt") serve as monitors to alert the brain to damage or

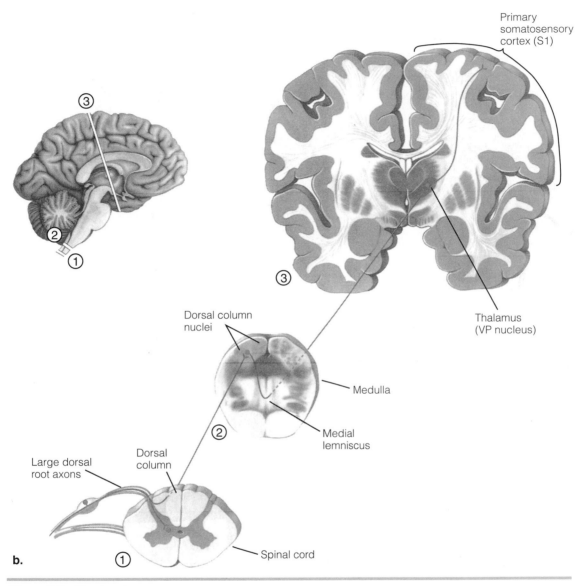

Figure 7.2 (Continued)

threat of damage. They can be mechanical or chemical, but are specifically activated by potentially damaging stimulation such as heat or cold, painful pressure or pricking, or chemical damage such as exposure to noxious chemicals. They are present throughout the body, but they are noticeably absent in the brain. This is how some types of brain surgery and brain mapping can be done while the patient is conscious and alert. **Proprioceptors** (derived from the Latin *proprius,* meaning "one's own") on skeletal muscles detect movement via degree of stretch, angle, and relative position of limbs. Proprioceptors on the hands help identify the shapes of objects via touch.

These somatosensory receptors synapse with neurons into two primary pathways that transmit information from the spinal cord to the thalamus (Figure 7.2). In each case, sensory information travels to the contralateral hemisphere from the point of origin. The first pathway, the **ascending spinal-thalamic tract,** carries sensory information related to pain and temperature and runs parallel to the spinal cord. It synapses over a wide region of the thalamus, and then to the somatosensory cortex. The second pathway is the **dorsal column medial lemniscal pathway,** which carries information pertaining to touch and vibration. It is so named because it is routed up the

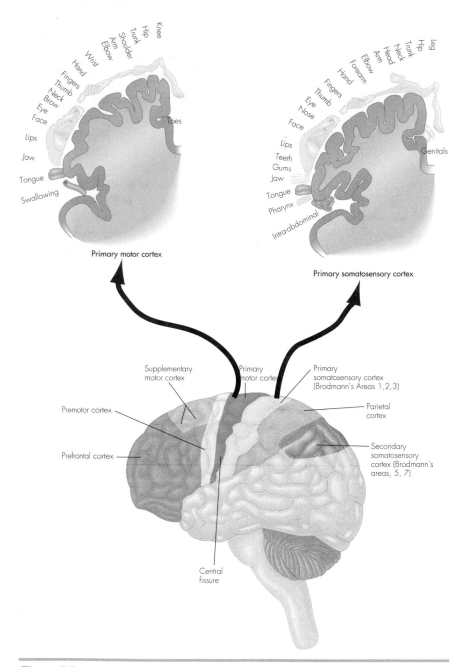

Figure 7.3 The homunculi from the primary motor and somatosensory cortexes. (Adapted from Kalat, J. W. [1998]. *Biological psychology* [6th ed., pp. 96, 227]. Pacific Grove, CA: Brooks/Cole.)

dorsal aspects of the spinal cord to a white matter tract termed the **medial lemniscus,** which courses through the contralateral side of the brainstem through the medulla, pons, and midbrain, and then up through the thalamus (ventral posterior nucleus) and on to the primary somatosensory cortex. All stimulation of the face is on a separate system through the large trigeminal nerve (cranial nerve V), which enters the brain through the pons.

The primary somatosensory cortex lies in the parietal lobe immediately posterior to the central sulcus on the post central gyrus (Brodmann's areas 1, 2, and 3; Figure 7.3). It is **somatopically organized;** that is, the distorted figure of the sensory homunculus mapped onto the primary somatosensory cortex represents the relative importance and distribution of touch in various areas of the body, rather than the actual size of the body part. Notice that the thumb,

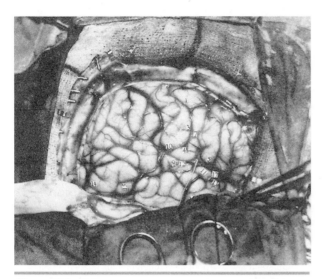

Figure 7.4 Penfield's electrical stimulation experiments. Penfield numbered sections of the open cortex of a conscious patient as he mapped the response to direct electrical stimulation to the brain. (From Case M. M., in Penfield, W. [1975]. *The mystery of the mind: A critical study of consciousness and the human brain, with discussions by William Feindel, Charles Hendel, and Charles Symonds* [Figure 4, p. 24]. Princeton, NJ: Princeton University Press, by permission.)

fingers, and face represent proportionately the largest areas. These are the areas of most sensitive and discriminating sensation in the body, having the largest proportion of touch receptors. The somatosensory system is organized contralaterally, with the left hemisphere processing tactile sensation from the right side of the body and vice versa. The work documenting the close correspondence of sensation to cortical mapping in the primary somatosensory cortex began in the early days of neurosurgery. In the 1940s, Wilder Penfield, a noted neurosurgeon at the Montreal Neurological Institute, started to use electrical stimulation to explore the functions of the cortex in patients undergoing neurosurgery for the relief of epilepsy. Applying electrical stimuli to different cortical areas in more than 1000 fully conscious patients, Penfield mapped motor, sensory, language, and memory functions (Figure 7.4).

From the primary somatosensory cortex, sensory information is then integrated at the next level in the secondary somatosensory cortex, which is immediately posterior (Brodmann's areas 5, 7). There, the individual properties of tactile stimuli such as shape, weight, and texture are combined to form the perception of single and whole percepts such as "pencil," "coin," or "key" that can be recognized by feel. Damage to this area may result in astereognosia, even though the person may readily recognize objects by sight. In this case, elementary powers of sensation are intact, but the person cannot recognize things placed in the hand contralateral to the lesion. Neuropsychologists usually test for

this problem by blindfolding the patient, placing an object in the hand, and asking the person to recognize and name it by touch only. Damage interrupting higher level somatosensory integration in the parietal area, particularly the right parietal lobe, may result in a problem variously referred to as *tactile suppression, tactile extinction,* or *tactile inattention.* In this instance of right parietal damage, a person does not report the sensation of touch on the left hand (that is, left-sided suppression) when the left and right hands are touched simultaneously, although he or she may accurately report a left-sided touch when that hand is touched in isolation. In this case, the problem involves sorting out competing tactile sensations. Left-sided touch is suppressed or extinguished when there is competing sensation from both sides of the body. Part of the Halstead–Reitan Neuropsychological Battery includes a sensory-perceptual examination that tests for finger agnosia, skin writing recognition, and sensory extinction in the tactile, auditory, and visual modalities (Reitan & Wolfson, 1993). Table 7.1 lists examples of somatosensory disorders.

Disorders of proprioception represent the second type of tactile disorder in that the sensory problem is one of recognizing the relative position of your own body in space, rather than the recognition of objects external to yourself. This is a problem of tactile integration, which is usually compromised by parietal lobe dysfunction. Because proprioceptors record from the stretching of muscle, what you are receiving as sensory information is feedback from your own motor movements. This sensory information then is available to feed back to fine-tune body movement. Normally, a combination of vision, the vestibular organs, and the proprioceptive sense supplies a **kinesthetic sense** of your physical body. Proprioception, like most elementary sensations, is so basic and automatic that you take it completely for granted unless it is disrupted or absent. Imagine, however, having no sense of where your hands and legs are, or even of your

---

Table 7.1 ***Examples of Somatosensory Dysfunction***

Astereognosis/tactile agnosia: inability to recognize an object by touch

Finger agnosia: inability to recognize or orient to one's own fingers

Paresthesia: spontaneous crawling, burning, or "pins and needles" sensation

Peripheral neuropathy: peripheral nervous system dysfunction causing sensory loss (for example, in diabetes)

Phantom limb pain: a feeling of pain in a nonexistent limb

Proprioceptive disorder: loss of body position sense

Tactile extinction/suppression/inattention: suppression of touch sensation on one side of body

Neuropsychology in Action 7.2

Phantoms of Feeling

by Mary Spiers

Phantoms are the experience of external sensory experience in the absence of available sensory input. This sounds strikingly like a hallucination. And perhaps had it not been for the widespread occurrence of phantoms felt by what are considered otherwise "rational" people, phantoms might have been considered psychosomatic experiences at best and psychotic episodes at worst. People most commonly think of phantoms in respect to phantom limb pain after amputation, but they can and do exist in any sensory modality. The interesting questions here are, How are phantoms experienced, and what are their causes? Finally, understanding phantoms may also provide some clues to understanding certain aspects of brain plasticity and reorganization.

Phantom limbs and phantom limb pain are most commonly associated with amputations. The amputee may feel a lost arm, feel that it swings in coordination with the other arm while walking, or experience it sticking out so much as to necessitate maneuvering through doors sideways. All the while, objective reality is shouting that it is not there. Cold, heat, pressure, itching, tickling, and sweat can all be experienced in the missing limb. Because as many as 70% of amputees experience pain in the amputated part, psychologists specializing in pain management are striving to understand causes and formulate treatments for this problem.

Phantoms may also be experienced in situations other than amputation and in senses other than tactile. Children born without limbs, people who have suffered paralysis after a spinal cord injury, and even women in labor who have had spinal anesthesia have also "felt" the presence of a limb. Some congenital amputees have reported being able to move nonexistent fingers or to experience the phantom emerge and disappear from consciousness. Phantom seeing and hearing can occur in the complete or partial absence of vision and audition. Auditory phantoms may be passed off as tinnitus, or ringing in the ears, but some people hear voices or music. Visual phantoms can also range from flashes of light and color to fully formed images of people and objects. In both cases, and perhaps a differentiating factor between these types of "hallucinations" and those experienced by schizophrenics, phantoms are quickly judged as separate from normal sensory-perceptual reality.

How can phantoms be described neurologically? Scientists know that phantoms emanate from central brain mechanisms rather than purely peripheral ones, although the exact mechanism for the production of phantoms is still a matter of some speculation. In the case of phantom limbs, amputations leave exposed nerve endings that heal

posture if your eyes are closed. In Oliver Sacks's case of the "Disembodied Lady" (Sacks, 1987), a young woman of 37, suffering a sensory neuritis, had the feeling of "losing" parts of her body if she could not see them; that is, she experienced the feeling of total disembodiment. Having no natural posture, her movements became a caricature of types, such as a dancer's pose. Quite the opposite problem is expressed in phantom limb pain. People with no external sensation entering the brain still have the curious experience of pain or other sensation. Neuropsychology in Action 7.2 explores this odd phenomenon.

Chemical Senses

Taste and smell evolutionarily are the oldest sensory systems. They work in concert, and to most people, they appear indistinguishable until a cold or other sinus condition congests and diminishes the sense of smell. People are likely to report that food does not "taste" so good or have as much flavor as usual, when it is actually blocked smell that is affecting the pleasurability of food. It is easy to experience this condition by just holding your nose and sampling different foods to see what "tastes" you actually experience. Taste and smell are also the least studied of the senses within neuropsychology and neuroscience. This neglect may be due, in part, to that other senses such as vision and audition are well developed in humans, and thus have overshadowed the chemical senses. The idea that the senses of taste and smell may be vestigial and no longer of any real adaptive use to modern humans has also probably contributed to the lack of interest. However, these chemical senses are enjoying a surge of research attention that is pointing to connections with emotional behavior, hormones, immunology, and identification of neurologic disease states.

TASTE

The tongue contains numerous **papillae** or bumps on which lie from one to several hundred taste buds consisting of between 50 and 150 taste receptor cells. The bundles of receptor cells resemble onions, with the cilia at the tips of the cells protruding into the surface of the pore.

as nodules called *neuromas*. Neuromas continue to generate neural impulses. For this reason, initial treatments focus on severing communication between the peripheral sensory input and the spinal cord. However, this does not obliterate phantoms. Consequently, as an attempted treatment, surgeons have blocked or cut spinal nerves, and then central pathways feeding the somatosensory cortex from the sensory relay station of the thalamus. But phantoms still exist. Traditional painkilling drugs are also largely ineffective, because phantom pain does not seem to arise from the same pain system.

From where in the brain do phantoms arise? Recent work in this area has led to rethinking about the supposed lack of plasticity of adult brains. A logical place to start is to understand what happens in the somatosensory strip when the corresponding sensory area on the body ceases to provide input. Researchers have done deep-brain electrode recordings on monkeys with an amputated finger. Surprisingly, sensory input from adjacent fingers remapped itself onto the somatosensory cortex so that it invaded the area previously serving the amputated finger. This remapping occurred within weeks of the amputation. Neuroscientist Timothy

Pons demonstrated this sensory strip encroachment in monkeys who had had their sensory nerves cut more than 12 years earlier. In this case, massive territorial invasion was seen; in one case, a hand and arm were now mapped onto the face. Recall that we made the point earlier that neurons, once severed, are for all practical purposes dead and unable to regenerate; only partially severed axons can resprout. At least, this has been the common wisdom. Also, no brain reorganization is expected after a certain critical period of development. However, in the case of phantoms, there is no damage to neurons in the brain; all the damage is peripheral. Somehow, healthy neurons are reorganizing themselves to take over an area of the brain that the body is no longer using. It is reasonable to expect that healthy brain neurons may more easily reorganize themselves than damaged ones. However, the mechanism by which this is done is still a mystery. One aspect that has puzzled scientists working on this problem is that if neurons were reorganizing themselves on the homunculus of the somatosensory strip itself, their growth would have to cover long distances. This mechanism seems unlikely, given that adult neurons can sprout over only short dis-

tances. One possible explanation is that instead of reorganization at the level of the somatosensory cortex, reorganization is occurring within the relay station of the thalamus, where all sensory inputs from touch, vision, and audition funnel through in a tight space. An axon merely has to reach across a narrow stream to remap a finger to the face or to even to the back. Odd as it may seem, this phenomenon is now being demonstrated in human amputees. Ramachandran (Ramachandran, Rogers-Ramachandran, & Steward, 1992) tested a teenager who had recently lost his left arm in an auto accident. As the boy sat blindfolded, Ramachandran touched various parts of his body with a cotton swab. When he stimulated various areas of his lip and lower face, the boy felt his missing thumb and fingers tingle. Sensations from his hand were now remapped onto his face. Because acupuncture has helped some people with phantom limb pain, it seems reasonable to speculate that knowledge of remapping may dampen pain if massage, acupuncture, or other means can be applied to the newly remapped areas of the body. In the case of this boy, odd as it may seem, face massage may alleviate left arm and hand pain.

Taste receptors are not neurons, but respond to the chemical qualities in food dissolved in saliva as they wash over the tips of the receptors. In the course of eating, taste receptors endure extremes of temperature, spicy food, and other chemical substances, which may cause damage. Perhaps because of this, taste receptors quickly wear out and are replaced on a cycle of about 10 days.

The traditional theory about how taste functions, presented in most general psychology textbooks, describes the ability of the tongue to discriminate four primary taste sensations: sweet, salty, sour, and bitter. This schema is based on specific taste bud receptor ability to detect the chemicals associated with each taste. For example, certain receptors are attuned to sodium chloride (NaCl) and other salty chemicals, and likewise for the remaining primary taste sensations. Some researchers have suggested a fifth taste, *umami* (derived from the Japanese, meaning "delicious"). Deliciousness is operationally defined by the activation of L-glutamate receptors that are attuned to glutamate-triggering substances such as monosodium glutamate (MSG). The primary tastes theory implies that, in any mixture, individual taste sensations, such as saltiness, are identified by specific saltiness receptor types and transmitted to the brain along dedicated pathways, where they are analyzed and labeled as salty. According to this theory, taste receptors of different types are grouped in various areas of the tongue; the tip is specific for sweetness and saltiness, the sides detect sourness, and the back is most sensitive to bitterness.

The competing pattern theory suggests that taste is best thought of as a pattern of sensation in which individual receptors can process information about more than one taste type. There is strong evidence that individual taste fibers are not exclusive to one taste sensation, although they may roughly focus on one type (Smith & Vogt, 1997). The suggestion from the pattern theory is that the experience of any particular taste, such as saltiness, is carried to the brain, because the fibers are activated to respond mostly to saltiness of the substance in the mixture. The implication is that taste receptors may have multiple potentiality, rather than being dedicated to respond to a specific chemical.

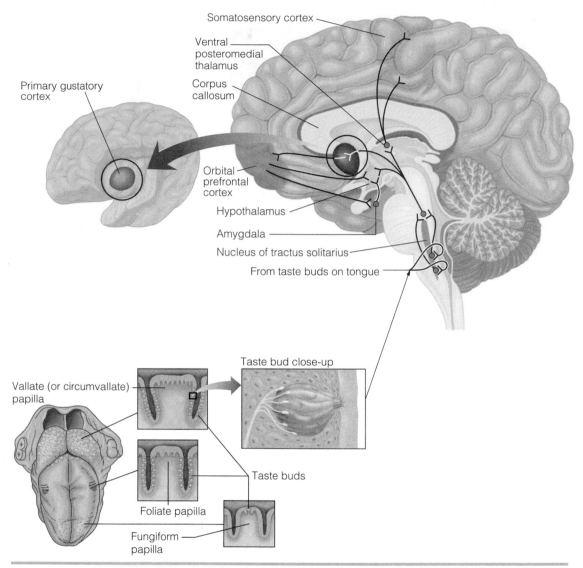

Figure 7.5 From taste buds to taste pathways in the brain. (Adapted from Kalat, J. W. [2004]. *Biological psychology* [8th ed., p. 210, Figure 7.18a, p. 212 Figure 7.19]. Belmont, CA: Wadsworth.)

Taste receptor cells synapse with sensory neurons that carry information via cranial nerves VII, IX, and X to the medulla of the brainstem (specifically the nucleus of the solitary tract), where they are relayed via the thalamus (ventral posterior medial nucleus) to the primary gustatory cortex (Figure 7.5). Additional projections run from the thalamus directly to the somatosensory cortex amygdala, hypothalamus, and orbital prefrontal cortex. The hypothalamus may code for pleasurability of food, because it contains neurons that respond specifically to sweetness of food (Rolls, 1986).

The function of taste appears to be drawing us to certain basic substances that the body needs and repelling us from potentially harmful chemicals. Certain receptors are attuned to sweet and salty foods, which the brain codes as pleasurable. Before the days of candy and salty fast foods, being drawn to sweet foods such as fruit provided needed nutrition. Salt contains the body's necessary sodium. It is also adaptive to be repelled by bitter foods, which might be poisonous, and by sour foods, which might be spoiled.

Disorders of taste are rare in comparison with disorders of smell, although as mentioned earlier, people may

---

Table 7.2 *Disorders of Taste*

Ageusia: inability to recognize tastes

Dysgeusia: distorted taste sensation

Phantogeusia: experience of a phantom or hallucinatory taste

Hypogeusia: diminished taste sensitivity

---

report disorders of smell as disorders of taste because the two systems interact in flavor perception. Taste disorders may range from a diminished sense of taste (hypogeusia) to a complete loss of taste (ageusia). Table 7.2 summarizes taste disorders. Phantogeusia is the experience of a taste "phantom" or hallucinatory taste. Taste phantoms often coincide with other disorders of taste. Most disorders of taste appear to be caused by a problem in the central perception of taste, rather than a problem at the level of the taste buds. For example, one of the more common reasons for taste distortion is medication usage. Other causes of taste dysfunction include head injury, upper respiratory infection, and in the case of phantogeusia, sometimes damage to the "taste nerve," the chorda tympani (cranial nerve VII) if it is injured during ear or dental surgery (see Cowart et al., 1997).

SMELL

Amble through a field on a summer afternoon, and the air is fragrant with smells of wildflowers, grasses, and aromatic herbs. Inhale and microscopic molecules of scent wafting through the air are gradually taken in by your relatively slow olfactory detection system. The aromas you detect and identify are, in part, a function of the ability of the odorant to dissolve in the moist mucous lining of the nose, but are also affected by age, sex, health, and brain injury.

Smell is the least understood sensory system, perhaps because scientists have considered it of little adaptive value to humans. Certainly, it is the oldest sensory system evolutionarily, and it appears much more crucial to animals such as bloodhounds and snakes, which are lower on the phylogenetic scale. What function does scent serve for humans? Is it a vestigial sense? Many people appear to function well in their lives having completely lost their sense of smell. However, the perfume industry is booming and aromatherapy is becoming a popular naturopathic approach to mood enhancement. This section examines the unique neuroanatomy of the primary olfactory system. Unlike other systems, olfactory neurons have regenerative qualities when

damaged. Finally, we also reflect on the potential implications of links among mood, memory, and olfaction.

Inhalation (but actually just a sufficient sniff is needed) sends molecules of scent traveling up to the roof of the nasal cavity. These odorants dissolve in the olfactory epithelium, a fine mucous lining consisting of odorant-binding proteins (OBPs), antibodies, and enzymes. Mucus is being continually produced; thus, the entire epithelium is replaced about every 10 minutes. Scent molecules bound to OBPs activate the fine, hairlike cilia of olfactory neurons waving within the olfactory epithelium. Researchers have discovered at least 500 to 1000 OBP genes that appear to be coded for different odorants. In humans, the epithelium is small, about half the size of a postage stamp (5–10 cm^2). Dogs, with their keen sense of smell, have an epithelium easily 10 times that of humans (100 cm^2), with 100 times the neurons per square centimeter. Olfactory neurons in the epithelium synapse with the right or left olfactory bulb through the thin cribriform plate of the skull, where the central olfactory pathway (cranial nerve I) originates. So whereas three cranial nerves subserve taste, smell has only one pathway.

The olfactory system is unique in several ways. Note that we have considered receptors when discussing other sensory systems. These receptors then synapse with dendrites of neurons. This is not the case with the olfactory system. The neurons themselves are directly exposed to the environment. The health of the epithelial layer, where the dangling neurons lie, is crucial because some viruses, such as rabies, take advantage of this direct route to the brain. This system is also interesting in that contrary to the notion that new neural cells do not form in adults, the olfactory neurons compose a uniquely "plastic" system, continuing to reproduce and replace themselves every 1 to 2 months throughout adulthood. The olfactory neurons, however, are susceptible to traumatic injury because they dangle through a opening in the skull, the cribriform plate. A blow to the head can easily sever these neurons. Although the neurons do regrow, they do not always reconnect with the olfactory bulbs (Figure 7.6).

The olfactory bulbs contain complex circuitry; the two bulbs even communicate with each other. Although the mechanism is not completely understood, microelectrode recordings show that various aromas produce identifiable spatial maps on the bulbs, and these mosaics may change even during the sniffing of an odorant. The plasticity of the system has suggested to scientists that experience with smell can easily modify the representational pattern of stimulation on the olfactory bulb. The map on the bulb projects to the areas of the brain that process and encode

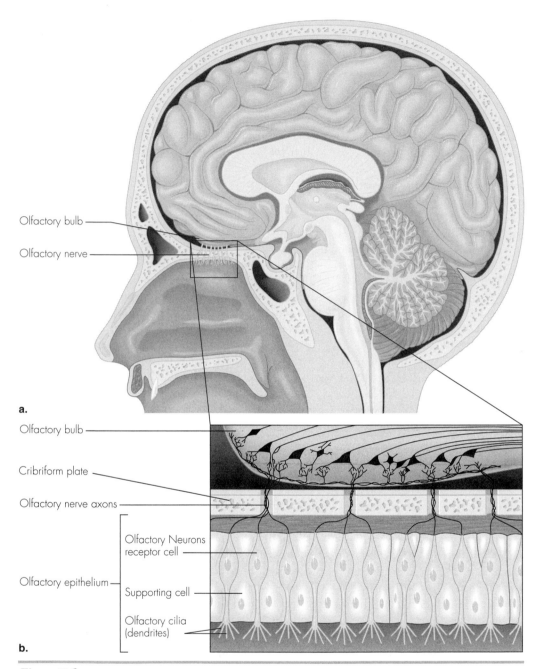

Olfactory bulb

Olfactory nerve

a.

Olfactory bulb

Cribriform plate

Olfactory nerve axons

Olfactory epithelium

Olfactory Neurons receptor cell

Supporting cell

Olfactory cilia (dendrites)

b.

Figure 7.6 Olfactory system. (a) Odorants are taken up via the olfactory neurons. (b) Close-up of olfactory neurons, which protrude through the cribriform plate. (From Kalat, J. W. [1998]. *Biological psychology* [6th ed., p. 205, Figure 7.22]. Pacific Grove, CA: Brooks/Cole.)

the scent. It appears that specific odors code specific patterns. It is unclear whether these coded representations are invariant, in other words, always stimulating the same brain areas, or whether learning can also feed back to modify scent maps when the same scent is later reintroduced.

Another unique aspect of olfaction is its pattern of projection into the brain. All other sensory systems first pass through the thalamus and then into the neocortex. However, the primary projections of the olfactory system innervate the limbic system directly through the amygdala and hippocampal formation. Olfactory information projects

Table 7.3 *Disorders of Smell*

Anosmia: total loss of smell

Dysosmia: distorted smell sensation

Phantosmia: experience of a phantom or hallucinatory smell

Hyposmia: diminished smell sensation

into these primitive areas of the brain before passing through the relay station of the thalamus, and then into the frontal cortex and onto other areas of the neocortex. Because of this connection, the effect of scent on emotion and mood is instantaneous and is most intensely processed preconsciously. Secondarily, scientists believe that parallel thalamic projections to the frontal lobes are responsible for conscious recognition of scent. The cortex can then elaborate and refine the perception of aroma. The hippocampus, although not a memory storage center, is responsible for processing and coding memories before they are stored in the neocortex. Together with the amygdala, these limbic system structures appear to be responsible for coding much of the emotional tone of memories. This neural pattern of projection into the brain reflects the ancient evolution of olfaction. Considering this brain anatomy, it is no wonder that smell is so strongly tied to emotional memory.

In the early part of the nineteenth century, Freud suggested that disorders of smell and specific psychological dysfunctions may be connected (for types of olfactory dysfunction, see Table 7.3). This idea remained largely unexamined until a relatively recent resurgence of interest in olfaction occurred as it relates to certain brain diseases such as Alzheimer's disease, Parkinson's disease, and schizophrenia. For some time, people have observed that decreased ability to smell (hyposmia) is associated with aging, and that both loss and distortion of smell (dysosmia) are associated with depression. With aging, the ability to perceive sour or bitter odors appears to diminish first, whereas the ability to detect pleasant smells such as sweetness may persist well into old age. Interestingly, recent work has shown that diminution of olfactory ability is an early sign of diseases of accelerated aging, such as Alzheimer's disease and Parkinson's disease (for example, see Doty, 1990). Also, schizophrenics often have a distorted sense of smell. Clinical neuropsychologists are now using scratch-and-sniff tests of odor identification and odor recognition threshold, such as the University of Pennsylvania Smell Identification Test (UPSIT) (Doty, Shaman, & Dann, 1984), to test for the presence of olfactory dysfunction in cases where clinicians suspect these diseases.

Partial or complete loss of smell is also a common occurrence after traumatic injury to the brain. As noted earlier, because the olfactory neurons dangle through the cribriform plate, they are easily damaged or sheared off by sudden movements of the brain in relation to the skull. Even though olfactory neurons can regenerate, they often do not reconnect to the olfactory bulbs because they are blocked by scar tissue.

Motor Systems

The sensory systems provide a window to the world, and the motor systems, in turn, provide the means of acting on the world. Whereas control of sensory systems occurs in posterior brain regions, the cortical control of movement is largely anterior. Movement takes several forms, including reflex actions, automatic repetitive actions such as walking, semivoluntary actions such as yawning, and voluntary actions such as deciding to pick up an object (Bradshaw & Mattingly, 1995).

Traditionally, scientists thought the motor system was organized hierarchically. Whereas sensory processing is thought to proceed in a bottom-up fashion, motor processing would follow a reverse path in a top-down manner. Sensory-perceptual processes build up from fragments analyzed in primary processing areas and are synthesized in secondary and higher order cortexes. Then information that directs motor processing comes into the system in the form of highly integrated sensory information from the **sensory association areas,** such as the parietal lobes, and the subcortical structures of the basal ganglia and the cerebellum. In addition, internally generated motivation for action also directs movement. The system then directs this information to areas of secondary motor planning and programming before sending it to the primary motor cortex. According to this hierarchy theory, the primary motor cortex sits at the top and funnels all information about movement to the body. However, a competing theory suggests that the system works in a parallel processing mode, with several motor processing circuits working in coordination with the primary motor cortex (Haines, 1997).

CORTICAL MOTOR PROCESSING

Several cortical areas of the motor system are involved in motor processing (Figure 7.7). The first of these is the primary motor cortex. The next three motor areas are often referred to as the secondary motor cortex and include the

Four Areas of the Motor Cortex

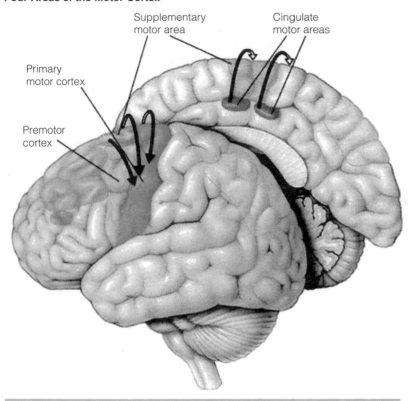

Figure 7.7 Cortical motor processing areas. (From Pinel, Biopsychology, 5th ed. Published by Allyn and Bacon, Boston, MA. Copyright © 1997 by Pearson Education. Reprinted by permission of the publisher.)

supplementary motor area, the **premotor area (PMA,** or **premotor cortex**), and the **cingulate motor area (CMA** or **cingulate motor cortex**). Finally, areas of the parietal lobes and the dorsolateral prefrontal cortex are areas of premotor planning.

The role of the **primary motor cortex** is to manage the fine details required to perform movement. The primary motor cortex lies in the precentral gyrus, or motor strip of the frontal lobes, just anterior to the central sulcus and the somatosensory strip. Neuronal input emanates from the secondary motor areas and from the somatosensory cortex. Neuronal output travels through the internal capsule, and on to descending tracts of the spinal cord, and ultimately to the muscles of the body. The primary motor cortex, like the somatosensory cortex, is somatopically (or topographically) mapped as a homunculus and allots area according to its degree of motor innervation (see Figure 7.3). If the primary motor cortex is stimulated directly, typically through microstimulation in the course of neurosurgery, corresponding muscles in the body move. For example, stimulating the thumb causes the thumb to twitch or jerk. If the motor homunculus is compared with the sensory homunculus, it is evident that there are many similarities in the cortical mapping for motor control and sensory processing of movement. For example, the acute sense of touch on the fingers is also related to fine finger dexterity. However, some areas have proportionately more motor control abilities, or vice versa, so the maps appear somewhat different. The motor cortex, like the somatosensory cortex, controls the contralateral side of the body. Damage or disease of the motor cortex results in **hemiplegia,** or the loss of voluntary movement, to the opposite side of the body. Hemiplegia is often a hallmark of stroke to the middle cerebral artery. So, for example, a common occurrence is to have a patient present with right-sided hemiplegia and difficulty speaking due to a left-hemisphere stroke.

The primary motor cortex and the somatosensory cortex are in reciprocal communication with each other through a reflex circuit. The primary motor cortex receives feedback from the somatosensory cortex about the effect of movement just initiated. So when your thumb moves across the page to turn it, the sensation of the contact of the thumb on paper is immediately sent to the somatosensory cortex and informs the primary motor cortex of the effect of its movement.

Each area of the **secondary motor cortex** has a slightly different role. The **supplementary motor area (SMA,** also **supplementary motor cortex,** or **medial premotor cortex)** functions in organization and sequential timing of movement. The internal intention to move is also a function of this area. The SMA lies on the dorsal and medial portion of each frontal lobe (in Brodmann's area 6). It is posterior to the prefrontal cortex and anterior to the primary motor cortex. The SMA receives input from the parietal lobes (posterior parietal association area), the somatosensory strip, the secondary somatosensory areas, and subcortically from the basal ganglia and the cerebellum. It also interconnects with the PMA. The SMA outputs to the primary motor cortex in both the ipsilateral and contralateral hemisphere. It also outputs back to the basal ganglia and the cerebellum (Bradshaw & Mattingly, 1995). It functions specifically as a planner of motor sequences. Like the primary motor cortex, it is also somatopically mapped to the musculature in the body; however, the mapping is not as tightly organized. Electrical microstimulation of the SMA elicits the urge to make a movement, or the feeling of anticipation of a movement (Bradshaw & Mattingly, 1995). Stimulation may also elicit muscle movement. But instead of the single-muscle flexion of the primary motor cortex, this stimulation activates groups of muscles and a sequence of movement, and it can activate bilateral movement (Haines, 1997).

Experiments with humans show a **dissociation,** or separation, between the functional contributions of the primary motor cortex and the SMA. In an early method of studying areas of brain activity, researchers injected radioactive xenon into the bloodstream. In this way, they could measure increased areas of brain blood flow, and thus brain neuronal activity, as they were occurring. When the researchers asked volunteers to make random finger movements, the primary motor cortex "lit up," but the SMA remained relatively silent. When the experimenters asked volunteers to make a sequence of movements with their fingers, such as drumming their fingers in a certain order, both the primary motor cortex and the SMA were active. Finally, when they asked the participants to only imagine and rehearse the movements in their minds, without doing anything, only the SMA was active (Roland, Larsen, Lassen, & Skinhølf, 1980). This offered strong evidence for the planning role of the SMA in sequential motor activities.

The PMA also plays a role in motor planning and sequencing and movement readiness. The PMA lies next to the SMA in Brodmann's area 6 of the frontal lobes. Whereas the SMA is more medial, the PMA is more lateral. The PMA receives neuronal input from some of the same general areas as does the SMA, but from slightly different places. For example, the PMA receives parietal input from posterior parietal areas, rather than parietal association cortex. The PMA receives input from the secondary somatosensory areas, rather than from both the primary and secondary somatosensory areas, and receives more cerebellar input. As stated earlier, it is also reciprocally interconnected with the SMA and projects to the primary motor cortex and the reticular formation (Haines, 1997). The PMA is also somatopically organized. In a general way, the PMA performs similar premotor planning functions as the SMA, such as the sequencing, timing, and proper initiation of voluntary movement, but it may function more in *externally* cued readiness for action, whereas the SMA provides more of an *internal* readiness cue (Bradshaw & Mattingly, 1995). For example, when runners line up for a race and hear the official say, "On your mark . . . Get set . . . Go," their PMA is most active between "Get set" and "Go." Studies with monkeys also indicate that the PMA is most active during this interval between *cue* and *go* (see Haines, 1997).

Less is known about the functioning of the third structure of the secondary motor cortex, the CMA, although it likely plays a role in the emotional and motivational impetus for movement. The CMA is a medial infolding of the frontal area of the cingulate gyrus. Recall that the cingulate gyrus plays a role in the limbic system. The CMA lies next to the cingulate gyrus. The CMA is organized somatopically in relation to the spinal cord. It projects both to the spinal cord and to the primary motor area. Damage to the CMA results in a lack of spontaneous motor activity (Bradshaw & Mattingly, 1995). This apparent apathy is neurologic in origin and not necessarily caused by a depressive state. People may be able to say what they can do or should do, but often do not translate this into action. Together with the SMA, the anterior cingulate also appears to play a role in the semantic premotor processing, or initiation, of speech.

Two additional cortical areas contribute to motor processing: the posterior parietal lobes and the dorsolateral prefrontal cortex. The posterior areas of the parietal lobes (Brodmann's areas 5 and 7) are important in coordinating spatial mapping with motor programming. These association areas receive input from the somatosensory cortex, the vestibular system, and the visual system. Integrated sensory information travels to the supplementary and premotor cortexes regarding the relative spatial position of the body and objects in space.

Much initiation for motor behavior and executive programming for movement originates in the higher association area of the **dorsolateral prefrontal cortex.** This area lies, functionally, in the prefrontal cortex, which is responsible for orchestrating and organizing many brain functions. The dorsolateral prefrontal cortex is not a "movement center" in and of itself, but it is instrumental in deploying movement. Much input to this area comes from the subcortical motor centers of the basal ganglia.

Testing Motor Functioning

Neuropsychologists are interested in assessing both simple and complex motor programming. Simple motor skills require little coordination, whereas more complex items tap into higher motor and cortical processes. Items involving gross-motor movement assess one of the most basic cortically mediated motor responses, such as a response to a single command: "Raise your right hand," or "Move your left leg." Motor speed can be qualitatively evaluated by asking someone to "Touch your thumb to your forefinger as quickly as you can," and fine-motor ability can be evaluated from asking, "Touch your thumb to each finger, one after the other." Examples of standardized motor tests include a measure of grip strength and finger-tapping speed, both from the Halstead–Reitan Neuropsychological Battery. The strength of grip test simply measures a person's ability to squeeze a hand dynamometer (Figure 7.8) as hard as possible. The Finger Oscillation or Finger Tapping Test requires a person to

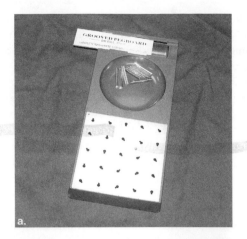

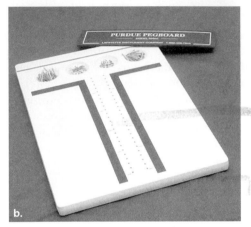

Figure 7.9   Neuropsychological tests of speeded motor coordination: (a) Grooved Pegboard Test; (b) Purdue Pegboard Test. (C/O Lafayette Instrument Company, Inc.)

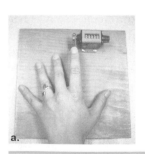

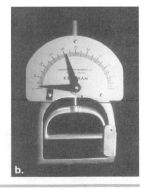

Figure 7.8   The Finger Tapping Test and Strength of Grip Test. (Courtesy Jeffrey T. Barth, University of Virginia, Charlottesville, VA.)

tap as rapidly as possible with the index finger on a small lever attached to a mechanical counter, alternating trials between the dominant and nondominant hand. It is generally expected that one's dominant hand would be both stronger and faster than the nondominant hand by about 10%.

Male individuals generally perform better on pure speed tests, whereas female individuals tend to show better performance on coordinated motor speed tests such as various pegboard tests that require one to insert, as quickly as possible, round or grooved pegs into slots with the dominant and nondominant hands (Figure 7.9).

Other motor tests integrate higher level cognitive processing, because they may, for example, require a person to shift between initiating and inhibiting behaviors (for example, "If I clap once, you clap twice." [Clap hands one time.] "Now, I clap twice, you clap once." [Clap hands two times.]). Neuropsychologists often examine graphomotor skills. The following items assess the ability to copy shapes with increasing degrees of difficulty. They involve the integration of visuoperception (input) and a complex motor response (output).

Example I

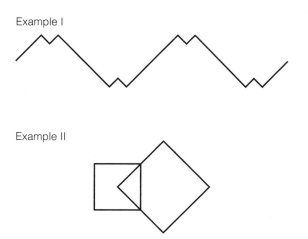

Example II

Disorders of Complex Motor Processing

A number of movement disorders may occur as a result of brain damage or disease. If the primary motor area in one hemisphere is damaged by stroke or injury, hemiplegia often results. Disorders of motor processing that go beyond the primary motor cortex can be classified under two main types: disorders of *when* to act and disorders of *how* to act. For example, the motor system instructs *when* to start and stop various behaviors. **Akinesia** is a difficulty in initiating and maintaining behavior. Patients with akinesia may be extremely slow to start or perform a movement, may become rapidly fatigued when performing repetitive movements, or may have problems in performing simultaneous or sequential movements. If a person continues in the same behavior, or constantly selects it in the presence of other choices, this is termed **motor perseveration,** another problem of *when* to act. In addition, if a person behaves inappropriately, displaying a motor response when it is unwanted, this is termed **defective response inhibition.** These examples of disorders of *when* to act can arise from a variety of cortical and subcortical lesions and disorders. For example, patients with Parkinson's disease show classic deficits in motor initiation and motor perseveration. People with this affliction often display a slow, shuffling

---

Table 7.4 *Examples of Motor Dysfunction*

Apraxia/dyspraxia: an inability or disability in performing voluntary actions

Akinesia: difficulty initiating and maintaining movement

Dyskinesia: uncontrolled involuntary movement

Chorea: involuntary, jerky, writhing, undulating "puppet-like" movements

Defective response inhibition: the inability to inhibit or an inappropriate motor response.

Hemiplegia: loss of voluntary movement to one half of the body contralateral to the affected motor strip

Motor perseveration: an inability to stop a behavior or series of behaviors

Tremor: involuntary shaking, usually of a limb; tremors may be resting or occur with intentional movement

---

gate when they walk and may "freeze" and be unable to move or back up when they enter a closet. People with Huntington's chorea often show jerky, undulating, "puppet-like" movements of their limbs and grimacing, writhing movements of their faces. (Parkinson's and Huntington's disease are discussed at length in Chapter 15.) Some examples of clinical motor dysfunction are described in Table 7.4.

Apraxia is the main type of disorder under the category of problems of *how* to act. Strictly defined, apraxia implies an absence of action, but neuropsychologists most often use it to describe a variety of missing or inappropriate actions that cannot be clearly attributed to primary motor or sensory deficits, or lack of comprehension, attention, or motivation. Thus, the term *apraxia* refers to an inability to perform voluntary actions despite an adequate degree of motor strength and control. The adjective "voluntary" is key to understanding this disorder. A patient may be able to spontaneously don a jacket, for instance, but be unable to do so on command. Therefore, family members who ask a patient to do something may perceive him or her as being oppositional or stubborn when, in fact, he or she does not control the skills required to perform the action. A typical type of task that is given if apraxia is suspected is to ask a patient to pantomime a goal-directed action or series of actions. For example, a person may be asked, "Show me how you would use a key to open a door." Depending on the type of apraxia, a patient may "misperform" this action in several ways.

There are several subtypes of apraxia, depending on a number of behavioral variables affecting movement and movement initiation. The types discussed in this chapter—limb-kinetic, ideomotor, conceptual, and

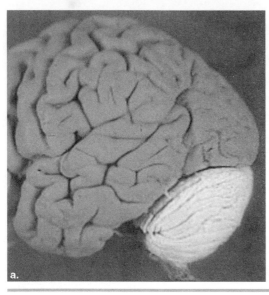

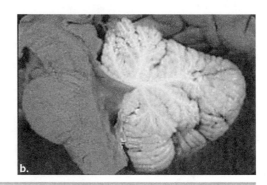

Figure 7.10   Two views of the cerebellum: (a) lateral view and (b) cutaway medial view. (Courtesy Mark DeSantis.)

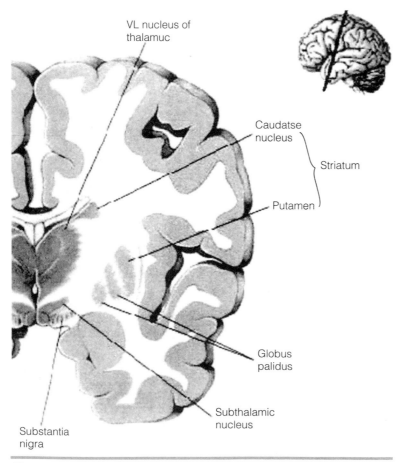

VL nucleus of
thalamuc

Caudatse
nucleus

Striatum

Putamen

Globus
palidus

Subthalamic
nucleus

Substantia
nigra

Figure 7.11   Basal ganglia. (Modified from Bear, M. F., Connors, B.W., &
Paradiso M. A. [2001]. *Neuroscience: Exploring the brain* [2nd ed., p. 389,
Figure 14.11]. Baltimore, MD: Lippincott Williams & Wilkins, by permission.)

dissociation (formerly ideational) apraxia—are the most frequently described.

People with **limb-kinetic apraxia** (also ideokinetic) appear clumsy and have poor motor control. In attempting to show how a key would be used, limb-kinetic apraxics may make large grasping motions, rather than fine thumb-to-forefinger movements. Because limb-kinetic apraxia is defined as a problem in executing precise, independent, or coordinated finger movements, people with this disorder are also likely to perform quite poorly on the finger-tapping (see Figure 7.8) and pegboard tests (see Figure 7.9). The theories regarding the brain areas implicated in limb-kinetic apraxia involve the corticospinal tract, basal ganglia, and the premotor cortex, as well as a larger frontoparietal circuit of motor control. A progression of gross- to fine-motor control can be observed with the myelinization of the corticospinal tract during development. As the corticospinal tract matures, children first grasp with the entire hand before being able to execute independent and coordinated finger movements. However, limb-kinetic apraxia goes beyond a corticospinal or basal ganglia deficit and involves aspects of grasping and fine-motor manipulation involved with the larger frontoparietal circuit (Leiguarda, Merello, Nouzeilles, Balej, Rivero, & Nogues, 2003).

Ideomotor apraxia involves difficulties in the execution of the idea of a movement, even though the knowledge of the action is preserved. For example, in response to a request to pantomime use of a key, the person may mistakenly use the index finger as the key (body part as tool error) or turn the whole arm in an unnatural fashion (movement orientation error). However, someone with ideomotor apraxia may be able to use a key correctly if it is put in the hand and should recognize the correct gesture if it is performed by someone else, or if given a choice, can match tools with correct actions. Lesions to the left parietal lobes are commonly associated with ideomotor apraxia of either hand. It is believed that the left parietal lobes have a special role in programming purposeful, skilled movements, especially in those who are left hemisphere dominant for language (Meador, Loring, Lee, Nichols, & Heilman, 1999).

With **conceptual apraxia,** in contrast, the *knowledge* of the action has been lost. For example, when asked to gesture how to use the key, the person may perform any number of vague movements. When given a key, he or she may try to use it as a pen or a toothbrush and, in addition, may not be able to pick out the correct gesture if shown by someone else. Conceptual apraxia is not associated with damage to any one area, but is related to wider loss of semantic knowledge of tools and actions. This problem may be seen in the early stages of dementia, such as Alzheimer's disease.

Dissociation apraxia (formerly ideational apraxia) involves impairment in an action sequence. This type of apraxia can be witnessed in a multistage request such as, "Show me how you would pour and serve tea." Actions may be performed out of order, although the individual actions themselves are correct. Disorders of an action sequence may be caused by executive or frontal lobe dysfunction and a possible dissociation of action programs from language.

In summary, the apraxias, as disorders of the *how* system of motor control, represent problems with the mental representation of actions. Although we present apraxia subtypes as independent entities, different types can occur together in the same person. The apraxias represent the most common type of motor problems treated by neuropsychologists, because they can occur due to a wide variety of cerebrovascular disorders (i.e., strokes), as well as with tumors or disease states, and the disability they produce interferes with many complex actions of daily life requiring higher cortical functioning.

THE CEREBELLUM AND MOTOR PROCESSING

The cerebellum permits seamless coordination and unconscious flow of movement. It coordinates reflex action and voluntary movement, is concerned with the timing of movement, and can differentiate movement frequency at a rate of 1/1000 of a second. The cerebellum aids in maintaining posture, balance, and muscle tone. It is also implicated in sequential aspects of motor learning, such as the steps required to learn to play the piano. The cerebellum is located posterior to the brainstem and inferior to the telencephalon (Figure 7.10) and reciprocally connects to the cortical sensory and motor systems, resulting in a constant feedback loop coordinating the two areas. Cerebellar motor disorders are most often caused by structural damage caused by trauma or stroke. They are characterized by irregular, jerky, and poorly coordinated movement. Muscle tone and strength, as well as motor resistance, may also decrease. Finally, in contrast with the resting **tremor** seen in Parkinson's disease patients, cerebellar patients show an intention tremor.

SUBCORTICAL MOTOR PROCESSING

Cortical motor processing is largely concerned with voluntary, conscious movement, whereas subcortical structures,

Neuropsychology in Action 7.3

Tourette Syndrome: Too Much Behavior

by Eric Zillmer

George was a patient I saw for neuropsychological evaluation. I knew that George, a 29-year-old left-handed man, was diagnosed with Gilles de la Tourette syndrome (TS), but I was not prepared for his odd behavior during my administration of the Category test. The Category test measures planning and reasoning. I asked George to match a stimulus to one of four targets. In essence, George had to figure out which abstract category the stimulus fit best. My responsibility was to present each stimulus figure, tell George whether he was correct, tell him when the category changed, and keep score. In total, more than 200 stimuli cards were presented, which fall into 7 categories. The first stimulus card was easy, and I told George his response, "two," was correct. As soon as I did so, he made a peculiar gesture, a kissing motion, in which he looked directly at me, raised his eyebrows, and shaped his mouth as if "blowing" me a kiss. If this were not odd enough, I was dumbstruck with George's behavior when I told him he had made an error. He made an obscene gesture commonly known as "flipping the bird"!

And so it went for the entire examination. When George was correct, he blew me a kiss, and when he made an error, he "gave me the finger." Like many neuropsychological tests, this one is staggered, so it becomes more and more difficult. This resulted in George making more errors toward the end, a total of 53. Midway through the examination, I decided to continue with the test, but I did ask George after the evaluation whether he knew he was engaging in these behaviors and if he was somehow angry with me. He informed me that he was aware of what he did, but that it seemed uncontrollable; "I just had to do it," he explained. He also told me that he was not angry with me and, in fact, enjoyed the testing and my company.

TS is a rare and fascinating disorder that has puzzled scientists for more than a century. TS occurs in less than 1% of the population. Symptoms include facial and bodily tics, usually progressing from the head to the torso and extremities, as well as repetitive verbal utterances, including coprolalia (uncontrollable cursing) in approximately 50% of the cases (Newman, Barth, & Zillmer, 1986). Onset of the disorder is typically before age 10; symptoms vary in intensity over time and may be exacerbated by stress. Most individuals with TS are male and left-handed.

The specific cause of TS is unknown, but the prevailing view is that there is a neurologic basis for the disorder, possibly involving subcortical structures that are responsible for motor coordination (Devinsky, 1983;

Bornstein, King, & Carroll, 1983). This view is supported by findings of a high incidence of motor asymmetries on clinical neurologic examinations and abnormal electroencephalographic and computed tomography scans (Newman, Barth, & Zillmer, 1986). However, no consistent or focalized neurologic deficits have emerged.

George, adopted in infancy, first displayed bizarre motor symptoms—jerking of his shoulders—at age 2. Later, he developed short barking sounds, repetitive movements of his facial muscles and arms, and finally, loud shouting of profanities. The bouts of impulsive and sometimes assaultive behavior became so difficult to manage in the classroom that George was taken out of school in the third grade. Subsequently, he was in and out of psychiatric institutions most of his life. He was in a state psychiatric facility when I evaluated him. He had been hospitalized because he threw a brick at a passing car and chased it with an ax. Somehow, he thought that passengers in the car were teasing him. Like George, many patients with TS display peculiar motor symptoms and psychiatric symptoms, including depression and impulsivity. Medications often help patients with TS so that, in most cases, they can lead a productive and symptom-free life.

---

namely, the basal ganglia and the cerebellum, function in a more automatic manner to regulate movement. The function of the basal ganglia in movement largely controls the fluidity of overlearned and "semiautomatic" motor programs (Bradshaw & Mattingly, 1995). The basal ganglia reciprocally connect to the PMA and the SMA via the thalamus. Also, an important brain circuit responsible for perceptual-motor learning and adaptation centers on the basal ganglia. Specifically, this circuit includes the caudate nucleus, putamen, and globus pallidus. The nuclei of the **striatal complex** (caudate and putamen) receive projected information from cortical sensory areas. From the striatum, information then funnels through the globus pallidus, and

then on to the thalamus, where it projects to the premotor and prefrontal areas (Mishkin, Malamut, & Bachevalier, 1984) (Figure 7.11).

Some well-known motor disorders are associated with neurochemical abnormalities that affect the basal ganglia—Tourette syndrome is one of these (Neuropsychology in Action 7.3) as well as Parkinson's disease, which specifically targets the substantia nigra, and Huntington's disease, which attacks the caudate nucleus. Although these two disorders attack structures within centimeters of each other, you can easily distinguish these motor disorders. You can recognize Parkinson's disease by its resting tremor and difficulty in initiating movement, whereas Huntington's disease patients show characteristic puppet-like jerking and grimacing choreic movements. The motor difficulties in these patients are prominent but exist within a larger constellation of symptoms. We discuss these two disorders and their specific motor impairments at length in conjunction with the discussion of subcortical dementia in Chapter 15. Tourette syndrome also is thought to affect the basal ganglia as well as other cortical structures.

Summary

The primary sensory areas receive afferent input through the relay station of the thalamus, except for olfaction, which receives input directly from the olfactory bulbs. In some sensory systems, such as touch and taste, primary sensory reception is completely crossed, coming entirely from the contralateral side of the body. In vision, the contralateral hemispace sends input to each hemisphere. In audition, information travels bilaterally. Olfaction has ipsilateral projection to the primary olfactory cortex.

Each sensory system has a primary receiving area in the cortex. In general, sensory information is represented in detailed one-to-one or pattern mapping onto the corresponding primary cortex. In vision, audition, and touch, these are, respectively, the retinotopic, tonotopic, and somatotopic maps. The primary mapping for the chemical senses is less well understood but likely occurs in a similar manner.

From the primary sensory cortices, where information is first labeled, it is then sorted and relayed to the secondary sensory processing areas. These areas are generally contiguous to the primary sensory areas. They receive preprocessed sensory information through reciprocal connections with primary areas. They do not receive sensory information directly. Secondary areas may process only specific qualities of sensory information in a parallel manner. In other systems, a distributed "maplike" representation may remain. As processing moves into tertiary or association areas, dense reciprocal interconnections both within and between sensory modalities are evident.

The motor system involves both cortical and subcortical areas of processing. The general stream of processing moves from subcortical and secondary motor areas to the primary motor area to output; however, there are many reciprocal interconnections. Some of the coordination and planning of movement occurs in the subcortical areas of the cerebellum and the basal ganglia. The three secondary cortical motor areas add fine planning, sequencing, and motivational aspects. The primary motor cortex, or motor homunculus, is responsible for managing the fine details of movement.

It would be difficult to imagine the behavioral oddities that disorders of specific sensory and motor systems present had not nature and odd twists of fate actually presented them. These include descriptions of sensory phantoms, distortions of chemical senses, and the odd disorder of "miswired" sensation termed *synesthesia*. Although these disorders can be connected to specific sensory modalities, it is at once evident that most afflictions do not stay within the bounds of a single system.

Critical Thinking Questions

- In what ways do the study of sensory-perceptual and motor disorders inform us about intact brain functioning? In what instances might the study of damaged brains lead us astray?
- Do conditions such as phantoms, neglect, and synesthesia represent altered states of consciousness? Explain.
- Does intact motor processing require intact sensory-perceptual processing? Explain.

Key Terms

Transduction	Somatosensory system	Thermoreceptors	Dorsal column medial lemniscal
Receptor cell	Proprioception	Nocioceptors	pathway
Agnosia	Mechanical receptors	Proprioceptors	Medial lemniscus
Tactile agnosia or Astereognosis	Chemoreceptors	Ascending spinal-thalamic tract	Somatopic organization

Kinesthetic sense
Finger agnosia
Paresthesia
Peripheral neuropathy
Phantom limb pain
Proprioceptive disorder
Tactile extinction/
    suppression/
    inattention
Papillae
Ageusia

Dysgeusia
Phantogeusia
Hypogeusia
Anosmia
Dysosmia
Phantosmia
Hyposmia
Sensory association
    areas
Premotor cortex or premotor
    area (PMA)

Cingulate motor area (CMA) or
    cingulate motor cortex
Primary motor cortex
Hemiplegia
Secondary motor cortex
Supplementary motor area
    (SMA) or supplementary
    motor cortex, medial
    premotor cortex
Dissociation
Dorsolateral prefrontal cortex

Akinesia
Motor perseveration
Defective response
    inhibition
Apraxia
Limb-kinetic apraxia
Ideomotor apraxia
Conceptual apraxia
Dissociation apraxia
Tremor
Striatal complex

Web Connections

http://www.ninds.nih.gov/disorders/chronic_pain/detail_chronic_pain.htm
The National Institute of Neurological Disorders and Stroke site on Pain: Hope through research.

http://www.pbs.org/safarchive/3_ask/archive/qna/3294_peppers.html
Linda Bartoshuk of Yale University discusses her research on supertasters.

http://www.cf.ac.uk/biosi/staff/jacob/teaching/sensory/olfact1.html
Tutorials on smell and what's new in olfaction research.

Chapter 8

VISION AND LANGUAGE

I am part of all that I have seen.

—*Alfred Lord Tennyson*

It is not often that we use language correctly; usually we use it incorrectly, though we understand each others meaning.

—*St. Augustine*

Visual Processing
Auditory and Language Processing

Neuropsychology in Action

Keep in Mind

■ Does vision operate as a bottom-up or top-down process?

■ What would it be like to no longer be able to recognize your friends by their faces?

■ What is the difference between primary auditory and visual processing and higher order processing?

Overview

The human visual and auditory systems cover more cortical area outside of their primary sites of processing than the sensory systems discussed in Chapter 7. Humans rely greatly on vision and hearing, and the areas of the cortex devoted to each reflect this. In the areas of visual and auditory processing, we progress to higher order functions such as visual object recognition, visuospatial processing, and speech and language that require an understanding beyond primary processing based on mapping of functions. This chapter discusses vision and audition from primary processing to higher integrative functions of vision and hearing. We also discuss representative disorders that can occur at each level of processing. As in Chapter 7, these include agnosias, or in the case of language, aphasias. In the visual system, we also take an in-depth look at the disorder of neglect as an example of a visuospatial problem, but also one that involves aspects of attention and consciousness.

Visual Processing

Vision is one of our most important senses. In addition to the occipital cortex, major portions of the temporal and parietal lobes are devoted to visual processing. Areas of the frontal lobes are involved in eye movement and higher processing of visuospatial working memory. The large areas devoted to vision reflect the human reliance on sight and visual processing. Visual information processing is also the most complex and best understood sensory systems of the brain. However, for all of the attention, there are still debates about how vision works.

No one "master processor" integrates all visual information into perceptible form. Recognition of surroundings, people, faces, and objects, though seemingly instantaneous, is the culmination of separate but locally connected visual-perceptual processes. As a prerequisite to recognizing a friend walking through a crowd, you must first have the necessary visual acuity, as well as adequate color and form perception. Visual acuity speaks to the ability to perceive light, contrast between light and dark, resolve a target, and have adequate visual fields. Receptors for form interpret shapes such as roundness or squareness, as well as orientation of lines to each other. Qualities of texture and color such as feathery and blue are processed

by yet other primary visual areas. Although somewhat overgeneralized, at a higher perceptual level, the ventral visual pathway to the temporal lobes serves as the "what" system largely responsible for object and face recognition. The dorsal pathway to the parietal lobes, or the "where" system, is specialized for spatial location. In building a visual percept, some of these processes operate in sequence, and others may operate in parallel. Although we discuss visual processing as a "bottom-up" process of analyzing rudimentary or local bits of information that are built up into coherent percepts, the issue of degree of impact of "top-down" or perceptual-driven processing on vision is an area of debate (Grill-Spector & Malach, 2004).

As complicated as this general characterization may be, the human visual system is actually much more sophisticated. In daily life you see under extremely "messy" visual conditions, through haze, from different perspectives, and from varying distances. Amazingly, visual perception of a tree stays constant, even though sometimes you may see it through a fog, sometimes in the shade, partially obscured, from the north, from a distance, or from underneath. Each time the image of the tree makes a different impression on your retina; yet, your brain's perception of "tree" remains constant. Obviously, you do not simply match templates for a particular tree—there would be so

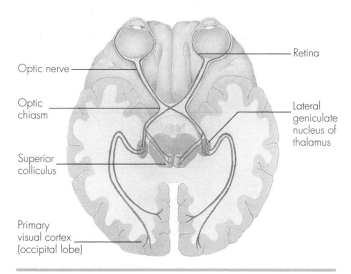

Figure 8.1 Visual pathways. The primary visual pathway partially crosses over at the optic chiasm. From there it routes through the thalamus to the primary visual cortex. (Reproduced from Kalat, J. W. [1998]. *Biological psychology* [6th ed., p. 174, Figure 6.6]. Pacific Grove, CA: Brooks/Cole.)

many as to soon overload the system. The visual-perceptual system must be highly flexible and sophisticated to accommodate a constantly changing visual landscape.

PRIMARY VISUAL PROCESSING

In a general way, the eye functions as a type of camera, mapping visual images on the retina and transmitting the inverted "picture" to a corresponding "retinotopic" map to the primary visual processing area of the cortex. But the eye is much more dynamic and complex in operation; it can constantly adjust focus and adapt to changing visual conditions, as well as extract information about images. The visual system operates via two types of photoreceptor cells. The rods and cones transduce the electromagnetic wavelengths of light energy and extract properties of objects. Cones, which detect wavelengths of color, are fewer, and center in the middle of the retina. The more numerous rods surround the cones and are attuned to the shades of gray we experience in low-light and nighttime conditions. Visual stimuli from the right side of space (that is, right visual field) activate receptors on the left side of each retina, and information from the left visual field activates right-sided receptors.

Visual information leaves the eye through the optic nerve's bundle of axons. The retina sends projections to at least 10 brain areas. Some of these areas, such as the pineal gland and the superchiasmic nucleus, are important in regulating long biological rhythms such as migration in birds and the circa-

dian rhythms of sleep and wakefulness. Others are involved in controlling eye movement. A small proportion of neurons from the optic tract synapse with the hypothalamus, and a proportion (10%) synapse with the superior colliculus in the midbrain tectum. However, the primary route, consisting of the largest number of axons, funnels information along the visual pathway to the occipital cortex (Figure 8.1). The route leaving the eye follows the optic nerve to the optic chiasm on the ventral surface of the brain, just anterior to the pituitary gland. There, information from both eyes joins and partially **decussates** (crosses over to the contralateral side). From then on, the left hemisphere processes information from the right visual field, and vice versa. In addition, information from the visual fields also reverses top to bottom. The lower portion of the visual field is now on top, close to the parietal lobes, and the upper portion is on the bottom, next to the temporal lobes. The optic tracts synapse with the thalamus in the dorsal portion at the lateral geniculate nucleus, then project to the occipital lobes.

Disorders of the visual system, along the pathway from the retina to the occipital lobes, depend on where along the pathway a lesion occurs. Because the pathway is topographically oriented, observing visual abilities gives a good clue to lesion location. Figure 8.2 shows a number of variants of visual difficulties, or **anopias,** possible with lesions to the optic pathways. If a lesion occurs anterior to the optic chiasm, effectively cutting off the visual input from one eye, the effect is blindness in one eye. Both visual

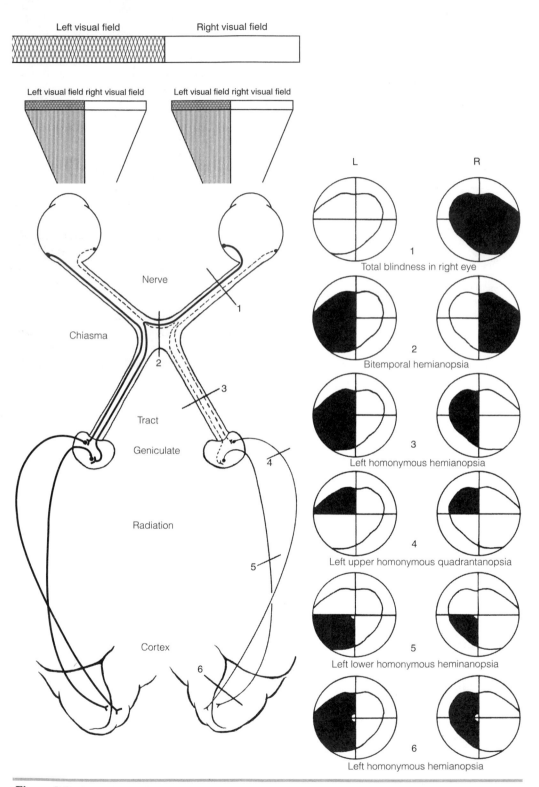

Figure 8.2   Visual field defects. Numbers indicate interruptions of visual pathways and their corresponding behavioral effects. In lesion 4, only the ventral temporal lobe fibers have been severed. In lesion 5, only the dorsal parietal lobe fibers have been severed. (Reproduced from Peele, T. L. [1977]. *The neuroanatomical basis for clinical neurology* [3rd ed.]. New York: McGraw-Hill, by permission.)

fields with full peripheral vision remain in the other eye. If, however, the optic nerve is cut posterior to the optic chiasm, the relay for one visual field in both eyes is destroyed. This condition is technically termed **homonymous** (same-sided) **hemianopia** (half blindness), and refers to partial blindness on the same side, or visual field, of each eye. The partial blindness is not related to a malfunction of the eye, but to the neural connection to the occipital lobes. This problem is also attributed to unilateral damage to the right or left occipital lobes. Often right- or left-homonymous hemianopia occurs as a result of hemorrhage, tumor, or trauma. The result of this condition can be quite hazardous. For instance, a person attempting to maneuver across a busy highway may not see traffic on the left side of his or her visual space. This condition is often compounded by other problems, for example, muscle weaknesses of the eyes that prevents a synchronized movement of the eyes across space.

Visual information reaches the occipital lobes after it has undergone early-stage processing at the level of the eye and as it passes through the thalamus. Early visual processing at the level of the occipital lobes corresponds to retinotopic areas that researchers have attempted to map out according to functional areas (generally labeled V1-V8). Although some functional areas are well understood, controversy remains for others. Areas V1-V3 appear to be best understood. Area V1 (visual area 1, formerly Brodmann's area 17) is also known as the **striate cortex,** because of its striated or banded appearance. It lies in the most posterior aspect of the occipital lobes, but a major portion of it extends onto the medial portion of each hemisphere. Functionally, this area is the primary visual cortex (Figure 8.3). The **secondary association,** or **prestriate cortex,** is contiguous and corresponds to functional visual areas V2 through V5. On the surface of the cortex these areas form donut-like rings around area V1. The responsibility for elementary visual interpretation lies in these visual areas, which process primary features of visual information such as light wavelength, line orientation, and features of shape. These represent the building blocks of the eventual composite image.

Area V1 contains the *retinotopic map,* which maintains the same topographic relations among visual elements as they are mapped on the retina. The primary purpose of this

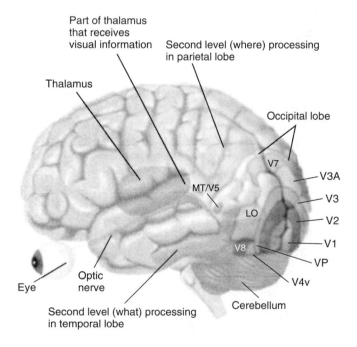

Figure 8.3 Cortical visual processing. Information relays from the thalamus to the primary visual cortex (Area V1). Visual information passes to the secondary areas of visual processing (V1–V8) where aspects of color, form, and motion are processed. From there it is analyzed in parallel streams through the ventral temporal ("What") and the dorsal parietal areas ("Where"). (Modified from Carlson, N., & Buskist, W. [1994]. *The science of behavior* [5th ed., p. 201]. Boston: Allyn & Bacon.)

area is to assemble and relay information to prestriate areas. In a reciprocal fashion, V1 also receives back projections from information processed by these visual areas within the occipital lobes and continues to play a role in maintaining spatial orientation between local bits of information. Area V2, which is closely related to V1, is also a visual preprocessing area, assembling and mapping information. Damage to area V1 causes cortical blindness, or hemianopia, in the opposite visual field. If area V1 is damaged in both hemispheres, complete blindness will occur. However, people with cortical blindness are sometimes able to indicate that a stimulus is present, that it has moved, or that it is in a certain location, even though they have no conscious ability to "see" in the conventional sense. This phenomenon is termed **blindsight.** Why does this happen? Although explanations are not definitive, part of the explanation may lie in that V1 may not be completely damaged or that some visual information, pertaining to motion, for example, may be processed outside of the striate (V1) cortex. However, the information is processed largely in an automatic or preconscious manner. No reports exist on the effect of damage to V2 alone. If V2 is damaged, V1 is also likely involved, because V2 encircles V1 like a donut. Blindness, in general, raises interesting questions about the plasticity of the brain. Neuropsychology in Action 8.1 examines what may happen to the occipital cortex in the absence of visual stimulation. As we discussed in Chapter 7, with phantom limb, the brain may reorganize itself in interesting ways.

The remaining functional visual areas in the occipital lobes (areas V3-V8) are organized into four parallel systems with reciprocal integration (Zeki, 1992). The four systems include motion, color, dynamic form (without color), and color plus dynamic form or shape. Area V3 appears specialized for dynamic form, or recognition of moving shapes, but does not code aspects of color. It has been postulated that area V4 is selective for the electromagnetic wavelengths of color, some aspects of line orientation, and form (color-and-form area). Area V5 (also called area MT) lies on the occipitoparietal juncture and receives input from a number of visual cortical areas. It contains visual motion detector cells that are specialized to respond to direction of motion. Columns of cells within the layers of the cortex are responsive to different directions. Damage that targets individual components of these secondary processors leads to specific deficits in visual behavior. For example, damage to V4 has resulted in **achromatopsia,** the complete loss of ability to detect color. People with this malady live in a black-and-white world. One man,

a successful painter of abstract art, experienced this as different from watching black-and-white TV (Neuropsychology in Action 8.2). V4 and V8 are contiguous to each other, and some have also attributed color processing to area V8. Lesions to area V5 result in a very different problem, **akinetopsia,** or the specific inability to identify objects in motion (Zihl, 1995). Damage to areas V3-V5 can result in a general inability to perceive form. In this situation, patients may be able to make a perfect copy of a drawing, but are totally unable to understand that the connection of lines corresponds to a specific shape or object.

In summary, the occipital cortex processes elementary aspects of vision. Although the functional types of processing are known, and some areas are mapped by currently understood functional location, elementary visual processing is still not completely understood. Some would suggest that visual processing, including color, proceeds in streams of processing that work in parallel fashion, rather than in localized or circumscribed structure-function maps. The next section further discusses the concept of processing streams.

HIGHER VISUAL PROCESSING: OBJECT RECOGNITION AND SPATIAL LOCALIZATION

Neuroscientists have identified at least 20 areas of secondary or higher visual processing. However, for the purposes of this discussion, we focus on the following topics: (1) how visual elements are integrated so that the viewer appreciates the pieces of vision as a coherent whole, or object; and (2) how objects are localized within a spatial framework. These two streams of visual processing are differentiated neuroanatomically, and they are often referred to as the "what" system, or ventral processing stream, of object recognition, in contrast with the "where" system, or dorsal processing stream, of object localization (Mishkin, Ungerleider, & Macko, 1983) (see Figure 8.3). The two anatomically distinct areas of the ventral and dorsal streams are probably coordinated through the thalamus (Petersen, Robinson, & Morris, 1987). In the first part of this section, we discuss the behavioral functions associated with object recognition and object localization and give an overview of the ventral and dorsal processing streams.

One of the best ways to understand the differences between the two systems is to examine the types of disorders that occur if each system is damaged. The disorders evident at this higher level of visual processing and perceptual integration involve the interaction of vision with

Neuropsychology in Action 8.1

Blindness: Helping Us See the Plasticity of the Brain

by Erin Abrigo

Does the brain's "visual" cortex lie dormant in the absence of visual input? Esref Armagan, a renowned Turkish painter, has been blind from birth. He impresses audiences all over the world with his realistic representations of objects and landscapes, complete with color, shadow, and perspective. Although visual input has never reached his brain, Mr. Armagan's occipital cortex has not atrophied, shrunk, disappeared, or even simply remained inactive over his 52 years without vision. In fact, research conducted at Beth Israel Deaconess Medical Center in Boston shows that while drawing objects that he had previously explored tactilely, his visual cortex becomes activated as if he were seeing. Current research on neuroplasticity is helping us to understand how we can explain "visual" cortex activation in a man who has never seen with his eyes.

Traditionally thought to handle only vision, research now suggests the occipital cortex can take on other duties ranging from somatosensory processing to verbal memory. In blind individuals, the occipital cortex is able to reorganize to accept nonvisual sensorimotor information. In an experiment using positron emission tomography scanning, occipital lobe activation was measured during tactile discrimination tasks in sighted subjects and in Braille readers blinded in early life. Blind volunteers showed activation of primary and secondary visual cortical areas during tactile tasks, whereas sighted control subjects actually showed reduced levels of regional cerebral blood flow in the visual cortex (Sadato, Ibañez, Deiber, & Hallett, 1996).

Further research suggests that disrupting the functioning of the occipital areas during tactile tasks leads to corresponding behavioral disruption in blind individuals. In a study conducted by Dr. Leonardo Cohen, early-blind and sighted volunteers read tactile symbols (Braille and embossed Roman letters, respectively) while transcranial magnetic stimulation (TMS) was applied to different scalp positions, transiently

disrupting the functioning of the corresponding cortical areas. In blind volunteers, TMS delivered over midoccipital regions resulted in increased errors in Braille reading as well as subjective accounts of distorted somatosensory perceptions. They reported missing dots, faded dots, extra dots, and dots that did not make sense. In contrast, midoccipital stimulation in sighted subjects did not produce significant effects on identification of embossed Roman letters or reports of abnormal perception of letters (Cohen, et al., 1997). This research suggests that the occipital or "visual" cortex is not only active during the processing of somatosensory stimulation but is functionally relevant during Braille reading for blind individuals.

Can neural plasticity also partially explain the widely recognized superior verbal memory abilities in the blind? A functional magnetic resonance imaging study conducted by Dr. Amir Amedi found occipital lobe activation during both verbal memory tasks and verb generation tasks in congenitally blind volunteers. During the same tasks, the extensive occipital activation was not observed in sighted volunteers. The results of this study suggest that, in the case of visual deprivation due to congenital blindness, the occipital lobe becomes involved during tasks that require verbal memory and may be related to the superior verbal memory skills reported in the blind. In fact, a functional role for the occipital cortex in verbal memory tasks is suggested by Amedi, as early visual cortex activity was correlated with verbal-memory scores (Amedi, 2003).

A growing body of evidence now contributes to the notion that brain regions traditionally associated with one sensory modality also participate in the processing of other senses. In this way, the occipital cortex may be viewed as being "metamodal," meaning that it is capable of adapting and changing in order to process information regardless of the sensory modality it receives. The occipital cortex may have evolved to

become the "visual cortex" simply because this region of the brain may be best suited for the processing of information supplied by vision; it may have qualities that provide it with strengths in processing spatial information using retinal visual information (Pascual-Leone & Hamilton, 2001). Because of neural plasticity, in the event of loss of visual input, the brain is able to adjust by recruiting the occipital cortex for use in another capacity, or by unmasking pathways that may already be present in the blind and sighted alike (Pascual-Leone & Hamilton, 2001).

From this collection of studies that suggest the "visual cortex" plays a role in tactile Braille reading and verbal memory in the blind, we now know that the human brain is capable of reorganizing itself and readily adjusts through adaptive recruitment of the occipital cortex. Advances in the understanding of this neuroplasticity have implications for the development of visual prosthesis aimed at restoring vision in the blind. Historic accounts of attempts at the restoration of vision have been largely unsuccessful, with some ending in depression and wishes to become blind again, presumably because of the reorganization that takes place in the cortex (von Senden, 1960). For example, when vision has been restored in patients, many have exhibited difficulties with depth perception, causing incapacitating fears of everyday activities such as crossing the street because of the inability to judge the proximity of oncoming cars. Despite cutting edge technology, restoration of functional vision through visual prosthesis without regard to the way blindness affects the brain is not likely to result in meaningful visual perception (Merabet, et al., 2005). Indeed, success in developing technology that will allow blind individuals to see will depend on the understanding of the neuroplasticity of the human brain and our ability to successfully communicate with the brain that has adjusted to blindness and that is readjusting to sight once again (Merabet, et al., 2005).

Neuropsychology in Action 8.2

The Case of Jonathan

I am a rather successful artist just past 65 years of age. On January 2nd of this year, I was driving my car and was hit by a small truck on the passenger side of my vehicle. When visiting the emergency room of a local hospital, I was told I had a concussion. While taking an eye examination, it was discovered that I was unable to distinguish letters or colors. The letters appeared "Greek" to me. My vision was such that everything looked to me as viewing a black and white television screen. Within days, I could distinguish letters and my vision became that of an eagle—I could see a worm wriggling a block away. The sharpness of my ability to focus was incredible. BUT—I AM ABSOLUTELY COLOR BLIND. I have visited ophthalmologists who know nothing about this color-blind business. I have visited neurologists, to no avail. Under hypnosis, I still can't distinguish colors. I have been involved in all kinds of tests. You name it. My brown dog is dark grey. Tomato juice is black. Color TV is a hodgepodge. (Sacks, 1995, p. 3)

And so begins Oliver Sacks's (1995) clinical tale of "The Case of the Colorblind Painter," the compelling tale of the artist Jonathan with cerebral achromatopsia, or total color blindness. Although the neuroimaging techniques of computed tomography or magnetic resonance imaging were negative, extensive neuropsychological testing by Sacks, a neurologist with an interest in neuropsychology, estimated the damage was to a small part of the secondary visual cortex of the occipital lobe. This specific injury, to an area no bigger than the size of a "bean," devastated this artist's life. The "wrongness" of everything was disturbing, even disgusting, and applied to every circumstance of daily life. He found foods disgusting because of their grayish, dead appearance and had to close his eyes to eat. But this did not help much, for the mental image of a tomato was as black as its appearance. Thus, unable to rectify even the inner image, the idea of various foods, he

turned increasingly to black and white foods—to black olives and white rice, black coffee, and yogurt. These foods at least appeared relatively normal, whereas most foods, normally colored, now appeared horribly abnormal. His own brown dog looked so strange to him that he even considered getting a Dalmatian (Sacks, 1995, p. 3).

Sacks describes an overwhelming sense of loss in Jonathan, who as a person had lost the sense of beauty of the world—particularly devastating to an artist whose whole world had been awash in a sea of color. Immediately after the injury, he was at times nearly suicidally depressed; he was fearful that he might lose more sight and was desperate in his hope that color would return. But within a month Jonathan began to show adaptation to his new condition. Two months after the accident, some of his agitation was calming down; he had started to accept, not merely intellectually but also at a deeper emotional level, that he was, indeed, totally color blind and might possibly remain so. His initial sense of helplessness began to give way to a sense of resolution—he would paint in black and white; indeed, he would live in black and white.

His first black-and-white paintings, done in February and March, gave a feeling of violent forces—rage, fear, despair, excitement—but these were held in control, attesting to the powers of artistry that could disclose, and yet contain, such intensity of feeling. In these two months, he produced dozens of paintings marked by a singular style, a character he had never shown before. In many of these paintings, there was an extraordinary, shattered, kaleidoscopic surface with abstract raging—and dismembered body parts, faceted and held in frames and boxes. They had, compared with his previous work, a labyrinthine complexity, and an obsessed, haunted quality—they seemed to exhibit, in symbolic form, the predicament he was in (Sacks, 1995, p. 14).

As time went on, Jonathan's paintings became less macabre and more vital. He

began sculpting and painting portraits, which he had not done before. Because he could only see in black and white, he became much more comfortable in the colorless world of the night. When he was not traveling, Jonathan would get up earlier and earlier, to work in the night, to relish the night. He felt that in the night world (as he called it) he was the equal, or the superior, of "normal" people: "I feel better because I know then that I'm not a freak . . . and I have developed acute night vision, it's amazing what I see—I can read license plates at night from four blocks away. You couldn't see it from a block away" (Sacks, 1995, p. 37).

Most interesting of all, the sense of profound loss, and the sense of unpleasantness and abnormality, so severe in the first months after his head injury, seemed to disappear, or even reverse. Although Jonathan does not deny his loss, and at times still mourns it, he has come to feel that his vision has become "highly refined" and "privileged"; he sees a world of pure form, uncluttered by color. Subtle textures and patterns, normally obscured for the rest of us because of their embedding in color, now stand out for him. He feels he has been given "a whole new world," to which the rest of us, distracted by color, are insensitive. He no longer thinks of color, pines for it, grieves its loss. He has almost come to see his achromatopsia as a strange gift, one that has ushered him into a new state of sensibility and being (Sacks, 1995, pp. 37, 39).

Jonathan changed in response to his damaged color system—so much so that he felt he had been able to develop extreme sensitivity to the colorless world. Interestingly, when someone suggested to him some time later that there might be a "cure," he was not interested. He was now comfortable with his new altered world and had trouble imagining anything else.

From "The Case of the Colorblind Painter," p. 3 in O. Sacks, An Anthropologist on Mars, © 1995 Alfred A. Knopf.

other sensory-perceptual and higher order systems such as attention, memory, and consciousness. The problem of visual object recognition is best illustrated by the **visual agnosias,** and the problem of spatial location can be considered by examining neglect.

The "What" and "Where" Systems of Visual Processing

The ventral processing stream is perceptually specialized for higher aspects of visual object recognition. It helps connect the visual perception of shape and form with the representation of that object's meaning. The ventral processing stream contains interconnected regions from the occipital lobes to the temporal lobes. The visual processing stream of the left hemisphere is more specific to recognizing symbolic objects such as letters and numbers. The left ventral occipital lobe shows increased blood flow when people process strings of letters (Snyder, Petersen, Fox, & Raichle, 1989). The right ventral system is more specific to the global recognition of objects and faces. Damage to this system can result in visual agnosia. The next section provides an in-depth discussion of the subtypes of visual agnosia (apperceptive and associate agnosia).

The dorsal processing stream is essential for visually localizing objects in space and for appreciating the relative relation of those objects to each other. Through reciprocal feedback to the motor system, this "where" system also helps in planning and coordinating motor movements. This stream of integrated structures connects the occipital to the parietal lobes. Disorders of this system contribute to right–left discrimination problems, constructional apraxia, and neglect.

Directional impairment, a form of spatial relations confusion, is usually referred to as a right–left discrimination problem. Patients with this kind of difficulty routinely get lost if left on their own, particularly in a new environment. An inability to perform voluntary actions, termed constructional apraxia, is the inability to perform actions that require three-dimensional movement, such as building a tower from blocks. (Apraxia is discussed in Chapter 7.)

Disorders of the "What" System: Apperceptive and Associative Visual Agnosia

Agnosia is derived from the Greek, *gnosis,* meaning "absence of knowing" and can occur in any sensory domain. In the modality of vision, people with **visual object agnosia** may fail to recognize objects at all, or in milder cases, confuse objects that they observe from different angles or in different lighting conditions. The term

prosopagnosia refers to the special case of inability to recognize people by their faces, even though the person can often recognize people by other means such as gait or tone of voice. People with visual agnosias can see. The disorder is less a pure sensory disorder than a higher perceptual disorder of "knowing." In *The Man Who Mistook His Wife for a Hat,* Oliver Sacks describes the affliction of Dr. P, a music teacher who can no longer recognize objects or people by sight. Presented with a red rose, Dr. P "took it like a botanist or morphologist given a specimen, not like a person given a flower. 'About six inches in length,' he commented. 'A convoluted red form with a linear green attachment.'" Dr. P was completely unable to name what he had in his hand until it was suggested to him to smell it. "'Beautiful!' he exclaimed. 'An early rose. What a heavenly smell!' He started to hum [the German tune] "*Die Rose, die Lilie. . . .*" (Sacks, 1987, pp. 13–14). Dr. P's affliction was that he was visually unaware of the totality or *gestalt* of objects. He could see and identify form and color but could not combine these aspects into a higher sense of meaning that is a rose. His only visual reality was a mechanistic identification of features. This is typical of how visual agnosia primarily involves the processes necessary for object recognition or object meaning while leaving intact elementary visual processes. Also, Dr. P's agnosia, as is usually the case, was modality specific. Although his visual knowing was impaired, a higher sense of knowing was available through sense of smell. Dr. P also had no problem in recognizing people by their voices.

Cognitive neuropsychologists often differentiate between **apperceptive visual agnosia** and **associative visual agnosia.** The essential difficulty in apperceptive visual agnosia is *object perception,* or the inability to combine the individual aspects of visual information such as line, shape, color, and form together to form a "whole" percept. They seem to see in bits and pieces, like the proverbial blind men feeling the elephant. Their brains are not synthesizing the entire picture. Associative visual agnosics have difficulty to varying degrees in assigning *meaning* to an object. Even though they can, for instance, recognize differences in form between pictures of a pair of scissors and a paper punch by matching the scissors to a like pair in a display of office objects (with which an apperceptive agnosic would have difficulty), they have lost the link between the visual percept and the semantic meaning. In both cases, if shown a pair of scissors, neither the apperceptive nor the associative agnosic can correctly name "scissors." But although the associative agnosic can pick out a pair of scissors, she or he shows difficulties not only in naming but in explaining or demonstrating the use for scissors.

This distinction provides a useful conceptual framework and is used here; but in practice, the line between apperceptive and associative agnosias becomes cloudy, partly because the brain damage likely to cause these problems is often widespread and overlapping.

Apperceptive Agnosia—At first glance, those individuals, like Dr. P., with the apperceptive form of object agnosia may be thought blind, because they tend to take no apparent notice of objects and people in their vicinity. But on closer examination, their sensory functions are clearly intact. Many people with this condition are aware that they can indeed see, but they have a problem correctly perceiving things. Curiously, others with apperceptive agnosia are strangely unaware of their condition. Only watching for a period of time might you catch them stepping over or avoiding objects. Awareness in this case is not an either/or phenomenon. Apperceptive agnosics may appear to disregard or show no concern for their problem until neuropsychological testing reveals it to them. For example, visual recognition tasks of the type shown in Figure 8.4, in which an object must be identified from fragments, is embedded, or is at an odd angle, are notoriously difficult. Apperceptive agnosics also have difficulty copying objects. Because they only "see" pieces, their drawings are likely to appear as a set of unconnected fragments focusing on the details rather than on the entire gestalt of the object.

The most common site of damage in apperceptive agnosia is the parieto-occipital area of the right hemisphere. Sudden insults to the brain are the most common cause, often from carbon monoxide poisoning, mercury intoxication, cardiac arrest, or stroke. In these cases, apperceptive agnosia does not usually occur in isolation without other visuospatial impairment, because these brain insults are likely to affect large areas of the cortex. Some cases of apperceptive agnosia are caused by bilateral cortical atrophy. If both hemispheres are involved, then the patient may have **Balint's syndrome,** which includes visual agnosia together with other visuospatial difficulties such as misreaching and left-sided neglect.

Associative Agnosia—Associative agnosia is differentiated behaviorally from apperceptive agnosia in that the primary difficulty is a loss of knowledge of the semantic meaning of objects. Conceptually, the person can "recognize" objects at a perceptual level by picking them out, or correctly copying them, but perception breaks down at a higher level of meaning. For example, some people have little apperceptive difficulty and can draw or copy pictures of objects in great detail but cannot name them (for example, see Rubens & Benson, 1971). As Figure 8.5

shows, after making an accurate rendition of a bird, the patient tentatively guessed it could be a "beach stump." This represents a pure form of associative agnosia, but many other patients also show aspects of apperceptive agnosia. For example, they may copy objects inconsistently, sometimes drawing them accurately and at other times making perceptual mistakes. However, whereas the perceptual mistakes of the apperceptive agnosic are likely to show inability to recognize the whole, the perceptual mistakes of the associative agnosic may show problems of either recognition of the whole or of the details of an object.

The research on the neurocorrelates of associative agnosia is confusing. A lateralized left hemisphere parieto-occipital lesion may be enough to cause an associative agnosia, although it can also occur in the presence of a unilateral right occipital lesion. Indeed, a number of structural areas may produce associative agnosia. Farah (1990) suggests the variety of sites that produce associative agnosia may lead to heterogeneous perceptual impairments. Because assigning meaning is such a high-level cortical process, different lesion sites producing a similar effect also speaks to the complexity of the perceptual-meaning system. We would venture, as have others, that, in general, the left hemisphere assigns meaning, whereas the right hemisphere governs the global aspects of perceptual integration.

As stated earlier, many patients show both apperceptive and associative aspects to their visual agnosia. For example, one artist who experienced a stroke resulting in bilateral medial occipital damage could name some objects but not others. Those he could name he could also draw well. But those he did not recognize, he could only mechanistically copy, feature by feature, first a square, then a circle, then connecting lines, without any inkling of what they represented (Wapner, Judd, & Gardner, 1978). In summary, the differentiation between apperceptive and associative agnosia is useful for descriptive and conceptual understanding, but it does not correspond to strict anatomic correlates that can be readily differentiated or dissociated.

Disorder of the "Where" System: Neglect

Certain types of brain damage can alter body experience. Damage to the right parieto-occipital or inferior parietal area is the most common site of damage for an odd type of inattention termed unilateral neglect, or simply neglect. (*Unilateral spatial neglect* has other aliases, such as *contralesional neglect, hemineglect, visuospatial* or *hemispatial agnosia,* and *visuospatial* or *hemispatial inattention.*)

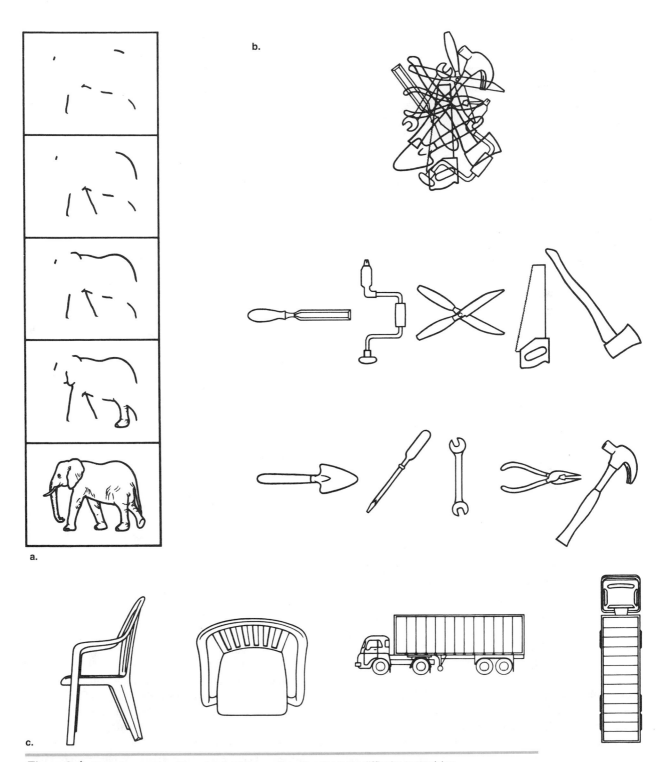

Figure 8.4 Tests for apperceptive agnosia. Apperceptive agnosics have difficulty recognizing (a) fragmented objects, (b) entangled object, and (c) objects seen from unusual views. (Modified from Bradshaw, J. L., & Mattingly, J. B. [1995]. *Clinical neuropsychology: Behavioral and brain science.* San Diego: Academic Press, by permission.)

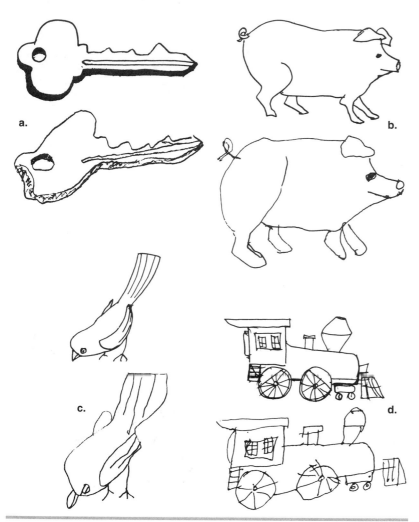

Figure 8.5 Drawings from an associative visual agnosic. These pictures were accurately drawn but mislabeled: (a) "I still don't know"; (b) "Could be a dog or any other animal"; (c) "Could be a beach stump"; (d) "A wagon or a car of some kind. The larger vehicle is being pulled by the smaller one." (Reproduced from Bauer, R. M. [1993]. Agnosia. In K. M. Heilman & E. Valenstein [Eds.], *Clinical neuropsychology.* New York: Oxford University Press, by permission.)

People with neglect lose conscious awareness of an aspect of spatial or personal space despite adequately functioning sensory and motor systems. Behaviorally, this problem may first look like the result of a right hemisphere stroke or lesion affecting the motor and somatosensory strips on the contralesional side. The left limbs may appear useless and hang limply. On closer examination, the arm or leg can clearly move and feel touch or pain—they are simply being ignored by the conscious mind. This failure of awareness extends beyond the body to the entire left hemispace from the perspective of the afflicted person. It

is not unusual for people with neglect to collide with objects and people on their left sides. Also, when reading, they may leave out the left side of words or pages. Their copied drawings focus on the right side of pictures. In one respect, neglect can be thought of as a forgetting or lack of conscious attention to the left side; but even more so, it is as if awareness is being *pulled* to the right. When trying to navigate, neglect patients frequently veer rightward and end up traveling in circles. The case study in Neuropsychology in Action 8.3 gives an in-depth illustration of the behavioral manifestations of unilateral neglect. Although

Neuropsychology in Action 8.3

Case Study: Neglect

by Mary Spiers

One of the first cases of pure spatial neglect was published by Paterson and Zangwill in 1944. Their patient was a healthy 39-year-old right-handed man who, because of an explosion, was hit by a projectile steel nut that penetrated his skull in the right parietal occipital area. "Stereoscopic X-rays of the skull (28.9.43) showed a metallic foreign body consisting of a hexagonal nut about 1 in. in diameter with a short length of screw-headed bolt projecting from its upper lateral surface" (Paterson & Zangwill, 1944, pp. 335–336). "The upper borders of the supramarginal and angular gyri on the right side were damaged on the surface and their deeper connection interrupted by the in-driven bone fragments to a depth of just over 1 in. The lesion was circumscribed and there was minimal contusional damage" (p. 337). The resultant difficulties, as you would expect, were largely confined to spatial and visual-perceptual functions. This man could perceptually recognize objects, identify colors, and discriminate right and left. He also had no problems in spatial depth perception and size constancy. But the patient himself alerted his doctors that he was having trouble finding his way through the hallways on the way to the bathroom and was having trouble reading the time. He said he had to read each hand of the clock separately and then figure out the time. Staff observed him to collide "with objects on his left which he had clearly perceived a few moments before. He was liable at table to knock over dishes on his left-hand side and occasionally missed food on the left of his plate. He commonly failed to attend to the left-hand page in turning the pages of a book and reading lines of disconnected words commonly omitted the first word or two" (Paterson & Zangwill, 1944, p. 339). On neuropsychological testing, when asked to draw, his figures showed a "piecemeal perception" typical of right hemisphere spatial problems. Interestingly, he could slowly recognize objects placed in his left visual field, but if two designs were presented simultaneously to the right and left visual fields, he did not acknowledge the left-sided design. In setting the time on a clock, he often transposed the minute hand from the left- to the right-hand side. In a pointing task, the authors arranged objects around the patient in a semicircle. "He was instructed to point to each object in turn. With eyes open no errors were made. With his eyes closed, on the other hand, there was at once a general shift toward the right-hand side. Thus when asked to point to the object on his extreme left the patient often pointed straight ahead" (Paterson & Zangwill, 1944, p. 339). Unlike other cases of neglect, this man did not neglect the left side of his own body, only his extrapersonal space.

This case presents an interesting problem of consciousness. How can this loss of awareness be explained? On one level, the patient was aware that he now disregarded the left side of space. This shows some insight into his problem. But on another level, no force of will could coax a full knowing of his left-sided spatial world.

not in this case, many people with neglect think that the left-sided part of their body does not belong to them. Protesting that it belongs to someone else, they may fail to dress half of the body, put makeup on only one side of the face, or simply treat the neglected parts as objects with no personal meaning. What mechanisms disable body and spatial awareness? We will return to this question after considering the neuropathologic and clinical presentation of neglect.

Neuropathology of Neglect—The classic picture of unilateral neglect that we have been discussing is most likely to occur with lesions in the right inferior parietal lobe or generally in the posterior regions of the cortex. As mentioned earlier, neglect cannot be solely attributed to sensory processing deficits, implying that lesions in the somatosensory strip are not enough to produce neglect. Neglect can also appear with other right hemisphere lesions, and much less frequently, with left hemisphere lesions. Other right hemisphere locations reported to produce neglect include a variety of subcortical structures, the majority of which implicate the thalamus.

Classic neglect produces an abrupt alteration of consciousness most commonly occurring as a result of a right parietal stroke, but sometimes coinciding with a traumatic brain injury. In any case, the manifestation is typically sudden and rarely seen in slow-growing tumors or disease processes. Temporary and reversible neglect may also occur in conjunction with seizures, electroconvulsive therapy, and intracarotid sodium amytal testing (Wada testing) (see Bradshaw & Mattingly, 1995). Neglect may also stand out against the background of widespread right hemisphere damage. In this instance, there are accompanying motor, sensory, or attentional problems. For example, a variety of neglect-type problems are associated with motor weakness. In these cases, awareness of left-sided stimuli may be less impaired, but neglect-type symptoms become evident with the inability to perform or sustain motor acts on the side contralateral to the lesion (see Heilman, Watson, & Valenstein, 1993). If we include all the subtypes and derivations, we can best conceptualize neglect as a syndrome or general classification for a number of related problems. However, we restrict this discussion to classical unilateral spatial neglect, caused by right hemisphere damage, which is the best example of the neglect phenomenon.

Clinical Presentation—In clinically evaluating cases of unilateral neglect, neuropsychologists must disentangle the contributions of spatial, motor, and attentional factors. This can only be done in a relative fashion, because each of these systems contributes a portion to a sense of body and spatial consciousness. For example, although investigators agree that a functioning attentional system is crucial to spatial awareness, unilateral neglect and severe inattention can be differentiated. With both problems there can be a failure to detect an object, such as an apple, that is placed in the left visual field. However, the inattentive person becomes aware of the apple if forced to orient to it, whereas the person with neglect may continue to insist that nothing is there. Neglect is also dissociable from visual field defects such as hemianopia, in which the person visually explores the left side of space (Hornak, 1992). Neglect may look similar to visual problems, but it is actually a problem at a much higher level of integration.

Because neglect is so obviously out of the range of ordinary experience, measures to test for it do not rely on norms, but rather on pathognomic signs. For example, we do not expect neglect to be evenly distributed in the population in the form of a bell-shaped curve, with only a few of us having no neglect, many of us having moderate neglect, and a few of us having profound neglect. Instead, we expect all people with normally functioning brains to be free of neglect. Therefore, the detection of neglect and neglect-like symptoms is fairly straightforward by observing performance on tasks such as drawings and line bisection tasks. Figure 8.6 shows several clinical examples of neuropsychological tasks performed by people with neglect. Notice that in the drawings the left side of the picture may be left out, sparse, or grossly distorted. In the line bisection and line cancellation tasks, the midpoint shifts to the right, leaving the left side of the line or the page empty.

It is clear that unilateral neglect patients do not consciously acknowledge stimuli in the left side of space. But does perception or a tacit recognition at an unconscious level exist? Clinical investigations suggest that it does. In an interesting series of studies, Vallar and his colleagues (Vallar, Sandroni, Rusconi, & Barbieri, 1991) tested autonomic responses such as galvanic skin conductance and brain response via evoked potentials. In each case, the patients with unilateral left-sided neglect failed to consciously recognize the presence of a stimulus presented to the right side, although autonomic testing demonstrated the patients were processing the stimulus implicitly at a preconscious level, without reaching awareness. Some clinical studies also suggest that people with neglect may implicitly process at a higher level, indicating acknowledgment of meaning or semantic awareness. In one of the first case studies to suggest implicit awareness in neglect, Marshall and Halligan (1988) gave their patient two pictures of a house, identical except for that in one the left side of the house was obviously burning. The patient did not acknowledge any discrepancies between the two houses when asked to describe the pictures, nor did she say they were different when forced to make a same–different choice. Curiously, however, when asked which house she would prefer to live in, she consistently chose the picture of the house that was not burning, although she could not explain or give reasons for her choice. It is as though, from her perspective, the only explanation she could give relied on an intuitive sense. Although not all neglect patients show this preservation of semantic knowledge (some actually chose the burning house; see Bisiach & Rusconi, 1990), studies using a variety of methodologies confirm that higher order processing of various types is possible in some patients with neglect (see Bradshaw & Mattingly, 1995).

Interestingly, the behavior of left unilateral neglect usually resolves somewhat over time if the damaged area remains stable. Afflicted people gradually begin to acknowledge stimuli on the left side of their bodily space. Tests of tactile recognition, in which the researcher touches one hand or the other while the patient is blindfolded, show that he or she is recognizing both hands. However, when both hands are touched at the same time in a specific test of double simultaneous stimulation, residual neglect is often evident in that the patient again suppresses or extinguishes perception of the left hand.

Neglect, as can be imagined, is notoriously difficult to treat in the beginning stages. Patients who do not acknowledge their problem and who may believe their left

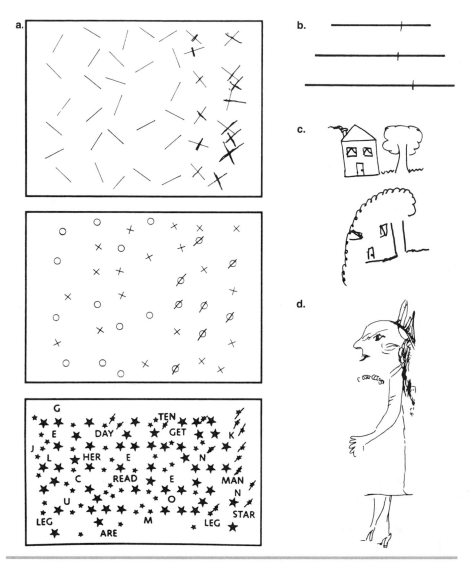

Figure 8.6 Performance of a patient with left-sided neglect. (a) Three cancellation tasks in which the left side of the page has been neglected. (b) A line bisection task that veers to the right of midpoint. (c) A copy of a house that is distorted on the right side. (d) Spontaneous drawing of a woman. (Reproduced from Bradshaw, J. L., & Mattingly, J. B. [1995]. *Clinical neuropsychology: Behavioral and brain science* [p. 128]. San Diego: Academic Press, by permission.)

side does not even belong to them are not motivated to pay attention to their left side. Rehabilitation methods often try to direct attention to the neglected side. Therapists may use various methods such as forcing attention to the left side via gradual movement of objects to the left, or even through the use of prism glasses. These methods do meet with some success, but often do not generalize to daily life.

Theories of Neglect—Two primary issues exist in conceptualizing neglect. The first issue is understanding the asymmetric presentation of neglect between the two hemispheres. Why is neglect more prevalent with right hemisphere lesions? Any theory of neglect must explain why the overwhelming majority of cases show left-sided neglect, and why right-sided neglect is so rare. The second issue relates to the higher order or "conscious" processing problem that is neglect. If neglect is thought of as a network problem rather than as a dysfunction of an individual system, it is easier to make sense of the variety of lesion sites that may produce neglect.

Research has established that the right hemisphere is more specialized for global spatial processing, whereas the left hemisphere has a propensity for decoding specific spatial features. Because the right hemisphere, and particularly the right parietal lobe, plays a role in understanding the gestalt or totality of space, disruptions there are more likely to upset global spatial awareness. Also, the right hemisphere plays a larger role in arousal and attentional levels, which are prime factors in many explanatory models of neglect. However, each of these problems can occur in isolation without the patient losing consciousness of the left side of space. As with the man described in Neuropsychology in Action 8.3, no force of will could coax a "knowing" of his spatial world on the left. Interestingly, it appears that patients may shift their "spatial axis" to the right so that midline is pulled or repositioned within the right side of space relative to the body (Mattingly, 1996). Marcel Kinsbourne (1993) has postulated that this strong rightward orientation is less a function of right hemisphere dysfunction per se than a release of inhibition that lets the left hemisphere assert dominance in the presence of a now weakened right hemisphere. Perhaps some of the prime areas damaged, rendering the right hemisphere spatially ineffective, are locations within the right parietal lobe having to do with personal spatial frames of reference. Body position with respect to space is always egocentric, although people may have multiple frames with respect to bodies, heads, or position in relation to environment. Animal studies support the contention that there are distinct neuronal centers for these spatial frames within the right parietal cortex (for example, see Anderson, Snyder, Li, & Stricanne, 1993).

Do these findings explain why the midline shift in neglect is nearly always to the right? Bradshaw and Mattingly (1995) suggest that each hemisphere plays a specific role in spatial body position processing. The left hemisphere focuses on features and is strongly rightward oriented. The right hemisphere takes a "global view." Normally, the two hemispheres hold each other in balance, but when certain spatial positioning aspects of the right hemisphere are damaged, the left hemisphere becomes overbearing, forcing a reorientation to the right side of space. According to this view, damage to the left parietal lobe produces no corresponding leftward shift because the spatial concerns of the left hemisphere are more feature oriented and language focused,

resulting in a "no specialized spatial position" sense within the left parietal lobes. If right neglect does occur, they suggest, together with other investigators (such as Ogden, 1985), that the focus of the left hemisphere lesion would be anterior to the parietal lobes. Unfortunately, partly because of the rarity of occurrence, no research has explained the mechanisms of right-sided neglect.

Understanding neglect is not only a problem of dominance and asymmetry, it is also an issue of conceptualizing the problem as a higher order network processing phenomenon. That unilateral neglect can occur with other nonparietal foci of damage is partial testament to this claim. We mentioned earlier that the region of the right inferior parietal lobe is the area most commonly damaged in cases of left unilateral neglect. As in other disorders discussed throughout this book, however, absence of function associated with a lesion does not necessarily imply that the lesioned area "contains" the function. Just as the hippocampus does not "contain" or store memory but is one of the most crucial links in memory processing and consolidation, the right inferior parietal lobe does not in itself contain "body mindfulness" but may be a crucial link. Neuroanatomically, left unilateral neglect also occurs with damage to a variety of subcortical structures, most notably the thalamus (see Bradshaw & Mattingly, 1995). It is reasonable to speculate that neglect results from a disconnection in higher order processing that involves the coordination of many second-order systems, such as visual processing, attention, memory, and possibly other systems.

A number of theories attempt to provide models for unilateral neglect. They are beyond the scope of this overview, and excellent reviews exist elsewhere (for example, see Bradshaw & Mattingly, 1995). Most models describe the process of body and hemispace cognition as including visual-perceptual processes, attention, and motor action. Mesulam's neural network model (for example, see Mesulam, 1985, 1990) is closely tied to neuroanatomic functioning. He identifies three major functional areas that must interact for the body–space system to work normally. Each of these areas corresponds to a cortical site. The parietal lobes control perceptual processing, the premotor and prefrontal cortices mediate exploratory-motor behavior, and the cingulate gyrus directs motivation. In turn, subcortical structures probably coordinate the orchestration of all three areas. The reticular formation directs arousal, and the thalamus (particularly the pulvinar of the thalamus) is postulated to focus and guide attention between spatial locations.

Summary—The visual processing system reflects both the complexity and the reliance of humans on our visual sense. We discussed both features and streams of visual processing. The primary visual system, which serves as a "feature analyzer," builds to the higher order systems of object recognition and spatial localization. Disorders such as visual agnosia and neglect provide good examples of how each of these systems may malfunction. However, with vision, there is much reciprocal networking between parallel systems, so what appears hierarchical may not be entirely so. What is discussed in a bottom-up fashion may also be affected by top-down processing. Currently, brain science has uncovered much of the structure and many of the functions of the visual road map through the brain. However, much work needs to be done in understanding how the brain accommodates to varying visual experiences that represent the same precept. With an expansion of functional imaging techniques, a better understanding of high-level integration of the fragmentary components of visual processing is occurring, especially in visual disorders, in which integration may be a product of systems beyond the visual system.

Auditory and Language Processing

The human auditory system is a crucial sensory system, because it is the pathway to language, a uniquely human development. This section examines the brain's control of auditory processing, speech, and language by exploring the brain structures believed to be principal in language functioning. Because no animal models of language exist, much knowledge of the neuropsychology of language links closely to knowledge about the behavioral effects of aphasia subtypes. Reliance on brain-damaged patients to delineate systems can be tricky because lesions may not indicate site of damage, and many aphasics are stroke patients with a fairly wide area of damage.

PRIMARY AUDITORY PROCESSING

Humans can detect a wide range of sound from the 30-Hz to the 20,000-Hz range. Difficulties in detecting the features of sound, such as how long a vowel versus a consonant sound might resonate, can result in higher level language disturbance. One theory of autism considers the idea that autistic people may not be tuned in to the frequency of human speech, but instead have a propensity for lower frequency environmental sounds such as

those made by machines. If human speech is an aversive and even fear-producing noise, then there would be a withdrawal from the sound of human speech. Many difficulties can emerge if the primary building blocks of sound detection and recognition are not intact.

The auditory system contains mechanical receptors designed to detect sound frequency. These hairlike receptors are located in the fluid of the long, coiled, snail-like *cochlea* of the inner ear. As the mechanical mechanisms of the middle ear respond to external sound waves, they cause vibrations in the fluid of the inner ear, thus vibrating the hairs of the auditory receptors. These receptors synapse with the auditory nerve. The auditory nerve from each ear projects ipsilaterally to the cochlear nuclei of the medulla. From there, each pathway branches to project auditory information to both the ipsilateral and contralateral superior olivary nuclei of the medulla. In this way, the auditory system differs from the visual system in that each hemisphere receives input from both ears, resulting in bilateral representation of sound. This may help the person localize sound in space. The auditory pathways then course through the lower brainstem and ascend through the thalamus, where they are projected to the primary auditory cortex (Figure 8.7).

The primary auditory cortex of each hemisphere lies deep within the temporal lobe, largely on the medial aspect of the superior temporal gyrus, within the valley of the lateral fissure. This area is commonly termed Heschl's gyrus and corresponds to Brodmann's area 41. Heschl's area is often larger in the right hemisphere, sometimes consisting of two gyri to the left's one gyrus. This cortical area processes the "fragments" of sound, much as the visual system processes individual visual stimuli. The primary auditory cortex is organized into frequency-specific bands that parallel the layout of auditory frequency ranges mapped on the cochlea (see Figure 8.7). In this way, a **tonotopic map** projects onto the auditory cortex, similar to the retinotopic map of the visual system. Because the cortical bands can respond to multiple frequencies, there is no strict one-to-one correspondence; rather, some bands are more attuned to certain frequencies than others. The primary auditory cortex processes several elements of sound. In addition to frequency, the features of sound include loudness, timbre, duration, and change.

HIGHER AUDITORY PROCESSING: SPEECH AND LANGUAGE

Speaking requires the ability to differentiate between speech sounds, or phonemes, such as vowels and consonants. For

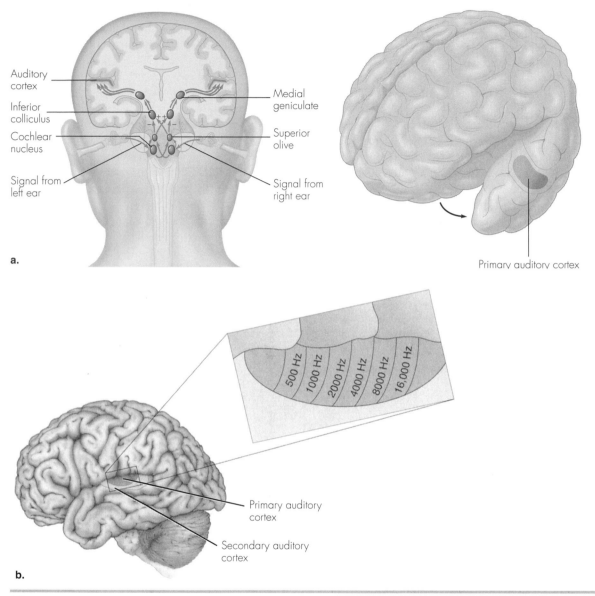

Auditory cortex

Inferior colliculus

Cochlear nucleus

Signal from left ear

Medial geniculate

Superior olive

Signal from right ear

a.

Primary auditory cortex

500 Hz 1000 Hz 2000 Hz 4000 Hz 8000 Hz 16,000 Hz

Primary auditory cortex

Secondary auditory cortex

b.

Figure 8.7 Pathway from the ear to the primary auditory cortex. (a) Each ear projects to the ipsilateral cochlea, and then projects to the primary auditory cortex in both hemispheres. (b) The primary auditory cortex is organized according to a tonotopic frequency map. ([a] Reproduced from Kalat, J. W. [1998]. *Biological psychology* [6th ed., p. 184, Figure 7.6]. Pacific Grove, CA: Brooks/Cole, by permission; [b] modified from Bear, M. F., Connors, B. W., & Paradiso, M. A. [1996]. *Neuroscience: Exploring the brain* [p. 303, Figure 11.28]. Baltimore: Williams & Wilkins.)

example, in French, the brain must hear the fine distinctions between the pronunciations of *tu* and *tous,* the sounds of which are not differentiated in English and only heard as *too.* Vowels have a slightly different frequency from consonants, and different consonants are differentiated from each other. Speech also requires the ability to produce intelligible speech output. Learning a language, as anyone who has tried to master a second language knows, involves much more than being able to understand and articulate words in a spoken fashion. Language also requires putting meaning to word fragments (morphemes), words, and groups of words (semantics). Another major

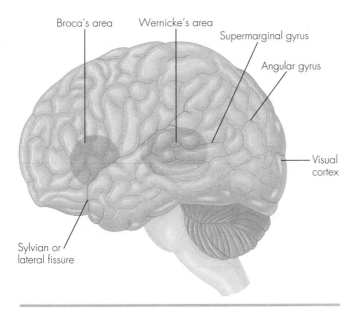

Figure 8.8 Major cortical language areas. In most people, the left frontal operculum, or Broca's area, is specialized for speech production, whereas Wernicke's area is specialized for speech comprehension. (Reproduced from Kalat, J. W. [1998]. *Biological psychology* [6th ed., p. 390, Figure 14.13]. Pacific Grove, CA: Brooks/Cole.)

requirement of language is knowledge of its syntax or grammatical rules. This requires learning information regarding subject–verb agreement (for example, "girls run"), how to use articles and propositions (for example, *the, to, but, if, and*), and how to put strings of words together to make meaningful sentences.

After the primary auditory cortex processes sound features, they are integrated into understandable speech sounds in the secondary auditory processing area commonly known as **Wernicke's area.** Wernicke's area lies on the posterior aspect of the superior temporal gyrus (see Figures 8.7 and 8.8). It includes the secondary auditory cortex and does not technically involve the adjacent primary auditory cortex (Heschl's gyrus). The secondary auditory processing area serves to connect sound from the primary auditory areas to word meaning stored in the cortex. This is an intermediate step to the full understanding of language. Additional cortical processing areas are required to integrate the comprehension of individual words into grammatically correct phrases and sentences, and to link spoken words with the written symbols of language necessary for reading comprehension. The supramarginal and angular gyri of the inferior parietal lobes are contiguous

to Wernicke's area, and the two are closely integrated. These higher association areas serve to bring together visual and spatial information from the occipital and parietal lobes with auditory information. The angular gyrus plays a role in reading comprehension by matching words and word sounds (phonemes such as the sound of /*ba*/) to written symbols of language (graphemes such as *b*).

Damage to the left hemisphere auditory processing areas results in the partial or total inability to decipher spoken words. This condition is known as **receptive aphasia, or Wernicke's aphasia.** However, people with receptive aphasia can often still recognize the emotional tone of language, because the speaker's intent, such as anger, sarcasm, or humor, is processed as voice intonation. Conversely, right hemisphere damage has the opposite effect: The patient accepts words at face value but loses the nuances of jokes and emotional intention. Another hallmark of right hemisphere damage is impaired harmonic and melodic ability. The ability to appreciate musical tunes may be completely eliminated. As an example of a problem with recognition of environmental sounds, one patient with a right hemisphere auditory processing deficit repeatedly had to have starters replaced in her car. She could no longer discriminate the difference in sound between the sound of the starter engaging and the sound of the engine turning over. Speech understanding, therefore, conveys word analysis, as well as emotional intentions, through tone of voice, pitch, intensity, and rhythm.

Expressive speech links to the **frontal operculum** (Broca's area), located in the left frontal lobe on the posterior portion of the third frontal gyrus (the inferior frontal gyrus). This area is adjacent to the facial area of the motor cortex. The inferior frontal gyrus is a premotor area of the frontal lobes, and thus is concerned with aspects of speech planning before output coordinated by the nearby motor strip. In addition to mediating the fluency of speech, Broca's area plays a role in the grammatical and syntactical arrangement of words. Wernicke's and Broca's areas are linked by a band of white matter fibers called the *arcuate fasciculus.* This allows for close communication between the two areas in expressive output. Words, whether from external sources or from the self, are picked out for meaning in Wernicke's area, and in parallel, the syntax of the phrase is constructed in Broca's area. This is possible because the arcuate fasciculus permits reciprocal interaction between the two areas (Yeterian & Van Hoesen, 1978). This interaction also makes logical sense, because syntax depends on the words used and the words selected also depend on the emerging syntax of the sentence (Bradshaw & Mattingly, 1995).

The basal ganglia and the thalamus have also been implicated in language functioning via their participation in a cortico-striato-pallido-thalamo-cortical loop (see Crosson, 1992). This loop, or perhaps set of loops, connects the language centers of the cortex to the putamen and caudate nucleus of the striatum, to the globus pallidus, to specific nuclei in the thalamus, and back to the cortical language centers. The current thinking regarding the function of these loops is that they play a role in regulating language; this role involves initiating language production more than constructing speech content (Crosson, 1992).

One hemisphere, usually the left, is dominant for speech. This means that the left cerebral cortex preferentially processes speech sounds, whereas the right processes nonspeech sounds. Not surprisingly, the functional dominance of the left hemisphere for speech corresponds to preferential treatment for speech sound processing in the larger planum temporale of the left hemisphere. After analysis of sound features, secondary auditory information, such as phonemes, is integrated in the planum temporale, in the temporal area adjacent to the primary auditory cortex (Brodmann's area 42). Although sound from each ear projects bilaterally, there

is an opposite hemisphere advantage; in this case, the left hemisphere preferentially processes sound from the right ear. Because the left hemisphere shows a preference for analyzing speech in most people, speech sounds processed through the right ear will be understood faster and more accurately than speech sounds processed through the left ear.

The left hemisphere also has a propensity for rhythm of both speech and music as it codes for the sequence of sounds. To check your left hemisphere dominance for rhythm, try keeping a metronome-like beat with your left hand and beat out the rhythm of a familiar tune, such as *Jingle Bells,* with your right hand. Most people find this easy if their left hemisphere, which controls their right hand, is dominant for rhythm. After doing this, try reversing what each hand is doing (right keeps the beat, and left taps out the rhythm) and see if you have more or less difficulty. The secondary auditory cortex of the right hemisphere, by contrast, is specific for aspects of tonality, including the melody of music and the intonation of speech, which is commonly referred to as *speech prosody.* The right hemisphere is adept at recognizing the relation between simultaneous sounds, such as the harmony of chords, or the musical interval between notes. It also shows an advantage for recognizing nonspeech or environmental sounds such as those made by machines and cars, as well as animals, birds, the pounding ocean surf, or a babbling creek.

The brain's asymmetry for language processing and production is an extension of speech processing. The left hemisphere specializes in processing word sounds, or morphemes; semantics; and the grammatical rules of language. The right hemisphere, long thought to be "mute," plays a role in the emotional intention of both vocalization and understanding. The right hemisphere may have no speech or understanding of grammatical rules; however, a number of people, and more women than men, have some bilateral representation of speech. The right hemisphere is nonetheless capable of considerable comprehension and expression. Although frank aphasia is rare after right hemisphere strokes, there can be linguistic impairments. These include a deficit in comprehending tone and voice, producing similar emotional tone, and understanding metaphors and jokes. We once examined a male adult patient who had undergone a complete left hemispherectomy. Although he was severely aphasic, he could communicate somewhat using "grunts." He was also able to curse, possibly because such communication is more emotional in nature and, therefore, partly controlled by the right hemisphere.

Table 8.1 *Aphasia Types*

Type of Aphasia	Fluency, Content	Repetition of Speech	Comprehension of Speech	Reading and Writing
Broca's	Confluent, agrammatical	Impaired	Normal	Agrammatical, misspelling
Wernicke's	Normal, word salad	Abnormal	Poor	Inaccuracies
Conduction	Normal fluency, phonemic errors	Abnormal	Relatively intact	Abnormal
Transcortical motor	Halting	Fluent	Normal	Reading normal, writing impaired
Transcortical sensory	Normal	Normal	Poor	Inaccuracies
Anomic	Normal fluency, word-finding errors	Normal	Normal	Normal
Global	Abnormal	Abnormal	Abnormal	Abnormal

In summary, the complexity of speech and language necessitates specific brain systems, which in most people are lateralized. Beyond the discrete cortical components controlling auditory reception (auditory cortices and Wernicke's area) and auditory speech production (Broca's area and motor cortex), language requires thought and, therefore, extensive interconnections to higher order planning and memory centers. The supramarginal gyrus and the angular gyrus of the parietal lobes are also important to integrating verbal aspects of language with the visual symbolic components involved in reading. Subcortical neural connections, including portions of the basal ganglia and the thalamus, also play a role in language. Finally, cerebral lateralization exists for various language functions.

APHASIA: A BREAKDOWN OF LANGUAGE

Aphasia is a disturbance of language usage or comprehension. It may impair the power to speak, write, read, gesture, or to comprehend spoken, written, or gestured language. Aphasia is a disturbance connecting speaking to thinking, and thus is differentiated from purely mechanical disorders of speech such as **dysarthria** or **speech apraxia** caused by paralysis or incoordination of the musculature of the mouth or vocal apparatus. Aphasic disorders also do not include pure mutism, that is, disturbances of language caused by severe intellectual impairment or loss of sensory input (such as deafness or inability to see words). Aphasias are most frequently caused by vascular disorders such as stroke or by tumor or brain trauma. Although cortical damage to the frontal and temporal areas of the left hemisphere causes most aphasias, damage to subcortical structures of the basal ganglia (specifically the corpus striatum) and the thalamus has also produced aphasia.

The two major types of aphasia are commonly referred to as Broca's aphasia and Wernicke's aphasia. Other classifications, subtypes, and combinations exist that may contain slightly different features or a mixture of some features of these two types (see Table 8.1). In seeing aphasia patients, it is quickly evident that few patients fit neatly into one classification or the other. This is not surprising, because brain lesions and preexisting brain anatomy for language varies among individuals, most notably between men and women. Many clinicians find it most useful to describe the features of the aphasia in behavioral terms, describing aphasia according to degree of fluency and the nature of the expressive and receptive problems involved. **Fluent aphasia** is characterized by fluent spontaneous speech with normal articulation and rhythm, or fluency in the repetition of words, phrases, or sentences. **Nonfluent aphasia** is difficulty in the flow of articulation, so that speech becomes broken or halting. **Expressive aphasia** is a disorder of speech output. Receptive aphasia implies a difficulty in auditory comprehension.

Often, patients experience not only a loss of spoken language but also a loss of written language and reading comprehension. Writing is one of the most complex language abilities. If it is disturbed as a result of impairment of the limb to produce letters and words, the disturbance is not thought to be a disorder of language. Rather, words, letters, or numbers may appear foreign or incomprehensible because of an inability to recall the form of letters. Attempts at writing may be filled with real or imagined letters that make no sense to others. With time and training, the person may be able to understand simple written language (for example, single words such as *bath* or *food*) but not more complex written language, such as sentences or paragraphs. The extent of the recovery in this and other areas largely depends on the degree of damage. Because reading comprehension is based on prior mastery of auditory language, deficits in reading (alexia) often accompany deficits in auditory comprehension. As with auditory defects, impairment in visual comprehension may involve a deficit in recognizing individual letters or words as being letters or words, or an impairment in attaching the correct meaning to the symbols written on a page. Deficits in writing are most often associated with lesions to the angular gyrus, a cortical association area that provides cross-modal integration of visual, tactile, and verbal information. Reading deficits (alexia) are frequently related to lesions of the left fusiform and lingual areas.

Broca's Aphasia

Broca's aphasia is an expressive, nonfluent aphasia characterized by difficulties in speech production but relatively adequate auditory verbal comprehension, as evidenced by the ability to follow spoken commands (such as, "Point to the cup"). Many forms of disorders of production exist, which can range from an inability to form words to an inability to place words together to form a spoken or written sentence. In simple expressive aphasia, the person knows what he or she wants to say but cannot find the words to say it. It is like continually experiencing a situation in which the word or words are on the tip of the tongue but are not quite connected to thought.

In mild cases of **anomia,** or word-finding difficulties, only a word or two here and there is lost, and the communication can proceed quite normally. In more severe cases, most or all words can be lost. This problem in word finding is one that virtually all expressive aphasics suffer. Even when the person produces words, he or she takes longer than normal to do so. Difficulty in finding a word often results in the person's deliberately "talking around" a word that approximates the intended idea when he or she cannot find the intended word. For example, an aphasic might say, "I looked through that long pipe thing at the stars" (that is, a telescope). Aphasics may also make phonetic or like-sounding errors, such as "I looked through that telephone at the stars," or semantic meaning–related errors, such as "I looked through that barometer at the stars."

Another problem experienced by many Broca's aphasics is one of **articulation,** or the ability to form phonetic sounds of vowels and consonants, which then are placed in different combinations to form words and sentences. People with severe deficits in articulating words often cannot produce simple sounds, even by imitation. If the

deficit in articulation is related to a motor impairment of the mouth, tongue, larynx, or pharynx, then it is not aphasia. The aphasic impairment is marked by the person's confusion or deficit in choosing the desired sound from all those available in his or her repertoire. This sometimes results in unintended strange-sounding syllables, words, or phrases (phonemic paraphasias) during the effort to speak, or in noises being produced rather than language. Those with Broca's aphasia may also show poor pronunciation and inappropriate speech rhythm, manifested by dysarthria, stuttering, and effortful speech.

Broca's aphasia most commonly occurs with lesions to the frontal operculum, but typically also includes lesions to the motor cortex (precentral gyrus or motor strip) and underlying white matter and subcortical structures of the basal ganglia. Aphasia appears to resolve quickly if the frontal operculum is the only structure involved, but it tends to be more persistent the more surrounding structures are damaged (Bradshaw & Mattingly, 1995).

Wernicke's Aphasia

Wernicke's aphasia is a receptive, fluent aphasia. This implies reduced comprehension of spoken language with the continued ability to produce speech. If you stop to imagine this odd situation, you can see that Wernicke's aphasics, in addition to not understanding what others say, may not be able to understand what they themselves are saying. This problem contributes to speaking in the form of a **word salad** of unconnected words and word sounds. This feature of Wernicke's aphasia is a deficit in putting words together in proper grammatical and syntactical form. This condition, more formally known as **paragrammatism** or **extended paraphasia,** refers to running speech that is logically incoherent, often sounding like an exotic foreign language. That is, the speech of a person with Wernicke's aphasia flows forth without hesitation and has appropriate intonation. Appropriate social interaction, such as speaking in turn and gesturing appropriately, remains intact. However, the words and phrases spoken are meaningless. Wernicke's aphasics usually do not realize their spoken language is meaningless to others (anosognosia for speech). It is as if they know exactly what is to be communicated, but their delivery is incoherent.

In mild cases of Wernicke's aphasia, only a word or two here and there sounds garbled or incomprehensible. In this case, communication can generally proceed because the person is able to grasp the essence of the intention based on the context within which the communication takes place. With moderate disability, the patient can understand part, but not all, of the communication. In severe cases, the patient may experience most or all speech as if it were nonsense syllables or a foreign language. It is not uncommon for others to misattribute behavior problems to people with receptive aphasia. Sometimes noncompliance is actually caused by the fact that the patient has misunderstood the communication in the first place. Thus, a patient may act as though a word was not heard at all (so-called word deafness) or as though only fragments of the word were heard. The most common defect, however, lies not in failing to recognize that a word was spoken, but rather in failing to attach meaning to the word. In some aphasics, comprehension of individual words is intact, but grammatical constructions are not.

Damage in Wernicke's aphasia includes the secondary auditory cortex (Wernicke's area) and some involvement of surrounding structures. These often include the supra-marginal and angular gyri and portions of the middle temporal gyrus.

O t h e r   A p h a s i a   S u b t y p e s

The classification of aphasias into receptive and expressive is a useful didactic tool, but many people with left hemisphere lesions have a combination of both symptoms, because of damage to the left middle cerebral artery, which serves both expressive and receptive areas. This section briefly reviews the symptoms of the various subtypes of aphasia beyond the more common Broca's and Wernicke's aphasias. Table 8.1 summarizes the behavioral features of the aphasias.

Conduction Aphasia—The behavioral hallmark of conduction aphasia is a problem in repeating what others say. This problem, obviously, may not become apparent except on formal testing. In ordinary conversation, expressive speech is fluent but marked with **phonemic paraphasias,** or errors of word usage of similar-sounding words (such as using the word *bark* for *tarp*). Comprehension is relatively well preserved but may suffer from minor errors. Reading aloud and writing are frequently impaired. Neuroanatomically, conduction aphasia is a result of separation of Broca's area from Wernicke's area by damage of the arcuate fasciculus, the connecting white matter fibers between the two areas. The damage may also include lesions to the posterior portions of the lateral fissure responsible for aspects of

reading and writing, specifically the supramarginal and angular gyri.

Transcortical Motor Aphasia—Clinicians can recognize transcortical motor aphasia by the patient's halting, nonfluent spontaneous speech; oddly, however, speech becomes fluent if the person merely repeats what another says. In many respects, except for the differences in repetition ability, this deficit resembles Broca's aphasia. Speech comprehension is unimpaired and writing may also suffer. Reading comprehension, however, is generally intact. Lesions to the area anterior or superior to Broca's area are associated with this aphasia type.

Transcortical Sensory Aphasia—Severe speech comprehension deficit marks transcortical sensory aphasia. Interestingly, despite being unable to comprehend speech, such aphasics can adequately repeat phrases and sentences presented to them. Lesions in the angular gyrus are the most likely culprits for this aphasia; thus, reading and writing are also affected.

Anomic Aphasia—A problem in word finding, or anomia, is the primary, and often only, difficulty in anomic aphasia. This aphasia is a frequent result of widespread brain impairment caused by conditions such as traumatic brain injury and dementias such as Alzheimer's disease. As people age, an annoying concomitant often reported is a difficulty in remembering people's names or being unable to retrieve a word that is just on the "tip of the tongue." The act of "word finding" seems to be one of the most easily affected aspects of expressive language. Witness even the problem of being "speechless" with anxiety. It is difficult, therefore, to distinguish what might be a temporary word-finding difficulty and a true aphasia.

Global Aphasia—Global aphasia is the most devastating of the aphasia subtypes because of its profound effect across all areas of speech functioning. There is marked disability in speech production, as well as speech comprehension. Reading, writing, and repetition are also impaired. This aphasia is caused by a massive lesion encompassing major portions of the left hemisphere.

Summary

The visual and auditory systems are two of the most important sensory systems for humans. Visual processing covers a wide cortical area beyond the occipital lobes when the meaning of visual material is considered. Likewise, auditory processing, because it also includes understanding and expression of the meaning of language, spreads out in a web that encompasses large portions of the cortex. One can conceptualize sensory-perceptual processing as a bottom-up process of sensory logic, because in each domain the brain seeks to make "sense" of incoming information. But, it is becoming more evident that we impose perceptions on sensory information from the top down as well. A fundamental question of consciousness is how the brain constructs perceptions of integrated wholes, such as an orange, for which you integrate the visual features with the smell and taste. Brain scientists are beginning to ask how the disparate local elements bind to form a unified experience. This is referred to as "the binding problem of consciousness."

A question related to the binding problem concerns how the brain accesses meaning. Some argue that meaning is specific within each sensory system. In other words, there exists a specific visual meaning, auditory meaning, or even olfactory meaning. If this meaning is lost, as in various sensory agnosias, the ability to access it through another sensory modality would be impossible. In discussing the senses, it is quickly evident that basic sensory perception is anatomically and functionally distinct. However, meaning lost in one sensory modality can often be accessed through another. Exactly how an integrated sense of meaning emerges remains unclear. Local interconnections may exist between sensory cortices or some sort of central integrative multimodal processor that allows multiple access from the sensory systems. Chapter 16 evaluates the problems of binding and how the mind constructs meaning. Neuropsychology and neuroscience are still wrestling with the larger questions of how this system operates. Functionally, however, knowing that sensory-perceptual agnosias are modality specific lets rehabilitation professionals seek alternative "routes" for accessing meaning when one system is damaged.

Critical Thinking Questions

▨ What does the neuropsychology of sensory-perceptual processing have to contribute to the idea that there is an objective reality related to object perception?

▨ How might it be possible to imagine or conjure up images in a sensory domains despite a lack of sensory input?

▨ Can one be "conscious" in one sensory domain but not in another?

Key Terms

Decussating	Akinetopsia	Receptive aphasia or Wernicke's	Anomia
Anopia	Visual agnosias	aphasia	Articulation
Homonymous	Visual object agnosia	Frontal operculum	Word salad
Hemianopia	Prosopagnosia	Aphasia	Paragrammatism or extended
Striate cortex	Apperceptive visual agnosia	Dysarthria	paraphasia
Secondary association or	Associative visual agnosia	Speech apraxia	Phonemic paraphasias
Prestriate cortex	Balint's syndrome	Fluent aphasia	
Blindsight	Tonotopic map	Nonfluent aphasia	
Achromatopsia	Wernicke's area	Expressive aphasia	

Web Connections

http://serendip.brynmawr.edu/bb
See the exhibits related to vision: blindsight, blind spot, and tricks of the eye.

http://neuro.caltech.edu/~seckel
Home page of illusions, perception, and cognitive science.

http://www.eyetricks.com
This site includes tons of optical illusion galleries, three-dimensional images, and brainteasers.

http://www.aphasia.org
This site provides information on aphasia from the National Aphasia Association.

http://www.nidcd.nih.gov/health/voice/adultaphasia.asp
This site provides information on aphasia from the National Institute on Deafness and Other Communication Disorders.

Chapter 9

MEMORY, ATTENTION, EMOTION, AND EXECUTIVE FUNCTIONING

It is abundantly obvious here that for longer than we can tell, the truth is immeasurably greater than all the tiny fragments we have so far been able to discover.

—Attributed to Pavlov by Luria (1947)

Everything should be made as simple as possible, but not simpler.

—Attributed to Albert Einstein

Memory Systems

Attention

Executive Functioning

Relation of Memory, Attention, and Executive Function

Neuropsychology of Emotional Processing

Neuropsychology in Action

9.1 Amnesia: The Case of N.A.

9.2 Executive Function Tasks

9.3 The Case of Phineas Gage

Keep in Mind

▪ What integrative and management functions do higher systems serve?

▪ If short-term memory is impaired, can information be learned and consolidated into storage?

▪ What are the similarities and differences of the models of attention?

▪ Is there a cognitive function that could be considered the highest function?

▪ What effects on behavior do disorders of "management" and "executive" functions have?

Overview

This chapter is devoted to higher functional systems that are not specific for sensory modalities. Language and visual perception (see discussion in Chapter 8) are also considered higher functional systems because their full expression depends on additional functional systems such as memory, attention, and executive functioning. However, language and visual perception emerge from sensory-perceptual systems; thus, it is easier to follow their progression when they are discussed with these systems. The sensory and motor systems represent the building blocks on which other systems are constructed and the raw material from which other systems draw; they are the most straightforward and best mapped systems. The systems we discuss in this chapter are integrated with the sensory-perceptual and motor systems but do not depend on any one modality. We refer to the systems here as higher order systems because, evolutionarily, the expression in humans is complex and highly integrated. Most of these systems can be thought of as background management systems. Their functions are important for learning, organizing, setting priorities, planning, self-reflection, and self-regulation.

The systems discussed in this chapter include the classic systems or modules of cognitive neuropsychology, namely memory, attention, and executive functioning. In addition, we consider the brain and mind expressions of emotional processing. For each system, we discuss the conceptual organization of the system, as well as known structure–function relations.

▪ Memory Systems

Memory forms the basis of experience and perceptions of self. It is dynamic and malleable. It allows people to travel back in time. How you see yourself, to a large degree, is a product of the experiences of your life, the lessons you have learned, and what you remember as being important. Even what you tell yourself to remember to do in the future must incorporate memory. Memory pervades most aspects of human experience. Stories of your personal and cultural past are stored in memory; thus, it is a necessary foundation of social communication. This section examines the various components of memory and what can happen when aspects of the memory system malfunction.

When memory is working fluidly, there is little need to notice it. But consider the question from a neuropsy-chological perspective: What do you lose if you lose your memory? One patient we evaluated, a man in his 70s with Alzheimer's disease, could not remember that his wife had died 2 years earlier. All his memories were still of her being there. Every time someone mentioned that his wife was dead, he relived the grieving experience. It is scary to imagine waking up and not knowing who you are, who your friends are, and what has happened in your life. Consider also what it might be like if you could not encode new information, if you could not remember what someone said 10 minutes ago, or if you could not register the information you needed to take a test or learn a new skill.

Memory is an umbrella concept, and it is impossible to say categorically that someone has an overall good or bad memory. It is simply not a single system. Memory is parceled into subsystems based on ideas of storage and processing. Neuropsychologists ask how the brain stores information over the long term and how it encodes, organizes, and then retrieves information from memory. In many disorders neuropsychologists treat on a daily basis, memory processing is at issue because memory is a "fragile" system, affected by many disorders, including most of the dementias, such as Alzheimer's disease, toxic conditions, loss of oxygen, and head injury.

Scientific understanding of normal memory processing in the brain has profited greatly from the study of people afflicted with various memory disorders, especially types of amnesia. However, the term *amnesia* can refer to more than one type of condition. The "soap opera" version of amnesia occurs when one of the characters gets hit on the head and promptly forgets who she or he is and all the specific episodes of her or his life. This character invariably wanders off to make a new life, including the development of a new identity. Perhaps, after a time, a startling event occurs (possibly another blow to the head) and the character's prior memory and identity floods back. This type of memory deficit is reminiscent of a psychiatric dissociative state caused by severe emotional trauma, but it is not what occurs with neurologic injury or disease.

Because neurologic patients acquire their memory problems in conjunction with a brain injury or disease, it is important to have terminology that marks the nature of the patient's memory before the event and the effect on memory after the event. **Anterograde amnesia** is the loss of the ability to encode and learn new information after a defined event (such as head injury, lesion, or disease onset). **Retrograde amnesia** is the loss of old memories from before an event or illness. For example, one of our patients, L.S., experienced a head injury as a result of a car accident and had moderate anterograde amnesia and mild retrograde amnesia. She had no memory of the car accident and only vaguely remembered the paramedics. She did remember being in the hospital emergency room. After the accident, she had difficulty learning new information (anterograde amnesia). She often forgot her physician's name, and when she returned to college, she found it hard to study and perform well on history tests for which she had to recall facts and dates. Her mild retrograde amnesia is evidenced by her memory for driving out of the grocery store parking lot, which was about five blocks from the accident. However, she remembered nothing else of the short time preceding the accident. Amnesias of this type are common in closed head injury (this condition is described further in Chapter 13). In general, anterograde (or a combination of anterograde-retrograde) amnesia is evident with brain injury. However, there are instances of retrograde amnesia with relatively spared anterograde learning and memory (Levine et al., 1998). Amnesia can be caused by a number of different problems and can take several forms. An example of a circumscribed lesion causing amnesia is the classic case of N.A. (Neuropsychology in Action 9.1).

A FRAMEWORK FOR CONCEPTUALIZING MEMORY SYSTEMS

Psychology textbooks typically describe memory as having three main divisions: sensory memory, **short-term memory (STM),** and **long-term memory (LTM).** Sensory memory is fleeting, lasting only milliseconds, but its capacity is essentially unlimited in what may be taken in. STM is of limited capacity (7 ± 2 bits of information) and degrades quickly over a matter of seconds if information is not held via a means such as rehearsal, or transferred to LTM. LTM, theoretically, is of unlimited capacity and is relatively permanent except for models that suggest that loss of information through forgetting is possible. Neuropsychologists are most concerned with LTM and its disorders because these are the problems most evidenced by patients. Often, STM, as measured by neuropsychological tasks, is intact even when there are deficits in LTM, although isolated disorders of STM exist. Neuropsychological conceptualizations of memory generally do not consider sensory memory; rather, it is thought of as a component of sensory processing.

Neuropsychology concerns itself with understanding how memory systems work in correspondence with known brain functioning. An important question concerns the possible existence of anatomically separate systems in the brain for such concepts as STM, LTM, explicit-implicit memory, and episodic-semantic memory. One way in which researchers can support the idea of separate structures is by showing a double dissociation between behaviors. Research can demonstrate strong evidence for different systems if a lesion in an area of the brain affects one system (LTM) but not the other (STM). Evidence is even stronger if researchers can show that a different lesion results in the opposite dissociation (affects STM but not LTM). This section focuses on conceptualizations of LTM and short-term working memory. We explore evidence for different memory subsystems, a division between STM and LTM, and between possible divisions of LTM such as separate declarative/explicit versus procedural/implicit systems. As we explore each subsystem, we also discuss disorders that affect that system.

Neuropsychology in Action 9.1

Amnesia: The Case of N.A.

by Mary Spiers

In 1960, N.A. was 22 years old and was a member of the U.S. Air Force. One day while working on a model airplane, he suffered an accident that would affect him for the rest of his life. His roommate, apparently in a playful mood, took a miniature fencing foil from the wall, tapped N.A. from behind, and as he turned around, thrust it forward. Unfortunately for N.A., the tiny foil penetrated the cribriform plate at the top of his nasal cavity and entered his brain. The foil pierced his third cranial nerve, but more important, it made a small lesion in the left dorsomedial nucleus of the thalamus. It was quickly discovered that N.A. was amnesic (retrograde) for the past 2 years. In addition, this minute injury left him with a devastating impairment in his ability to register new verbal memories (anterograde amnesia).

In meeting him, the casual observer may not initially suspect there is anything wrong. N.A.'s intelligence quotient (IQ) is in the high average range and he exhibits good social skills. Furthermore, he is friendly, polite, and has a good sense of humor. But after talking with him for a few minutes, it becomes apparent that he does not remember details of just a few minutes ago. If he is distracted by a passing thought or a passing car, the thread of conversation is lost. He has little recollection of the day's events. If you meet again the next day, he probably will not remember you or what transpired in your previous meeting with him.

N.A. likes to keep his room exactly the same at all times and spends much time obsessively arranging things. He becomes upset at his mother if she moves the telephone or one of his model airplanes. He likes things exactly the same so he has a better chance of finding them. Only after a long period and much repetition does he remember something. If N.A. saw you every day, after a period of time he might recognize you, but still might not know your name. He has only a sketchy memory of events that have transpired since 1960. For example, he has a vague idea that Watergate was a political scandal in "Washington or Florida" but recalls no other details. Because N.A.'s injury is in the left dorsomedial nucleus, he shows more verbal than visual memory deficits. Interestingly, when he had to learn a new route from his house to the Veterans Administration

hospital for therapy, even after 4 years he was unable to form a spatial map. He found his way much like an adult returning to a childhood neighborhood after years of absence. As pieces of the visual scenery popped up before him, he decided if the landmark looked familiar and turned accordingly. This haphazard approach of seeing things sometimes required him to back up or retrace his steps until something looked familiar.

N.A. recognizes that he has memory problems and is not confused. He knows who he is and where he is, but may not know the day or year. As would be suspected, he has little social life. In a sense, he remains stuck in time. Most of his memories are from the 1950s. When he fantasizes, he thinks of Betty Grable. He does not know of the people or events since then. However, N.A. remains optimistic about his situation and rarely uses notes because he wants to work on his memory.

This case demonstrates that even a very small lesion, strategically placed, can cause a devastating problem of memory. Kaushall, Zetin, and Squire (1981) have reported the complete case of N.A.

LONG-TERM MEMORY

A problem that is inherently confusing in studying memory is the multiple terms scientists use to describe the possible subcomponents of LTM. Cognitive psychologists, neuropsychologists, neurologists, and the lay public use various, and sometimes conflicting, terms. For example, when referring to LTM, the lay public often thinks of the ability to remember information from the distant past. However, neuropsychologists are referring to the specific ability to register information (encode), organize the information in a meaningful way (storage), and recall or recognize the information when needed (retrieval). According to this definition, LTM is the ability to learn and retain *new* information. **Remote memory,** by contrast, concerns memory for long-past events.

Various theoretical conceptualizations parcel LTM into subsystems (Figure 9.1). Squire (Squire & Cohen, 1984; Squire & Butters, 1992) and other investigators advocate for a structural–functional difference between declarative and nondeclarative memory.

Declarative memory is explicit and accessible to conscious awareness. **Nondeclarative memory** is usually implicit, and a person demonstrates it via performance. Squire and Butters (1992) maintain that the domain of nondeclarative or **procedural memory** is that of rules and procedures, rather than information that can be verbalized, although nondeclarative memory has not been clearly operationally defined and often includes a hodgepodge of tasks such as motor skills learning, mirror reading, and verbal priming. Schacter (1987) differentiates between **explicit** and **implicit memories.** Recall or

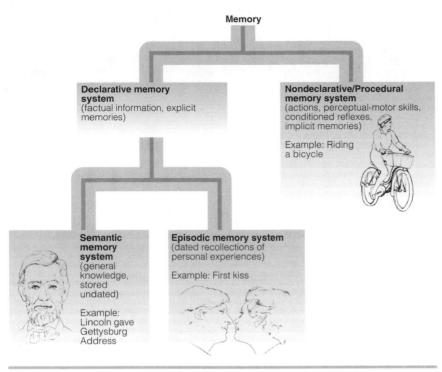

Figure 9.1   Long-term memory (LTM) taxonomy. Theories of anatomically separate LTM stores have included the noted distinctions. (From Weiten, W. [1998]. *Psychology: Themes and variations* [p. 291, Figure 7.28]. Pacific Grove, CA: Brooks/Cole.)

recognition, through verbal or nonverbal means, directly indicates explicit memories. Conscious awareness is usually implied, as is intention to remember. People demonstrate implicit memory by means in which conscious awareness is not always necessary, such as implicit priming, skill learning, and conditioning. Yet another possible distinction within LTM is between semantic and episodic memory. Researchers consider both of these to be forms of explicit or declarative memory. Tulving (1972) introduced the distinction between an **episodic memory,** which refers to individual episodes, usually autobiographical, that have specific spatial and temporal tags in memory, and **semantic memory,** which refers to memory for information and facts that have no specific time tag reference. For example, remembering the details and events of your first date involves episodic memory, whereas remembering the definition of a word relates to semantic memory. With semantic memory, the context in which the memory was encoded is generally not present. Thus, most of us do not remember the specific setting and people involved when we learned the name of the first president of the United States.

The most neuroanatomically defensible division between LTM systems is that of declarative/explicit and nondeclarative memory systems. Some also use the terms *declarative* versus *procedural* or *explicit* versus *implicit* in a nearly synonymous manner. There is much debate over the existence of separate episodic and semantic systems; in fact, although researchers first described these two systems as clearly distinguishable conceptually, they now consider the systems to overlap with other memory concepts.

Declarative Memory

One of the first questions that come to mind when people begin thinking about memory is, "Where is memory stored in the brain?" This often implies the search for a "center" for memory storage in the brain. It also implies that if this center is removed, then all memory is removed. This would be like erasing the entire hard disk of a computer. (Please note that the brain does not operate like a computer; in fact, brains build computers!) If all remote memory were removed from the brain, a person would be unable to remember his or her language, facts, episodes, names of people, or any other information previously encoded. From studies of brain-injured individuals, we know that this does not happen. People may lose pieces of remote memory, but their brains are not "erased." There is no one memory storage center. Rather, most neuropsychologists think of memory as being ultimately stored in the area where it was first processed (for example, see Squire, 1987). This would imply, for example, that auditory memories are stored in primary, secondary, or auditory association areas, and likewise for other functional systems.

The function of the declarative memory system is to process information in such a way as to tag it or consolidate it for storage in the brain. According to this model, when new declarative learning is occurring, information from various cortical areas funnels into the structures responsible for declarative memory. After it is processed, return neural pathways transmit information back to specific cortical areas.

Declarative Model of Encoding and Retrieval—Tulving and coworkers (1994), based on neuroimaging studies of healthy individuals, developed a model of memory encoding and retrieval, Hemispheric-Encoding-Retrieval-Asymmetry (HERA). The model proposes that the prefrontal (dorsolateral) region of the left hemisphere is primarily involved in episodic encoding, whereas the prefrontal area of the right hemisphere is prominently activated for retrieval of episodic information. Subsequently, a comprehensive review of 275 positron emission tomography (PET) and functional magnetic resonance imaging (fMRI) studies by Cabeza and Nyberg (2000) provided partial support for the model. Analysis of these neuroimaging studies showed that the left prefrontal region activated in verbal episodic encoding while retrieval of episodic information was right-lateralized (prefrontal region) for both verbal and nonverbal contents. In contradiction with the prediction based on the HERA model, encoding of nonverbal information yielded bilateral and right-lateral prefrontal activation. Other regions activated during episodic retrieval included temporomedial, parietal, medial parietotemporal, temporal, occipital, and cerebellar areas, highlighting the multiplicity of regions and circuitry involved in memory retrieval. Unlike episodic retrieval, the recall of semantic information is dependent on the left prefrontal area for both verbal and nonverbal information (Cabeza & Nyberg, 2000). Similar to episodic retrieval, other brain regions are involved in semantic retrieval including temporal, anterior cingulate, and cerebellar regions.

Declarative Consolidation—Three major interconnected constellations of brain structures play a role in consolidating information into LTM. The first memory centers around the *medial temporal lobes*, the second around the *diencephalon*, and the third in the *basal forebrain*.

The medial temporal structures, which are important for long-term declarative memory, center around the hippocampus and medial temporal lobe. The well-documented case of H.M. (Milner, Corkin, & Teuber, 1968; Scoville, 1968) best exemplifies what occurs when these structures are damaged. In 1953, at the age of 27 years, H.M. underwent brain surgery to reduce intractable seizures. The surgery involved bilateral removal of the hippocampus and portions of the surrounding area, which included the hippocampal formation (Figure 9.2). The hippocampal formation, or hippocampal complex, includes the hippocampus, the dentate gyrus, and the subiculum. In cross section, the hippocampus has a distinctive "sea horse" shape. Information funnels into the hippocampus via the entorhinal cortex. In addition, the perirhinal and parahippocampal cortexes adjacent to the hippocampal formation are believed to have a role in memory. At the time of H.M.'s surgery little was known regarding the effects of such surgery on memory. After the surgery, despite the preservation of above-average intelligence, he was profoundly amnesic for new learning (anterograde amnesia), both episodic and semantic. He was able to recall old memories and facts, but new learning was no longer possible. STM was preserved in that he could retain new information for a few minutes. However, this information could not be consolidated into long-term storage. If he met someone and then the person left, he would not have any memory of the meeting a few minutes later. As a result, if he met the person again, it was as if they had met for the first time. H.M.'s amnesia was even more profound than N.A.'s, in that he also had difficulty learning new visuospatial information.

The preservation of old memories with medial temporal damage suggests that memories are not stored in the hippocampus; rather, this structure appears to be involved in the movement of new information into long-term storage. PET and fMRI studies (Cabeza & Nyberg, 2000) show that the left medial temporal region activates during the encoding of verbal material, whereas bilateral activation is evident for processing of nonverbal contents. Damage to the hippocampus can significantly disrupt declarative memory, but the extension of damage to the entorhinal and parahippocampal regions produces even more severe and long-lasting amnesia.

The specific functions of the regions of the medial temporal lobe are not fully known, but research suggests that they make differential contributions to memory. For example, the visual association cortex shows significant projections to the perirhinal cortex, whereas the parietal cortex projects to the parahippocampal cortex. These structures appear to play specific roles in visual recognition and

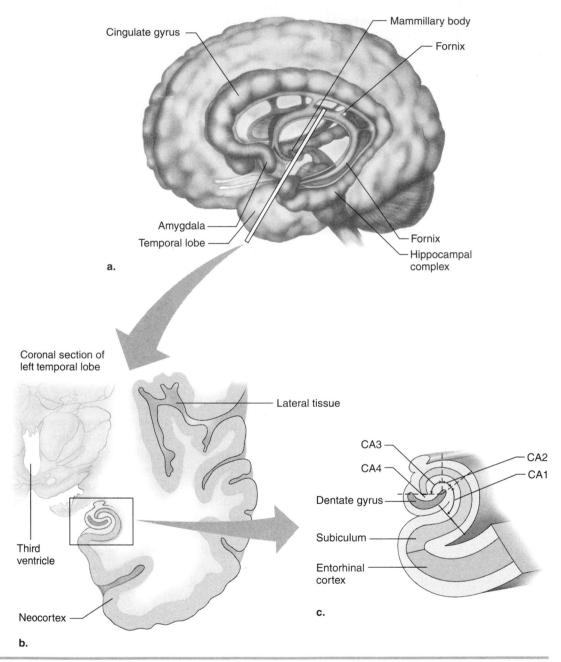

Figure 9.2   The hippocampal complex. (a) The hippocampal complex is located on the medial surface of the temporal lobe. (b) A coronal section shows the hippocampus as a deep infolding of the temporal lobe. (c) A close-up shows the structures in relation. The hippocampus consists of four parts (CA1-CA4). The pathway to the hippocampus from the cortex leads through the entorhinal cortex. ([b] Adapted from Pinel, P. J., & Edwards, M. [1998]. *A colorful introduction to the anatomy of the human brain* [p. 169, Figure 10.1]. Boston: Allyn & Bacon, by permission; [c] adapted from Burt, A. M. [1988]. *Textbook of neuroanatomy* [p. 488, Figure 20.7]. Philadelphia: W.B. Saunders, by permission.)

spatial memory, respectively (Squire & Knowlton, 2000). The hippocampus appears to have a special role in memory tasks that require the relating or combining of information from different cortical sources, such as the relation of specific objects or events in time and space.

The structures of the diencephalon involved in memory center around specific nuclei of the thalamus and the mammillary bodies of the hypothalamus (Figure 9.3). The thalamus consists of several nuclei, with the dorsal medial nucleus of the thalamus the most often implicated in memory disorders. Although the dorsal medial nucleus is involved in memory consolidation, there are suggestions that it may also assist in the initiation and monitoring of conscious retrieval of episodic memories (Wenk, 2004). Damage to the dorsal medial nucleus is often implicated in Korsakoff's syndrome and in some cases of specific amnesia, such as N.A.'s case (see Neuropsychology in Action 9.1). Korsakoff's syndrome is a consequence of chronic alcoholism associated with vitamin deficiency (thiamine). As a result, degeneration of the thalamic dorsomedial nucleus and the mammillary bodies occurs. Patients with Korsakoff's syndrome exhibit significant anterograde and retrograde amnesia, although certain forms of nondeclarative memory (for example, procedural memory) are preserved. Moreover, there are cases of damage specific to the diencephalon region resulting in amnesia, such as N.A.'s case (see Neuropsychology in Action 9.1).

The basal forebrain is the third area implicated in long-term declarative memory processing. As described in Chapter 5, this area is a subcortical part of the telencephalon surrounding the inferior tip of the frontal horn and is strongly interconnected with limbic structures; some neuroscientists consider it part of the limbic system (for example, see Crosson, 1992). The basal forebrain represents a major source of cholinergic output to the cortex. Some investigators have suggested that extensive damage of basal forebrain structures may be needed to affect memory (Zola-Morgan & Squire, 1993); thus, looking at the contributions of an individual nucleus to memory is probably not as profitable as regarding the system as a network. Because of its location surrounding the inferior tip of the frontal horn and that the inferior communicating artery perfuses this area, stroke easily affects the basal forebrain. This area is important to memory not only for the nuclei within but for the fibers that traverse the area. The basal forebrain also contains numerous connections to the mediotemporal area.

The basal forebrain structures implicated in memory include the nucleus basalis of Meynert, the medial septal nucleus, the nucleus of the diagonal band of Broca, and the substantia innominata (Figure 9.4). The nucleus basalis of Meynert includes a group of large neurons in-

terspersed within the substantia innominata. The substantia innominata is a gray and white matter area that separates the globus pallidus from the inferior surface of the forebrain. It interconnects with the frontal, parietal, and temporal cortexes. An important tract coursing through the substantia innominata is the ventral amygdalofugal pathway, which connects the amygdala to the dorsal medial nucleus of the thalamus. The medial septal nucleus lies at the precommissural end of the fornix and projects to the hippocampus through the fornix. It most likely affects memory when damage disrupts information flow to the hippocampus. The nucleus of the diagonal band of Broca is a white matter and cell body area located near the nucleus basalis. It also projects to the hippocampus through the fornix. Researchers think these structures are important cholinergic memory structures.

The major declarative memory system is the Papez circuit. Papez originally proposed that this looping pathway was specific for emotional processing. He noticed that the clinical presentation of intense emotional symptoms in animals with rabies (derived from Latin meaning "rage") was associated with lesions in several limbic system structures, specifically the hippocampus. Today, researchers know this loop has more to do with consolidating information in memory than as a primary emotional processor. Information from the cortex and higher cortical association areas enters the circuit through the cingulate gyrus, moves to the parahippocampal gyrus, and then into the hippocampus through the hippocampal formation. The major output system of the hippocampal formation is the fornix. It contains nearly 1 million fibers and is comparable in size with the optic tract (Nauta & Feirtag, 1986). The fornix rises out of the hippocampal complex and arches anteriorly under the corpus callosum. The fornix relays information to the mammillary bodies (specifically the medial mammillary nucleus) of the hypothalamus. From there information is projected to the anterior nucleus of the thalamus along the mamillo-thalamic tract, from where it then goes to the cingulate gyrus to complete the circuit. Figures 9.2 and 9.5a show the anatomic location of the structures, and Figure 9.5b presents a schematic of the loop.

It is readily apparent by examining amnesia cases such as H.M. and N.A. that a break in the memory consolidation circuit can disrupt memory in a manner similar to direct removal of the hippocampus, which neurologists typically consider the most crucial structure in the system.

Nondeclarative Memory

The term *nondeclarative memory* does not refer to a discrete memory system as much as it acknowledges that some

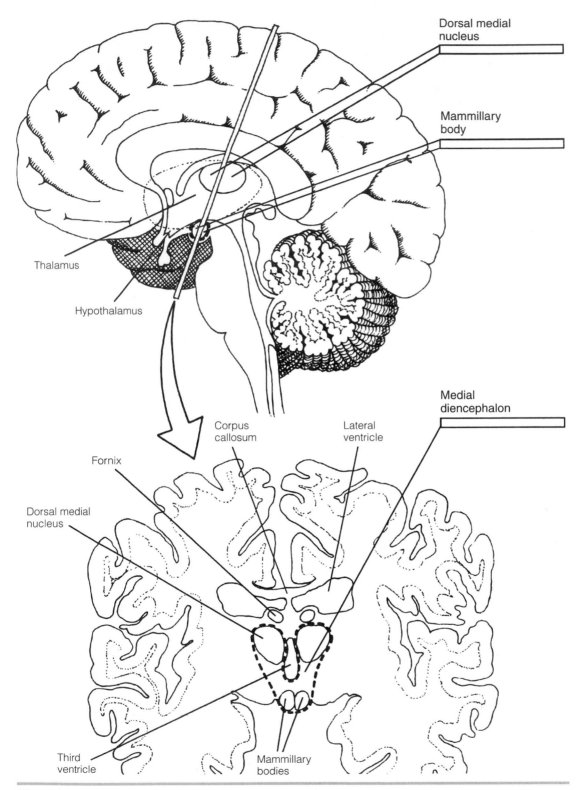

Figure 9.3   The medial diencephalon, comprising the mammillary bodies and the dorsal medial nucleus of the thalamus, is located on both sides of the third ventricle. (Adapted from Pinel, P. J., & Edwards, M. [1998]. *A colorful introduction to the anatomy of the human brain* [p. 175, Figure 10.4]. Boston: Allyn & Bacon, by permission.)

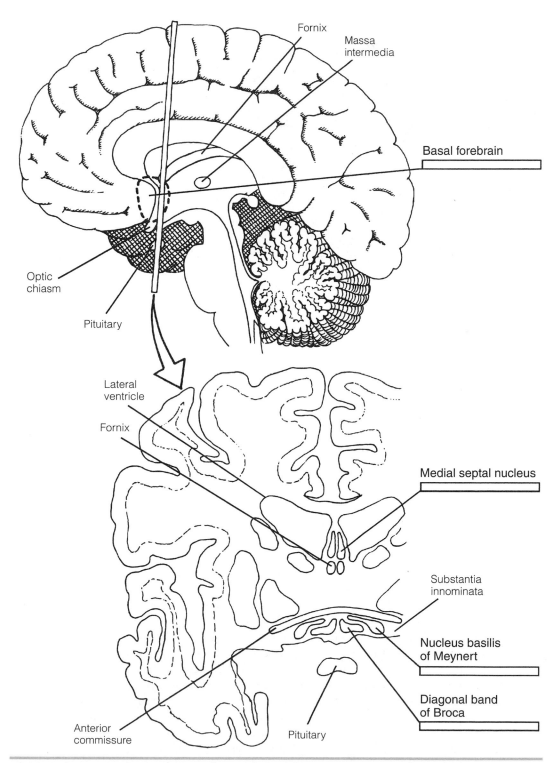

Figure 9.4 The basal forebrain consists of a set of structures at the base of the forebrain. The four structures implicated in memory include the medial septal nucleus, the nucleus basilis of Meynert, the nucleus of the diagonal band of Broca, and the substantia innominata. (Adapted from Pinel, P. J., & Edwards, M. [1998]. *A colorful introduction to the anatomy of the human brain* [p. 177, Figure 10.5]. Boston: Allyn & Bacon, by permission.)

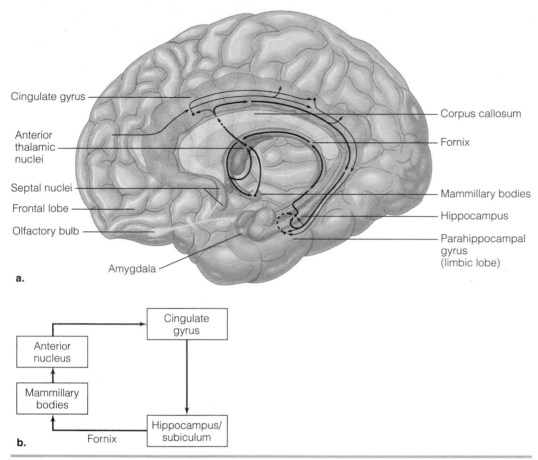

Figure 9.5 The circuit of Papez. (a) The circuit of Papez in the limbic system. (b) A schematic representation of the circuit of Papez. The pathway proceeds from the hippocampus to the mammillary bodies (MB) via the fornix. It then projects to the anterior nucleus (AN) of the thalamus, around the cingulate gyrus, and back to the hippocampal complex. ([a] Reproduced from Kalat, J. W. [1998]. *Biological psychology* [6th ed., p. 324, Figure 12.1]. Pacific Grove, CA: Brooks/Cole, by permission; [b] reproduced from Crosson, B. [1992]. *Subcortical functions in language and memory.* New York: Guilford Press, by permission.)

memory functions operate outside the limbic circuitry of explicit or declarative memory. Researchers have variously referred to the opposite of limbic circuitry–based memory as "habit memory" (Mishkin, Malamut, & Bachevalier, 1984), "procedural memory" (Cohen, 1984), and "implicit memory" (Graf & Schacter, 1985). The variety of memory functions this term encompasses most likely reflects a collection of different abilities, not necessarily mutually exclusive, and perhaps dependent on different processing systems. For example, implicit memory implies influence by prior experience without conscious awareness of the event. Procedural learning concerns the learning of procedures, rules, or skills manifested through performance rather than verbalization, although conscious awareness may aid procedural learning. Because these

terms do not by themselves encompass the entire range of nondeclarative memory, researchers prefer the less specific term (see Squire, 1994). Neurologists also know that a single lesion cannot erase all nondeclarative memory, as it may for declarative new learning. Although it is premature to present a neuroanatomic classification scheme, scientists can describe some aspects of nondeclarative memory with respect to brain structures, particularly subcortical basal ganglia areas.

Researchers observing H.M. noticed that despite severe amnesia for declarative information, H.M. improved with practice on certain perceptual motor tasks (Milner et al., 1968; Scoville, 1968). He was learning, with practice, without conscious recognition of this learning. If his amnesia had been total, examiners would have expected that each presentation of the task would be performed as if it were brand new. One area of nondeclarative memory involves perceptual motor adaptation and skills acquisition. Many amnesiacs, such as H.M., show a normal learning curve as they practice the pursuit rotor and reverse mirror-reading tasks. The pursuit rotor requires the examinee to keep a stylus on a spinning disk, much like having to hold a place on a record on a turntable. Reverse mirror reading requires an individual to trace a maze while looking at it through a mirror. Perceptually, amnesiacs also show normal adaptive behavior when wearing visual prisms. Because prisms distort visual input, simple acts such as reaching for an object are misdirected at first. The visual motor system must quickly learn to "retune" the system so that it again correctly targets reaching according to the new visual information. Interestingly, amnesiacs can do this performance learning and adaptation despite severe declarative amnesia. However, amnesiacs do not show normal nondeclarative skill learning for all tasks. For example, investigations (Gabrieli, Keane, & Corkin, 1987; Xu & Corkin, 2001) of H.M.'s performance on a complex, nondeclarative, problem-solving task (Tower of Hanoi) did not find evidence of consistent improvement across learning trials or mastery of the task.

Further support for a nondeclarative memory system is provided by the differential performance of patients with amnesia, Huntington's disease, and Parkinson's disease on a measure of serial reaction-time skill learning (Schacter & Curran, 2000). The patients were required to press one of four keys when illumination occurred above a key. The patient groups were not aware that there was a repeating sequence of illumination; yet, across learning trials, the patients with amnesia demonstrated improved performance as evidenced in decreased key press reaction times. In contrast, patients with Huntington's and Parkinson's diseases showed impaired learning. Subcortical striatal pathology is central to both Huntington's and Parkinson's diseases, suggesting the involvement of this region in serial reaction-time learning. Functional imaging studies have confirmed that serial reaction-time skill learning is supported by the striatal region and circuitry. Other regions that exhibit learning-related changes during serial reaction-time skill learning primarily involve the neocortex (primary motor, supplementary motor, premotor, parietal and occipital cortices). These changes suggest that serial reaction-time learning involves changes in perceptual and motor areas supporting visually guided movements (Schacter & Curran, 2000).

Researchers also noticed that severely amnesic patients with Korsakoff's syndrome showed a phenomenon known

as **implicit priming.** For example, in the word stem completion priming paradigm, a list of words is first presented (for example, *church, parachute, clarinet,* and so on). Because of the severe amnesia, the person's memory is poor when examiners demand recall in a declarative task. Examiners then give patients three-letter word stems (for example, *chu____, par____, cla_____*) and ask them to make a word by completing the stems. "Primed" patients with Korsakoff's syndrome were more likely to complete the stem with a word they had already seen than were unprimed examinees, despite the same level of declarative amnesia for the words. Perceptual priming also appears in the quicker recognition of fragmented objects (such as those presented in Chapter 8 for testing apperceptive agnosics) or of words (see Figure 9.6 for examples of priming stimuli). Similar to patients with Korsakoff's syndrome, amnesic patients with damage to medial and diencephalic brain areas often show unimpaired implicit perceptual priming.

Perceptually based implicit priming is associated with decreased activity of the posterior neocortex. It has been theorized that the decreased activation of the posterior neocortex reflects a reduction in neural resources needed to process the content when it recurs, because a visual trace remains from the original presentation of the material (Squire & Knowlton, 2000). Notably, implicit priming is

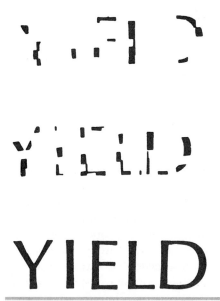

Figure 9.6 Amnesiacs who have deficient declarative memory may still have intact implicit memory as they demonstrate by quickly recognizing fragments of previously presented words. (Reproduced from McCarthy, R. A., & Warrington, E. K. [1990]. *Cognitive neuropsychology* [p. 302, Figure 14.3]. San Diego: Academic Press, by permission.)

not synonymous with recognition memory (identification of target stimuli when presented with other nontarget stimuli). Recognition memory appears to involve the encoding of phonetic or semantic declarative information, whereas priming depends on the visual features of the presented content. In addition, different brain systems are believed to support the two types of memory. An example of recognition memory would be asking a person to memorize a list of words, and then presenting the words, at a later time, randomly interspersed with other nonpresented words. The person is then asked to identify the words initially learned. Identification of the words originally learned provides a measure of recognition memory. Case studies show that patients with lesions of the visual extrastriate region demonstrate deficits of visual perceptual priming but intact recognition memory. Patients with amnesia show the opposite pattern.

Another form of implicit learning is that of "artificial grammar." Individuals are presented seemingly random strings of consonants without awareness that the organization of these strings reflects a complex set of rules. The individuals are then informed that the consonant strings were generated in accordance with a set of rules. After this explanation, they are exposed to a list of grammatical and nongrammatical consonant strings and are asked to judge which strings were formed by the same set of rules. Patients with amnesia perform the task as well as healthy participants, even though they have no memory for the consonant strings used during the training. In addition, patients with basal ganglia disease (for example, Parkinson's disease) are also able to perform artificial grammar tasks, indicating that striatal pathology is not involved in this form of memory. Research suggests that the posterior neocortex may support the performance of artificial grammar tasks, leading some investigators to pose that this type of learning may reflect priming or perceptual processing (Schacter & Curran, 2000; Squire & Knowlton, 2000).

The simplest form of nondeclarative memory involves classic or associative learning. This type of memory is evolutionarily much older and generally operates on the basis of learned associations. Researchers can demonstrate that even animals whose hippocampus has been removed can learn simple stimulus–response associations. For example, planaria can learn a light–shock pairing and recoil from the light when they subsequently encounter it alone. This suggests that some basic and primitive aspects of associative conditioning are operating. Human amnesiacs produced corroborating evidence for this associative learning. Amnesiacs who meet a doctor on one occasion do not remember the doctor's name on the next meeting. But, amnesiacs who have been pin-pricked by their doctor while shaking hands during their first meeting, often withdraw their hand when the doctor extends his or her hand at a second meeting even though they may not consciously recall the association between shaking hands with the doctor and being pricked by a pin.

Whether the same brain circuitry governs all aspects of nondeclarative memory is not fully understood. However, evidence suggests that structures supporting nondeclarative memory are probably evolutionarily and ontologically older and more primitive. We stated earlier that even simple animals without a hippocampal system can learn associative information. Also, preverbal babies show perceptual-motor learning. Infants between 2 and 5 months of age quickly learn that they can kick to move a mobile attached to one leg (Rovee-Collier, 1993). Many brain structures involved in movement, including the cerebellum, the basal ganglia, and the motor strip, are implicated in motor learning. The cerebellum aids in sequential motor learning such as the steps required in learning the piano. The basal ganglion is an important brain circuit responsible for perceptual-motor learning and adaptation (Figure 9.7). We discuss this circuit in

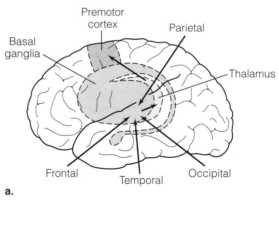

a.

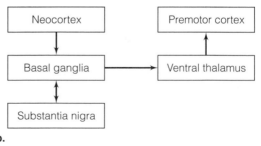

b.

Figure 9.7 (a) The circuitry of nondeclarative perceptual-motor learning. (b) Schematic of information flow from the neocortex through the basal ganglia to the premotor cortex. (Adapted from Petri, H. L., & Mishkin, M. [1994]. Behaviorism, cognitivism and the neuropsychology of memory. *American Scientist 82*, 30–37, by permission.)

Chapter 7 (see the section "Subcortical Motor Processing"). Specifically, this circuit includes the caudate nucleus, putamen, and globus pallidus. The nuclei of the striatum (caudate and putamen) receive projected information from cortical sensory areas. From the striatum, information then funnels through the globus pallidus, and then on to the thalamus, where it projects to the premotor and prefrontal areas (see Figure 7.11) (Mishkin, Malamut, Bachevalier, 1984). Behaviorally, Huntington's disease best portrays the effect of caudate nucleus dysfunction of the basal ganglia. Huntington's disease develops as a progressive subcortical dementia (see Chapter 15 for a thorough description), but caudate nucleus degeneration is the hallmark of Huntington's disease and is one of the first structural changes that computed tomography scans identify. The atrophic imaging change appears at the onset of the choreiform movement disorder. The effect of this change appears to target perceptual-motor learning tasks. In a series of studies spearheaded by Nelson Butters (for review, see Squire & Butters, 1992), patients with Huntington's disease showed a dissociation in performance from patients with Korsakoff's syndrome, amnesia, and Alzheimer's disease. On declarative verbal memory tasks, patients with Huntington's disease performed relatively better than patients with Korsakoff's syndrome and Alzheimer's disease. However, on motor learning tasks, the two cortically impaired groups outperformed the patients with Huntington's disease. This double dissociation in functioning prompted the initial suggestion for separate cortical and subcortical memory structures. Since that time, animal studies and imaging studies with healthy participants performing motor learning tasks have added evidence for the role of the basal ganglia in implicit memory.

SHORT-TERM MEMORY AND WORKING MEMORY

> There seems to be a presence-chamber in my mind where full consciousness holds court, and where two or three ideas are at the same time in audience, and an ante-chamber full of more of less allied ideas, which is situated just beyond the full ken of consciousness. Out of this ante-chamber the ideas most nearly allied to those in the presence chamber appear to be summoned in a mechanically logical way, and to have their turn of audience.
>
> —*Francis Galton* (1883)

A moment in time. In the case of amnesiacs such as H.M. and N.A., this is everything they had. But healthy people also travel from moment to moment in a "presence-chamber" of the mind, using this workspace to assemble information for storage and to connect and reconnect information retrieved from LTM, to solve problems or to make new associations. The difference is that N.A. could no longer connect moments and store aspects of the present as new memory in LTM. The limited capacity and short time frame of STM does not accommodate more than a few thoughts, ideas, or bits of information at a time. As new bits arrive, they may take the place of others or simply degrade. If there is no linkage between STM and LTM, STM floats as an island with only a small area of possible habitation.

Researchers interested in memory have debated the question of the relation of STM to LTM. Cognitive tasks illustrate that the two appear to measure different areas of memory. STM is a limited-capacity, rapid-access, input-and-retrieval system analogous to computer RAM (random-access memory). LTM has unlimited capacity but with a restricted rate of input and retrieval much like ROM (read-only memory). The two systems are also coded differently. STM uses phonologic coding, relying on an acoustic code, whereas LTM heavily uses semantic coding, or the associative meaning value of information to be remembered (for review, see Baddeley, 1986). Even though the two seemingly measure different aspects of memory functioning, a unitary view of memory functioning would argue that LTM depends on STM. That is, these two systems are viewed as two components of one system linked in a serial fashion; thus, information entering LTM must inevitably flow through STM. In contrast, a separate system view would argue that LTM and STM are dissociated, so someone could have an LTM deficit with intact STM, whereas another person could have an STM deficit but maintain adequate LTM. Patients with amnesia with severe LTM deficits often show intact STM. On formal testing, they can repeat increasingly longer series of digits and perform well on other tasks presumed to test STM. However, other patients have a specific STM deficit with preserved LTM. This is some of the most convincing evidence that STM and LTM are anatomically separate.

Patients with a pure STM deficit are rare. However, researchers have reported cases with exactly this problem (for example, see Shallice & Warrington, 1970; Basso, Spinnler, Vallar, & Zanobio, 1982). Shallice and Warrington (1970) reported the case of K.F., a patient who suffered a left posterior temporal lesion that left him with a greatly reduced STM capacity for verbal information. He had a profound

STM deficit, having a digit span length of about two, rather than the usual seven bits of information. He also demonstrated conduction aphasia whereby he could not repeat sentences. Surprisingly, K.F. showed a normal verbal learning curve with practice, indicating intact storage of information in LTM. It is difficult to reconcile K.F.'s performance with theories posing that verbal STM and LTM use the same anatomic structure, but in different ways. K.F.'s performance also challenges models that serially link STM and LTM and, conversely, provides support for models that postulate that verbal STM and LTM are separate or parallel systems.

The notion of STM as a component of LTM has gradually given way to ideas that now refer to **working memory** (Baddeley, 1986) as a distinct system encompassing some of the capacity limitations of STM, but that is a dynamic system also influencing aspects of attention and executive functioning. Several distinctions differentiate STM (sometimes called short-term span) from working memory. First, a cognitive (mental) representation of information is held "on line" in temporary store (similar to STM). Second, the cognitive representations are subjected to some form of mental manipulation or transformation. Third, attentional and inhibitory control is necessary for the protection of the on-line cognitive representations, manipulations, and transformations from external or internal inference. Fourth, the cognitive manipulations or computations often involve using information drawn from long-term storage. To understand working memory, consider the following: You are presented a multiplication problem to solve mentally such as multiplying 234 by 354. When performing this problem, you will hold a mental representation of the problem in short-term storage. As you maintain this mental representation while performing the necessary computations to solve the problem, you will need to intensely concentrate and, at the same time, block out any internal or external stimuli that could disrupt your focus. Simultaneously, you will draw from LTM the appropriate multiplication facts and the mathematical operations needed to solve the problem. Because of the dynamic and effortful cognitive processes involved in working memory, Moscovitch and Winocur (2002) believe that it would be more aptly named "working-with-memory."

Alan Baddeley's (2001, 2002) seminal research and theorization has substantially enhanced our understanding of working memory. Working memory is integral to a wide range of cognitive tasks from reading to math to problem solving. Baddeley initially conceptualized working memory as involving three components (Figure 9.8). The **central executive** is an attention-controlling system; it supervises and coordinates slave systems and is the proposed

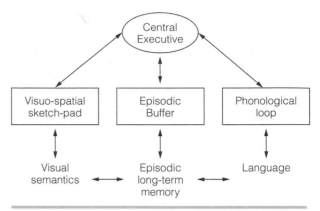

Figure 9.8   A simplified representation of Baddeley's working memory model. (Adapted from Baddeley, A. [2002]. Fractionating the central executive. In D. T. Stuss & R. T. Knight [Eds.], *Principles of frontal lobe functioning* [p. 256, Figure 16.4]. New York: Oxford University Press, by permission.)

deficit in Alzheimer's disease. The attention-controlling functions of the central executive system involve focusing, shifting, and dividing attention and interfacing with LTM. There are also two modality-specific "slave" systems. The **articulatory phonologic loop** stores speech-based information and is important in the acquisition of vocabulary. The **visuospatial sketch pad** manipulates visual and spatial images. Recently, Baddeley (2000, 2002) extended the model to include a fourth component, the **episodic buffer** (see Figure 9.8). The episodic buffer is a temporary and limited capacity storage system whose posited function is to hold and integrate information of *different* modalities (for example, visual and auditory) through linkage with LTM. The central executive controls this buffer and uses conscious awareness as a primary retrieval strategy. For example, if you are asked to recall a series of numbers presented in word form, and you are able to categorize the numbers into meaningful groups based on associations in long-term storage, memory recall will be enhanced. Thus, if numbers are visually presented in *word form*—fourteen, ninety-two, nineteen, forty-one—and you draw from LTM the numeric representation of historically significant dates and group the numbers as 1492 (Columbus discovers America) and 1941 (beginning of the World War II), you have integrated verbal and visual information through linkage with associative information held in LTM.

Neuropsychologically, the phonologic loop and the visuospatial sketch pad link to lateralized modalities in the brain and to frontal lobe executive processes. The phonologic loop involves auditory-verbal processing and depends on language-based left hemisphere processes. Likewise, the visuospatial sketch pad is associated with the

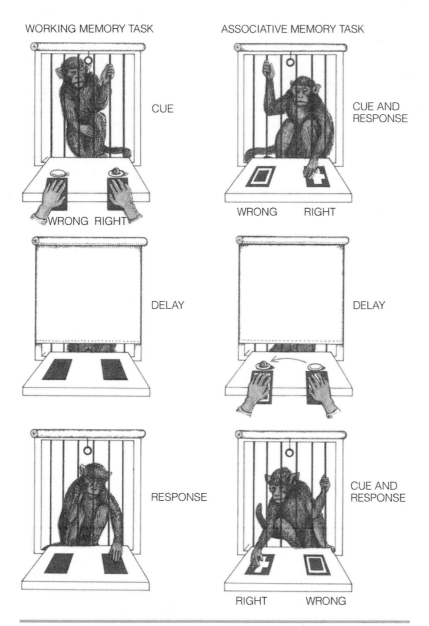

WORKING MEMORY TASK

ASSOCIATIVE MEMORY TASK

Figure 9.9 In Goldman-Rakic's working memory task (left), the target food stimulus is placed and the monkey must remember the position during a brief delay. This contrasts with an associative long-term memory task (right) in which the monkey has to learn the association of the plus sign with food. (Courtesy Patricia J. Wynne/Tody Press; from Goldman-Rakic, P. [1993]. Working memory and the mind. *Mind and brain: Readings from Scientific American* [p. 69]. New York: W. H. Freeman, by permission.)

right hemisphere. The neural substrates that support the episodic buffer remain to be identified, although frontal architecture is believed to play a crucial role (Baddeley, 2002). Goldman-Rakic's (1988) groundbreaking work in primate models of working memory points to the dorsolateral prefrontal cortex as the area that holds information "on

line" while it is processed. In these studies, Goldman-Rakic tested monkeys' abilities to recall the position of food in one of two food wells after a short delay of several seconds. Figure 9.9 shows the general paradigm of the study. Simultaneous recordings from neurons in the dorsolateral prefrontal area continued to fire during the delay until the action of food selection was completed. Since Goldman-Rakic's work, PET and fMRI studies have supplied confirmation in humans that the prefrontal cortex activates during working memory tasks (Jonides et al., 1993; Smith, Marshuetz, & Geva, 2002). For example, based on neuroimaging research, Petrides (1998) has identified two areas of the prefrontal cortex that are involved in support of working memory. The first area, the ventrolateral prefrontal cortex (Brodmann's areas 45 and 47/12), activates when dynamic (strategic) retrieval of information from posterior brain regions is required; that is, when there is a conscious effort to retrieve specific information in accordance with the individual's intentions and plans. Thus, the ventrolateral cortex is actively involved in the selection, comparison, and judgment of information held in memory. In contrast, the mid-dorsolateral frontal cortex (Brodmann's areas 46 and 9) activates when information is to be maintained on line for the purpose of monitoring and manipulation. Jointly, these two areas provide the foundation for higher order processes involved in the planning and organization of behavior.

The move from conceptualizing STM as a storage capacity system to that of working memory as a dynamic, integrated system entailing both lower and higher order processes highlights the interrelated nature of brain systems. Other memory processes such as prospective memory (the memory for future intention), temporal memory (memory for information in time order), and source memory (memory for context) also rely on frontal lobe and executive functioning processes. The next section discusses attention, a major higher function that is essential to the efficiency of mental processing.

Attention

> Everyone knows what attention is. It is the taking possession of the mind in clear and vivid form of one out of what seem several simultaneous objects or trains of thought.
>
> —*William James* (1890)

Moving about the world, people confront a flood of information that the nervous system cannot treat equally. Your brain must target or "spotlight" specific material to process and tune out the irrelevant information. For example, when you stop to talk to a friend in a hallway, you may hear competing sounds of others talking and people walking down the corridor. You may also be preoccupied by your own inner thoughts. Nonetheless, if you "pay attention," you can orient to a small sample of the incoming information and ignore most of the other input. In this way, attention operates as a gateway for information processing. Attention allows orienting to, selecting, and maintaining focus on information to make it available for cortical processing.

The neuropsychology of attention historically has been a confusing subject because there are so many subsets of attentional processing and many possible definitions of attention. The term *attention* can refer to a general level of alertness or vigilance; a general state of arousal; orientation versus habituation to stimuli; the ability to focus, divide, or sustain mental effort; the ability to target processing within a specific sensory arena (such as visual attention or auditory attention); or a measure of capacity. Researchers have also asked whether attention implies a general state of cortical tone or energy, or functions as a network or set of specific structures or networks within the brain. Attentional processing does not imply a unified system, and most researchers now view it as a multifaceted concept that implies multiple behavioral states and cortical processes that various subsets of cerebral structures control.

In many types of brain dysfunction, efficiency of the brain to process information diminishes. Sometimes people cannot sustain attention to one particular stimulus for longer periods or cannot select information (selective attention) from competing sources. This impairment may be minimally present and detected only through formal neuropsychological testing, or may be profound and easily noticeable by any observer.

Neuropsychological theories of attentional processing (for example, see Mesulam, 1981; Posner & Petersen, 1990) usually consider the role of the reticular activating system (RAS) in cortical arousal, subcortical and limbic system structures (particularly the cingulate gyrus) in regulation of information to be attended to, the posterior parietal lobe system in focusing conscious attention, and the frontal lobes in directing attentional resources. They also give the right hemisphere prominence as an attentional processor. Theorists have not yet worked out any one-to-one correspondence between levels of attentional behavior and brain structures or networks. Rather, they can describe general subsets of brain systems related to attentional functioning.

SUBCORTICAL STRUCTURES INFLUENCING ATTENTION

The RAS regulates the level of cortical activation or arousal—a necessary first step in attentional processing.

With its genesis in the midbrain and its ability to project to large cortical areas, the RAS sets a general cortical tone. Researchers can observe and categorize this arousal into brain wave types (beta, alpha, theta, and delta) by their frequency as measured by an electroencephalograph (EEG). In a general way, sensory input "charges" the RAS. If the brainstem is processing sensory input, the RAS maintains high cortical activation. However, lack of sensory input does not necessarily make one drowsy. In fact, even with constant sensory input there can be habituation. Those who live on a noisy street grow accustomed to the sound, but a sudden silence will cause the brain to orient to the change in sound patterning. Daily biorhythms of 90 minutes of relatively higher and lower alertness also cycle throughout the day, and circadian rhythms control the sleep/wake cycle through the RAS. We discuss these changing levels of cortical tone further in our discussion of sleep (see Chapter 16). If a person is awake and alert, general level of arousal is more of a background issue than a central one in the neuropsychology of attentional processing. However, the RAS also plays a role in anticipatory responding. Researchers have hypothesized that the RAS may send a preparatory signal to the cortex to alert it to receive stimuli, and thus put it in a heightened state of readiness to receive. Lesions to the RAS can result in lowered alertness or coma. Chapter 13 discusses coma in greater detail.

Neuroscientists are also identifying the role of other subcortical structures in attention. Although the precise functions that these structures play in attentional functioning remains to be specified, several interpretations have been posed. Moreover, these regions do not operate in isolation from one another or from other subcortical and cortical structures. For example, support of sustained attention is ascribed to the right fronto-parietal-thalamic neural network (Sarter, Givens, & Bruno, 2001). With regard to selective visual attention, the thalamus, basal ganglia, and superior and inferior colliculi play a supporting role. The thalamus receives activation from the reticular formation and projects this arousal to the cortex. Moreover, the thalamus serves to select and relay information from subcortical regions to the cortex and, conversely, conveys cortical neural signals to subcortical regions. Through its gating function, it is in position to influence the selectivity of attention (Cohen, 1993). The superior colliculus of the midbrain plays a role in the reflexive movement of the eyes and head when orienting to visual stimuli, whereas the inferior colliculus is implicated when orienting to auditory stimuli. Researchers have historically attributed motor functions to the basal ganglia, but increasingly are recognizing their role in cognitive operations. Posner and DiGirolamo (1998) pose that the basal ganglia is involved in shifting or switching sets, and thus is a component of the act of orienting to stimuli.

THE CEREBRAL CORTEX AND ATTENTION

The attentional issues of most interest to human neuropsychology generally concern the higher levels of attentional processing coordinated by the cerebrum, including focused attention, the ability to alternate and divide attentional processes, and the ability to sustain attention. **Focused attention** is the ability to respond and pick out the important elements or "figure" of attention from the "ground" or background of external and internal stimulation. Focused attention also implies a measure of concentration or effortful processing. A basketball player who can concentrate on making a free throw, while tuning out the crowd, is a good example of high focus. However, even the most ordinary event of noticing requires cognitive focus. People are frequently called on to alternate and divide attention in the course of daily activities. For example, a receptionist who must switch back and forth between answering the phone and talking with customers must use **alternating attention** while mentally holding a place to return to the other activity. **Divided attention** requires partialing out attentional resources at the same time rather than switching back and forth, however quickly. A good example is driving a car, listening to a radio, and talking with a passenger. Researchers have debated whether divided attention is, in fact, possible, or whether people just manage to shift their attention quickly between different stimuli. However, evidence indicates that people can divide attention to some degree. *Sustained attention* is the ability to maintain an effortful response over time. It is related to the ability to persist and sustain a level of vigilance. People who work as air traffic controllers or on assembly-line jobs must have excellent abilities for sustaining attention.

Attention can be further characterized by task or information-processing demands. Tasks that are routinely processed or overlearned can be performed automatically with minimal conscious thought. Automatic processing places minimal demands on attentional resources, and since processing demands are low, other tasks can be performed concurrently. In contrast, new, unfamiliar, or conflicting tasks require the conscious deployment of mental operations. Controlled processing involves the execution of mental operations in a linear or serial manner with a significant allocation of attentional resources. Parallel processing of additional tasks is generally not possible (Cohen, Aston-Jones, & Gilzenrat, 2004). An experienced driver

Table 9.1 *Disorders That Show Prominent Attentional Dysfunction*

Attention-deficit/hyperactivity disorder

Neurologic disease
    Multiple sclerosis
    Alzheimer's disease
    Parkinson's disease

Head trauma

Seizure disorders

Metabolic disorder
    Hypoglycemic encephalopathy
    Hyperthyroidism

Psychiatric disorders
    Depression
    Mania
    Schizophrenia

Right hemisphere stroke: unilateral neglect

does not need to attend to the mechanics of driving while conversing with a passenger, because eye, hand, and foot movement associated with driving are well-practiced or "habitual." A person driving for the first time must commit considerable attention to the mechanics of driving and will find conversing with a passenger to be not only difficult but highly disruptive.

The disruption of attention is a common complaint of patients who have a variety of disorders. Table 9.1 provides a partial listing of disorders that include attentional dysfunction as a prominent component of the symptom pattern. The range of disorders illustrates that attentional dysfunction is easily compromised by neurologic, metabolic, and psychiatric disorders. Fatigue, or inability to sustain attention to an activity, frequently appears across a number of more generalized neuropsychological disorders. Patients with neurologic disease, as well as patients who have suffered focal or generalized brain insults, often describe mentally wearing out when engaged in tasks that require persistent effortful attention. People with affective disorders frequently report attention and concentration problems. Depressed people often describe drifting off or "spacing out," so that even when driving they may miss an exit. Mania is associated with concentration problems of another sort. Manic people may become so energetic with a relentless "flight of ideas" passing through their minds that they cannot accomplish anything, because they cannot concentrate on one thing at a time. Attentional deficits are also a common concomitant of schizophrenia. These include perseveration of thought

and action, inability to disengage attention, problems in sustained attention or vigilance, distractibility, and an almost random tendency to orient to both external and internal stimuli. This set of deficits may cause the loose associations in thought processes that schizophrenics commonly show. Close to half of schizophrenics show no galvanic skin conductance response (SCR), which is ordinarily considered an orienting response to novel sensory stimuli (Dawson & Nuechterlein, 1984). Neuropsychologists call this subgroup of schizophrenics *electrodermal nonresponders.* Nonresponders are more likely to show the negative symptoms of schizophrenia including apathy, emotional and social withdrawal, and blunted affect. Nonresponders are also more likely to have cortical atrophy than schizophrenic galvanic skin responders. Interestingly, the failure of a psychophysiological skin conductance orienting response to sensory stimulation comes against a background of chronic elevation of autonomic responses, which implies a generalized hyperarousal in this subgroup. Some investigators suggest (see Cohen, 1993, for review) that the attention deficit in schizophrenia may be a primary cognitive dysfunction.

MODELS OF ATTENTION

A myriad of models have been developed to conceptualize attentional functioning. Each model represents a different theoretical orientation, type of attention, method of study, and degree of empirical verification. We present the individual models that Mesulam, Posner, and Mirsky developed in order to provide familiarity with neuropsychological conceptualizations of attentional functioning.

Mesulam's Model of Spatial Attention

Mesulam (2000) presents a model of selective, spatial attention that has enhanced our understanding of neuropsychological manifestations of patients exhibiting symptoms of attentional neglect. Based on clinical and empirical research, Mesulam poses that a neural network involving the frontal, parietal, and cingulate cortices supports spatial attention to the extrapersonal world (Figure 9.10). Each of these regions makes a differential contribution to spatial attention. The parietal region generates an internal spatial representation (sensory map) of the extrapersonal environment, whereas the cingulate cortex assigns and regulates motivational and emotional significance to extrapersonal elements (Gitelman et al., 1999; Kim et al., 1999). The frontal cortex, particularly the frontal eye fields (Brodmann's area 8) and surrounding areas, modulates and coordinates motor programs for exploration,

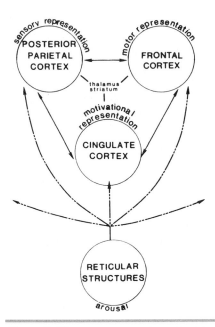

Figure 9.10 A theoretical schematic of the attentional system. (From Mesulam, M. M. [1985]. *Principles of behavioral neurology*. Philadelphia: E. A. Davis; reprinted from Cohen, R. A. [1993]. *The neuropsychology of attention* [p. 334, Figure 14.2]. Reprinted by kind permission of Springer Science and Business Media.)

scanning, foveating, fixating, and manipulating (reaching) extrapersonal stimuli. Spatial attention requires the integrity of these three cortical areas, as well as their interconnections with one another and with subcortical regions in the thalamus and striatum. The model thus conceptualizes spatial attention in terms of sensory representation, motivational importance and expectancy, and motor response.

Recently, Mesulam's model (Nobre, Coull, Maquet, Frith, Vandenberghe, & Mesulam, 2004) was extended to spatial attention to information held within working memory. Research participants underwent neuroimaging (fMRI) while performing a spatial working memory task and a spatial orientation task. The former task required the orientation of attention to internalized representations of previously encoded stimuli, and the latter required attentional orientation to extrapersonal stimuli. Neuroimaging demonstrated that both tasks recruited overlapping networks involving the occipital, parietal, and frontal cortices. While both spatial tasks activated the superior parietal lobe, only the right inferior parietal cortex was selectively activated during extrapersonal attentional orienting. With regard to the frontal lobes, orienting to extrapersonal stimuli activated the premotor and dorsal prefrontal cortex, while more anterior prefrontal regions

were selectively engaged in orienting attention to internally represented stimuli. Previous research has associated these anterior prefontal regions with working memory operations. Overall, the findings suggest that overlapping neural networks are involved in orienting attention to external and internal spatial representations.

Lesions in any of the neural components supporting spatial attention can lead to **hemispatial neglect,** that is, a failure to attend to the contralateral visual field. Hemispatial neglect generally relates to right rather than left hemisphere injury, suggesting hemispheric asymmetry in the support of spatial attention. The right hemisphere appears specialized for control of spatial attention across the visual field, whereas the left hemisphere's control is primarily limited to the contralateral right side visual field.

Posner's Anterior and Posterior Attention Model

Michael Posner presents a model of attention from the perspective of cognitive psychology and neuroscience. He poses that attention can be defined by three major functions: (1) orienting to events, particularly to locations in visual space; (2) achieving and maintaining a vigilant or alert state; and (3) orchestrating voluntary actions (Fernandez-Duque & Posner, 2001). Each attentional function is, in turn, supported by separate neural networks, namely, orienting, vigilance, and executive networks (Table 9.2). Moreover, these attention-neural networks operate interactively with each other and other cortical and subcortical regions.

Table 9.2 *Posner's Attention Networks*

Attention Networks	Functions	Neural Correlates
Posterior orienting system	Orienting to stimuli	
	Disengage attention from a stimuli	Temporoparietal, superior temporal, superior parietal
	Move to a stimuli Engage new stimuli	Superior colliculus Thalamus
Vigilance attention system	Achieving and maintaining an alert state	Right frontoparietal
Anterior or executive attention system	Orchestrating voluntary actions	Anterior cingulate, lateral and orbitofrontal prefrontal cortex, basal ganglia, thalamus

When visually orienting to an event in the environment, three basic cognitive operations—disengage, move, and engage—activate. Attention is first disengaged from the current event of focus and then moved to the new point of focus, where attentional resources are engaged. The operations of disengage, move, and engage are linked to the parietal, midbrain, and thalamic region, respectively. Accordingly, the visual orienting system is termed the **posterior attention system.** This system plays a role in conscious attention to portions of your visuospatial field and directs the attention of your eyes to a point in space. The posterior parietal lobe mediates conscious attention to spatial targets, the midbrain superior colliculus plays a role in moving the eyes from one position to another, and the pulvinar of the thalamus helps select and filter important sensory information for processing. The orienting system is also activated in covert orientation. *Covert orientation* refers to the spatial engagement of attention to a target without moving the eyes or the head. For example, if you fixate your eyes on an object, you can also attend to a peripherally located object without moving your eyes or head.

Posner initially ascribed the disengage function to the superior parietal lobe. However, lesion studies showed that disruption of the disengage function was often associated with lesions in the temporoparietal junction or superior temporal lobe. This difference was resolved by the discovery that lesions of the temporoparietal junction or superior temporal regions impair the ability to disengage from a stimulus, and then shift attention to a new or novel stimulus (Posner & Fan, in press). In contrast, lesions of the superior parietal lobe disrupt voluntary shifts of attention following a cue or when searching a visual target.

There are indications that the orienting system is modulated, in part, by the cholinergic neurotransmitter ACh (acetylcholine). ACh is produced by the nucleus basalis of the brain forebrain and innervates many cortical areas, including the parietal lobes. Research with primates shows that lesions of the nucleus basalis disrupt the disengagement of attention from an ipsilesional cue to engage a target contralateral to the side of the lesion (Fernandez-Duque & Posner, 2001).

Patients with lesions to the right posterior orienting system frequently fail to attend to the opposite visual field, a condition referred to as hemispatial neglect. As discussed previously, hemispatial neglect is not a sensory deficit to visual input, but rather a failure to attend to half of the visual field (Figure 9.11). Posner (Posner & Petersen, 1990) describes this as a problem of engaging, moving, and disengaging focus to objects in the contralateral field

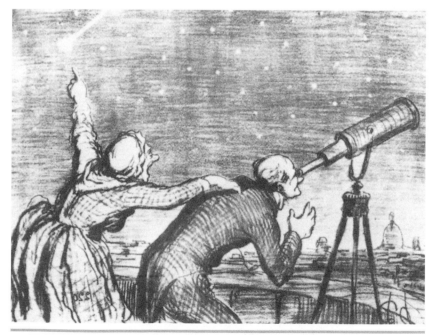

Figure 9.11   A case of hemispatial inattention. (From Honoré Daumier, M. [1858]. Babinet prevenu par sa portiere de la visite de la comete. *Le Charivari.* Courtesy of Museum of Fine Arts, Boston, MA. Reprinted from Cohen, R. A. [1993]. *The neuropsychology of attention* [frontispiece]. New York: Plenum Press, by permission.)

of vision. In this view, the system does not direct the eyes and the brain to engage the left side of space, or to disengage attention from the right side of space.

The **vigilance attention system** mobilizes and sustains alertness for processing high-priority targets and is important to attentional functioning. For example, if you were involved in an aerial search for survivors of a boating accident, you would have to maintain a high level of alertness and preparedness to identify a survivor in the expanse of the ocean. In addition, you would need to avoid processing irrelevant information (external or internal) to avoid distraction. The neural network supporting the vigilance system includes the right frontal and parietal regions of the brain. The neurotransmitter norepinephrine, produced by the locus ceruleus of the midbrain, is implicated in achieving an alert state and maintaining attention over time (Fan, McCandliss, Sommer, Raz, & Posner 2002).

The **anterior** or **executive attention system** controls and coordinates other brain regions in the execution of voluntary attention. A hierarchy exists for attentional processing, with the anterior system passing control to the posterior system as needed. The executive attention system orchestrates higher order cognitive functions such as task switching, inhibitory control, conflict resolution, error detection, attentional resource allocation, planning, and the processing of novel stimuli. A number of cortical and subcortical substrates support the executive attention network, although Posner has focused much of his research and theorization on the anterior cingulate and lateral prefrontal cortex (Posner & DiGirolamo, 1998). One of the primary functions of the anterior cingulate relates to the monitoring and resolution of conflict between operations occurring in different brain areas (Posner & Fan, in press). For example, if an overlearned (automatic) response to a stimulus is to be inhibited in favor of a less salient response, the anterior cingulate provides the top-down control necessary to initiate the operations of inhibition and response selection. Similarly, the anterior cingulate activates when a task requires error detection. Thus, if you were proofreading a recent paper that you had prepared for a class, the anterior cingulate would be active with regard to identifying errors in the text.

Often, the lateral prefrontal cortex and anterior cingulate are jointly activated, depending on the nature of the presented demand or task. The involvement of the lateral prefrontal cortex in the executive attention system relates to its role in holding mental representations of specific information in temporary memory. This set of cognitive operations is consistent with the definition of working memory. The Stroop test (1935) illustrates the roles of the

anterior cingulate and lateral prefrontal cortex in executive attention. One of the trials of the Stroop test presents the examinee with the words *red, green,* and *blue* printed in an incongruous color. For example, the word *red* is printed in green type. Reading is an overlearned (automatic) behavior for most adults, and when written text is presented, decoding occurs quickly and automatically. In contrast, naming the color of objects is a less rapid and automatic process. When the words *red, green,* and *blue* are presented in incongruous color, reading the word is the salient response. If you are asked *not* to read the words, but to name the incongruous color of the printed words, significant conflict is produced. The anterior cingulate activates, as discussed earlier, to provide the top-down inhibitory control and response selection. The lateral prefrontal region holds the mental representation of the "rule" ("Name the color, don't read the word.") in working memory to guide the process.

Although norepinephrine and ACh are implicated in the support of the alerting and orienting systems, respectively, dopamine is considered the primary neural modulator of the executive or anterior attention system (Fernandez-Duque & Posner, 2001). Disorders that involve disruption of dopaminergic modulation (for example, schizophrenia) frequently demonstrate dysfunctions of executive attention. Furthermore, administration of a dopamine agonist to patients with lesions of the frontal lobes improves performance on measures of executive function (McDowell, Whyte, & D'Esposito, 1998).

Mirsky's Elements of Attention Model

Allen Mirsky (National Institute of Mental Health, Bethesda, MD) developed a neuropsychological model that identifies the possible elements of attention and relates these elements to neuropsychological measures and the underlying neural systems. Mirsky (1996) proposed that there were three elements of attention: focus-execute, sustain, and shift. A battery of neuropsychological measures considered sensitive to attentional functioning was compiled (Table 9.3) and administered to adult neuropsychiatric patients and healthy control participants. The test data revealed four factors, three of which corresponded with the elements of attention proposed by Mirsky, and an additional element that was labeled encode. Subsequently, the battery was extended to healthy children with measures appropriate to the younger age-group. Once again, four factors were identified, each similar to the elements of attention identified in the adult studies.

Table 9.3 *Mirsky's Elements of Attention*

Subject Group	Factor 1: Focus-Execute	Factor 2: Shift	Factor 3/5: Sustain/Stable	Factor 4: Encode
Adult	WAIS-R Digit Symbol, Stroop test, Letter Cancellation, and TMT-A and -B	WCST	CPT	WAIS-R Digit Span and Arithmetic
Child	WISC-R Coding and Digit Cancellation	WCST	CPT	WISC-R Digit Span and Arithmetic
Supporting substrata	*Focus:* Inferior parietal and superior temporal cortexes *Execute:* Inferior parietal and corpus striatum	Prefrontal cortex	Rostral midbrain structures and brainstem	Hippocampus and amygdala

Note: WAIS-R = Wechsler Adult Intelligence Scale-Revised (Wechsler, 1981); Stroop Test (Stroop, 1935); Letter Cancellation = Letter Cancellation Test (Talland, 1965); TMT-A and -B = Trail Making Test Parts A and B (Reitan & Davison, 1974); WCST = Wisconsin Card Sorting Test (Grant & Berg, 1948); CPT = Continuous Performance Test (Rosvold, Mirsky, Sarason, Bransome, & Beck, 1956); WISC-R = Wechsler Intelligence Scale for Children-Revised (Wechsler, 1974); Digit Cancellation (Mirsky, 1995).

Source: Adapted from Mirsky (1995, 1996).

The four elements of attention, and their hypothesized supportive neural substrates, are presented in Table 9.3. In brief, the four elements are described as follows:

1. **Focus-execute attention** involves selective attention and rapid perceptual-motor output.
2. **Shifting attention** describes the ability to move or change attentional focus in a flexible and adaptive manner.
3. **Sustained attention** pertains to the attention function of vigilance.
4. **Encode attention** specifies the capacity to briefly maintain information in memory (that is, "on line") while performing other related computations or actions.

Recently, a fifth component of attention, **stable,** was identified, and represents the consistency of attentional effort. The five elements of attention are believed to be supported by relatively distinct neuroanatomic regions (see Table 9.3) that interconnect to form an attention system. The distribution of the attention system throughout the brain is widespread. Accordingly, the attention system is quite vulnerable to disruption when brain injury is sustained; yet, it is also resilient. A specific attention function may be compromised by injury, but undamaged neural regions can provide some degree of compensation.

Mirsky's model has enhanced our understanding of the potential difference in attentional regulation of various clinical groups. Chapter 11 discusses the application of Mirsky's model to the investigation of the attentional processing of children with attention-deficit/hyperactivity disorder (ADHD).

The attention systems and structures presented here are skewed toward visual attentional processing because this is the best understood and most widely studied sensory processing system in relation to attention. Interestingly, studies of auditory spatial attention, similar to visuospatial attention, have been found to recruit the parietal cortex (Kim et al., 1999). There is agreement that, at a cortical level, the right hemisphere, particularly the parietal and frontal regions, plays a central role in attentional control. Subcortically, the anterior cingulate, thalamus, colliculi, and basal ganglia contribute to attentional functioning. These cortical and subcortical regions do not operate independently, but rather perform their functions via interconnecting neural systems.

Executive Functioning

Compared with all other areas of the cortex, the prefrontal lobes are unique in organization and function. For more than a century, controversy, confusion, and speculation have existed over the function(s) of the frontal lobes. Speculation has included conceptualizations of the frontal lobes as structures that are "silent" (having limited function), support a singular or global function (for example, abstract thinking), or underpin different classes of behaviors (for example, impulse control, judgment, creativity, emotional regulation, and moral judgment). The functions of the temporal, parietal, and occipital lobes follow straightforward principles of organization built around sensory system processing. In contrast, frontal lobe pathology does not result in primary disorders of sensation or perception, motor disability, memory, or language. Rather, the frontal lobes, by virtue of their interconnections with almost all other brain regions—including the brainstem; occipital, temporal and parietal lobes; limbic regions; and subcortical areas—serve to guide, direct, integrate, and monitor goal-directed behavior (Anderson, 2002; Anderson, Levin, & Jacobs, 2002). If the brain is a symphony, the frontal lobes act as the conductor—guiding, coordinating, and directing the separate sections of the orchestra to produce a harmonious and integrated musical performance.

The terms *frontal lobe functioning* and *executive functioning* are often used interchangeably. Although the terms overlap, the former suggests that presented behaviors are *directly* linked to the frontal lobes, whereas the latter connotes a class of behavioral manifestations that may be directly or *indirectly* related to frontal lobe functioning. Because of the significant afferent and efferent connectivity of the frontal lobes with other brain regions, disruption to any one these connecting systems can produce pathologic behaviors similar to those caused by direct frontal damage. For example, lesions to the caudate nucleus of the basal ganglia can result in pathologic behaviors similar to those seen with dorsolateral prefrontal damage. Although the term *executive functioning* does not denote a specific anatomic basis for behavior, it does implicate the frontal cortex and its interconnective neural circuitry. Both terms converge in the conceptualization of cortical functions that relate to the directing, controlling, and managing of behavior, that is, higher order supervisory brain computations. Functions attributed to the executive system include planning, flexible problem solving, working memory, attentional allocation, inhibition, and at the highest levels, the self-monitoring and self-assessment of behavior. Clearly, executive functioning refers to sets of higher order behavior, rather than a single type of behavior. Likewise, executive functioning is not limited to cognitive processes, but is intimately involved in emotional and social behavioral regulation. In fact, lesions of the prefrontal regions, and associated subcortical regions linked to emotional and social functioning, can produce some of the most devastating impairments. Executive functioning impairments become more evident in the most complex aspects of human conscious activity, or those activities of higher problem solving, reasoning, abstraction, critical self-awareness, and social interaction that make us human.

DEVELOPMENT OF EXECUTIVE FUNCTIONS

The maturation of executive functions is crucial to psychological adaptation and adjustment across the life span

(Eslinger, Biddle, & Grattan, 1997). Initially, our understanding of the development of executive functions lagged behind that of the maturation of other cortically supported functions such as intelligence. As discussed earlier, the lag was partially related to the belief in neuropsychology that prefrontal functions did not begin to emerge until late childhood or early adolescence. Although this belief delayed the initiation of active study and research of childhood executive functions, significant progress has been evident since the early 1980s. Accordingly, we preview here some of the advances in our understanding of the development of executive functions.

Empirical studies (Levin et al., 1991; Welsh, Pennington, & Groisser, 1991) suggest that basic executive functions develop early in life and follow a protracted, multistep trajectory to maturity in adulthood. The early appearance of rudimentary executive functions and the later development of more complex functions, such as abstract reasoning and judgment, parallel the lengthy development of the prefrontal cortex. Interestingly, the emergence of rudimentary executive functions correlates with the periods of maximum synaptic density of the frontal lobes. However, more complex functions continue to evolve long after maximum synaptic density is reached, and reflect a host of other developmental advances such as synaptic pruning and sculpting, axonal myelination, and neurochemical and neurophysiologic changes.

Important advances in understanding the development of executive functions are due to the remarkable investigations of Goldman-Rakic (1987a,b), Diamond (1991), and others. Goldman-Rakic has studied the relation of prefrontal development to the emergence of the cognitive operation of **object permanence,** that is, the capacity to store in memory a representation of an object that is removed from view for the purpose of guiding future behavior. Using a delayed response task (see Figure 9.9), the experimenter required rhesus monkeys to maintain in memory the spatial location or features of an object over delays ranging from 0 to 10 seconds. By the age of 2 to 4 months, the rhesus monkeys could perform the memory tasks at delay intervals of 2 to 5 seconds. During this 2- to 4-month period, researchers observed maximum synaptic density in the prefrontal lobes of the rhesus monkeys. The corresponding period of synaptic density in the human infant occurs between 8 and 24 months (Huttenlocher, 1990). The latter time interval also correlates with the infant's ability to perform a delayed response task (Neuropsychology in Action 9.2), suggesting that the executive function of working memory has emerged.

Diamond (1991) conducted a series of infant studies that have helped clarify the development of executive

Diamond (1991) has adapted a number of tasks that Jean Piaget initially used in studying cognitive development to investigate executive functions. In her study of infants, Diamond endeavored to relate the development of executive functions to the maturation of the underlying frontal circuitry.

Contiguous Object Task

The contiguous object task involves the use of a transparent box that is open at the top (Figure 9.12). The experimenter places a toy block behind the wall of the box and prompts the infant to pick up the toy block. Infants of 7 months can reach the block behind the wall if a single straight movement is required (frame A). However, if the placement of the block necessitates a two-directional reach (two sequential movements), the infant cannot accomplish these movements until approximately 10 months (frame B). Also, at younger than 10 months, the infant cannot inhibit the reflexive grasping of the edge of the box when his or her hand comes in contact with it.

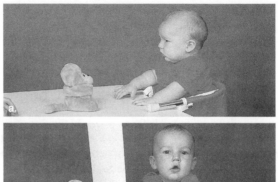

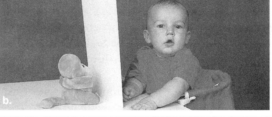

Figure 9.13   Hidden object task. (a) The infant is gazing at a toy. (b) The toy is shielded by a screen and the infant does not search or reach for the object. (© Doug Goodman/Photo Researchers, Inc.)

Hidden Object

Piaget noted that the infant 5 to 7 months old would not reach or search for an object hidden from view; that is, "out of sight, out of mind."

The hidden object task involves showing the infant a toy, and then covering it with a blanket or placing a screen in front of it to block the child's view (Figure 9.13). Diamond's research suggests that the 5- to 7-month-old infant does, in fact, realize that the object is hidden, but cannot demonstrate this knowledge by executing a motor response. That is, the infant is unable to organize and execute a means–end action sequence such as removing the blanket from the hidden object. However, by 7.5 to 8 months old, the infant is capable of executing the necessary action sequence.

A not B (Delayed Response Task)

The A not B task involves placing two "wells" in front of the infant (Figure 9.14) in which a toy can be hidden. The infant observes the researcher hide a toy in one of the wells, and then after a short period (2–5 seconds) is allowed to reach for the toy. Then the researcher hides the toy in the opposite well, and after a delay again allows the infant to reach for the toy. An infant younger than 8 months will reach for the well that contained the previously retrieved toy, even

Figure 9.12   Contiguous object task. (a) Single, straight-line reach for the block. (b) Two-directional reaching movement for the block. (Reproduced from Diamond A., & Gilbert, J. [1989]. Development as progressive inhibitory control of action: Retrieval of a contiguous object. *Cognitive Development, 12,* 223–249. Presented by Diamond, A. [1991]. Neuropsychological insights into the meaning of object concept development. In S. Carey & R. Gelman [Eds.], *The epigenesis of mind: Essays on biology and cognition* [p. 72, Figure 3.2]. Hillsdale, NJ: Erlbaum, by permission.)

a.   b.

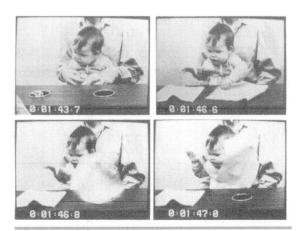

Figure 9.14 A not B task. (top) The infant is gazing at the toy in the well. In the following frames, the infant continues to gaze at the well holding the toy, yet lifts the cover from the well that contained the toy on the previous trial. (Reproduced from Diamond, A. [1991]. Neuropsychological insights into the meaning of object concept development. In S. Carey & R. Gelman [Eds.], *The epigenesis of mind: Essays on biology and cognition* [p. 86, Figure 3.4]. Mahwah, NJ: Lawrence Erlbaum Associates, by permission.)

Detour Reaching Task

In the detour reaching task, the experimenter requires the infant to detour around a barrier to reach and retrieve an object. The task involves a small transparent box that the experimenter places in front of the infant with one of its sides open (Figure 9.15). If they can see the toy through an open side, infants 6.5 to 7 months of age will reach in to retrieve a toy. However, if the experimenter places the toy directly in the child's view, but behind a closed side, the infant repeatedly and unsuccessfully tries to reach through the closed side. The infant is unable to inhibit reaching straight for the toy. Also, the infant is unable to raise the box with one hand and reach at the same time with the other hand. In Figure 9.15, the child has lifted the box and is establishing a direct line of sight to the toy. As one hand moves down to reach into the box (second frame), the other hand holding the box also moves down. At this point (third frame), the toy is in the child's direct line of sight through the top of the box. The child withdraws her hand from the opening and tries, unsuccessfully, to reach for the toy through the closed top of the box. Between 8 and 12 months, the child develops the ability to look through one side of the box while reaching through another side. Similarly, the child can raise the box with one hand, and simultaneously reaching in with the other.

though he or she has seen the researcher place the toy in the opposite well.

In Figure 9.14, the infant has already successfully retrieved the toy from the well to the viewer's right. The researcher then placed the toy in the opposite well. In the first two frames (top left and right), the infant is looking at the well containing the toy. However, when allowed to reach for the toy, the infant uncovers the well that contained the toy on the previous trial (bottom left and right). Success on this task requires the emergence of working memory capability and the ability to inhibit a previously reinforced response.

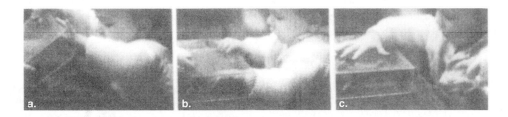

Figure 9.15 Detour reaching task. (a) The child has lifted the box and is looking in at a toy. (b) As the child begins to reach for the toy, the box lowers. The toy is now in the child's line of sight through the top of the box. (c) The child removes the hand from the box and tries to reach for the toy through the top of the box. (*Society for Research in Child Development Abstracts, 3,* 78, as presented in Diamond, A. [1991]. Neuropsychological insights into the meaning of object concept development. In S. Carey & R. Gelman [Eds.], *The epigenesis of mind: Essays on biology and cognition* [p. 90, Figure 3.5]. Mahwah, NJ: Lawrence Erlbaum Associates, by permission.)

inhibitory control and other functions as they relate to the maturation of the frontal cortex. She presented infants from 5 to 12 months old with tasks involving detour reaching, contiguous objects, hidden objects, and delayed response (A not B task) to determine the emergence of frontal functions (see Neuropsychology in Action 9.2). Her findings demonstrated that the ability to inhibit reflexive reactions to contact (elicitation of the grasp reflex when touching an object) and to combine two or more actions into a behavioral sequence develops between the 5th and 9th months of life. These two functions are contingent on the maturation of the supplementary motor cortex (SMC) of the frontal lobes.

Between 8 and 12 months of age, an infant develops the ability to inhibit a response that is primed for release, and to relate information over time delays and spatial separation. The infant's successful performance of the delayed response task (A not B) and the detour reaching task, respectively, reflects the development of the ability to relate information across time and space. The performance of these tasks requires inhibitory control and working memory capabilities, functions that the dorsolateral prefrontal cortex support (Goldman-Rakic, 1987b). Finally, the ability of the infant to simultaneously coordinate two different movements emerges between 8 and 12 months of age. That is, the infant can execute an action with one hand and simultaneously perform a different action with the other. These hand movements require both coordination and inhibition of movements. That is, the action of each hand must coordinate with the other, but each is inhibited from performing the same movement as the other. This complex set of actions requires the maturation of the corpus callosum that joins the SMC areas of each hemisphere. The interhemispheric communication of the SMC regions is necessary for coordinating bilateral actions.

Other researchers (Denckla, 1996; Pennington, 1997b) have also made notable contributions to the identification of emerging childhood executive functions. For example, Welsh and coworkers (1991) have traced the development of executive functions in healthy children, ages 3 to 12, and young adults. The investigators determined that subjects achieved adult-like performance at three different age levels: 6 years old, 10 years old, and during adolescence. Simple functions, such as visual search (searching an array of stimuli for targets), emerge early, followed by the more complex inhibitory skills, and finally, the most advanced abilities as demonstrated in complex planning. Age-related changes in the development of the executive functions of working memory, inhibition, and cognitive flexibility have been identified for healthy preschool

(Espy, Kaufmann, Glisky, & McDiarmid, 2001) and elementary school (Archibald & Kerns, 1999) children. There are suggestions that some executive functions unfold in a gradually progressive manner, whereas others move toward maturity in a stepwise, or staged fashion. Furthermore, executive function performance does not appear to correlate significantly with intelligence, supporting the proposition that these two cognitive constructs are relatively independent from each other.

Similarly, Culbertson and Zillmer (1998a, 1998b, 2005) used the Tower of London-Drexel University (TOL^{DX}) test to assess age-related changes in the **executive planning** of healthy children and children with ADHD. Executive planning, as assessed by the TOL^{DX}, involves the development of a "mental template" to guide the sequential movement of colored beads across three pegs to match a pattern presented on the examiner's model (Figure 9.16). The examiner asks the child to replicate a series of bead patterns of increasing difficulty while adhering to specific problem-solving rules. The goal is to solve each pattern in a minimum number of moves without violating the rules. Children who fail to plan, or plan superficially, require additional moves to reproduce the target patterns.

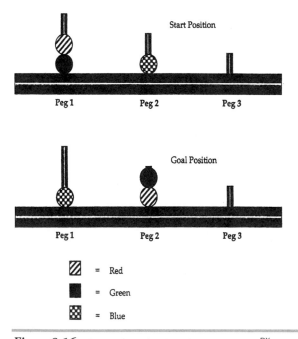

Figure 9.16   Tower of London-Drexel University (TOL^{DX}) test: start and goal positions. (Reproduced from Culbertson, W. C., & Zillmer, E. A. [1998]. The Tower of London: A standardized approach to assessing executive functioning in children. *Archives of Clinical Neuropsychology, 13,* 289. Copyright © 1998 Elsevier Science, Ltd. Reprinted with permission of the authors and the publisher.)

Culbertson and Zillmer selected children with ADHD for study in an effort to determine whether deficits in executive planning were associated with the disorder (see Chapter 11 for a discussion of ADHD). The researchers hypothesized that the ADHD children would perform less efficiently on the TOL^{DX}. Figure 9.17 shows the TOL^{DX} total move scores of the two groups of children.

Noteworthy is the steady improvement in executive planning from 7 to 12 years of age, with the healthy and ADHD children groups showing a parallel trajectory. However, the children with ADHD, as predicted, performed in a significantly less efficient manner than the healthy children. The poorer TOL^{DX} performance of ADHD children is consistent with emerging research (Pennington, 1997b) suggesting that the disorder is developmental in origin and potentially a consequence of impaired executive functions. Further analysis of the chil-

dren's TOL^{DX} performance showed the following results for the younger children, both healthy and those with ADHD: (1) spent less time planning before attempting to solve the bead patterns, (2) solved fewer bead patterns in a minimum number of moves, and (3) violated a greater number of problem-solving rules than the older healthy and ADHD children. Clearly, the maturation of executive planning involves the advance of a number of component cognitive skills.

Recently, Anderson (2002) reviewed factor analytic studies pertinent to the development of executive functioning of childhood and adolescent populations. Despite differences in executive measures used, participants sampled, and ages represented, similar executive factors were identified to include planning, impulse control, concept reasoning, and response speed. Integrating these findings with the recent conceptualizations of executive functioning reported by Alexander and Stuss (2000), Anderson proposed four developmentally sensitive executive function domains: attention control (selective attention, inhibitory control, sustained attention, and monitoring of executed plans), information processing (fluency, efficiency, and speed of output), cognitive flexibility (shifting between response sets, profiting from mistakes, developing alternative strategies, dividing attention, and multitasking), and goal setting (planning, organization, conceptual reasoning, and strategic problem-solving). Using this framework, a developmental trajectory of executive functions is proposed (Figure 9.18). Attention control undergoes significant maturation during infancy and early childhood, with adult levels of functioning reached by

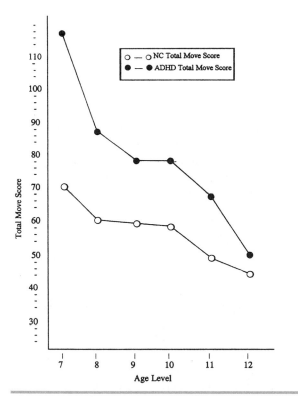

Figure 9.17 Mean Tower of London-Drexel University (TOL^{DX}) test total move score by age level for attention-deficit/hyperactivity disorder (ADHD) and normal control (NC) children. (Reproduced from Culbertson, W. C., & Zillmer, E. A. [1998]. The Tower of London: A standardized approach to assessing executive functioning in children. *Archives of Clinical Neuropsychology, 13,* 291. Copyright © 1998 Elsevier Science, Ltd. Reprinted with permission of the authors and the publisher.)

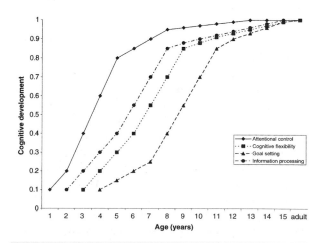

Figure 9.18 Developmental trajectory of executive functions. (Reproduced from Anderson, P. [2002]. Assessment and development of executive function during childhood. *Child Neuropsychology, 8,* 78, by permission.)

middle childhood. Despite somewhat different trajectories, information processing, cognitive flexibility, and goal-setting functions achieve maturation by the end of middle childhood. However, developmental refinement continues into mid-adolescence and early adulthood.

A more recent meta-analysis of relevant studies of executive/frontal development (Romine & Reynolds, 2005) reported that abilities such as planning, verbal fluency, and inhibition of perseveration demonstrated pronounced increases between 5 and 8 years of age. Developmental increases were evident across all executive functions between 8 and 11 years of age. Small incremental changes were noted between 11 and 14 years of age for the inhibition of perseveration and set maintenance. Planning and verbal fluency functions continue to develop throughout adolescence and into early adulthood. The two reviewed meta-analyses indicate that executive functions reach maturity at different points during development. It should be remembered that the development of executive functions is, in part, contingent on the maturation of other brain regions and neural systems that support attention, language, emotions, and memory.

Research has also focused on the relation between the development of emotional regulation and maturation of the frontal region. Bell and Fox (1994) have found that changes in EEG activation associated with emotional expression appear early in infant development. When a stranger approached, 10-month-old infants exhibited right frontal EEG activation, but the opposite pattern was evident when the mother approached—that is, greater left frontal activation. Similarly, infants who appeared sad or distressed, as assessed by facial expressions, showed greater right frontal activation, whereas those expressing joy demonstrated greater left frontal activation. Of importance was the finding that comparable frontal EEG activation patterns continue to be evident in childhood and adulthood (Davidson, 1994).

Case studies of children who sustained damage to the frontal cortex provide further insight into frontal lobe development and the regulation of emotional, moral, and social behavior. In a review of cases with varying ages of lesion onset (ranging from prenatal to age 16), Eslinger and colleagues (1997, 2004) found that the children demonstrated impairments in emotional regulation and interpersonal relations, regardless of the age at which the damage occurred. Both immediate and delayed deficits were observed, suggesting that the development of socioemotional regulatory control was ongoing. The progressive emergence of delayed deficits indicated that the damaged frontal system could not negotiate the increasing cognitive, social, and emotional demands of adolescence and adulthood. For example, a boy who suffered damage to his right frontal lobe at age 3 appeared to recover fully, although the mother did note alterations in his personality after the insult. During his early school years, he demonstrated problems in visuospatial performance, attentional focus, impulse control, and establishing friendships. By adolescence, he exhibited limited facial expressions and modulation of voice, interrupted the conversation of others, had not developed friendships or dated, and often failed to understand the gist of intended communications. His social deficits reflected an inability to empathize or reciprocate emotionally with others, to understand social cues and the pragmatics of language, and to accurately evaluate his own social strengths and weaknesses.

FRONTAL-MEDIATED FUNCTIONS AND DYSFUNCTIONS

There is increasing evidence that the frontal lobes, interacting with cortical and subcortical circuitry, support relatively distinct but overlapping functions. Five primary circuits have been identified—although evolving research suggests that there may be at least two additional circuits (Middleton & Strick, 2001). These circuits project from different regions of the frontal lobes to designated regions of the basal ganglia and return via specific thalamic nuclei. The five neural circuits (Saint-Cyr, Bronstein, & Cummings, 2002) and their cortical origination are skeletomotor (motor and premotor regions and parietal somatosensory cortex), oculomotor (frontal and supplementary eye fields), dorsolateral prefrontal (dorsolateral prefrontal cortex), orbitofrontal (consists of two subcircuits that originate in the lateral and medial frontal cortex), and anterior cingulate (anterior cingulate cortex).

We focus on the three circuits that are often implicated in neuropsychological and neuropsychiatric disorders. However, before we begin, several caveats are in order. The frontal lobes are, as previously discussed, richly interconnected with other cortical and subcortical regions of the brain. Thus, the student should *not* consider the functions attributed to the frontal circuits to be solely localized or mediated by a specified region or circuit. The finding that damage to different regions of a circuit can produce executive dysfunction comparable with that evident when the frontal lobes are directly involved speaks to this caution. It is probably more accurate to describe the different frontal circuits as contributors, often major, to the mediation of certain types or forms of behavior. Second, a review of relevant studies shows that differential processing biases for content (for example, verbal versus nonverbal), modality, and types of mental operations are ascribed to left versus right frontal architecture. However, there are notable exceptions to the putative specificity of right versus left prefrontal systems. For example, verbal semantic retrieval and episodic encoding activates the left prefrontal region, whereas episodic retrieval instigates right prefrontal computations (Cabeza & Nyberg, 2000). Moreover, it is not unusual to find bilateral activation of the frontal cortex for a given task, suggesting complementary processing. Thus, care needs to be exercised when assuming a one-to-one correspondence between task content, input-output modality, or mental process recruited and the implicated anterior laterality (left versus right). Third, despite significant research and study, we do not fully understand the functions of the frontal systems, nor do researchers and clinicians agree on the functions that are associated with the different frontal circuits or regions.

Dorsolateral Circuit

The first circuit, dorsolateral prefrontal, is involved in higher order cognitive operations. Often, this circuit is labeled the "executive" circuit; however, with our realization that executive functioning is implicated in the mediation of emotional, motivational, and social behavior, we consider the functions of each of the three circuits to be executive in nature. A sample of functions attributed to the dorsolateral circuit includes working memory, cognitive flexibility, maintenance of behavioral sets, selective and sustained attention, generation of strategic and divergent responses, verbal and nonverbal fluency, planning and organization, inhibitory control, abstract reasoning, memory search and retrieval, temporal-spatial "tagging" (binding time and spatial context to episodes), self-monitoring, insight, and judgment. Furthermore, the dorsolateral circuit participates in emotional-motivational behavior, such that damage to the region may precipitate depressive symptoms, although these symptoms are more frequently associated with damage to the ventromedial prefrontal region. The depressive symptoms associated with the dorsolateral prefrontal cortex are characterized by decreased initiative, apathy, indifference, psychomotor retardation, and social uneasiness (Anderson & Tranel, 2002). This depressive presentation differs from clinical depression by the absence of vegetative functions, negative cognition, and dysphoria. Some patients with dorsolateral damage demonstrate a decreased capacity to empathize with others, although this impairment is more frequently associated with disruption of the orbitofrontal circuit (Anderson & Tranel, 2002). The dorsolateral and orbital circuits may play complementary roles in empathic processing, with the former mediating the cognitive aspects of empathy, and the latter mediating the emotional elements (Eslinger, 1998).

Luria (1990) gives an example of the cognitive difficulties of Patient U, who suffered from a progressive frontal lobe tumor:

Patient U is presented the problem: *One ABC book and one pen cost 37 cents. One ABC book and two pens cost 49 cents. How much do one ABC book and one pen cost separately?*

The patient repeats the problem correctly but does not begin to solve it.

(Dr. Luria): *What should you do to solve the problem?*
(U): "37 and 49. . . . then it's 86 all in all. . . ."
(Dr. Luria): *What did you add them for?*
(U): "To learn how much they paid all in all."
(Dr. Luria): *What should you do next?*
(U): "Next. . . . I don't know what next. . . . There is nothing else. . . ."

In order to draw the patient's attention to the final question and help him distinguish the main solution elements, the statement is presented in writing in the form of the following equations:

One ABC book + one pen = 37 cents
One ABC book + two pens = 49 cents

(Dr. Luria): *How much do one ABC book and one pen cost separately?*

Patient U reads the equation, draws a line underneath and writes down the result of simple summation:

"Two ABC books + three pens = 86 cents" saying, "I've learned how many pens and ABC books, how much everything costs."

It is evident that our attempt to show the difference between the two equations and to prompt the proper logical sequence ended in failure. . . . [T]he investigator gives him the initial element of the respective logical chain.

(Dr. Luria): *First 37 cents were spent, then 49 cents. What is the difference accounted for?*
(U): "It is accounted for by one pen! Then, 49 − 37 = 1 pen."
(Dr. Luria): *What should you learn?*
(U): "How much do an ABC book and a pen cost separately."
(Dr. Luria): *So?*
(U): So, a pen costs 12 cents. Now an ABC book. . . . 49 − 24 = 25 cents. One ABC book costs 25 cents. (Luria, 1990, pp. 106–107)

In the above example, Patient U knows the arithmetic operations necessary to solve problems but cannot discern the important aspects of the problem without external structure. In fact, at first, he cannot initiate any response. His first, rather impulsive response is simply to sum the numbers. He rigidly adheres to this strategy and is too cognitively inflexible to think of other possibilities. However, when he is guided, when the interviewer provides the important aspects of the problem for him, he can arrive at the correct answer. According to Stuss and Benson (1986), Patient U's primary programs for math algorithms are intact, and they act in a fairly automatic or stereotyped manner. Unless organized by higher order executive functions, problem-solving behavior becomes chaotic—sometimes failing to initiate, sometimes having no logical sequence, or sometimes perseverating on the first problem-solving strategy that comes to mind.

Joaquin Fuster (2002, 1997) has developed a theory of prefrontal functioning that focuses significantly on the role of the dorsolateral cortex. He poses that the overarching function of the prefrontal architecture is the temporal organization of behavior, that is, the development and implementation of action sequences across time. Temporal organization of behavior extends to all voluntary behavior including skeletal, ocular, speech, and internal cognitive processes such as logical reasoning (Fuster, Van Hoesen, Morecraft, & Semendeferi, 2000). Four cognitive processes support the temporal organization of behavior: attention, working memory, preparatory set, and monitoring. These four cognitive processes are based on the functional cooperation of the prefrontal cortex and the subcortical and other cortical structures and circuits.

- Attentional control relates to the cooperative activation of the dorsolateral (selective, sustain, and orienting of attention), anterior cingulate (motivation and drive aspects of attention), and orbital (inhibitory control and filtering) cortices.

- Working memory encompasses the processes dedicated to the maintenance and manipulation of information held in short-term storage to guide behavior. This function is supported by the dorsolateral prefrontal areas. Working memory provides a retrospective function in temporal organization. Its retrospective function relates to the temporary retention of mental representations of environmental (sensory) information pertinent to goal-directed behavior. For example, you need to hold "on line" the instructions for a test if you are to perform it correctly. The temporal organization of behavior requires both retrospective memory and the preparation for action.

- Preparatory motor set involves the preparation, timing, and instigation of relevant goal-directed motor behaviors. Once again, the dorsolateral cortex is implicated in the support of this function. Patients with frontal lateral lesions often demonstrate deficits in planning due to a failure to prepare for or to initiate a series of actions to achieve a goal. In essence, preparatory set

can be viewed as a failure in prospective memory, or memory for future action.

- Response monitoring determines whether current goal-directed behaviors should be maintained or modified. This is important since sensory processing and motor output operate across time, and environmental changes may occur that warrant alterations in goal-directed behaviors. Both the dorsolateral cortex and the anterior cingulate are implicated in the support of response monitoring.

These four functions support the diverse cognitive functions attributed to the dorsolateral prefrontal cortex. Notably, Fuster recognizes that the dorsolateral cortex functions in concert with other cortical and subcortical circuitry in the support of behavior.

Orbitofrontal (Lateral and Medial) Circuit

The orbitofrontal circuit is involved in the mediation of emotional and social responses. Initially, neuropsychologists considered inhibitory processes as a primary function of the orbitofrontal cortex. Converging research has altered this notion in that each region of the prefrontal cortex plays a role in behavioral inhibition (Roberts, Robbins, & Weiskrantz, 1998). However, the inhibitory processes of the orbitofrontal circuit are relatively specific to the regulation of emotional and social behavior.

Impulsive, poorly modulated, and contextually inappropriate behavior results when orbitofrontal inhibitory functioning is impaired. For instance, one of our patients, a man in his 50s, provides a classic example of impulsivity after a frontal lobe injury. Before his injury, T.J. was a successful businessman who traveled around the region making sales calls. One day, after the injury, he was to arrive at our office within a major medical center at 9 A.M. He drove around the parking garage trying to find a parking space. Unsuccessful in finding an empty spot, he became frustrated. Finally, he was stuck behind a car whose driver was waiting for someone else to back out. Impulsively, T.J. rammed the car ahead of him. Relating this story, T.J. expressed dismay at himself for acting in a way he felt was wrong. Yet, he felt that at the moment, he just could not help himself.

Patients with orbitofrontal damage can show a range of negative or poorly modulated emotionality. Often, irritable, angry, depressive, or manic-like emotions are prominent. Paradoxically, some patients exhibit a blunting or dampening of affective responsivity and reduced initiative. Accompanying characteristics of social disinhibition may include crude, coarse, and tactless behaviors.

Neuropsychology in Action 9.3

The Case of Phineas Gage

by Mary Spiers

In 1848, Phineas Gage was a 25-year-old foreman employed by the Rutland and Burlington Railroad. On an autumn day in Vermont, he and his crew were blasting through a rocky section when an accidental explosion sent a long metal bar, a tamping iron, shooting through his head. The pointed end of the rod entered under his left cheek and exited near the top middle of his skull, near the coronal and sagittal sutures. The rod was launched with such force that it landed 30 meters away from him. Amazingly, although Gage was knocked flat, he was able to get up and walk to the ox cart on which he sat while being driven into town. During the ride he chatted and made an entry into his logbook. Because he survived such a freakish accident, the case of Phineas Gage is arguably one of the most famous in the early history of neuropsychology.

Before the accident, Gage was seen as well balanced emotionally and mentally, healthy and active. Immediately after the accident, he fought postinjury infection to recover physically. He could walk and converse, recognized his friends and family, and appeared rational. To some he seemed fully recovered. But changes in his behavior soon emerged. His physicians noted, "Remembers passing and past events correctly, as well as before the injury. Intellectual manifestations feeble, being exceedingly capricious and childish, but with a will as indomitable as

ever; is particularly obstinate; will not yield to restraint when it conflicts with his desires" (Harlow, 1868, cited in Macmillan, 1996, p. 246). As time went on, this behavior did not abate but endured. Six months later, his physician, John Martin Harlow, summarized his condition:

> The equilibrium or balance, so to speak, between his intellectual faculties and his animal propensities, seems to have been destroyed. He is fitful, irreverent, indulging at times in the grossest profanity (which was not previously his custom), manifesting but little deference for his fellows, impatient of restraint or advice when it conflicts with his desires, at times pertinaciously obstinate, yet capricious and vacillating, devising many plans of future operation, which are no sooner arranged than they are abandoned in turn for others appearing more feasible. A child in his intellectual capacity and manifestations, he has the animal passions of a strong man. Previous to his injury, although untrained in the schools, he possessed a well-balanced mind, and was looked upon by those who knew him as a shrewd, smart businessman, very energetic and persistent in executing all his plans of operation. In this regard his mind was radically changed so decidedly that his friends and acquaintances said he was "no longer Gage." (Harlow, 1868, cited in Macmillan, 1996, p. 247)

Gage certainly suffered extensive damage to his left frontal lobe and probably also suffered damage to his right frontal lobe. Damasio and colleagues (Damasio, Grabowski, Frank, Galaburda, & Damasio, 1994) have attempted to reconstruct the trajectory and site of damage based on three-dimensional computer modeling of the brain and skull. Their best estimate is that the tamping rod impacted "the anterior half of the orbital frontal cortex . . . the polar and anterior mesial frontal cortices . . . and the anterior-most sector of the anterior cingulate gyrus" (p. 1104). Some right hemisphere damage was also implicated. It is interesting that Harlow implied Gage could no longer "execute" his plans. Many behaviors Gage exhibited are characteristic of people who have problems of executive functioning. Although his basic abilities to process information were intact, he showed low frustration tolerance and impulse control and a loss of ability to structure and follow through on plans—so much so, in fact, that he was seen as a changed person.

Source: The historical references for this case were summarized from Macmillan, M. (1996). Phineas Gage: A case for all reasons. In C. Code, C. Wallesch, Y. Joanette, & A. R. Lecours (Eds.), *Classic cases in neuropsychology* (pp. 243–262). Sussex, United Kingdom: Psychology Press, by permission.

There is often a disregard for rules of social decorum and restraint; an excessive involvement in pleasure seeking; a minimal tolerance for frustration; a lack of sensitivity to future outcomes, both positive and negative (Bechara, Tranel, & Damasio, 2000); and a diminished or lost capacity to empathize with others (Chow & Cummings, 1999; Lichter & Cummings, 2001). Consequently, patients with orbitofrontal damage are prone to make poor, and sometimes disastrous, life decisions (poorly conceived business ventures). Moreover, antisocial actions may result and lead to criminal or legal difficulties (Zald & Kim,

2001). As in the tragic case of Phineas Gage (Neuropsychology in Action 9.3), family members and friends often report that the "personality" of the patient, subsequent to orbitofrontal damage, has undergone significant change.

As you read the description of behaviors associated with orbital frontal damage, you might have noted the similarity between many of the behaviors associated with orbitofrontal damage and those exhibited by individuals with the diagnosis of "psychopath or sociopath" (currently, the diagnoses of psychopath and sociopath have been replaced by the diagnosis of antisocial personality disorder (*Diagnostic and Statistical Manual of Mental Disorders,* Fourth Edition [DSM IV], 1994). In fact, the similarity between the two conditions prompted the labeling of the orbitofrontal behavioral syndrome as **"pseudopsychopathic"** or **"acquired sociopathy"** (Blumer & Benson, 1975; Damasio, Tranel, & Damasio, 1990). Unlike the true psychopath or sociopath, the patient with orbitofrontal damage experiences remorse for inappropriate actions (Knight & Stuss, 2002) and does not demonstrate the intentional viciousness or planning with regard to committing antisocial acts (Zald & Kim, 2001).

With large lesions, particularly bilateral to the orbitofrontal region, stimulus-bound behaviors or **environmental dependency syndrome** may be evident. Stimulus-bound behaviors or environmental dependency syndrome subsume a group of actions (utilization behavior, imitation behavior, grasp reflex, and manual groping; Archibald, Mateer, & Kerns, 2001) that are emitted without voluntary intent as the result of the loss of frontally mediated inhibitory control. This loss of inhibitory control enables external stimuli to directly trigger thoughts and actions. For example, **utilization behavior** relates to use of a presented object without intent or regard for the context. Thus, if pajamas are presented to a patient with orbitofrontal damage, she or he may undress and slip into the garment, although the act is not "willed" or appropriate to the setting (for example, disrobing in the presence of others).

Several theoretical explanations have been posed to account for the social deficits associated with orbitofrontal damage. First, the orbitofrontal circuit is intimately involved in the support of the capacity to empathize with others. The diminishment or loss of the capacity for empathy appears to preclude an emotional appreciation of others, an essential prerequisite of social sensitivity and reciprocal interactions. Second, Damasio and colleagues (Damasio, 1994, 1998; Bechara, Tranel, & Damasio, 2000, 2002) hypothesize that the orbitofrontal cortex (ventromedial) participates in the attachment of autonomic "tags" to events that, in turn, bias response selection. These autonomic tags are termed *somatic markers* and represent "gut" reactions that covertly or overtly influence behavior. Specifically, somatic markers are visceral-autonomic signals as to the valence (desirability or undesirability) of choices or decisions learned through previous experiences with similar or related events. They assist in decision making by rapidly tagging those options that have been associated with positive outcomes, and they eliminate those alternatives that are likely to be associated with negative outcomes. They are particularly influential

when a presenting issue is novel or when uncertainty exists as to the immediate or long-term consequences of available decision or judgment options. In real-life situations, we frequently encounter decision-making demands in which the presenting situation is unfamiliar and/or uncertainty exists regarding which responses will or will not bring about desired consequences. In such situations, we rely on a conflation of past knowledge, cognitive abilities, and intuition (hunch, "a sense," or "best guess"). The latter reflects a conscious awareness of somatic biasing, although such effects need not be conscious. Support for the somatic marker hypothesis is evident in studies (Bechara, Tranel, Damasio, & Damasio, 1996; Bechara et al., 2000) showing that patients with bilateral orbitofrontal damage (ventromedial) do not generate an SCR (indexing autonomic activity) when viewing emotionally arousing stimuli (pictures). Similarly, these patients are able to recall these emotionally arousing images, but do so without the concomitant autonomic response. The latter suggests a disruption of the coupling of memory content and somatosensory states. These patients are not emotionless and are capable of evoking simple somatic states in response to emotional stimuli. However, their ability to generate and couple complex somatic states to events necessary for the guidance and constraint of decision making and judgment is impaired.

Third, Rolls's (1998, 2002) research with nonhuman primates and humans suggests that the orbitofrontal cortex is specialized for rapidly altering behavior in response to changing reinforcement contingencies (reward, nonreward, and punishment). The alteration of behavior in response to changing reinforcing consequences is not restricted to motor actions, but also pertains to emotional and social behavior. The orbitofrontal cortex is uniquely suited for its involvement in emotional-social processing because of its significant anatomic connections (direct and indirect) with the primary and association sensory cortices and limbic regions. Thus, the orbitofrontal cortex plays a crucial role in rapidly learning, modifying, and relearning behavioral responses to changing contextual signals, particularly those of a social nature. Rolls (2002) views emotions as a form of response elicited by reinforcing contingencies. In social situations, reinforcing contingencies are continually being exchanged and updated based on the presentation of interpersonal stimuli and the association of these stimuli with reward and punishment. As a function of this exchange, preexisting responses are maintained, altered, or extinguished, and new responses are learned. With orbitofrontal damage, the capacity to rapidly alter and learn emotional and related responses in the face of changing contingencies is impaired. Consequently, emotional and social behaviors lack contextual regulation as evidenced by in impulsive, rigid, or inappropriate responses.

Interestingly, individuals with orbitofrontal (ventromedial) lesions can demonstrate a relatively unimpaired neuropsychological profile when administered traditional measures of executive functioning, perception, intelligence, memory, and language. Paradoxically, their social, vocational, and economic lives are often in shambles. The case of EVR (Barrash, Tranel, & Anderson, 2000) portrays the consequences of such damage.

At age 35, EVR underwent resection of a bilateral orbitofrontal meningioma. To achieve complete removal, orbital and lower mesial frontal cortices were excised along with the tumor. Profound personality changes ensued. Although his marriage had previously been stable, he divorced his wife of many years and quickly entered into a second, short-lived marriage. Whereas formerly he had had a keen business sense with considerable financial success, postsurgically he entered into a series of disastrous business ventures over a brief period of time. He had been a respected community leader, but since the tumor resection he has never been able to maintain employment and now lives in a sheltered environment. Despite generally superior intellect, memory, and social knowledge by formal neuropsychological assessment, in real life he manifests severe defects in decision making, ability to judge the character of others, and in his abilities to plan activities on a daily basis and into the future. (p. 356)

The finding that traditional executive measures fail to identify the deficits of patients such as EVR has prompted the development of measures that are potentially more sensitive to dysfunctions associated with orbital damage. Illustrating this advancement is the "gambling task" that Bechara and colleagues (2002) developed. The measure provides a facsimile of decision-making in real life with regard to the weighting of potential rewards and punishments and the uncertainty of outcomes. The gambling task consists of four decks of cards (A, B, C, and D). The patient can select from any deck, and with each selection receives a reward (accrual of money) or penalty (loss of money). Two of the decks are "disadvantageous" because they provide large rewards, but periodically assign unpredictably large penalties. Continued selection from the disadvantageous decks culminates in a net loss. The two advantageous decks provide smaller rewards and penalties and, if repeatedly selected, result in a net gain. Healthy subjects, over time, show a response pattern beginning with a random selection from the four decks to a preference for the two advantageous decks. In contrast, the patients with ventromedial lesions did not develop this preference pattern and, in fact, were more likely to choose the high-risk decks. Moreover, the SCRs of the healthy and ventromedial subjects were monitored during the performance of the gambling task. Initially, the healthy subjects generated SCRs as they won or lost money. Subsequently, as they gained experience with the decks, they began to generate SCRs *before* the selection of any of the cards. These SCRs were more pronounced before picking a card from a disadvantageous relative to an advantageous deck. In contrast, the patients with ventromedial damage did not generate SCRs before selecting cards and continued to show a preference for the disadvantageous decks. These findings suggest that decision making is guided by somatic signals that are generated in anticipation of future consequences. With damage, insensitivity to the future consequences of behavior often results (Wagar & Thagard, 2004).

Anterior Cingulate Circuit

The anterior cingulate is a relatively large neural substrate with widely distributed interconnections to other cortical and subcortical regions, implicating its functional involvement in neural circuits that support behavior. Not surprisingly, it is implicated in both cognitive and affective/motivational processing (Devinsky, Morrell, & Vogt, 1995). The anterior cingulated is believed to support a number of overlapping functions, including response monitoring, error detection, conflict resolution (incompatible competing responses), inhibition when prepotent (primed) responses are to be overcome, selective and divided attention, and motivation or drive behavior. Debate continues over whether the major role of the anterior cingulate relates to the monitoring or regulation of neural processing. Neuroimaging and event-related potential studies (Barch, Braver, Sabb, & Noll, 2000; Van Veen & Carter, 2002) show involvement of the anterior cingulate when (1) competing responses vie for release; (2) an error occurs in performance; or (3) a presented task is difficult, novel, complex or ambiguous. Moreover, its activation often precedes or co-occurs with the activation of other neural substrates. This latter activation pattern suggests that the anterior cingulate may monitor and coordinate the engagement or amplification of control by other neural systems. The purpose of this engagement or amplification of control is to ensure efficient or optimal goal-directed performance (MacDonald, Cohen, Stenger, & Carter, 2000; Miller & Cohen, 2001).

The proximity and interconnectivity of the anterior cingulate and orbitofrontal regions suggests that they may interact in support of executive functioning. Ullsperger and von Cramon (2004) pose that both are implicated in monitoring and decision-making behavior. The two regions appear to play complementary roles, with the rostral anterior cingulate implicated in monitoring self-generated actions and in signaling the need to quickly alter neural processes to ensure optimal goal-directed motor performance, whereas the orbitofrontal cortex monitors the outcome of goal-directed actions by external consequences. The external consequence of action is, in turn, used to guide future decision making. Thus, the anterior cingulate appears to be involved in the monitoring and alteration of ongoing actions, and the orbitofrontal cortex monitors the external consequences of these actions to guide future actions.

Although the role of the anterior cingulate in response inhibition is often stressed, it appears also to play an important part in the initiation of behavior. For example, when confronted with conflicting response options, the anterior cingulate participates in both the suppression of inappropriate responses and the initiation of appropriate ones (Cabeza & Nyberg, 2000). Its role in initiating behavior is further indexed by its activation when an individual is confronted with tasks that require semantic generation, episodic memory retrieval, and working memory. In addition, evidence exists that the anterior cingulate may be selectively activated when an individual's movements are "willed" (volitional), as contrasted with actions that are determined by external stimuli. The effects of bilateral anterior cingulate damage dramatically illustrate the role of the anterior cingulate in behavioral initiation. With bilateral anterior lesions, the patient may experience "akinetic mutism" or "abulia." **Akinetic mutism** refers to a syndrome involving profound apathy, reduced or absent verbal or motor behavior, a sense of psychological "emptiness," reduced response to novelty, and indifference to pain, hunger, or thirst. **Abulia** refers to a similar, although less severe syndrome of apathy, indifference, and minimally spontaneous verbal and motor activity (Lichter & Cummings, 2001). Damage to the orbital frontal cortex has also been associated with akinetic mutism; however, research (Bechara, Tranel, & Damasio, 2002) suggests that the damage has to extend into regions of the anterior cingulate and/or basal forebrain for the syndrome to be evident. Duffy and Campbell (2001) describe the following case of akinetic mutism:

One patient, after a gunshot wound to both frontal lobes, was essentially inert when left alone. When questioned, he related an awareness of personality change. He denied boredom and described it as a "loss of motivation" in that he entertained numerous ideas for activities but felt no impetus to act on them. His facial expression was one of casual indifference, and he would often respond with simple gestures instead of speaking. (p. 118)

Clearly, this patient portrays the amotivational state that characterizes akinetic mutism.

Relation of Memory, Attention, and Executive Function

Memory, attention, and executive function represent relatively distinct processes, although in some cases, there is disagreement whether a particular attentional or memory process is better classified as an executive function (for example, working memory). Clearly, these processes are inter-related, but specifying the exact nature of this inter-relation is hindered by our limited understanding of these domains, divergent definitions and conceptualizations, and varied theoretical perspectives. When experts from the fields of memory, attention, and executive function were asked to specify the behaviors denoted by the term *executive function,* no less than 33 different terms were generated with only 40% agreement for 6 of the terms (self-regulation, sequencing of behavior, flexibility, response inhibition, planning and organization; Eslinger, 1996). Nonetheless, there is some agreement that executive functions represent overarching controlling, organizing, integrating, and supervising computations. Attention and memory processes are subject to varying degrees of executive orchestration depending on the nature and type of attention and memory processes involved. From a neuroanatomic perspective, memory, attention, and executive functions are served by relatively distinct, yet interconnected and overlapping, neural systems. Neuroimaging investigations demonstrate that different neural systems support executive, attention, and memory functions; yet, these neural systems coactivate in the performance of many executive, attentional, and memory tasks, indicating shared or distributed processing. Furthermore, the inter-relation of these functions is evident when one realizes that executive functions would be of little value if memory systems did not operate to register, store, and enable the retrieval of life experiences and knowledge, and if attentional systems did not support the processing of relevant or critical environmental and body events. Jointly, attention, memory and executive functions play a central role in thinking, reasoning, problem solving, language, and emotional and social behavior. Finally, human experience involves the capacity to represent and relate past, present, and future events. Attentional systems are necessary for the processing of relevant ongoing and novel events, memory systems for the symbolic maintenance of these experiences over time, and executive functions for the generation, guidance, and evaluation of behavior necessary to attain future goals (Eslinger, 1996).

As you reviewed the effects of damage to the attentional, memory, and executive systems, you likely realized that there is typically either a direct or indirect disruption of emotional functioning. A review of Phineas Gage's case (see Neuropsychology in Action 9.3) clearly portrays the profound disruption to emotional regulation, arousal, and style that damage to the brain can engender. It is emotion that gives direction, drive, and value to our personal and social behavior. Emotions intimately affect that which we attend to, remember, and strive to achieve (goals). It is to this fundamental aspect of human behavior that we now turn.

Neuropsychology of Emotional Processing

Brain processing of emotion is an area that neuropsychology has largely ignored until recently. This neglect is partly a holdover from philosophical traditions of rational empiricism and from conceptualizations of the body and brain as being machine-like. People saw emotions as peripheral to understanding cognition, as being of a lower order of evolutionary development, perhaps even vestigial. In other words, humans had evolved to become rational, logical beings somehow above emotion. Moreover, it is difficult to study subjective feeling states. Such research is not straightforward, as is presenting a visual or auditory stimulus and recording activation of corresponding brain regions. Also, animal models can provide only limited information, because they cannot verbalize their feelings, and researchers must rely on motor behaviors to infer the expression of emotions as rage and fear. The emotional repertoire of humans is enormous, subtle, and much more complicated than a response to external threats to physical safety, such as embodied in the fight-or-flight response.

Today, science views emotions as necessary for higher evolutionary adaptation. In the television show *Star Trek* (and its spinoffs), the ultralogical characters Mr. Spock, Data, and Seven of Nine show that being human entails having "emotional equipment." People who are out of touch with emotions and who have autistic-like qualities—like Temple Grandin, who describes herself as an "anthropologist on Mars" in Oliver Sacks' book of the same name (1995)—have expressed a sense of alienation from other humans on these grounds. Humans live in a social context where self-understanding and social skills are some of the most crucial factors in determining success in society. Witness the surging interest in "emotional intelligence," which stresses the ability to understand mood and emotion in self and others, to understand self and one's own character, and then to act effectively on that knowledge. Researchers suggest that emotional intelligence accounts for just as much or more variance in determining success in life as traditionally measured general cognitive intelligence.

One of the more interesting questions related to understanding emotions is to ask whether emotional processing is a type of cognitive processing that the cortex initiates, or whether emotion emerges without conscious thinking, and only secondarily becomes labeled. This dichotomy is a variation on an old debate emanating from the early twentieth century. The **James–Lange theory** of emotion, promoted by American psychologist William James and Danish psychologist Carl Lange (Lange, 1922), postulates that people consciously experience emotion as a reaction to physical sensory experience. That is, we feel fear because our hearts are racing; we are sad because we are crying. Although others saw this as an overstatement, the James–Lange theory does insist that sensory and cognitive experiences were intimately entwined and inseparable from each other. In other words, if all the physical sensations of fear disappeared, so would the cognitive experience of fear. The opposing theory of the time was the **Cannon–Bard theory** (Cannon, 1927). Walter Cannon, and later Philip Bard, argued that the conscious emotional experience is separate from bodily sensation or expression. Although today most scientists agree that cognitive experience of emotion corresponds to sensory experience, much variation exists among types of emotion, emotional intensity, and individual variation.

Joseph LeDoux (1992, 1996) describes emotion as a subjective state of awareness and suggests that only because people have a cortex can they label emotion and think about it, rather than just react to it as other animals might. Someone walking along in a forest might be startled by something that looks like a snake. It is adaptive if the mind signals the body in an immediate response of danger. Some scientists suggest that certain emotional responses, such as reactions to certain movements and noise, may be genetically "hardwired" as a protective mechanism. According to LeDoux (1996), after that initial lower order automatic processing, the cortex receives and further processes the information, perceiving the object as a snake or a stick, weighing options, and directing the body to take further action. The competing view argues that the person must first recognize something cognitively as a threat for the emotion to develop. LeDoux and others have amassed convincing research suggesting that basic fear conditioning can occur without a cortex. Some animals with their cortex removed still show basic fear responses. In this scenario, thought does not necessarily precede emotion. However, in addition to subcortically initiated emotion, is it also possible to initiate an emotional response just by thinking? Certainly the experience of most people would confirm this. Considering an upcoming speech, thinking about running into a snake, feeling socially embarrassed, or anticipating a joyful reunion can all produce emotional responses in the body separate from immediate external threats or joys. This section examines both subcortical and cortical contributions to emotional behavior.

BRAIN ORGANIZATION OF EMOTION

Emotions involve complex physiological, cognitive, and motor (action) processes that are supported by multiple cortical-subcortical architectures and circuitries. Different and overlapping interconnected regions are involved in processing varied emotions, a clear indication that there is not a single "emotional system." Yet, these subsystems are collectively referred to as the "limbic system" of the brain. The Papez's circuit (see Figure 9.5) was initially proposed as the supporting system of emotional processing. Subsequently, MacLean (1949, 1952) extended the system to include the amygdala, orbital prefrontal cortex, and regions of the striatum. Advances in neuroscience do not fully support these earlier conceptualizations of the limbic system because we now realize that the hippocampus is more intimately involved in nonemotional memory processing, whereas the amygdala and related structures play a greater role in emotional processing. The two regions work in a complementary manner depending on the event being processed. For example, patients with damage to the amygdala without co-occurring hippocampal damage do not demonstrate a learned fear response to a conditioned stimulus. However, the patients are able to recall that the conditioned stimulus was associated with an unconditioned stimulus during training. In contrast, patients with the opposite lesion profile (damaged hippocampus + preserved amygdala) exhibit a fear response to the conditioned stimulus without memory of the conditioned and unconditioned pairing (Armony & LeDoux, 2000). Thus, one region appears to underpin the learning of the declarative content (context), whereas the other supports the emotional learning associated with the event.

Investigations of the effects of emotion on memory retention provide further evidence of the complementary relation of the hippocampus and amygdala. Studies (Cahill & McGaugh, 1998; McGaugh, 2004) of animals and humans show that the degree of activation of the amygdala during encoding of emotionally arousing material (positive or negative) correlates significantly with subsequent recall of the material. That is, as amygdala/emotional arousal increases, the retention of declarative information improves. It has been hypothesized that the amygdala enhances the consolidating processes of the hippocampus, and thus strengthens the retention of the declarative learning. However, there is a limit to this enhancing effect. With excessive or chronic emotion, memory retention can actually be impaired. High levels of adrenocortical hormones released during stress may account for this impairing effect.

Primary Emotions

Primary emotions are automatic, preorganized, arise from sensory experience, and are processed through the limbic system before or parallel to being recognized consciously. Emotions such as fear, disgust, surprise, anger, and joy appear to be universal, because people express and recognize them across all cultures of the world. Damasio (1994) suggests that these emotions are innate and primarily controlled by the amygdala and anterior cingulate of the limbic system. As we have discussed, sensory information first funnels through the thalamus, is relayed to the cortex, and then travels to the subcortical limbic system. Because of this anatomy, the general consensus was that conscious perception of an emotion preceded emotional limbic response. But LeDoux, who has studied fear conditioning, has suggested that projections from the thalamus to the amygdala provide a "shortcut" allowing the amygdala to process information directly, bypassing the cortical loop. This allows for an immediate, automatic, preconscious, and unconscious emotional response.

Fear is a well-researched primary emotion. In the hope that the knowledge of fearful emotions can aid in treating secondary emotions, such as human anxiety and post-traumatic stress disorders, Joseph LeDoux, who has done extensive work in the area of fear conditioning with animals, has studied how primary fear interacts with memory. The neuroanatomy of the primary conditioned-fear response centers on the amygdala. Fearful behaviors are easily conditioned to a tone via shock, trauma, or loud noise. Researchers have long known that severing connections between the subcortical areas of the brain and the cortex does not eliminate the conditioned-fear response. Therefore, the learning and maintenance of fear conditioning must occur in the subcortical structures. Researchers then demonstrated that lesioning the amygdala in certain places did interfere with fear conditioning.

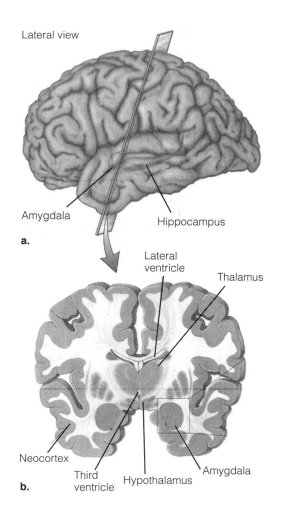

Lateral view

Amygdala

Hippocampus

a.

Lateral ventricle

Thalamus

Neocortex

Third ventricle

Hypothalamus

Amygdala

b.

Most notably, if they destroyed the central nucleus of the amygdala, animals no longer showed an autonomic fear response when presented with a tone (which previously had been associated with shock). The expected increase in heart rate, respiration, and vasodilation did not occur. LeDoux concluded that the cortex is not necessary to condition fear, but the amygdala is crucial. He then showed that the sensory information reaches the amygdala via two routes. The first or direct route (thalamo-amygdala circuit) sends sensory information to the thalamus, which, in turn, transmits it to the amygdala. The second or indirect route (thalamo-cortico-amygdala), involves the transmission of sensory information to the thalamus and then to the cortex. After cortical processing, the information is returned to the thalamus, which directs it to the amygdala. The more direct route allows for rapid, although relatively imprecise, appraisal of the threat potential of a sensory event. The indirect route is slower but provides a more detailed representation of the event (Armony & LeDoux, 2000). Once the input is processed by the amygdala, it is transmitted via the central nucleus to various brain regions that instantiate autonomic, attentional, perceptual, cognitive, and behavioral response (Figure 9.19).

As noted earlier, primary emotions are processed without conscious awareness. This does not mean that processing of the emotional stimuli is not ultimately realized at a cortical level. Rather, the emotional state can

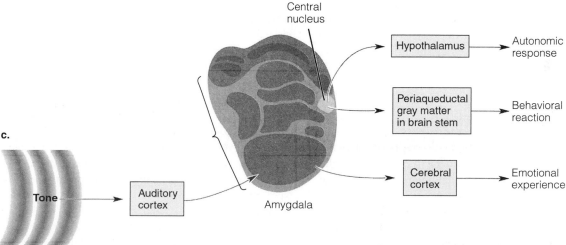

c.

Central nucleus

Hypothalamus → Autonomic response

Periaqueductal gray matter in brain stem → Behavioral reaction

Cerebral cortex → Emotional experience

Tone → Auditory cortex

Amygdala

Figure 9.19 The amygdala and fear conditioning. (a) A lateral view showing the amygdala through the temporal lobes. (b) A coronal section showing the amygdala. (c) A close-up of the nuclei of the amygdala showing the pathways of the conditioned fear response to emotional auditory stimuli. ([a, b] Reproduced from Bear, M. F., Connors, B. W., & Paradiso, M. A. [1996]. *Neuroscience: Exploring the brain* [pp. 444, Figure 16.5]. Philadelphia: Lippincott Williams & Wilkins, by permission; [c] reproduced from Bear, M. F., Connors, B. W., & Paradiso, M. A. [1996]. *Neuroscience: Exploring the brain* [pp. 445, Figure 16.6]. Philadelphia: Lippincott Williams & Wilkins, by permission.)

be triggered before there is conscious awareness. Support has been provided for the involvement of the amygdala in the unconscious mediation of learned emotional responses. For example, Morris, Ohman, & Dolan (1998) presented healthy participants with two angry faces, one face (CS+) paired with a noxious stimuli (unconditioned stimulus, white-noise burst), and the other face (CS−) displayed without aversive stimulus pairing. After the conditioning training, the faces were presented to the participants either masked or unmasked. Masking enables a stimulus to be processed, but without conscious awareness of the stimulus. The participants were instructed to press a button if they saw an angry face. None of the participants reported perceiving the masked faces, whereas all identified the unmasked faces. A measure of emotional evocation (skin conductance) revealed that the CS+ face produced a significantly greater emotional response than the CS− face for both the masked and unmasked conditions. Moreover, PET neuroimaging showed significantly greater activation of the amygdala for the presentation of the CS+ face relative to the CS− face, regardless of whether it was masked or unmasked. That is, fear learning was evident with and without conscious awareness. Interestingly, the right amygdala showed greater activation to the masked CS+ face, while the activation of the left amygdala was enhanced for the unmasked CS+ face. This finding suggests greater involvement of right hemisphere regions in unconscious emotional facial processing, whereas left hemisphere regions appear preferentially involved in conscious or cortically mediated emotional processing.

Damage to the amygdala can adversely impact on cortical processing of emotions. In essence, it leaves higher cortical processing bereft of important input. Exemplifying this negative impact is a study (Adolphs, Tranel, & Damasio, 1998) of patients with complete bilateral amygdala damage. These patients were presented facial pictures and asked to rate the degree of positive/negative emotions represented by each face and the degree of approachability and trustworthiness of the person represented by the face. When contrasted to patients without lesions of the amygdala, the patients with bilateral amygdala damage rated the faces as expressing more positive emotions and as more approachable and trustworthy. This positive bias was particularly evident for faces considered to be most negative. The investigators pose that the positive bias related to the role of the amygdala in processing threatening and aversive stimuli. The loss of this input to cortical regions resulted in a shift to more positive ratings and increased approachability/trustworthy judgments by the bilateral amygdala group.

Fear learning is not limited to subcortical amygdala action (direct sensory conditioning). For example, one can learn to fear a wild animal, such as a lion, without experiencing an attack by the animal. Support for involvement of the amygdala in fear learning without experiencing a noxious event is provided by Phelps and colleagues (2001), as well as other investigators. In Phelps' study, participants were informed that the presentation of a specific stimulus (blue square) would be associated with a shock, whereas a second stimulus (yellow square) would not. Neither stimulus was ever paired with a shock. Yet, when the shock-specific stimulus was presented, there was significant activation of the amygdala, insular cortex, anterior cingulate, premotor cortex, and striatum. A measure of fear evocation (skin conductance) confirmed a fear response with the specified stimuli. The investigators pose that the insular cortex was central to the transfer of a cortical representation to the amygdala. Thus, fear learning was produced by an imagined or anticipated cognitive representation without actual contact with a negative sensory event. Clearly, fear learning can involve both subcortical and cortical processes.

Secondary Emotions

Secondary emotions require higher cortical processing, and according to Damasio (1994), this processing is orchestrated by the prefrontal cortical networks. There is also a hemispheric asymmetry to higher emotional processing. People acquire secondary emotions through learning and experience. The perception of these states is highly personal and individual. Social emotions such as embarrassment, pride, shame, and anxiety are highly dependent on learning and interact with one's cognitive perception of the social environment as it pertains to oneself. Secondary emotions do not necessarily imply a separate "feeling" experience in the body. The feeling of emotional experience remains linked through the limbic system. The difference is that secondary emotions are generated through higher cortical processes and arrive at the limbic system over a different route from that taken by primary emotions generated through sensory experience. Once in the limbic system, the brain processes the experience of primary and secondary emotions in a similar manner.

Secondary, or social, emotions mediated by the cerebral hemispheres show lateralization of functioning. If a face is considered closely, you soon see that it is not symmetric. In 1902, before the days of computer morphing, the German scientist Hallervorden (cited in Borod, Haywood, & Koff, 1997) cut pictures of faces in half at the midline. Taking the left half, he recreated the whole face by using the original and its mirror image. He did the same with the right half. Among other descriptors, he saw right-sided faces as more "lucid," "sensible," and "active," and left-sided faces as more "perceptive" and "affective." Because the right hemisphere controls the left side of the lower face, and vice versa, lateralized facial differences in emotion basically reflect the activity of the contralateral hemisphere. The general consensus across subsequent studies confirms some of the early observations in that the left side of the face (left hemiface) is more emotionally expressive than the right hemiface. In general, the right hemisphere seems to be dominant for emotional expression (for a review of the literature, see Borod, Haywood, & Koff, 1997). The picture, however, is not completely cut and dry. Faces have an amazingly complex ability for emotional expression. The amount of space devoted to facial control on the motor homunculus attests to this. Just in variations of smiles, there may be more than 18 different types. Psychologist Paul Ekman has described the cocktail party smile, the smile of relief, and the miserable smile, to name just a few. Some theorize that each hemisphere may be specifically attuned to emotional type. Perhaps positive emotions emanate from the left hemisphere and negative emotions from the right (for review, see Borod, Haywood, & Koff, 1997). The structure–function picture for emotion is complex, but many neuroanatomic theorists continue to assert that the right hemisphere plays the major integrative role in emotional processing. People with right hemisphere damage caused by stroke are usually less accurate at producing emotions compared to those with left-sided damage or healthy control individuals (Borod, 1993).

Observations of neurologically impaired patients have provided clues to an interesting issue in emotional processing, the anatomic differences between spontaneous and posed smiles. Posed facial expression appears largely controlled by contralateral cortical structures in the motor cortex. Spontaneous smiles and laughter, however, appear to be largely a function of subcortical limbic system structures, including the cingulate gyrus, thalamus, and some structures of the basal ganglia (such as the globus pallidus). Left hemisphere stroke patients, with damage to the left motor cortex, have difficulty smiling for the camera because their facial muscles malfunction in response to the brain command to produce a willful or social smile. The smile pulls to the left. A quite different picture emerges if the person laughs spontaneously. The smile appears natural. The limbic system and other subcortical structures, including the basal ganglia, control the spontaneous smile (Figure 9.20). In any person, an observer can easily see a difference between these two types of

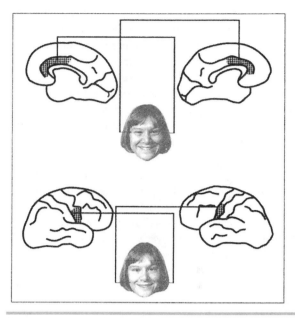

Figure 9.20 The limbic cortices control a spontaneous smile (top), whereas the motor cortex controls a posed smile (bottom). (From A. R. Damasio, *Descartes' Error,* New York: Putnam's, 1994, p. 141.)

smiles. The true smile of enjoyment activates the orbicularis oculi muscles around the eyes; a fake smile does not. Another way of describing this is that smiling eyes show an activated limbic system. People with subcortical disorders, such as Parkinson's disease, show the opposite problem of stroke patients. Although they can show willful emotion, much of their spontaneous emotion is dampened by a "masklike" face.

An area of research that has increased our understanding of cortical involvement in emotionality centers on the consequences of frontal damage. As reviewed earlier, damage to the frontal cortical system can result in a wide range of emotional and behavioral dysfunctions. Some specificity in the type of emotional dysregulation produced can be traced to whether the dorsolateral, orbital, or medial frontal region is preferentially damaged. In addition, certain regions of frontal damage leave cognitive processes relatively unimpaired, as verified by neuropsychological assessment, but result in significant social and emotional deficits. This pattern is often evident in patients who have experienced damage to the ventral and medial prefrontal cortices. Studies of the ventromedial cortex indicate that this region is implicated in emotional decision making (O'Doherty, Kringelbach, Rolls, Hornak, & Andrews, 2001), recognition of emotions as represented in voice and facial expressions (Hornak, Rolls, & Wade, 1996), and processing of fear and anger (Blair, Morris, Frith, Perrett, & Dolan, 1999; Vuilleumier, Armony, Driver, & Dolan, 2001). Anatomically, the ventromedial prefrontal cortex is interconnected with the hypothalamus, brainstem, amygdala, ventral striatum, and basal forebrain. These regions have been implicated in the mediation of attention, memory, and other cognitive functions in the processing of emotions.

Recently, an investigation (Kawasaki et al., 2005) sought to determine whether the ventromedial prefrontal cortex was involved in the processing of different categories of emotions. Electrophysiologic monitoring via implanted electrodes allows for the assessment of neuronal responsiveness. However, because of ethical constraints, this method is generally not condoned for use with healthy individuals. Therefore, the investigators identified patients with epilepsy who had electrodes implanted in the ventromedial prefrontal cortex to monitor their epilepsy. The epileptic foci of these patients did not involve the ventromedial prefrontal region. The patients were presented emotional scenes of different emotional valence and arousal. Three categories of scenes (pleasant, aversive, and neutral) of high and low levels of emotional arousal were used. More than 200 neurons in the left and right ventromedial prefrontal regions were monitored. Results of the study showed that approximately 60 neurons in the left and right ventromedial prefrontal cortices participated in encoding the emotional significance of the visual scenes. These neurons were selective for pleasant and aversive scenes, with the largest number being responsive to the aversive scenes. The investigators hypothesize that the ventromedial prefrontal cortex, in coordination with other interconnected cortical-subcortical regions, participates in associating visual stimuli with emotion and with the recognition (awareness) of this emotion.

Emotional dysfunction often appears in conjunction with neurologic disorders, sometimes as normal reaction to loss of function, and sometimes as a direct result of brain dysfunction. For example, depression is a common reaction to a life-altering injury or disease, but depression is also common in people with cortical dysfunction and some subcortical disorders such as Parkinson's disease. As discussed earlier, a frontal executive system called amotivational syndrome often appears behaviorally as indifference, apathy, or depression. On the other side of the emotional spectrum, euphoria or inappropriate labile emotional responses can occur with frontal and subcortical syndromes.

Summary

The systems presented in this chapter represent the highest level of brain integration. They depend on the input of processed sensory information and, to a large extent, manage, organize, manipulate, and store this information for further use. Many of the processes of these systems operate automatically or unconsciously without apparent verbal awareness. Subcortical brain regions control many "unconscious" processes. The more explicit and, therefore, more seemingly conscious aspects of higher order processing are represented in the cortical areas, most notably the frontal lobes. Cortical functions mediate our interactions with the external environment and support those behaviors that we consider to be "willed" or volitional.

This chapter, as well as the previous chapters, provides the foundation for the clinical issues and disorders presented later in this book. Whereas here we have considered functions and disorders by subsystem, we next examine cases of disorders that cut across functional areas.

Critical Thinking Questions

▓ Do the higher cognitive functions discussed in this chapter represent more intelligent thought processes than those functions discussed in previous chapters? Explain.

▓ The memory, attention, and executive function systems interact. How would you explain this interaction?

▓ Do disorders of executive functioning represent a greater disability for humans than sensory-perceptual and motor disorders? Why or why not?

▓ Do emotions represent a higher cognitive function or a lower basic function? Explain.

▓ Are there advantages to multiple brain memory systems as contrasted to a single memory system?

Key Terms

Anterograde amnesia
Retrograde amnesia
Short-term memory (STM)
Long-term memory (LTM)
Remote memory
Declarative memory
Nondeclarative memory
Procedural memory
Explicit memory
Implicit memory
Episodic memory

Semantic memory
Implicit priming
Working memory
Central executive
Articulatory phonologic
  loop
Visuospatial sketch pad
Episodic buffer
Focused attention
Alternating attention
Divided attention

Hemispatial neglect
Posterior attention system
Vigilance attention system
Anterior or executive attention
  system
Focus-execute attention
Shifting attention
Sustained attention
Encode attention
Stable attention
Object permanence

Executive planning
Pseudopsychopathy
Acquired psychopathy
Environmental dependency
  syndrome (stimulus-bound)
Utilization behavior
Somatic markers
Akinetic mutism
Abulia
James–Lange theory
Cannon–Bard theory

Web Connections

http://www.lycaeum.org/drugs/other/brain
Mind-Body—great source for links to topics related to theories of the mind.

http://www.nimh.nih.gov/events/prfmri2.htm
Working Memory—site provides graphics for three-dimensional MRI reconstruction of the subject's brain, including parietal and frontal areas, while holding a series of letters in working memory.

http://www.exploratorium.edu/memory/index.html
Memory Web Site—features online exhibits and articles and lectures on memory. Page also shows demonstration of memory for common objects such as a penny. The page asks the user to click on the penny that actually looks like one.

Part Three

DISORDERS OF THE BRAIN

Chapter 10

DEVELOPMENTAL DISORDERS OF CHILDHOOD

Sometimes even to live is an act of courage.
　　　　　　　　—*Seneca* (died a.d. 65), Letters to Lucilius

Vulnerability and Plasticity of the Developing Brain
Child and Adult Brain: Structural and Functional
　　Differences
Specific Developmental Disorders

Neuropsychology in Action

Overview

This chapter focuses on childhood developmental disorders that result from genetic and chromosomal alteration, and early environmental insults. Although these disorders can be traced to disruption of early brain development, the effects of the disruption persist throughout childhood, adolescence, and adulthood. We first discuss the vulnerability and plasticity of the young brain, then compare the child and the adult brain. These topics are particularly significant in evaluating and predicting the immediate and long-term effects of brain insult or injury. Next, we examine a number of developmental disorders to highlight the often disabling consequences of anomalies in brain development. The disorders reviewed include hydrocephalus (HC), Turner's syndrome (TS), Williams syndrome (WS), and fetal alcohol syndrome (FAS). We discuss these developmental disorders for prevalence and manifestations, pathogenesis and neuropsychological assessment, and current interventions to halt or ameliorate the negative effects of early neural disruption.

Vulnerability and Plasticity of the Developing Brain

The brain may fail to develop structurally and functionally as a consequence of inborn (genetic and chromosomal) anomalies and environmental insults. Brain disorders, such as **phenylketonuria (PKU),** a genetic metabolic disorder, can be inherited or result from alterations of cellular material, as evident in TS. Environmental causes relate to damaging agents (such as alcohol) that preclude, alter, or halt natural brain development. The degree to which a brain can recover from damage is complex and not fully understood. Neuroscientists do know, however, that the plasticity of the brain allows for recovery of function under certain conditions.

Teratogens are agents that, if introduced or present during certain periods of prenatal development, can produce central nervous system defects. The defects can include **agenesis,** the failure of an organ to develop, or **dysgenesis,** the abnormal development of an organ. Furthermore, the damaging effects of the teratogens can be focal or diffuse, and can result in minimal to complete loss of function. Examples of potential teratogens are general diseases (such as rubella, influenza, and mumps), sexually transmitted diseases (such as syphilis, AIDS, and genital herpes), drugs (such as alcohol, cocaine, barbiturates, and vaccines), environmental toxins (such as mercury, carbon monoxide, lead, and polychlorinated biphenyls [PCB]), and radiation (such as from x-rays and exposure to radioactive materials).

The precise impact of the teratogen on the unborn fetus varies with the nature of the insult and its proximity to a particular period of rapid brain growth, the genetic makeup of the child/mother, the quality of the intrauterine environment, and the "dosage" and extent of exposure (Spreen, Risser, & Edgell, 1995). The prenatal brain appears most vulnerable to morphologic damage during early organogenesis (weeks 2–8). Resultant malformations are often so severe that the embryo is spontaneously aborted or presents at birth with conditions incompatible with life (Anderson, Northam, Hendy, & Wrennall, 2001). Although the probability of massive malformations decreases during later periods of gestation, the brain continues

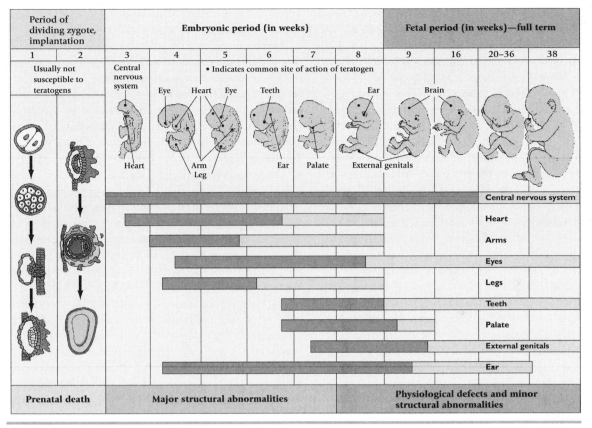

Period of dividing zygote, implantation		Embryonic period (in weeks)						Fetal period (in weeks)—full term			
1	2	3	4	5	6	7	8	9	16	20–36	38

Figure 10.1 Gestational periods that developing organs or structures are most susceptible to teratogenic effects. The dark bands indicate the most sensitive periods, whereas the light bands specify periods when each organ or structure is less sensitive to teratogens, although damage may still occur. (Reproduced from Moore, K., & Persaud, T. [1993]. *Before we are born: Essentials of embryology and birth defects* [4th ed., p. 130]. Philadelphia: WB Saunders.)

to be vulnerable to damage throughout pregnancy (Figure 10.1). For example, disruption of cell migration (16–20 weeks) is associated with **polymicrogyria,** whereas **porencephaly** relates to perturbations at a later point (5–7 months) of gestation. Damage during later gestational periods of cell proliferation and growth often results in disruption that is more limited to specific cellular layers, structures, or circuitry. However, generalized brain dysfunction may also occur depending on the nature of the insult. Cortical cellular migration, myelination, dendritic arborization, and synaptogenesis continue for significant periods after birth. Damage during these periods can also lead to differential impairment of cognitive and behavioral functions.

To exemplify the hazards of prenatal exposure to toxins, we will review one of the heavy metals that is relatively well studied, and the impairing effects of which are increasingly being identified. Inorganic lead may be one

of the most widespread neurotoxins in the world due to its presence in gasoline, paint, and industrial plants. Fortunately, there has been a significant decrease in reported lead blood levels in the United States due to the elimination of lead from gasoline and the banning of lead from interior house paints. Specifically, the average lead blood level of U.S. residents has decreased from an average of 15 μg/dL (micrograms per deciliter) to 2 μg/dL since the mid-1990s (Canfield, Gendle, & Cory-Slechta, 2004). Children continue to be exposed to lead through both older and substandard homes painted with lead-based paint, contaminated soil, and water (lead pipes) (Nigg, 2006). Currently, the major source of exposure for pregnant women is the industrial/work setting.

Of significance, cross-sectional and longitudinal studies have shown that the injurious effects of lead exposure may occur at lower levels than previously deemed safe. As a result, there has been a decrease in blood lead levels considered nonhazardous by the Centers for Disease Control and Prevention and the World Health Organization. Before 1991, the safe blood lead level threshold was ≤25 µg/dL, whereas the current standard is ≤10 µg/dL. Yet, there is growing evidence that even this blood level threshold may be too high, as evident in the finding of cognitive and behavioral impairments after blood lead levels of ≤10 µg/dL, leading some investigators (Canfield, Henderson, Cory-Slechta, Cox, Jusko, & Lanphear, 2003) to propose that an even lower standard is warranted. At higher levels, there is clearer evidence regarding the negative impact of lead exposure on intellectual functioning; however, the findings for the negative effects of lower levels of exposure on intelligence are less definitive. That is, not all studies (for review, see Kaufman, 2001) report a decrease in intellectual performance at lower levels of exposure, and many report only small reductions, and often these reductions are related more to postnatal relative to prenatal lead exposure (Koller, Brown, Spurgeon, & Levy, 2004). Notably, many of these studies fail to control for potential confounding factors (namely, mother's intelligence quotient [IQ], education level, socioeconomic level, prenatal care, and use of other substances) that could account for lower IQ scores.

Recent longitudinal and cross-sectional studies of children exposed to prenatal lead that have controlled for potentially confounding variables report a reduction in intellectual performance. For example, Schnass and colleagues (2006) observed children with prenatal lead exposure (pregnant mothers' average blood lead levels were 8 µg/dL) through their first 10 years of life. The average lead blood level for the children during their 1st to 5th years of life was 9.8 µg/dL, and the level was 6.2 µg/dL when the children were 6 to 10 years of age. The investigators determined that lead exposure at approximately 28 weeks gestation was negatively related to intellectual performance. That is, the higher the maternal blood lead level, the lower the child's assessed postnatal intelligence. A dose–response analysis indicated that the most significant impact on intelligence occurred within the first few micrograms of blood lead levels. The investigators concluded that prenatal lead exposure has a lasting and negative impact on intellectual development.

Similarly, in an earlier well-controlled study (Ris, Dietrich, Succop, Berger, & Bornschein, 2004) of children exposed to prenatal lead, the effects on specific cognitive and motor skills were examined. Neurocognitive assessments during childhood showed that the children demonstrated deficits in attentional control, fine-motor speed and dexterity, and visuoconstructive abilities. More alarming was the finding that the children's deficits in attentional control and visuoconstructive skills continued to be evident when they were assessed as adolescents.

Empirical studies with animals suggest that lead exposure disrupts the mesocorticolimbic dopamine and glutamate neurotransmitter brain receptors, particularly those receptors in the nucleus accumbens of the basal ganglia. Other structures that have been implicated are the frontal cortex, hippocampus, amygdala, and cerebellum (Ris et al., 2004). However, the precise disruption of brain structure and function remains to be clarified.

Dangers to the developing brain are not limited to prenatal teratogens. Potential dangers also threaten the perinatal process of birth, including anoxia, medications introduced during labor and delivery, and mechanical injury to the skull and brain caused by trauma during delivery. Intracranial hemorrhage and tissue damage are recognized results of mechanical injury associated with the birthing process (Spreen, Risser, & Edgell, 1995). Babies of low birth weight are at particular risk for central nervous system damage. Furthermore, a wide range of potential dangers threaten postnatal development. Traumatic head injury, toxins, radiation, malnutrition, tumors, infections, and stroke all can cause significant injury to the developing brain. Yet, there is resilience to the damaged brain related, in part, to protective factors such as a responsive, nurturing, and stimulating postnatal environment.

The term *plasticity* refers to the enduring changes in neural activity that accompany learning, or the recovery of behavioral functioning after brain injury or disease (Frackowiak, 1996). Neuroscientists hypothesize that the brain's plasticity is greatest during developmental periods when synaptic density is highest; that is, when excessive numbers of synapses exist, many of which have not committed to function. These periods of maximum synaptic density differ across cortical regions due to differential rates of neuromaturation. For example, the window of plasticity for the visual cortex is smaller than for the prefrontal cortex. In the former case, synaptic density extends until 5 years of age, whereas in the latter case, maximum density extends into late childhood (Huttenlocher, 1999; Huttenlocher & Dabholkar, 1997).

Initially, neuroscientists believed that the likelihood of recovery from a brain insult was greater if the injury occurred earlier rather than later in development. They later named this principle the **Kennard principle** in honor of its originator, Margaret Kennard (Kolb, Gibb, & Gorny, 2000). The Kennard principle suggests that the immature brain is more plastic than the mature brain. Some forms of insult do appear to follow this principle; for example, children with early focal brain injury often demonstrate milder and less extensive cognitive and emotional impairments than adults with comparable lesions (Anderson, Northam, Hendy, Wrennall, 2001). However, the opposite effect is also evident. That is, earlier brain lesions, particularly if generalized, can have a pervasive impact on developing functions. In some cases, the early injury may initially appear to have minimal effect if the cognitive or behavioral functions that the damaged region subserves do not emerge until a later point in development. As this development point is reached, significant functional impairments emerge. For example, the effects of early damage to the auditory cortex may not be fully evident until language skills fail to develop.

Some authors have proposed (Anderson, Northam, Hendy, Wrennall, 2001; Kolb, 1995) that the effect a lesion has on the developing brain varies with the age at insult. Lesions occurring before age 1, including prenatal development, typically correlate with more global and lasting impairment than later injuries. Some degree of neural reorganization and sparing of function is possible with lesions occurring between 1 and 5 years of age, depending on the nature, severity, and region of damage. During this period, most cortical regions reach maximum synaptic-dendritic density. Finally, injuries after age 5 generally predict minimal recovery of function. Thus, there appears to be a "window" for optimum recovery extending from the toddler through the preschool years. However, not all studies support this set of generalities. For example, Bates (1999), in a review of studies, concluded that worse outcomes were associated with damage occurring between 5 and 12 years of age as contrasted with injury during the prenatal period and subsequent early childhood years. Clearly, a simple linear association between age of damage and cognitive and behavioral outcomes does not exist.

Child and Adult Brain: Structural and Functional Differences

Neuroscientists are learning more and more about the maturation of the central nervous system. An important realization is that the child's brain differs in many significant ways from the adult brain. This section discusses several of these differences to clarify this basic, though often forgotten, principle of the relation between brain and behavior.

The brain of the adult is anatomically, physiologically, and functionally mature, whereas that of the child is still developing. Accordingly, the effects of lesions to the immature and mature brain differ significantly. In the

former case, injuries disrupt the acquisition of developmental abilities; in the latter case, previously acquired abilities break down (Eslinger, Biddle, & Grattan, 1997). With the achievement of brain maturity, greater stability and predictability of behavior is evident. In comparison, the cognitive and behavioral functions of the developing brain can vary dramatically. This variability depends on the current developmental stage and on the nature and quality of the child's social-psychological-physical environment.

With lesions of the mature brain, assessing the degree of functional loss and potential for recovery often involves examining the adult's premorbid history. Young children have an obviously abbreviated history from which to draw variables necessary for prediction. Likewise, the young child has not developed a host of higher order functions such as reading and writing, thus severely hindering efforts to determine which functions are spared or compromised, both in the present and in the future.

Many pathologic signs of adult brain injury are developmentally appropriate if the developing child exhibits them (Bernstein & Waber, 1997). For example, the primitive neural reflexes of the infant are obviously normal, but in adulthood, they are signs of frontal lobe or related neural damage. Likewise, early childhood damage to one cortical region may impact the development of other brain regions—a phenomenon not consistently observed with adult injury. For example, Eslinger and coworkers (1997) report that childhood lesions to the left prefrontal cortex can disrupt development of the right prefrontal regions, an effect these researchers did not observe with comparable damage to the mature brain.

One of the most striking examples of how the child's brain contrasts with that of the adult's is the differing response to lesions in the language areas of the left hemisphere. Young children who experience such injury rarely show aphasia. Moreover, most children with early left hemisphere damage acquire language abilities within the lower end of the average range (Stiles, 2000). In contrast, adults subject to similar lesions show a high prevalence of aphasic disorders and recovery is often less robust. Investigators initially attributed the difference to the brain's plasticity, and they posed that language transferred to the opposite hemisphere. However, the transfer of language to the right hemisphere is at a cost due to the finding that many of the affected children show visuospatial deficits and significant declines in intellectual performance. Researchers attributed the functional loss to a "crowding" effect. That is, language "crowds" into right hemisphere at the expense of other cognitive functions.

The posing of a transfer and crowding effect to account for the differences in language functioning of childhood versus adulthood damage is being challenged. Emerging research suggests that the relationship between early hemispheric damage and language performance differs for young children as compared to adults with similar injury. In a series of studies (Bates & Roe, 2001; Stiles, 2000; Stiles, Bates, Thal, Trauner, & Reilly, 1998), the language development of children with either early left or right unilateral damage was examined. During the initial assessment, when the children were between 10 and 17 months of age, the majority of children were delayed in early language acquisition. Noteworthy was the finding that receptive language deficits were more common in the children with *right* hemisphere rather than with left hemisphere injury. Furthermore, children with damage specific to the left temporal injury were delayed in word production, but they performed within the normal range on measures of comprehension and gestures. This profile is the opposite of adults with left posterior injury, in whom language production is spared whereas comprehension is impaired. In contrast, children with right hemisphere damage demonstrated visuoconstructive and emotional comprehension and expression deficits similar to those demonstrated by adults with comparable damage. These findings suggest that language acquisition is supported by widely distributed brain regions of both hemispheres, and thus allows for the development of alternative pathways for neural mediation of language. In contrast, there is greater neural specificity to the regions supporting spatial and affective processes. Accordingly, the visual constructive and emotional deficits associated with injury during early childhood are more likely to be similar to those demonstrated by adults (Stiles, 2000). With age and commitment of brain regions and circuitry to language and other abilities, the brain is less able to reorganize and redistribute functions to accommodate to injury. However, brain plasticity is evident in adulthood, although greatly constrained.

The impact of adult injury is generally apparent soon after the lesion occurs, whereas the effects of injury to the immature brain are less straightforward. Studies of primates suggest that early lesions to the prefrontal and temporal cortexes can produce both immediate and delayed presentation of impairments. Goldman-Rakic (1987a,b) conducted a series of studies to investigate the effects of damage to the prefrontal cortex. Lesions in the prefrontal dorsolateral region of the brain of mature monkeys impaired performance on a delayed response task (see Figure 9.9), whereas infant monkeys with comparable lesions did not show immediate impairment. However, as the infant monkeys matured, a significant deficit emerged in delayed response performance. In contrast, lesions of the prefrontal orbital cortex produced delayed response deficits

regardless of age at injury. Thus, age and region of prefrontal cortex damage interacted to determine immediate or delayed impairment.

Similarly, case studies of children (Eslinger et al., 1997; Tranel & Eslinger, 2000) with early prefrontal damage suggest that immediate and delayed impairments of cognitive and socioemotional executive functions can result. The emerging deficits in adolescence and early adulthood appear most prominent in the development and regulation of socioemotional behaviors such as social awareness, interpersonal sensitivity, perspective taking, friendship skills, and close emotional relationships. These emerging deficits appear more disruptive to adjustment than similar deficits that occur in adulthood. The relation of immediate and late-appearing deficits of age, affected hemisphere, specific cortical region of damage, and other mediating variables remains unclear and warrant further study.

Our discussion of the vulnerability and plasticity of the brain, as well as its difference from the adult brain, serves as a basic framework for understanding the neuropsychological assessment of childhood disorders. William Culbertson presents a case study of the effects of an early frontal tumor and its subsequent cognitive impact (Neuropsychology in Action 10.1).

Specific Developmental Disorders

This section reviews several groups of neurodevelopmental disorders that neuropsychologists frequently treat. These include abnormalities of anatomic development, genetic and chromosomal disorders, and acquired cerebral insults and diseases. We discuss a sample disorder from each of these groups to acquaint the student with the clinical presentation, neuropsychological pathogenesis, and treatment of the disorder. The first disorder, HC, frequently co-occurs with many other disorders of anatomic malformation. Next, TS is one of the most commonly seen chromosomal disorders. We follow with a discussion of WS, a unique genetic disorder that continues to spawn research because of its neurocognitive profile. Finally, FAS is a relatively common and destructive disorder. Of the four disorders developmental disorders, FAS is completely preventable.

ABNORMALITIES OF ANATOMIC DEVELOPMENT

Many conditions exist that reflect anomalies of neurodevelopment. Hynd, Morgan, and Vaughn (1997) divide these disorders into five groups (Table 10.1). Each category reflects a malformation of brain tissue with concurrent disruption

Case Presentation

S.B. is an 8-year-old girl who was referred for neuropsychological evaluation after neurosurgical removal of a right frontal tumor. The evaluation was sought to determine her current levels of cognitive functioning, establish a baseline for monitoring her recovery, and provide appropriate educational and management recommendations. The referral for evaluation was made 2 months after surgery.

During second grade, S.B. began to complain of headaches. These headaches became increasingly frequent and intense. Initial medical consultations did not identify the basis for her headaches. Subsequently, her academic skill levels began to decline. Her headaches failed to abate and were accompanied by vomiting. She experienced at least one night seizure. She was referred for neuroimaging (magnetic resonance imaging and computed axial tomography). The neuroimaging studies showed a massive ($7 \times 5 \times 6$ cm) nonfiltrating right frontal lobe tumor. Subsequently, S.B. underwent neurosurgery for the excision of the tumor. Her postsurgical recovery was uneventful, and neither adjunctive radiation nor chemotherapy was recommended.

Since the surgery, S.B. has continued to experience headaches, although these are less frequent and intense than in the past. She fatigues quickly, appears to sleep more, and seems to struggle with sustaining attention to tasks. Her parents have witnessed no major sensory, motor, or cognitive alterations since her release from the hospital. Similarly, no major changes or alterations in personality or social interactions have been observed. She continues to be viewed by her parents as an active, energetic, and socially adept child.

Before the tumor, S.B.'s developmental and medical history was unremarkable. She was an average student who was well liked by her teachers and peers. At the time of the evaluation, S.B. had returned to school on a reduced day schedule and was making steady but slow academic progress. Her teacher reported inattentiveness, impulsivity, disorganization, and high levels of minor motor activity as areas of concern.

Behavior Observed During Assessment

S.B. is a dark-haired, well-developed child who was appropriately attired in contemporary garb for the assessment. Her surgical scar was clearly evident in the anterior region of her skull. She did not appear to be concerned by the visibility of the scar to others. She related in a friendly, talkative, and spontaneous manner. Her verbal responses tended to be overly detailed, poorly organized, and often tangential in nature. However, her thinking was reality oriented, and emotional responses were appropriate to the evaluative context. She was prone to fatigue quickly and to report that she was developing (or had developed) a headache. Accordingly, a number of relatively short sessions were required to complete the assessment.

S.B. was motorically active across assessment sessions. This activity included fidgety and restless behaviors and actions such as fiddling with her hair, the zipper on her jacket, objects on the desk, and a piece of thread pulled from her shirt. It was not uncommon for her to sing or hum as she worked on tasks. She was quick to reach out and manipulate test materials as they were placed in front of her. Similarly, she would often try to initiate her performance of the assessment tasks before the examiner could complete the directions for the tasks.

When presented with new or difficult tasks, S.B. was prone to state, "I won't be able to do this," or to seek assistance. Her sense of self-efficacy appeared limited, as evident in frequent requests for feedback on the adequacy of her performance (such as, "How many did I get right?" "Did I miss any?"). Her tolerance for frustration was limited, and support and coaxing was often necessary to maintain her comfort and performance.

S.B. did not consistently monitor the accuracy of her performance, resulting in needless errors. She encountered difficulty with drawing/copying tasks due, in part, to a quick and uncritical approach. Her pencil grasp (right hand) was unusual in that the barrel of the pencil rested on her ring finger.

Neuropsychological Assessment

S.B.'s teacher completed rating scales pertinent to her observations of S.B.'s in-class behavior. The teacher provided elevated ratings (clinical range) on subscales sensitive to deficits in working memory, planning and organization, organization of materials, and self-monitoring. The parents also completed rating scales related to their observations of S.B.'s behavior. Their ratings showed clinical elevations on subscales assessing inattention, hyperactivity, restless-impulsive behaviors, psychosomatic complaints, and poor organization of materials. Borderline clinical ratings were presented for problems with inhibition, working memory, planning and organization, and self-monitoring.

S.B.'s intelligence was determined to be within the average range, with a nonsignificant discrepancy between verbal and performance intelligence. Her verbal subtest scores fell within the average range without any significant individual strengths or weaknesses. In contrast, her performance subtest scores ranged from significantly below average to above average. Her above-average performance was evident on a subtest assessing her ability to determine the appropriate sequence of social stimuli. Below-average performance was demonstrated on subtests assessing visual attention to details and visuoconstructive abilities (block design construction and puzzle assembly). Her achievement in reading, mathematics, and

(continued)

(*continued*)

spelling was found to be consistent with her assessed level of intelligence.

S.B.'s working memory for verbal contents (mental arithmetic, repeating digits backward) was age appropriate. Similarly, when learning a list of words across repeated trials, she demonstrated an age-appropriate learning curve and unimpaired memory recall. However, the introduction of an alternative list of words for learning revealed interference from the originally encoded list (words from the first list intruding into her recall of the second list of words). Although her verbal fluency (letter and semantic) performance was within the average range, her design fluency performance fell within the impaired range.

Deficits were also evident when judging the spatial orientation of lines, imitating sequences of movement in space, drawing familiar objects (for example, bicycle), and copying developmental visuomotor forms. Furthermore, she demonstrated an impaired level of performance when rapidly shifting between numbers and letters. Her fine-motor dexterity with her dominant and nondominant hand was below age expectancy, with significant impairment evident for her nondominant left hand.

S.B.'s performance on measures of sustained attention demonstrated poor attentional and inhibitory control. Although she demonstrated age-appropriate performance on an executive task assessing abstract abilities and cognitive flexibility, she significantly faltered on a second measure assessing executive planning and problem solving.

Commentary

The impact of a major tumor on the developing brain can result in a myriad of cognitive, emotional, and social deficits/excesses. Factors mediating the effects of the tumor are the child's stage of development, nature and extent of the insult, cognitive resources (for example, intelligence), form of postsurgical treatment (radiation and/or chemotherapy), and the availability and quality of supportive services. Despite the multiplicity of outcomes, a number of sequelae are associated with right anterior damage, including poorly organized narrative discourse, inattention/distractibility, disruption of working memory, disinhibition, visual construction skill deficits, limited nonverbal fluency, and impaired monitoring. Moreover, memory disruption secondary to inattention and interference effects is frequently evi-

dent. Executive planning and problem solving can be markedly impaired. In contrast, cognitive functions associated with left frontal circuitry can be relatively well preserved. S.B.'s pattern of neuropsychological performance is consistent with compromised cognitive functions supported by right anterior brain circuitry.

S.B.'s neuropsychological strengths and weaknesses were presented to the parents. It was stressed that it was too early in her recovery to determine precisely which deficits would persist or resolve, but her progress should be monitored carefully, particularly because the impact of anterior damage is often not fully evident until adolescence. Recommendations were developed to aid school personnel in providing appropriate educational modifications and interventions. An evaluation by a physical therapist was recommended. The parents were further advised that if S.B.'s inattention, impulsivity, and minor motor activity did not improve over time, they should consult with her neurologist to determine the feasibility of introducing psychostimulant medication. Supportive group therapy/counseling with children who had undergone treatment for brain tumors was recommended.

---

of function. Several of these malformations are incompatible with life (for example, **anencephaly** and **hydranencephaly**), whereas others do not necessarily compromise the child's survival, but do significantly impair or alter neuropsychological functioning. In many cases, a given disorder may have multiple causes; in others, the pathogenesis is quite specific. However, the origin of most of the disorders is undetermined.

The extensiveness and severity of damage to the developing brain tends to reduce life expectancy of children with anatomic brain malformations. Surviving children show a high rate of mental retardation, speech and language delays, learning disabilities, motor impairments, physical anomalies, and epilepsy. Children with severe and global neuropsychological deficits often require lifelong supervision and assistance. We turn first to HC, a relatively frequent anomaly of the brain that can result in minimal to severe neuropsychological deficits.

Hydrocephalus

Clinical Presentation and Incidence—Hydrocephalus (HC) can occur during any developmental period and seriously damages the developing brain, disrupting both subcortical and cortical functions. This condition results from an excessive accumulation of cerebrospinal fluid (CSF) in the brain's ventricles (Figure 10.2). The increased volume of CSF produces a concomitant increase in intracranial pressure and expansion of the ventricles. As the ventricles expand, cerebral tissue is compromised and the cranium distorts. If untreated, the child may die or suffer severe mental retardation. The actual incidence of HC is unknown because it is frequently associated with other congenital disorders. However, it is estimated that 27 per 100,000 newborns suffer from the condition (Kolb & Whishaw, 1996). The incidence of HC of mixed causes appears to be greater for boys (62%) than girls.

Neuropathogenesis—HC is a disorder that occurs secondary to other pathologic events or processes. This pathogenesis can be of prenatal, perinatal, or postnatal origin. Congenital (prenatal) disorders such as spina bifida, Dandy–Walker malformation, Arnold–Chiari malformation, and stenosis of the aqueduct of Sylvius often result in HC (see Table 10.1). Of these congenital disorders, **spina bifida** is most frequently associated with HC (Mataró, Junqué, Poca, & Sahuquillo, 2001). The most common cause of perinatal and postnatal HC is **intraventricular hemorrhage (IVH)**, a condition that occurs in premature infants (see later). Other causes of HC, both prenatal and postnatal, include infections (meningitis and encephalitis), vascular abnormalities, tumors, cysts, traumatic brain injury, and other disease processes (Erickson, Baron, & Fantie, 2001; Fletcher et al., 1996).

Physiological Dynamics—Any one of three underlying causes can produce an abnormal increase in the volume of ventricular CSF. These causative factors include oversecretion of CSF, obstruction of CSF passages, and impaired absorption of CSF (Greenberg, Aminoff, & Simon, 2002; Fletcher et al., 1996). Oversecretion of CSF is rare and is generally a consequence of a secreting tumor of the choroid plexus, the primary producer of CSF in the lateral ventricles.

The second cause of HC occurs within the ventricular system and involves obstruction of the CSF pathways as a result of congenital malformation, tumors, or scarring. HC of this etiology is termed **obstructive** or **noncommunicating HC** (Brookshire, Fletcher, Bohan, Landry, Davidson, & Francis, 1995; Marino, Fine, & McMillan, 2004). The aqueduct of Sylvius, also called the cerebral aqueduct of the third ventricle, is the most commonly obstructed ventricular pathway, because of its long, narrow structure. Conditions obstructing the aqueduct of Sylvius include: (1) congenital narrowing (stenosis) of the aqueduct; (2) a thin membrane lying on the aqueduct; (3) constriction of the aqueduct by pressure from an adjoining tumor; and (4) herniation of the cerebellum and displacement of the fourth ventricle, as in Arnold–Chiari malformation (Hynd et al., 1997). However, the pathogenesis of obstructive or noncommunicating HC may be idiopathic (unknown), and research findings suggest that different familial forms may exist (Hynd & Willis, 1988).

The third form of HC results from disrupted reabsorption of CSF into the bloodstream caused by obstruction in the basal subarachnoid cisterns or in the arachnoid villi (Fletcher et al., 1996; Marino et al., 2004; see Figure 10.2).

When spina bifida is excluded, the most common cause of HC in early development is IVH, a condition that, until relatively recently, occurred in 40% to 50% of premature infants with birth weights less than 1800 g (Mataró et al., 2001; Willis, 1993). Recent medical advances have reduced the incidence of IVH to 20% for premature infants (Fletcher, Dennis, & Northrup, 2000). IVH is a result of breathing problems or pressure on the brain during the delivery process causing vessels in the germinal matrix (area around the ventricles) to rupture and bleed into the ventricles. Blood and cellular debris clog the arachnoid villa (which is responsible for reabsorbing CSF into the bloodstream) and CSF volume and pressure increase, although its outward flow into the spinal canal is not blocked. HC of this form is known as **nonobstructive** or **communicating HC.**

Obstructive or noncommunicating HC is a congenital disorder that develops early in gestation and is associated with an ever-expanding impact on subsequent brain development. In contrast, nonobstructive or communicating HC is primarily a consequence of perinatal and postnatal insults to a brain that heretofore had developed normally.

Impact of Hydrocephalus on the Developing Brain—If unchecked, HC has a devastating impact on the developing brain and skull (Figure 10.3). As CSF volume increases, the ventricles progressively enlarge in a posterior to anterior direction with corresponding disruption of brain anatomy and function. The ventricle lining suffers focal damage, cerebral blood vessels distort and become dysfunctional, neurons are injured, and the concentration of neurotransmitters and cerebral fluid alters (Del Bigio, 2004; Dennis & Barnes, 1994). Increasing pressure extensively damages the underlying white matter of the brain. Specifically, the corpus callosum stretches and thins (hypoplasia), midline projection fibers that connect the hemispheres to the diencephalon and caudal regions stretch and distort, the internal capsule (fanlike white fibers separating regions of the basal ganglia and dorsal thalamus) displaces, and the periventricular white matter (white matter adjacent to the lateral ventricles) is damaged (Dennis & Barnes, 1994; Ewing-Cobbs, Barnes, & Fletcher, 2003). Furthermore, the cortical mantle thins, often damaging the cerebral cortex and compromising cognitive functions. Because of the posterior-to-anterior progression of HC, the cognitive and motor functions supported by the posterior cortical regions, cerebellum, and midbrain structures with their connecting white matter tracks are most compromised

Table 10.1 *Anatomic Disorders*

Malformation	Description	Clinical Manifestations
Abnormalities of bulk growth		
Micrencephaly	Subnormal brain size associated with abnormally small head (<2 SD below mean for age and gender)	Size of face near normal; folded scalp, possible epilepsy, and most typically intellectual retardation
Megalencephaly	Abnormally large brain from overproduction of cerebral parenchyma. Males > females	Associated with mental subnormality, normality, or (hypothetically) giftedness. Epilepsy may occur.
Dysplasias of cerebral hemispheres		
Holoprosencephaly	Two hemispheres fail to develop. A large fluid-filled cavity results. No interhemispheric fissure present. 1:13,000 live births	Faciocerebral dysplasias, cebocephaly, apnea spells, severe mental retardation, hypotelorism, and other systemic deformities. Usually incompatible with life.
Agenesis of the corpus callosum	Complete or partial failure of the corpus callosum to develop. Males > females	Occasionally asymptomatic or found in association with spina bifida, facial and ocular deformities, micrencephaly, and hydrocephalus. Epilepsy and mental retardation may occur.
Malformations of the cerebral cortex		
Agyria/pachygyria	Smooth lissencephalic surface of brain. Few coarse gyri may be present	Commonly found in association with agenesis of corpus callosum, micrencephaly, epilepsy, severe mental retardation, and early death
Polymicrogyria	Development of many small gyri. Microscopically, they may form an overlapping folded cortex	Found in association with learning disabilities (dyslexia), severe mental retardation, and epilepsy. Also appear asymptomatically
Focal dysplasia	Focal abnormalities in the cortical architecture usually consisting of disordered cells and layering of cortex	Reported in cases of epilepsy and learning disabilities (dyslexia)
Malformations associated with congenital hydrocephalus		
Dandy-Walker malformation	Malformation of the cerebellum associated with a dilation of the fourth ventricle. Males > females	Hydrocephalus, agenesis of the corpus callosum, Klippel-Feil and DeLange syndromes, and severe psychomotor retardation

(Mataró et al., 2001). As a result, children with HC frequently exhibit deficits in nonverbal (especially visuospatial) and motor performance.

As the ventricles continue to distend, the cerebral hemispheres mold into a balloon shape. Because sutures in the cranium of the fetus and infant have not yet fused, increasing pressure enlarges the skull to accommodate the increased CSF volume. Once the sutures close, however, cranial volume is invariant, and the HC develops further at the expense of brain tissue (Rowland, Fink, & Rubin, 1991).

Most children with symptoms of HC receive a **shunt** (see Figure 10.3). This medical procedure drains excessive CSF away from the ventricular system into the stomach. A shunt that fails, or needs adjustment, may necessitate additional surgeries during the child's life. Each surgery increases the risk for ventriculitis, or infection of the ventricles. Furthermore, introducing the shunt involves causing a lesion to the brain, generally of the parietal lobe of the right hemisphere. The shunt track can irritate the surrounding brain tissue and increase the potential for seizures (Willis, 1993).

Although cognitive, motor, and sensory (visual) impairments frequently associate with HC, the precise symptom presentation is highly individualistic. The period of developmental onset, the presence of other congenital disorders and anomalies, surgery to introduce or adjust a shunt, and the nature of the child's environmental context are several variables that affect the array, severity, and form of symptoms the child will experience.

Malformation	Description	Clinical Manifestations
Malformations associated with congenital hydrocephalus *(continued)*		
Arnold-Chiari malformation	Congenital deformation of the brainstem and cerebellum	Congenital hydrocephalus, spina bifida, and severe psychomotor retardation
Stenosis of the aqueduct of Sylvius	Obstruction of the aqueduct and CSF circulation	Often insidious onset of symptoms associated with hydrocephalus. Shunted children may suffer learning/behavioral problems. Nonverbal IQ < verbal IQ
Abnormalities of the neural tube and fusion defects		
Spina bifida occulta	Usually asymptomatic lesion discovered incidentally	Can be associated with lipoma, dermal sinuses, and dimples
Spina bifida cystica	Spinal defect that includes a cyst-like sac that may or may not contain the spinal cord	Hydrocephalus a frequent complication. Cognitive deficits related to extent of hydrocephalus. Arnold-Chiari malformation not uncommon
Cranium bifidum and encephalocele	Fusion defects of skull referred to as *cranium bifidum;* myelomeningoceles or meningoceles on the skull are referred to as *encephaloceles.* Males < females	Many associated difficulties with hydrocephalus including ataxia, cerebral palsy, epilepsy, and mental retardation
Anencephaly	Vault of skull absent and brain represented by vascular mass. Face is grossly normal. 1 male: 4 female	Condition incompatible with life
Hydranencephaly	Cerebral hemispheres replaced by cystic sacs containing CSF	Difficult initially to distinguish from hydrocephalus. Hypnoatremia, eye movement disturbances, and death
Porencephaly	Large cystic lesion develops on the brain. May occur bilaterally or unilaterally	Occasionally asymptomatic but typically associated with mental retardation, epilepsy, and other neurodevelopmental malformations

Source: Modified and updated from Hynd, G., Morgan, A., & Vaughn, M. (1997). Neurodevelopmental anomalies and malformations. In C. Reynolds & E. Fletcher-Janzen (Eds.), *Handbook of clinical child neuropsychology* (2nd ed., p. 45). New York: Plenum Publishing Corporation. Reprinted by kind permission of Springer Science and Business Media.

Neuropsychological Assessment—Neuropsychological assessment of the child with HC focuses on clarifying both spared and compromised functions. The extent and degree of impaired or spared cognitive functions differ for each child. In general, greater overall impairment of higher order cognitive abilities accompanies more advanced cases of HC. However, interaction of HC with other moderating variables, such as age, intelligence, and socioeconomic status, potentially can lead to differential effects on cognitive functioning.

Before widespread use of the shunt, only a fourth of untreated HC children survived to adulthood, and many survivors were profoundly retarded (Hynd, Morgan, & Vaughn, 1997). In contrast, the cognitive performance of early shunted children is significantly higher, spanning the range of abilities from below to above average

(Willis, 1993). Some investigators suggest that children with HC uncomplicated by other structural disruptions (such as multiple shunt operations or Arnold–Chiari malformation) are likely to demonstrate less impairment of overall cognitive ability (Erickson, Baron, & Fantie, 2001). Yet, even in cases of relatively preserved overall intelligence, children with shunted HC frequently demonstrate deficits in visual-perceptual, visuospatial, motor (fine and gross), and memory performance (Ewing-Cobbs, Barnes, & Fletcher, 2003; Scott et al., 1998). The deficits in the visual-perceptual, visuospatial, and visuomotor domains are related to the disruption of the posterior cortical regions, cerebellum, corpus callosum, and other white matter pathways, whereas poor motor skills are believed to be a consequence of damage to the cerebellum, basal ganglia, motor strip,

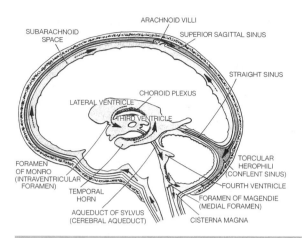

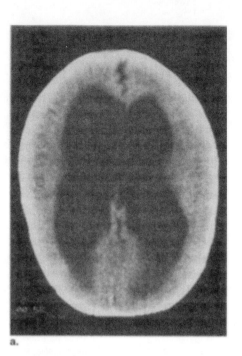

Figure 10.2 Ventricles of the human brain. (Reproduced from Gilman, S., & Newman, S. W. [1996]. The cerebrospinal fluid. *Manter and Katz's essentials of clinical neuroanatomy and neuropsychology* [9th ed., p. 260, Figure 81]. Philadelphia: F. A. Davis, by permission.)

and connecting white matter pathways (Erickson, Baron, & Fantie, 2001).

The memory deficits associated with HC include poor recall of both verbal and nonverbal contents. However, debate continues over which memory processes (encoding, retrieval, or consolidation) are impaired (Erickson, Baron, & Fantie, 2001). A singular profile of strengths and deficits associated with HC is not likely to be identified because of the multiple and widely distributed neurosubstrates that support memory processes. Rather, different memory profiles will likely be identified that reflect the specific neural memory systems that are impacted, the severity of damage, the stage of brain development at the onset of the disorder, and a host of other mediating variables.

HC may also affect the development of other important cognitive abilities and skills. For example, children with HC tend to demonstrate age-appropriate word recognition, but markedly lower reading comprehension, math computation and problem solving, and writing skills. Even HC children of average to above-average intelligence are likely to demonstrate this disparity (Dennis & Barnes, 1994; Ewing-Cobbs, Barnes, & Fletcher, 2003). Similarly, HC children often exhibit relative strengths in speech and language production. Yet, even though their language is fluent and well structured, 28% to 41% of the children exhibit an atypical communication style termed **"cocktail party syndrome" (CPS)** (Mataró et al., 2001). This communication style is characterized by excessive verbiage that lacks clarity, organization, and relevance—a form of speech that resembles the "fluent, but empty" speech patterns associated with receptive aphasia, a communication disorder that involves impaired

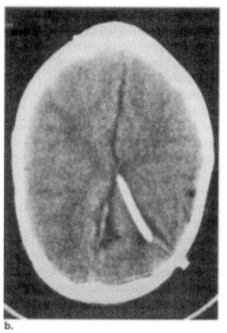

Figure 10.3 Computed tomography (CT) images of child with hydrocephalus. (A) Child at 3 months of age with unshunted hydrocephalus. Note the significantly enlarged ventricles. (B) The same child at 4 years 8 months with shunt in left hemisphere (white line, bottom right). (Reproduced from Anderson, V., Northam, E., Hendy, J., & Wrennall, J. [2001]. *Developmental neuropsychology: A clinical approach* [p. 193, Figure 6.4]. Philadelphia: Taylor & Francis, by permission.)

language comprehension. Interestingly, deficits related to understanding and expressing abstract language are associated with HC and are believed to contribute potentially to the development of CPS. On a more positive note, many children who demonstrate CPS develop a more appropriate communication style with increasing age.

A particularly interesting finding concerns the relation of cognitive functioning to early- and late-occurring HC. Children with prenatal obstructive HC are prone to exhibit average verbal and language abilities, but below-average visuospatial and visuomotor abilities. This profile is similar to that of the nonverbal learning disability syndrome (see discussion in Chapter 11). In contrast, children with HC resulting from perinatal and postnatal insults (such as IVH) are more likely to show comparable verbal and performance abilities, although both generally fall within the low-average range (Willis, 1993).

The integrity of the executive functions of children with HC has received less empirical attention than other cognitive domains. *Executive functions* refer to a wide range of higher order mental processes related to the generation, integration, control, and evaluation of goal-directed behaviors that are supported by the frontal and frontal-cortical-subcortical networks of the brain (see Chapter 9). Preliminary studies of executive performance in children with HC have identified executive deficits of attentional allocation and control, concept formation, planning, cognitive flexibility, response inhibition, and self-regulation (Fletcher, Dennis, & Northrup, 2000; Willis, 1993).

Importantly, poor executive performance by children with HC does not necessarily implicate damage or disruption in the frontal cortex. For instance, in a recent study (Anderson, Anderson, Northam, Jacobs, & Mikiewicz, 2002), the executive performance of children with HC, PKU, and frontal focal lesion and healthy control children was examined. Both the HC and frontal lesion groups performed poorly, relative to the healthy control children, on an executive measure sensitive to visuocontructive, planning, and organization skills (Rey Complex Figure; Rey, 1941, translated by Corwin & Bylsma, 1993). These findings leave unanswered the extent to which the poor executive performance of the HC group related to visuospatial, motor, or executive planning/organizational deficits, or some combination of these deficits. Because of the posterior-to-anterior progression of damage associated with HC, posterior cortical and subcortical structures, as well as white matter pathways, are generally disrupted before the frontal structures. This posterior disruption can, in turn, result in the transmission of distorted or incomplete visuospatial and/or motor input to the frontal system. Thus, the poor performance of the HC group could reflect an "executive deficit" engendered by anomalies of nonfrontal structures and pathways, rather than actual damage to the frontal lobes. Additional empirical study is needed to clarify the specific contributions of different neurosubstrates to the executive deficits of children and adolescents with HC.

Treatment—The prognosis for children with HC was dire before the development of shunting. However, the advent of shunting has markedly increased the number of children who both survive and escape the significant destruction of their cognitive functioning. Children with HC uncomplicated by the presence of other anomalies who receive early shunting often exhibit few, if any, cognitive impairments. **Ultrasonography,** a procedure that uses sound waves to image internal structures, enables medical personnel to identify HC in utero. This procedure allows for measurement of the ventricular expansion that precedes the later enlargement of the cranium. From birth until age 2, HC is fairly easy to diagnose because the cranium quickly enlarges, developmental delays are evident, and eye movement abnormalities are present (Hynd, Morgan, & Vaughn, 1997).

GENETIC AND CHROMOSOMAL DISORDERS

This section explores genetic and chromosomal disorders. Advances in the study of genetics, such as the mapping of the human genome, are accelerating at an exponential rate. More than 100 genetic and chromosomal disorders have been identified that, if untreated, can produce significant neuropsychological and physical deficits (see Table 10.2 for examples). A multitude of factors can disrupt the genetic blueprint that defines the developing child. Genetic disorders can be a consequence of **single-gene, chromosomal, parental imprinting,** or **molecular cytogenic anomalies.** A discussion of the disorders associated with each of these genetic abnormalities is beyond the scope of this chapter. Accordingly, we focus on neurodevelopmental disorders associated with chromosomal abnormalities.

Chromosomal disorders are a consequence of the malformation, deletion, addition, and/or dislocation of chromosomal material during the development of the oocyte or spermatocyte, or during conception and germination of the egg (Marino, Fine, & McMillan, 2004; Spreen, Rissell, & Edgell, 1995). As a result, a genetic defect occurs even though the family history is negative for the disorder. However, there are some families who have a history of chromosomal disorders, suggesting direct genetic transmission from the parent to the offspring.

Table 10.2 *Genetic and Chromosomal Disorders*

Genetic	Chromosomal
Adrenoleukodystrophy	Angelman's syndrome
Friedreich's ataxia	Cornelia de Lange's syndrome
Galactosemia	Down's syndrome
Hyperphenylalaninemia	Fragile X syndrome
Krabbe's disease	Klinefelter's syndrome
Lafora's disease	Prader-Willi syndrome
Lesch-Nyhan disease	Sotos' syndrome
Mucopolysaccharidosis	Trisomy X syndrome
Phenylketonuria	Tuberous sclerosis complex
	Turner's syndrome
	Williams syndrome

Source: Harris, J. C. (1995). *Developmental neuropsychiatry, vol. II: Assessment, diagnosis, and treatment of developmental disorders.* New York: Oxford University Press, by permission.

Chromosomal abnormalities can affect either **autosomes** or **sex chromosomes.** Autosomal abnormalities generally produce more severe birth defects than sex chromosome disturbances. More than 50% of first-trimester miscarriages are due to chromosomal defects. In addition, congenital and cognitive deficits are frequently a consequence of this class of genetic disorder (Marino, Fine, & McMillan, 2004). We discuss two chromosomal disorders: TS and WS. TS is the consequence of a missing or abnormal X sex chromosome, whereas WS is produced by a submicroscopic deletion on autosome 7. Studies of these two disorders have significantly advanced our understanding of the neuropsychological effects of disturbances to the developing brain.

Turner's Syndrome

Background and Clinical Presentation—In 1938, Turner presented a syndrome characterized by a failure to develop secondary sexual characteristics, short stature, webbed neck, and **cubitus valgus** (an increased carrying angle at the elbow). The disorder was subsequently named **Turner's syndrome (TS).** A previous case of the disorder had also been reported by Otto Ullrich (1930); therefore, the syndrome is occasionally known as Ullrich–Turner syndrome. TS was recognized as a chromosomal disorder affecting female individuals in 1959, when Charles Ford and colleagues identified a missing X on the 45th chromosome. The **karyotype**—a visual representation of the configuration of a chromosome—is designated as 45,XO,

although there are other variations (see Web Connections section later in this chapter).

Consistent with Turner's earlier description of the disorder, an essential characteristic of TS is gonadal dysgenesis, as evident in either the absence of the ovaries or the presence of **vestigial ovarian streaks.** Short stature is another distinguishing characteristic, with achieved height often falling between 4 feet 6 inches and 4 feet 10 inches (Powell & Schulte, 1999). Physicians often identify infants with TS at birth due to characteristic edema of the hands and feet and loose skin folds at the nape of the neck. In childhood, physicians observe webbing of the neck, low-set ears, shield chest, deformed nails, cardiac and kidney malformations, and other features. Table 10.3

Table 10.3 *Physical and Medical Problems of Turner's Syndrome*

Anatomic Abnormalities	Cardiovascular
Short stature	Aortic narrowing
Webbed neck	Mitral valve prolapse
Cubitus valgus	Septal defect (defect of the wall separating chambers of the heart)
Broad chest	
Prepubertal ovarian failure	Partial anomalous venous blood return
Growth	**Renal**
Decreased mean birth weight	Horseshoe kidney (abnormal tissue connecting the kidneys) or ptotic kidney (abnormal location in the pelvis)
Lack of pubertal growth spurt	
Skeletal	
Curvature of the spine	Unilateral failure to develop or underdeveloped kidney
Genu valgum (knock-knee)	
Wrist deformity	Unilateral double ureter
Short hand and feet bones	**Lymphatic**
Craniofacial	Dilation of the lymph vessels
Premature closure of the skull sutures	Congenital swelling of the hands/feet
Small jaw	**Hair and Skin**
Strabismus (cross-eyes)	Low posterior hairline
Inner ear defects	Multiple moles
Malrotation of ears	Finger/toenail deformities
High arched palate	

Source: White, B. J. (1994). The Turner syndrome: Origin, cytogenetic variants, and factors influencing the phenotype. In S. H. Broman & J. Grafman (Eds.), *Atypical cognitive deficits in developmental disorders* (p. 185). Mahwah, NJ: Lawrence Erlbaum, by permission.)

presents a sample of the physical characteristics and medical problems associated with TS. A distinctive cognitive profile for TS has been proposed and is discussed later in this section (see Neuropsychological Assessment).

Incidence and Comorbidity—TS is one of the most common chromosomal disorders, with an estimated female incidence rate of 1 in 2500 to 5000 births (Berch & Bender, 2000). Researchers believe it occurs at conception, and 99% of the affected fetuses spontaneously abort. The life expectancy of individuals born with TS is not affected, although a number of physical conditions accompany the disorder (see Table 10.3).

Frequent comorbid conditions of TS are learning disabilities and early symptoms of an attention-deficit/hyperactivity disorder (ADHD). Also, some researchers have suggested that female individuals with TS are prone to depression, feelings of inadequacy, difficulty in concentrating, poor peer relationships, and anxiety over sexuality and relationships with male individuals. The factors that account for these difficulties are unclear, but the small stature and sexual limitations of the individual with TS likely contribute to social difficulties and negative emotionality.

Chromosomal Defect and Turner's Syndrome—TS is the result of an anomaly of the female sex chromosome. The XX chromosome defines the developing embryo as female. In TS, the second X is either missing (monosomy X or 45,XO) or otherwise abnormal in formation or location. A wide variety of karyotypes appear in liveborn TS children, with 45,XO evident in approximately 50% of the cases. **Isochromosome,** the duplication of one arm of the X chromosome with the loss of the other arm, constitutes 10% to 20% of cases. **Mosaic karyotypes** appear in 30% to 35% of children with TS (Temple, Carney, & Mullarkey, 1996). The mosaic karyotypes are characterized by the presence of normal chromosomes in some cells (46,XX) and abnormal chromosomes in others (Temple & Marriott, 1998). The mosaic karyotype, 45,X/46,XX, is associated with milder and less pervasive anomalies than the other karyotypes.

At birth, these children exhibit few distinguishing features, and short stature may be the first presenting symptom. In contrast, the small X-ring karyotype appears to increase the risk for mental retardation, smaller head size, and greater growth-related retardation than the other TS karyotypes. Note, however, that the TS physical phenotype occasionally appears in children with apparently normal karyotypes.

Neuropathogenesis—Neuroimaging studies provide support for right hemisphere (particularly posterior region)

involvement in the pathogenesis of TS. In an earlier magnetic resonance imaging (MRI) study of TS and healthy control children, Reiss and coworkers (1995) determined that the ratios of gray to white matter for the right temporal and parietal areas were significantly lower for the participants with TS. In a more recent study (Brown et al., 2002) of children and adolescents with TS, MRI showed bilateral decreases in parietal gray and occipital white matter and increased cerebellar gray matter. Moreover, a positron emission tomography (PET) study (Elliott, Watkins, Messa, Lippe, & Chugani, 1996) of children with TS demonstrated significant bilateral parietal region hypometabolism (reduced metabolism) relative to a healthy control group. The researchers also observed a trend toward hypometabolic activity of the occipital region. They hypothesized that the visuospatial and mathematic deficits associated with TS stemmed from parieto-occipital hypoactivation. Other regional differences in brain volume or neuroactivation of patients with TS have been identified in the hippocampus, lenticular nucleus, thalamus, temporal cortex, and insula (Murphy et al., 1993, 1997). However, reduced tissue volume or atypical activation patterns for parietal and parieto-occipital areas are the most consistent findings across neuroimaging studies.

Although posterior brain regions have received the greatest empirical attention, increasing attention has focused on the frontal system as it relates to executive performance associated with TS. Neuropsychological studies have shown that individuals with TS demonstrate deficits in verbal fluency, planning and organization, impulsive regulation, strategic memory organization, cognitive flexibility, and attentional control (Buchanan, Pavlovic, & Rovet, 1998; Romans, Roeltgen, Kushner, & Ross, 1997; Temple, Carney, & Mullarkey, 1996). Haberecht and colleagues (2001) subjected children and adolescents with TS and healthy control participants to function MRI (fMRI) while performing an executive function task, namely, a visuospatial working memory task. The children and adolescents with TS showed poorer performance than healthy control participants on the visuospatial working memory task. Moreover, fMRI showed significant bilateral hypoactivation (relative to healthy control participants) of the dorsolateral prefrontal cortex, caudate, and inferior parietal cortex while performing the working memory task. The authors hypothesized that the working memory deficits of TS relate to disruption of the frontal-striatal and frontal-parietal executive circuits.

In a more recent study (Tamm, Menon, & Reiss, 2003), children and adolescents with TS and healthy volunteers underwent fMRI while performing a measure of executive **inhibitory control.** The TS and healthy groups did not, contrary to prediction, differ in their inhibitory performance. Yet, the TS group was found to show activation of additional regions of the superior and middle prefrontal cortices not demonstrated by the healthy control group. The authors conclude that patients with TS demonstrate altered (possibly compensatory) prefrontal cortical functioning with regard to response inhibition. Overall, neuroimaging studies have contributed to our understanding of the brain-behavior relations of TS, but much remains to be discovered.

Neuropsychological Assessment—Originally, it was believed that mental retardation was a common concomitant of TS. However, ongoing studies (Powell & Schulte, 1999) have demonstrated that the intellectual functioning of children with TS is generally within the low-average to average range. A smaller proportion of children fall within the below- or above-average range of intelligence (Swillen et al., 1993). Often, verbal intelligence exceeds performance intelligence. That is, children with TS, when performing intellectual measures such as the Wechsler scales (1997, 2002, 2003), tend to achieve higher scores on verbal language–related scales (for example, vocabulary) as contrasted with performance scales (for example, block design) that assess visual-perceptual and visuomotor abilities.

Several researchers have suggested that children with TS demonstrate a relatively distinct neurocognitive profile. The profile is characterized by intact verbal abilities in contrast with deficits in visuospatial, visuomotor, and arithmetic performance (Romans et al., 1997; Temple & Marriott, 1998). Table 10.4 summarizes the types of visuospatial and visuomotor deficits identified. Note that these deficits are generally associated with right parietal or diffuse right hemisphere dysfunction. Several investigators have drawn a parallel between the neurocognitive profile of TS and that of the nonverbal learning disability syndrome (see discussion of the NVLD syndrome in Chapter 11). Alternatively, Pennington and Smith (1983) contend that the performance of individuals with TS suggests diffuse brain injury, rather than injury specific to either the right or left hemisphere. Increasingly, investigators are realizing that children with TS are at greater risk for the development of specific neurocognitive deficit patterns (such as preserved verbal abilities and visuospatial weaknesses), but these deficits are not universal for all children with TS.

Developmental Course—The incidence of prematurity for children with TS (45,XO) is high, with more than 25% of the infants born 2 to 4 weeks early, and approximately

Table 10.4 *Visuospatial and Visuomotor Deficits Associated with Turner's Syndrome*

Dysfunctions of:

Arithmetic	Mental rotation	Visual discrimination
Design copying	Motor learning	Spatial working memory
Directional sense	Part-whole perception	
Extrapersonal space		Visual sequencing
Left-right discrimination	Route finding	Visual-motor integration
	Spatial reasoning	
Maze performance		Visual memory

Source: Buchanan, L., Pavolic, J., & Rovet, J. (1998). A reexamination of the visuospatial deficit in Tuner syndrome: Contributions of working memory. *Developmental neuropsychology* (pp. 341-367). Mahwah, NJ: Lawrence Erlbaum, by permission.)

30% born more than 4 weeks before their due dates (Harris, 1995). The body length of the infant at birth is below average. Measures (blood assays) of **gonadotropins** assist in diagnosing the disorder. In the female individual, gonadotropins are hormones that stimulate the functions of the ovaries. The majority of children with TS are diagnosed before school age.

During the preschool years, children with TS are described as immature, overactive, distractible, and having difficulty sustaining attention. With increasing age, activity appears to slow, and many children with TS later become normally active or hypoactive. Young children with TS do not exhibit behavioral problems and are generally accepted by and involved with peers. However, by school age, the peer interactions of many children with TS lessen and involvement in solitary activities increases. Temperamentally, children affected with TS tend to be compliant, unassertive, and conforming in their interactions with caretakers and peers. Peer interactions, however, continue to decline during the elementary and middle school years, and many youngsters with TS report feelings of loneliness and alienation (Powell & Schulte, 1999; Swillen et al., 1993). With the onset of adolescence, teenagers with TS date less frequently and are involved in fewer romantic and sexual relationships than their peers. Some investigators suggest that they may not be proficient at reading social cues, which negatively affects their efforts to relate to peers. Growth retardation, physical anomalies (such as webbing of the neck), medical problems, social difficulties, and an awareness of their sexual difference likely contribute to diminished self-esteem

(Bender, Linden, & Robinson, 1994). In light of these factors, it is not surprising that teenagers with TS are at risk for development of anxiety, insecurity, and depression. Despite deficits in the visuospatial and visuomotor areas, most children affected by the disorder (90%) attend regular school programs, although they may need remedial interventions. Moreover, because of the physical problems associated with the condition (see Table 10.3), individuals with TS often need ongoing medical monitoring and services. On a more encouraging note, TS does not preclude the establishment of stable personal relationships, marriage, or gainful employment.

Treatment—It is essential that adolescents with TS receive estrogen therapy because of their gonadal dysgenesis. Without proper medical interventions, youngsters with the disorder do not mature sexually, which can cause significant distress. Furthermore, the short stature associated with TS often requires growth hormone therapy. Psychological or counseling services may be needed, because the risk for teasing and lack of peer acceptance appears high for children with TS (Powell & Schulte, 1999; Rovet, 1993). Children and adolescents with TS who demonstrate inattention, impulsivity, and hyperactivity encounter significant difficulties within the classroom. Specialized educational interventions and, in many cases, the introduction of psychostimulant medications may assist the student. In addition, spatial, executive, and academic weaknesses (mathematics) must be addressed to ensure appropriate academic progress. Chapter 11 explores additional educational recommendations relevant to the needs of the child with TS (see the Nonverbal Learning Disability Syndrome section).

Williams Syndrome

WS is an intriguing and enigmatic disorder. The disorder is characterized by physical abnormalities and low intellectual functioning, yet presents an uneven cognitive profile of relatively preserved strengths and distinct weaknesses. Our understanding of the disorder is rapidly increasing due to the surge in significant research since the mid-1980s.

Background and Incidence—In 1961, Williams, Barratt-Boyes, and Lowe described a neurodevelopmental disorder characterized by unusual facial features, cardiovascular defect, hypercalcemia, and mental retardation that subsequently was designated as **Williams syndrome (WS).** The disorder is also referred to as Williams–Beuren syndrome because of the contributions of Beuren and colleagues (1964) to the understanding of the medical features of WS. Advances in genetics and molecular biology reveal that WS is associated

with a submicroscopic genetic deletion on chromosome 7 (band q11.23). WS equally affects male and female individuals and does not appear to be overly represented in any specific ethnic groups. The disorder is relatively rare and occurs at an estimated incidence rate of 1 per 20,000 to 50,000 live births (Dykens, 2003; Karmiloff-Smith, 1997).

Clinical Presentation—WS is a unique neurodevelopmental disorder characterized by a recognizable pattern of dysmorphic facial features, cardiovascular and physical abnormalities, mental retardation, specific cognitive profile, and distinct personality.

Table 10.5 presents a number of the physical and medical features associated with WS (Morris & Mervis,

Table 10.5 *Physical and Medical Conditions Associated with Williams Syndrome*

Visual and Ocular	Gastrointestinal	Renal
Stellate or lacy iris	Infant feeding difficulties	Kidney structural abnormalities
Hyperopia (farsighted)	Colic	Renal artery stenosis
Abnormal binocular vision	Vomiting	Recurrent bladder infections
Strabismus	Failure to thrive	Enuresis
	Constipation	Urinary frequency
Auditory/Voice	Chronic abdominal pain	
Chronic otitis media	Umbilical and inguinal hernias	**Dental**
Sound hypersensitivity (hyperacusis)	Obesity (adult)	Small, widely spaced teeth
Hoarse, low pitched		Malocclusion
	Musculoskeletal	Enamel hypoplasia
Cardiovascular	Hyperextensible joints	
	Muscle hypotonia	
Supravalvar pulmonic stenosis	Nocturnal leg pains	
Peripheral pulmonic stenosis	Compensatory posture	
	Kyphosis, lordosis, and scoliosis	
Generalized arteriopathy	Joint contractors	
Hypertension	Stiff, awkward gait	
Metabolism/Growth	Muscle hypertonia (Adult)	
Hypercalcemia		
Precocious puberty		
Short stature		

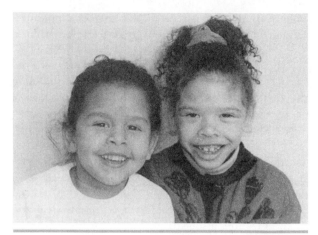

Figure 10.4 The distinctive facial features of a 7-year-old child with Williams syndrome (right) and her normally developing 4-year-old sister (left). (Reproduced from Morris, C. A., & Mervis, C. B. [1999]. Williams syndrome. In S. Goldstein & C. R. Reynolds [Eds.], *Handbook of neurodevelopmental and genetic disorders in children* [p. 558, Figure 24.2]. New York: Guilford Press, by permission.)

1999). The distinctive facial dysmorphia of the child with WS (Figure 10.4) has been called "elfin" due to a broad brow, puffy eyes, a stellate or lacy iris pattern, a small upturned nose, a broad nasal bridge, full cheeks, a wide mouth, prominent lips and ears, and small, widely spaced teeth. As the child ages, the face narrows, the nose tip broadens, and asymmetry of facial features is common.

Cardiovascular anomalies, particularly **supravalvar aortic stenosis (SVAS),** are common. SVAS refers to the abnormal narrowing of the walls of the aorta, potentially leading to cardiac pathology. Approximately 65% to 75% of children and adults with WS are afflicted with SVAS (Morris & Mervis, 1999). Although aortic stenosis is of significant concern, other arterial systems (for example, renal) are also affected. Because of the generalized arteriopathology associated with WS, ongoing medical monitoring and treatment are warranted.

During infancy and childhood, the **hypercalcemia** (excessive calcium in the blood) of WS contributes to feeding disturbances, vomiting, failure to thrive, constipation, and chronic abdominal pain. Individuals with WS are highly sensitive to sounds **(hyperacusis),** and young children demonstrate an exaggerated startle response to noise (Hagerman, 1999). Similarly, older individuals with WS are often aware of sounds that others fail to detect and complain that certain sounds produce a sense of apprehension. Children with WS are prone to distractibility and hyperactivity, and

the extent to which hyperacusis contributes to these disturbances remains unclear.

Young children with WS exhibit **hypotonia,** whereas older children and adults have problems with **hypertonia.** Joint instability and **joint contractures** adversely affect fine- and gross-motor movements. Due to poor muscle tone and joint anomalies, children with WS demonstrate delays in motor development; a stiff, awkward gait; and abnormal posture.

Genetic Defect and Williams Syndrome—The microdeletion of chromosome 7q11.23 can be transmitted by either parent, and the resulting physical and cognitive features of the disorder vary depending on the size of the deletion (Morris & Mervis, 1999). Seventeen genes have been identified in the 7q11.23 region that potentially relate to WS. The specific genes deleted and size of the deletions are believed to affect the particular constellation of features that can be exhibited by individuals with WS. Several of these 17 contiguous genes are associated with specific features of the WS phenotype. Of these genes, deletion of the **elastin** *(ELN)* gene has received the greatest support as pathogenic to WS (Schultz, Grelotti, & Pober, 2001). ELN is an important connective tissue protein found in the skin, ligaments, organ walls, and walls of arteries. The ELN deletion is believed to account for a number of the physical anomalies associated with WS (see Table 10.5), particularly those related to the cardiovascular system. Currently, the chromosomal test **fluorescent in situ hybridization (FISH)** is the primary tool for determining whether an individual is afflicted with WS. Using this technique, 97% to 100% of individuals with WS demonstrate the deletion of the *ELN* gene (Morris & Mervis, 1999).

The second identified gene, LIM-Kinase *(LIMK1),* is a protein kinase that appears important in axon guidance during brain development (Osborne & Pober, 2001). It is hypothesized that deletion in the *LIMK1* gene is associated with the significant visuospatial and visuospatial construction deficits demonstrated by individuals with WS. A third implicated gene, syntaxin 1A *(STX1A),* is a protein found in the membrane of cells, particularly neurons, and is necessary for neurotransmitter release. Hyperactivity and other behavioral problems of individuals with WS are hypothesized to relate to the deletion of this gene. Finally, the deletion of three other genes—*GTF2I* (general transcription factor 2-I), *GTF2IRD1* (general transcription factor 2-I repeat domain containing protein 1), and *CYLN2* (cytoplasmic linker 2)—may be associated with the mental retardation associated with WS. *GTF2I* and *GTF2IRD1* are believed to be involved in the regulation of gene expression, and *CYLN2* is thought to perform linkage functions within the neurons (Osborne & Pober, 2001). Notably, the discussed linkage of individual gene deletions to the specific features of WS awaits future research for verification. Likewise, little currently is known of the functions of the remaining genes located at 7q.11.23 with regard to the WS phenotype.

Anatomic Brain Anomalies—Neuroimaging studies (Reiss et al., 2000; Schultz, Grelotti, & Pober, 2001) have reported a reduction in the overall brain volume of individuals with WS, although regional brain reductions were not uniform, with preserved volume of the temporal-limbic structures, cerebellum, and gray matter noted. Furthermore, Reiss and associates (2000) found that the decreased volume was primarily in the white matter, although there was significant loss of gray matter evident in the right occipital lobe. There were also indications of greater posterior (occipitoparietal) than anterior volume loss. These anatomic differences are consistent with the cognitive profile of relatively preserved language and impaired visuospatial abilities demonstrated by individuals with WS.

Likewise, cytoarchitectonic studies of individuals with WS have shown abnormal auditory cell packing density and neuronal size in the temporal lobe (Brodmann's area 41), suggesting hyperconnectivity of the auditory cortex (Galaburda & Bellugi, 2000; Holiger, McMenamin, Sherman, & Galaburda, 2001). This finding may be related to the relatively spared auditory functions (language and music) and unusual reactions to auditory stimuli such as hyperacusis (Levitin, Cole, Chiles, Lai, Lincoln, & Bellugi, 2004).

Neuropsychological Profile—The neuropsychological profile associated with WS includes a unique constellation of abilities, skills, and interests. This profile includes intellectual impairment, relatively preserved language skills, increased attention to facial processing, visuoconstructive skill weaknesses, significant interest and relative proficiency in music, and high levels of sociability.

*General Intellectual Performance and Language Abilities—*Individuals with WS frequently demonstrate mild-to-moderate mental retardation; there is appreciable variability in intellectual performance, with cognitive scores ranging from significantly below average to low average (Robinson, Mervis, & Robinson, 2003). Particular weaknesses are often evident in higher order conceptual reasoning and problem solving (Levitin et al., 2004). Generally,

measures of verbal intelligence reveal higher levels of functioning than measures of nonverbal intelligence, particularly if visuospatial abilities are assessed.

Language skills are consistently reported to be an area of relative strength for individuals with WS. Particular verbal strengths are evident in vocabulary development, phonologic processing, auditory short-term memory, auditory working memory, and verbal fluency (Robinson et al., 2003; Volterra, Caselli, Capirci, Tonucci, & Vicari, 2003). In the normal population, language and global intelligence are generally highly correlated with each other. Yet, the language abilities of individuals with WS are often more advanced than would be predicted by their cognitive ability performance. Increasingly, however, research shows that certain aspects of the language development associated with WS are far from normal. Specifically, anomalies in the development of semantics, complex syntax, grammar, pragmatic language (Laws & Bishop, 2004), and comprehension of nonliteral language (Sullivan, Winner, & Tager-Flusberg, 2003) are evident. Furthermore, indications exist that the precursors of language, as well as formal language, develop later and in different ways in children with WS relative to healthy children. For example, the precursor to naming objects is referential pointing; yet, Mervis and Bertrand (1997) found that naming precedes referential pointing for young children with WS. Moreover, joint attention, another precursor of normal language development, is significantly reduced in toddlers with WS compared with healthy peers of comparable mental and chronologic age (Karmiloff-Smith, Brown, Grice, & Paterson, 2003). The emergence of formal language in children with WS is delayed approximately 2 years as contrasted with healthy children of a similar age (Morris & Mervis, 1999). Furthermore, the onset of novel two-word combinations is even more delayed, ranging from 26 to 50 months of age. However, once language emerges, it develops at an increasing rate, often more rapidly than in children with other neurodevelopmental disorders such as **Down's syndrome** (Mervis & Robinson, 2000). The language of adolescents and adults with WS continues to be an area of relative strength, although language attainment is not comparable with that of healthy adolescents and adults.

A number of studies have indicated that children with WS differ in the manner in which they acquire language. For example, a series of recent studies (Robinson, Mervis, & Robinson, 2003; Volerra et al., 2003) has determined that children with WS rely more heavily on auditory working memory and short-term phonologic memory in language acquisition, particularly grammar, than typically developing children. Similarly, children with WS, relative to matched control children, show greater proficiency in encoding language via phonologic relative to linguistic-semantic features. Overall, these findings suggest that language, although a relative strength for children with WS, is less advanced than typically developing children of the same age and is possibly acquired by different cognitive processes.

Facial Processing—The facial processing abilities are recognized as another unique aspect of the cognitive profile associated with WS. Children with WS spend an inordinate amount of time focusing on the faces of others. For example, in a relatively recent study (Mervis et al., 2003), infants and toddlers (8–43 months old) with WS demonstrated greater attention to and focus on the face of others relative to that of healthy children. Moreover, normal to near-normal performance has been reported (Deruelle, Mancini, Livet, Casse-Perrot, & de Schonen, 1999; Karmiloff-Smith, 1998) for individuals with WS on standardized measures of facial recognition (for example, Benton Facial Recognition Test; Benton, Hamsher, Varney, & Spreen, 1983). Yet, facial recognition appears to be accomplished by different cognitive processes for WS relative to healthy control individuals. Specifically, typically developing children focus more on the configuration of facial features for recognition, whereas those with WS rely primarily on the features of the face for identification (Karmiloff-Smith et al., 2003).

Visuoconstructive Skills—Despite a relative strength in facial processing, visuoconstructive abilities are generally significantly impaired relative to the global intellectual ability of individuals with WS. Two areas of visuoconstructive, drawing and replication of block patterns, have been examined extensively. The performance of individuals with WS in drawing or copying geometric or familiar forms (for example, a person) is significantly poorer than that of healthy children (matched for chronologic or mental age) or children with Down's syndrome (matched for chronologic and mental age) (Klein & Mervis, 1999; Morris & Mervis, 1999). The drawings of children and adolescents with WS are often unrecognizable (Figure 10.5), with the components or parts of the drawn object scattered over the page and unconnected. Thus, the drawings reveal deficits in global organization and spatial integration. Interestingly, the drawings of children and adolescents with Down's syndrome are recognizable, although simplified (see Figure 10.5). That is, the global organization and integration of the

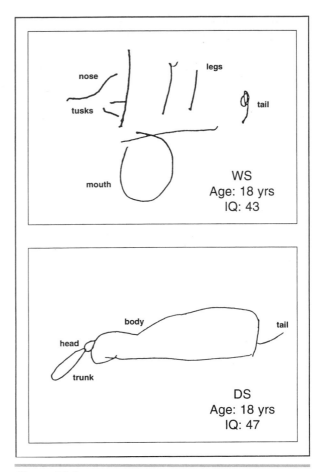

Figure 10.5 Drawings of an elephant by an adolescent with Williams syndrome (WS; top) and an adolescent with Down's syndrome (DS; bottom). (Reproduced from Temple, C. [1997]. *Developmental cognitive neuropsychology* [p. 154, Figure 4.6]. Philadelphia: Psychology Press Ltd., by permission.)

drawings of the children with Down's syndrome are relatively preserved.

Similarly, the ability of children and adolescents with WS to replicate structures (for example, a tower) or geometric designs with blocks is poorer than that of matched control participants. That is, the performance of children and adolescents with WS is often below that of healthy children matched for mental age, children with mental retardation of mixed etiology, and children with Down's syndrome. The WS groups struggle with maintaining the overall organization or configuration of the block structures/designs, whereas the other matched groups demonstrated significantly less difficulty in spatial-motor organization (Farran & Jarrold, 2003; Morris & Mervis, 1999).

Visuoconstructive tasks require that visuospatial information be processed and transmitted to the frontal system for action. Although the spatial deficits of WS have been associated with disturbances of the posterior regions of the brain, the impact of the disorder on the executive action system and interconnecting pathways remains to be elucidated. For example, Atkinson and associates (2003) presented a WS and a healthy control group of children with three executive measures sensitive to the inhibition of a prepotent response—holding in abeyance a response that is primed for release. The children with WS, in contrast with the healthy children, showed a diminished ability to inhibit a prepotent spatially directed response. Yet, the two groups demonstrated comparable performance related to inhibiting a pictorial-verbal (nonspatial) response. Although executive dysfunction is suggested, the basis of the deficit remains unanswered. As the authors correctly conclude, the inhibitory deficit may relate to a disturbance of the dorsolateral frontal region, parietal region, and/or interconnecting pathways of the two systems.

A potentially confounding factor in the studies of the visuospatial processing of individuals with WS is presented in Table 10.5. Children with WS frequently experience visual sensory deficits such as binocular disorders, poor visual refraction, and decreased visual acuity. Thus, the visual sensory deficits associated with WS may account for, or contribute to, poor visuoconstructive performance. To test this possible confound, Atkinson and colleagues (2003) have investigated the relation of visual sensory deficits to visuospatial and visuoconstructive performance. Approximately 50% of the children and adolescents sampled for study exhibited some form of visual sensory deficit. The children and adolescents were administered a battery of tests sensitive to visuospatial and visuoconstructive abilities. The results demonstrated a negligible relation between the occurrence of visual sensory deficits and severity of spatial deficits. Accordingly, the visuospatial and visuoconstructive deficits associated with WS do not appear to relate to visual sensory impairments.

As discussed previously, individuals with WS demonstrate a local rather than global bias in face processing. A similar processing bias is proposed to account for, at least in part, the visuoconstructive deficits associated with WS. However, Farran and Jarrold (2003), based on a review of research of visual-perceptual and visuoconstructive performance of individuals with WS, conclude that individuals with WS are capable of global processing depending on the nature of the task introduced. Specifically, individuals with WS show a global processing style on tasks of visual perception, but rely on a local processing approach with tasks requiring visuoconstruction. That is, they rely on local processing when task performance involves the manipulation and construction of spatial elements. If the elements of the task are spatially invariant, and mental-motor manipulation is not required, they are able to use a global processing approach. Unfortunately, this interpretation does not account for the local preference of individuals with WS in facial processing.

Dorsal versus Ventral Processing—Because of the significant deficits in visuospatial relative to facial processing, neuroscientists and neuropsychologists have sought to determine whether the disparity represents a dissociation between the ventral and dorsal streams of visual processing. The ventral stream ("what" processing; see Chapter 8) conveys visual object and face recognition to the temporal lobes, whereas the dorsal stream ("where" processing) carries information to the parietal lobes necessary for the processing of spatial relations. Using tasks sensitive to ventral and dorsal processing, investigations (Atkinson et al., 1997, 2003) have shown that WS is generally associated with deficits in dorsal relative to ventral processing, although a number children and adolescents with WS show equally poor performance on both types of tasks. Thus, there appears to be a subgroup of individuals with WS who demonstrate deficits in processing tasks supported by the dorsal stream, and another group who show deficits consistent with dorsal and ventral stream disruption.

Recently, a National Institute of Mental Health (NIMH)–sponsored study (Meyer-Lindenberg et al., 2004) investigated the dorsal and ventral stream activation of individuals with WS of normal intelligence. WS and control participants underwent neuroimaging (fMRI and MRI) while performing visual tasks requiring dorsal or ventral stream activation. The performance of the WS group with dorsal stream items showed isolated hypoactivation in the parietal portion of the dorsal stream. Control and WS participants did not differ in activation when processing ventral stream items. Furthermore, structural MRI revealed a reduction in gray matter volume in an area immediately adjacent to the parieto-occipital intraparietal sulcus for only the WS group (Figure 10.6). Analysis determined that the hypoactivation of the dorsal stream could be attributed to impaired input from this isolated region. Clearly, the findings of the neuroimaging study are consistent with the deficits of individuals with WS on measures of visuospatial processing.

Musicality and Williams Syndrome—WS is associated with enhanced interest, involvement, and proficiency in music.

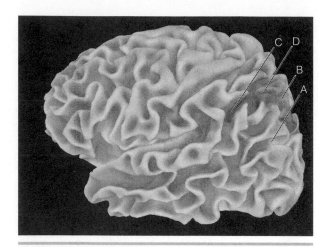

Figure 10.6 A three-dimensional magnetic resonance image rendering of the white matter of individuals with Williams syndrome. A small anomaly (A) of the occipitoparietal region that may disrupt the "downstream" activation of the "where" dorsal stream. The regional activation of the dorsal stream is evident in visuospatial processing of location (B) and construction (C). D represents regional overlap. (Karen Berman, M.D./NIMH.)

Those with WS are as proficient at reproducing music, show comparable levels of achievement in music, and spontaneously produce rhythmic sequences as often as typically developing individuals of the same age. Furthermore, individuals with WS are more musical than Down's syndrome and autistic individuals. Specifically, individuals with WS spend more time listening to music, show more interest in music-related activities, are more accurate in their reproductions of music, and play original music and rhythms more frequently those with other neurodevelopmental disorders (such as Down's syndrome and autism). Furthermore, individuals with WS demonstrate a greater emotional response to music than other groups. For example, one child with WS began to weep with she heard a couple of notes played at a Mozart concert. The girl's reaction was so strong that she had to leave the concert. When she tried to return, she once again began to weep. She later noted, "There are two kinds of Mozart: the kind that hurts and the kind that does not hurt" (Levitin et al., 2004, p. 238).

Sociability and Emotionality—Children and adolescents with WS are characterized as highly sociable, interpersonally sensitive, and empathetic. They tend to be overly happy and friendly, yet are also prone to irritability (which appears to abate with age) and moodiness. They are known to approach and speak indiscriminately with others and

to be excitable, restless, and inattentive. In addition, they experience high levels of anxiety, worry, fearfulness, and somatic complaints. They are significantly more anxious than children with other neurodevelopmental disorders (for example, Down's syndrome) (Morris & Mervis, 1999), mental retardation of mixed etiology, and healthy developing children (Dykens, 2003). Although they are proficient at understanding the feelings of others, they find it difficult to recognize their own fears (Lai, 1998). Interestingly, in contrast with healthy children, they do not show an age-related reduction in their fears.

Despite their social interest and affability, children and adolescents with WS are not fully accepted by peers because of their indiscriminate approach to others, immaturity, and communication differences. The basis of their overfriendliness and sociability is unclear, but it is believed that their extreme focus on the faces of others may play a role in shaping these characteristics (Mervis et al., 2003). In a recent study (Meyer-Lindenberg et al., 2005), the amygdala activation of individuals with WS and healthy control participants was investigated. The participants underwent fMRI while processing faces portraying threatening feelings (anger and fear) and threatening scenes (for example, burning building). The amygdala is implicated in the support of a number of emotion-related functions, including the monitoring of environmental events for danger. For healthy control participants, the amygdala showed greater activation when processing threatening faces than threatening scenes. The participants with WS showed the opposite pattern of greater activation for threatening scenes relative to faces. The investigators hypothesize that the underactivation of the amygdala to threatening faces may account for the diminished fear of strangers and social disinhibition demonstrated by individuals with WS. That is, the decreased activation may indicate an attenuation of normal social fear or apprehension. In contrast, the greater activation of the amygdala to threatening scenes may underpin their high rates of nonsocial anxiety, worry, and fears.

Treatment—The first few months of the infant's life can be quite trying for the parents and the infant. Infants with WS often feed poorly, vomit frequently, experience reflux, and fail to thrive. Hypercalcemia contributes to these gastrointestinal disturbances, requiring medical attention and dietary restrictions. When a child is identified with WS, a comprehensive examination should be undertaken due to the increased probability of medical complications, particularly cardiovascular disease.

Motor delays, muscle weakness, and hip contractures become increasingly evident as the child moves into his or her toddler/preschool years. Orthopedic and physical/occupational services are often needed to address these problems. Although verbal skills are an area of relative strength for children with WS, the precursors to formal language, and the emergence of formal language itself, are delayed or disturbed, warranting speech and language interventions.

The hyperacusis associated with WS may be a significant problem for the child. Accordingly, environmental modifications to reduce or alleviate the occurrence of loud and disturbing noises are needed. For example, the child might be removed from the classroom in advance of a fire drill and placed in a room where the sound of the fire alarm is muffled or be allowed to use ear plugs or ear phones. Interestingly, as discussed earlier, individuals with WS often enjoy and show relative proficiency in the area of music (Hopyan, Dennis, Weksberg, & Cytrynbaum, 2001).

During the preschool and elementary school years, the child often warrants special or remedial educational services because of general cognitive delays. These children frequently demonstrate greater success in reading and spelling relative to math and handwriting. The academic interventions used for children with nonverbal learning disability syndrome (see Treatment of Nonverbal Learning Disability Syndrome in Chapter 11) are generally recommended for children or adolescents with WS (Hagerman, 1999). Behavioral modification techniques and psychostimulant medication may be warranted to address poor attentional focus, distractibility, and impulsivity. Social skills training is important to facilitate social acceptance by peers because of their overfriendliness and indiscriminate approaching of others. The child or adolescent may need to learn verbal self-protective skills to cope with teasing or abuse by peers.

As discussed earlier, individuals with WS often experience disruptive anxiety, depression, and other psychiatric issues. They can profit from psychotherapy due, in part, to their verbal strengths. Often, medications addressing anxiety or depression are needed to augment treatment; however, careful monitoring by medical professionals is imperative for those individuals with cardiovascular disease or other significant medical issues.

ACQUIRED DISORDERS

The number of agents, events, and processes that can potentially injure the prenatal and postnatal brain is staggering. Environmental toxins, radiation, infections, anoxia, malnutrition, tumors, and traumatic head injuries can result in anomalies of the developing brain. Of these agents, traumatic head injuries, such as concussions, lacerations, and contusions, are the cause of most brain damage in children and adolescents. Regardless of the nature of the insult, a one-to-one relation between brain disturbance and behavior is not evident. The prediction of functional outcomes is contingent on a host of factors including: (1) age at which the lesion is incurred; (2) type, severity, and status (static or progressive) of the lesion; (3) premorbid personality and intelligence of the child; (4) quality and timeliness of medical attention; and (5) accessibility of acute and long-term services.

FAS is a specific condition that reflects the devastating effects of prenatal exposure to alcohol. Initially, it was suspected that impairments associated with FAS were restricted to mothers who chronically abused alcohol or were "binge" drinkers. Increasingly, it is being realized that the prenatal embryo/fetus is at risk even with social drinking.

Fetal Alcohol Syndrome

Clinical Features—Fetal alcohol syndrome (FAS) is a long-lasting and debilitating disorder recognized in the medical and neuropsychological fields since the early 1970s. Lemoine, Harrowsseau, Borteryu, and Menuet (1968) are credited with being the first to describe the effects of alcohol on a group of children with alcoholic parents. Jones, Smith, Ulleland, and Streissguth (1973) later identified the anomalies and characteristics that have come to define FAS.

Children with FAS frequently exhibit intrauterine growth retardation; characteristic facial features of widely spaced eyes, shortened length of eyelids, elongated midface, flattened nose, underdeveloped upper lip (Figure 10.7), and deficits associated with central nervous system involvement (Streissguth, 1997). Central nervous system deficits include **microcephaly** (abnormally small head), infantile irritability, seizures, tremors, poor coordination, poor habituation (difficulty in tuning out repeating stimuli), and reduced muscle tone. In addition, below-average intelligence, inattention, hyperactivity, learning disabilities, and poor behavioral regulation commonly characterize children with FAS (Mattson, Riley, Gramling, Delis, & Jones, 1998; Kerns, Don, Mateer, & Streissguth, 1997). Although FAS is one of the most well-known causes of mental retardation, not all children affected with it are retarded. Table 10.6 presents frequently identified physical and medical characteristics associated with FAS.

Children who are exposed to alcohol in utero, but who fail to exhibit growth deficits or other physical abnormalities of FAS, may still show functional impairments similar

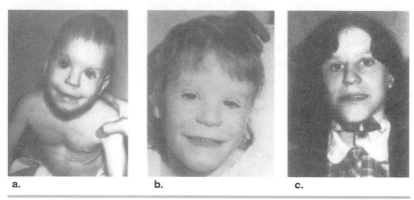

Figure 10.7   The facial features of the developing FAS child (a–c): Unique features are the widely spaced eyes, shortened length of eyelids, low nasal bridge, short and flattened nose, elongated midface, and thin upper lip. ([a, b] Reproduced from Hanson, J. W., Jones, K. L., & Smith, D. W. [1976]. Fetal alcohol syndrome: Experience with 41 patients. *Journal of the American Medical Association, 235*[14], 1459, by permission of the American Medical Association; [c] reproduced from Streissguth, A. [1997]. *Fetal alcohol syndrome* [p. 53]. Baltimore: Paul Brookes, by permission.)

to those of FAS. That is, the exposed children may manifest sensory and sensorimotor impairments, speech and language delays, cognitive and learning weaknesses, and regulatory deficits such as inattention, impulsivity, and hyperactivity (Jacobson, Jacobson, Sokol, Martier, & Ager, 1993). These features are called **fetal alcohol effects (FAE)** or **alcohol-related neurodevelopmental disabilities (ARND).**

Incidence—Estimates of the incidence rate of FAS in the general population range from 1 to 3 per 1000 live births. Researchers consider the incidence significantly higher, possibly two to three times greater, if children with FAE are included (Streissguth & Connor, 2001). The incidences of FAS and FAE among alcoholic mothers (chronic users) are markedly greater, with estimates of 25 per 1000 and 90 per 1000, respectively (Jenkins & Culbertson, 1996).

Neuropathogenesis—FAS is a consequence of alcohol use by the pregnant mother during the baby's prenatal development. The relation of the teratogenic effects of prenatal alcohol exposure to intake (amount, frequency, and drinking patterns), period of brain development, and maternal health/lifestyle variables during pregnancy remains poorly understood.

The teratogenic effects of alcohol, as revealed in animal and human studies, suggest a continuum of negative effects determined, in part, by a dose–response relation, that is, increasing amount and frequency of alcohol ingestion correlates with greater injurious effects (Korkman,

Kettunen, & Autti-Rämö, 2003). The children of mothers who consumed relatively low levels of alcohol are less likely to exhibit either physical or structural stigmata, but they may still experience behavioral disturbances, social maladjustment, and cognitive deficits (Mattson et al., 1998). At the most severe end of the continuum, characterized by excessive alcohol abuse, there is a significantly greater risk for the development of the full-blown FAS.

Although the risk to the developing embryo/fetus is much greater for pregnant mothers who chronically abuse alcohol or frequently "binge" (multiple drinks consumed in a relatively short period), the point in brain gestation that alcohol is introduced appears to have a differentially damaging impact. Alcohol exposure appears to cause greater damage to the developing brain during the early months of gestation (first trimester). However, the greatest disruption occurs when the exposure spans the entire pregnancy (Carmichael Olson et al., 1997). There are indications that the introduction of alcohol during the stage of brain neurogenesis (weeks 6–18th week) may disturb cortical cell migration, resulting in global cognitive deficits, whereas later prenatal exposure produces cognitive deficits that are more circumscribed in nature. Fraternal twin studies suggest that genetic factors may play a role in determining the vulnerability of the embryo/fetus to FAS. That is, maternal alcohol use can significantly affect one twin more than the other twin, despite their sharing the same prenatal environment. Other factors, such as the mother's health, psychiatric status, and lifestyle (for example, cigarette smoking and abuse of

Table 10.6 *Physical and Medical Conditions Associated with Fetal Alcohol Syndrome*

Growth

Decreased fat tissue

Prenatal and postnatal growth deficiency

Cardiac

Atrial septal defect (defect in the wall between the atria)

Ventricular septal defect (defect of wall between the ventricles)

Craniofacial

Abnormally small jaw in adolescence

Microcephaly (abnormally small head)

Ptosis (droopy eyelid)

Short upturned nose

Shortened eyelid length

Underdeveloped lip features

Underdeveloped upper jaw

Skeletal

Altered palm crease patterns

Cervical spine abnormalities

Foot position defects

Joint alterations

Skeletal *(continued)*

Pectus excavatum (abnormally depressed sternum)

Tapering terminal fingers, deformities of finger/toenails

Union of the radius and ulnar bones

Other

Abnormal thoracic cage

Abnormally small eyes

Anomaly of the sex organs

Cleft lip and/or cleft palate

Dental malocclusion

Epicanthal folds

Excessive hair in infancy

Hearing loss, protuberant ears

Hernias of diaphragm, umbilicus, or groin

Myopia, strabismus (cross-eyes)

Renal deformity

Small teeth with faulty enamel

Strawberry hemangiomata (blood-filled birthmarks or benign tumors of small blood vessels)

Source: Harris, J. C. (1995). *Developmental neuropsychiatry, vol. II: Assessment, diagnosis, and treatment of developmental disorders* (p. 362, Table 12.1-1). New York: Oxford University Press, by permission.)

other substances) and how efficiently she metabolizes alcohol appear related to the risk for development of FAS/FEA (Streissguth & Connor, 2001).

An often neglected but important factor mediating the phenotypic expression of FAS/FEA is the postnatal social environment (particularly the home) of the child. The FAS/FEA child is often raised by a mother who is coping with the stresses of alcoholism and the demands of parenting a child. Children of alcoholics are subject to high levels of neglect, abuse, inconsistent parenting, and out-of-home placements. The extent to which adverse environmental events shape and exacerbate the cognitive-emotional-

behavioral disturbances of the child with FAS/FEA remains poorly understood (Streissguth & Connor, 2001).

Originally, researchers thought more severe neuropsychological deficits were specific to FAS. However, increasing evidence indicates that children, adolescents, and adults with FAE can display comparable functional deficits (Connor, Sampson, Bookstein, Barr, & Streissguth, 2000; Korkman et al., 2003). In one study (Mattson et al., 1998), for example, children with FAS and FAE underwent a comprehensive neuropsychological evaluation. The assessment results showed that both groups, relative to healthy control children, demonstrated impairment in language skills, verbal learning and memory, academic performance, fine-motor speed, and visuomotor integration skills. Of significance was the finding that children with FAE showed a pattern of deficits comparable with those of FAS children, except in the areas of visuomotor integration and nonverbal concept formation. In a more recent study of adults with FAS and FEA (Connor et al., 2000), both the FAS and FEA groups were found to be significantly impaired on a number of measures of executive function. Thus, individuals with a history of prenatal alcohol exposure are likely to demonstrate significant neuropsychological deficits, even though they appear physically normal.

Investigators have identified a number of neuroanatomic alterations in the brains of FAS/FEA children that reflect the destructive impact of alcohol on the developing brain. Specifically, children with the disorder present with dysgenesis or agenesis of the corpus callosum, hippocampal damage, reduced basal ganglia volume, cerebellar anomalies, expanded ventricles, and reduction in white matter (Archibald, Mateer, & Kerns, 2001; Kaemingk & Paquette, 1999; Streissguth & Connor, 2001). The high proportion of FAS children with microcephaly indicates that brain size is reduced. Wass and colleagues (2001) studied living fetuses exposed to alcohol with ultrasound sonography and identified a reduction in size of the frontal cortex. Executive dysfunctions (Kaemingk & Paquette, 1999) consistent with disturbances of the frontal circuitry have been identified. Similarly, studies of animals exposed to prenatal alcohol report a wide range of brain anomalies, including reduction in brain weight and volume, and structural disturbances or loss of neurons, dendritic spines, and subcortical and cortical white matter circuitry (Chen, Maier, Parnell, & West, 2004).

Neuropsychological Assessment—Children with FAS/FEA exhibit a broad spectrum of neuropsychological deficits. In addition to mental retardation, common FAS/FEA deficits are evident in attentional regulation, response inhibition, complex problem solving, spatial and object memory, language skills, verbal learning and memory, speed of information processing, consistency of task performance, cognitive flexibility, planning, and academic performance (Korkman, Kirk, & Kemp, 1998; Mattson, Riley, Delis, Stern, & Jones, 1996; Streissguth, Barr, Bookstein, Sampson, & Carmichael Olson, 1999). Furthermore, the array of deficits that accompany FAS/FEA often exceeds what would be predicted based on level of intelligence, suggesting that limited cognitive ability is not the sole basis for these impairments (Kerns et al., 1997). Thus, multiple cognitive domains of functioning are vulnerable to in utero alcohol exposure including intellect, language, learning and memory, and executive functions (Lee, Mattson, & Riley, 2004).

Interestingly, the ratings of parents and teachers suggest that the primary behavioral difficulties of children with FAS/FEA relate to attention deficits and social problems (Streissguth & Connor, 2001). Empirical support for the observations of parents and teachers regarding the poor attentional regulation associated with FAS/FEA is growing (Lee, Mattson, & Riley, 2004; Mattson, Lang, & Calarco, 2002). Moreover, there are indications that poor attention may be a more sensitive marker of prenatal alcohol exposure than either low global intelligence or facial stigmata (Mattson & Riley, 2000).

The myriad of behavioral, adaptive, and neuropsychological characteristics of the child with FAS/FEA signals the need for a multidisciplinary approach to assessment. Clearly, a comprehensive neuropsychological evaluation is needed to identify and interpret the cognitive, behavioral, and adaptive dysfunctions that characterize the child. Because of the increased risk for cardiac, skeletal, and other physical conditions (see Table 10.6), a medical consultation is certainly warranted. Finally, contingent on the child's presenting issues, the evaluative services of a speech and language pathologist, educational specialist, social worker, and occupational/physical therapist may be warranted.

Developmental Course—Longitudinal studies (Streissguth, 1997) have revealed that the cognitive, behavioral, and adaptive deficits of FAS/FEA children do not fully resolve with age. Thus, the negative effects of intrauterine exposure to alcohol generally endure. Infants with FAS/FEA often present with low birth weight, feeding and sleep disturbances, poor habituation, and high levels of irritability (Jenkins & Culbertson, 1996). By 4 years of age, deficits appear in gross- and fine-motor skills, attention, memory, academic achievement, and reaction time. In addition, **enuresis** (age-inappropriate bedwetting) and communication disorders are quite frequent. By elementary school age, attention-deficit/hyperactivity disorder (ADHD)

symptoms of inattention, impulsivity, and hyperactivity, coupled with poor organization, communication deficits, behavioral problems, and disturbances of basic functions (sleeping, eating, and elimination) disrupt the adaptive efforts of FAS children (Steinhausen, Willms, & Spohr, 1993). Cognitive deficits, microcephaly, small physical stature, and poor socialization skills often interfere with peer acceptance. Children affected by FAS/FEA with significant intellectual and learning deficits are often identified in their preschool or elementary years and provided with early special education services.

With the advent of adolescence, communication disorders and disturbances of basic functions decline, although other cognitive and behavioral deficits persist. Reports that teenagers with FAS/FEA tend to manifest high rates of antisocial behaviors and substance abuse are of considerable concern. Unfortunately, the multiple cognitive, behavioral, and adaptive deficits of FAS/FEA appear to continue into adulthood.

Treatment—It goes without saying that the best form of treatment for an acquired disorder is prevention. Avoiding or significantly reducing alcohol consumption during pregnancy eliminates or reduces the risk for FAS/FEA to the unborn child. Although public awareness discourages many mothers from drinking during pregnancy, the alcoholic mother is of special concern. The physician, or other personnel who encounter a pregnant women who abuses alcohol, should immediately apprise her of the risk to the fetus. In addition, the mother should be informed that emerging research indicates that children of mothers who appreciably reduce or cease drinking during the first or second trimester are at a reduced risk for development of FEA/FAS (Korkman et al., 2003). A referral to persons or agencies that can assist the mother in altering her drinking behavior is a priority. Furthermore, the finding that FAS/FEA children often experience high levels of neglect, abuse, inconsistent parenting, and out-of-home placements should prompt an assessment of the family's need for therapeutic, social, and economic assistance.

Children with FAS/FEA who are mentally retarded generally require specialized educational services either within the public schools or in a residential setting, depending on the severity of retardation and particular learning needs of the child. Higher functioning children affected by FAS/FEA, despite average or above-average intelligence, may also need supplemental or specialized educational services due to specific cognitive and achievement weaknesses (Kerns et al., 1997). Furthermore, children with FAS/FEA with communication deficits should have appropriate speech and language therapy. Behavioral management systems are often needed within the home and school, particularly if the child also displays symptoms of ADHD. Medications can be introduced to help regulate the child's ADHD, particularly if the symptoms of inattention, impulsivity, and hyperactivity significantly disrupt the child's learning, family, and peer relationships. Social skills training may help improve peer acceptance. The aforementioned interventions must be continued into adolescence and modified in accordance with the changing learning and behavioral needs of the teenager.

Summary

The developing brain is vulnerable to a myriad of insults that can lead to damage and dysfunction. Yet, a degree of plasticity allows limited compensation, or return of function, after cerebral insults. However, the dynamics of this recovery process remain poorly understood. The clinical presentation, neuropathogenesis, neuropsychological assessment, and treatment of HC, TS, WS, and FAS illustrate the complex brain–behavior relations that define each of these neurodevelopmental disorders.

Critical Thinking Questions

- In light of the devastating effects of many of the genetic and chromosomal disorders, do you think that potential parents should seek genetic counseling before having children? Explain.
- In recent years, an increasing number of teratogens have been identified in the environment. Are our children at greater risk for brain anomalies than children of earlier generations? Why or why not?
- What steps can be taken to prevent FAS?
- What do the neuropsychological profiles associated with TS and WS tell us about the organization of the brain?

Key Terms

Phenylketonuria (PKU)
Teratogens
Agenesis
Dysgenesis
Polymicrogyria
Porencephaly
Kennard principle
Anencephaly
Hydranencephaly
Hydrocephalus (HC)
Spina bifida
Intraventricular hemorrhage (IVH)

Obstructive or noncommunicating hydrocephalus
Nonobstructive or communicating hydrocephalus
Shunt
"Cocktail party syndrome" (CPS)
Ultrasonography
Single-gene disorders
Chromosomal disorders
Parental imprinting disorders
Molecular cytogenic anomalies
Autosomes

Sex chromosomes
Cubitus valgus
Turner's syndrome (TS)
Karyotype
Vestigial ovarian streaks
Isochromosome
Mosaic karyotypes
Inhibitory control
Gonadotropins
Williams syndrome (WS)
Supravalvar aortic stenosis (SVAS)
Hypercalcemia
Hyperacusis

Hypotonia
Hypertonia
Joint contractures
Elastin
Fluorescent in situ hybridization (FISH)
Down's syndrome
Fetal alcohol syndrome (FAS)
Microcephaly
Fetal alcohol effects (FAE) or alcohol-related neurodevelopmental disabilities (ARND)
Enuresis

Web Connections

http://www.patientcenters.com/hydrocephalus
Hydrocephalus Center—provides information about hydrocephalus and its treatment.

http://gslc.genetics.utah.edu/units/disorders/karyotype
Genetic Science Center at the University of Utah—presents karyotypes for a number of genetic disorders including TS and WS.

http://www.turner-syndrome-us.org
Turner's Syndrome Society of the United States—facts and information on TS.

http://www.williams-syndrome.org
Williams Syndrome Association—provides information on the identification and treatment of individuals with WS.

http://www.nofas.org
National Organization of Fetal Alcohol Syndrome—page dedicated to raising the public awareness of FAS; includes definition and strategies for working with children with FAS.

Chapter 11

LEARNING AND NEUROPSYCHIATRIC DISORDERS OF CHILDHOOD

Youth, even in its sorrow, always has a brilliancy of its own.
—*Victor Hugo, Les Miserables (1862)*

Learning Disabilities

Pervasive Developmental Disorders

Disruptive Behavioral Disorders

Tic Disorders

Neuropsychology in Action

11.1 Genetics of Learning Disabilities

11.2 Case Study of an Adolescent with Asperger's Syndrome

11.3 Case Study of a Child with an Attention-Deficit/Hyperactivity Disorder

> ### Keep in Mind
>
> ■ What are the specific neurocognitive assets and deficits of children with verbal and nonverbal learning disabilities?
>
> ■ Can a nonverbal learning disability directly disrupt a child's socioemotional adjustment?
>
> ■ Is Asperger's syndrome a separate disorder, or merely high-functioning autism?
>
> ■ What treatment interventions are effective for children with attention-deficit/hyperactivity disorder (ADHD)?
>
> ■ Why is there such a high rate of comorbidity among ADHD, Gilles de la Tourette's syndrome, and obsessive-compulsive disorder?

Overview

This chapter discusses learning, pervasive developmental, disruptive behavioral, and tic disorders of childhood. These four classes of disorders can significantly disrupt a child's developmental progression and adaption and often coexist with other conditions that further compromise the child's functioning. Although the pervasive developmental disorders occur less frequently, the impact of these conditions is profound, generally precluding self-sufficiency and independence and necessitating lifelong supervision.

The developmental disorders reviewed in Chapter 10 are often considered biological rather than psychological in origin because prominent anatomic brain defects and physical anomalies often accompany the disorders. Moreover, the cause of these disorders is generally traceable to genetic/chromosomal defects or prenatal disruption. In contrast, the causes of childhood learning and neuropsychiatric disorders are not as easily linked to congenital anomalies. Accordingly, theorists have often proposed psychological factors as determinants of these disorders. However, ongoing research and advances in neuroimaging are providing evidence that brain disturbances may, in fact, play a prominent role in the etiology of both learning and neuropsychiatric disorders.

This chapter examines, in detail, specific disorders that represent learning, pervasive developmental, disruptive behavioral, and tic disorders. The first disorder, dyslexia, has received considerable attention because of the importance of reading skills in our technologically advanced society. The second disorder, nonverbal learning disability syndrome (NVLD), reflects a major contribution of neuropsychology to the study of learning disabilities. Byron Rourke (1989), through his extensive research, has identified a specific pattern of neurocognitive assets and deficits that differentiates the NVLD from reading disabilities. The third disorder, autism, is a pervasive developmental disorder that has attracted a voluminous body of research. Despite this research, the cause and brain–behavior relations of autism remain poorly understood. We then review attention-deficit/hyperactivity disorder (ADHD), one of the most prevalent childhood disruptive behavioral disorders, comprising about 50% of the population of child psychiatric clinics (Cantwell, 1996). Similar to autism, ADHD is the focus of considerable research that transverses diverse fields of study. Neuropsychology and related fields have identified a number of brain–behavior relations of ADHD that are enhancing our understanding of the pathogenesis of this disorder. Finally, we examine Gilles de la Tourette disorder, a childhood tic disorder, that waxes and wanes in severity and presentation over time.

Learning Disabilities

Learning disabilities adversely affect the ability of the child to communicate and meet the challenges of education. Children with learning disabilities constitute between 7% and 15% of the school population (Gaddes & Edgell, 1993) and are one of the largest childhood groups referred for neuropsychological services (Culbertson & Edmonds, 1996). Controversy persists regarding the definition, diagnosis, etiology, and remediation of learning disabilities.

Generally, professionals define learning disabilities as impairments of one or more academic skills that cannot be accounted for by sensory or motor deficits; mental retardation; emotional disturbance; or environmental, cultural, or economic disadvantage (Hooper, Willis, & Stone, 1996). Common learning disabilities involve impairment of reading (**dyslexia),** arithmetic (**dyscalculia),** and written expression (**dysgraphia).**

Verbal learning disabilities, such as dyslexia, have received significantly more research and theoretical attention than the NVLD, which focuses on deficits in mathematics. We discuss dyslexia to help clarify, by contrast, the NVLD. An expanded coverage of the NVLD follows. This emphasis acknowledges the greater disruptiveness of the NVLD to the child and the availability of a specific neuropsychological model to guide identification and treatment of the disorder (James & Selz, 1997).

VERBAL LEARNING DISABILITY: DYSLEXIA

Dyslexia may be acquired by insult to a previously normal functioning brain or be developmental in origin. With acquired dyslexia (often referred to as *alexia*), the patient, before brain insult, possessed reading skills. However, after the insult, this ability is partially or fully lost.

In contrast, developmental dyslexia characterizes a limitation in the ability to *acquire* reading skills. Historically, the diagnosis of dyslexia has involved evidence of a significant discrepancy between the child's current reading achievement and grade level or intelligence. The discrepancy models that contrast reading to grade level or intelligence are currently under challenge, and alternative criteria for classification are being proposed (Siegel, 2003; Van den Broeck, 2002).

Dyslexia is a prevalent disorder, as evident in the finding that approximately 4% to 9% of school-age children are affected, with boys outnumbering girls 3 to 2 (Culbertson & Edmonds, 1996; Pliszka, 2003; Rumsey, 1996a). Similar to other developmental disorders, dyslexia tends to run in families, suggesting a genetic etiology. As Bruce Pennington reports in his discussion of the genetics of learning disabilities (Neuropsychology in Action 11.1), a child with parents affected with dyslexia is eight times more likely to exhibit the disorder than children of parents who are not reading disabled.

Visual Processing Model of Dyslexia

Despite a long history of research and investigation, the study of dyslexia continues to be fraught with divergent diagnostic criteria, putative classifications, and a myriad of theoretical explanations. However, a review of the research and theoretical models demonstrates increasing convergence on two basic subtypes. The first subtype encompasses children with significant reading deficits caused by possible visual and visual-perceptual anomalies, whereas the second relates to children whose reading impairment stems from auditory-language dysfunction. Reflecting this division are two forms of dyslexia: "surface" and "deep." **Surface dyslexia** refers to impaired whole-word reading and an unimpaired ability to sound out words, whereas **deep dyslexia** involves intact whole-word reading and impaired ability to sound out words. The former suggests an impairment of orthographic skills, and the latter, an impairment of phonologic skills.

In studies of the visual domain, researchers have examined eye movements and speed of visual processing (Eden, Stein, Wood, & Wood, 1995; Stein, 2001). Specifically, reading-disabled children and adults show slower flicker fusion rates when presented images of low spatial density and contrast (brightness). **Flicker fusion rate** is the speed at which two separate visual images fuse into a single image when rapidly presented. The magnocellular visual system controls the processing of this form of visual input, prompting the magnocellular-deficit theory of dyslexia.

The magnocellular-deficit theory centers on the two visual pathways of the human visual system, namely, the magnocellular and parvocellular pathways. Each of these pathways processes information from the retina and, in turn, transfers the information to the visual cortex for further processing (Figure 11.1). The **magnocellular visual system** consists of large cells that are located in the inferior region of the lateral geniculate bodies and are highly sensitive to movement, rapid stimulus change, low contrast, and spatial location. The **parvocellular visual system** involves smaller cells that are located dorsally in the lateral geniculate bodies and are responsive to stationary objects, color, high contrast, and fine spatial details (Birch & Chase, 2004; Skottun & Parke, 1999). The former system is activated during rapid **saccadic eye movements,** whereas the latter system is stimulated during eye fixation and is involved extensively in discriminating and identifying printed/written symbols. In reading, the individual makes a series of brief fixations, separated by saccadic eye movements. Neuroscientists hypothesize that the magnocellular visual system inhibits the parvocellular system at the time of each saccade, ensuring that the previous eye fixation image is terminated. In dyslexia, the magnocellular visual system may fail to appropriately inhibit the parvocellular system, resulting in a prolonged afterimage that interferes with reading; that is, letters seen in one fixation blur into the next fixation.

Neuropsychology in Action 11.1

Genetics of Learning Disabilities

by Bruce Pennington Ph.D., Department of Psychology, Director of Developmental Cognitive Neuroscience Program, University of Denver, Denver, CO

When I finished graduate school in clinical psychology in 1977, considerable controversy existed about the validity of the construct of learning disabilities. Some claimed the construct was a middle-class myth to excuse the poor performance of some children. Another possibility, offered by the psychoanalytic paradigm that dominated clinical work at that time, reduced learning problems to largely unconscious motivational problems. One of my supervisors only half-jokingly interpreted problems with addition as representing conflicts over oral issues, problems with subtraction as representing castration anxiety, and so on. Partly because I had minored in cognitive development in graduate school, I was quite curious about whether learning disabilities existed, and if they did, how to understand and treat them.

Serendipity played a major role in focusing my curiosity. My first job after graduate school was to help with a longitudinal study of children with abnormal sex chromosome numbers (the 45X, 47XXX, 47XXY, and 47XYY karyotypes) initiated by Dr. Arthur Robinson, a pediatric geneticist. These children had been observed since birth, and they were now of school age. It soon became clear that these children had higher rates of learning disabilities than either their siblings or children with abnormal numbers of sex chromosomes in only some of their cell lines (mosaics). Most interestingly, the type of learning disability a child exhibited was largely karyotype specific. These children provided strong evidence that some learning disabilities were influenced by genetic factors, and that different genetic factors affected different aspects of cognitive development and academic skill.

Suddenly, a whole new vista opened on the question of how valid the construct of learning disabilities was. The fact of differential genetic cause for at least some learning disabilities convinced me of their validity, and also gripped me with an intense curiosity to understand in detail how the genetic alteration lead to the alteration in cognitive development. It was clear to me that one of the missing links in this causal chain was the brain, and so I set out to learn all that I could about neuropsychology, as well as genetics. My new question was, How do the genetic alterations change brain development to cause specific changes in cognitive development? I also wondered whether genetic influences on learning disabilities were rare and limited to infrequent syndromes, such as abnormalities in sex chromosome number, or if they played a substantial role in learning disabilities that currently had no known cause.

An opportunity to answer this second question soon presented itself. Herbert Labs and Shelley Smith, both medical geneticists, invited me to help with their study of familial dyslexia by helping to define its cognitive phenotype. They had taken quite seriously Hallgren's (1950) classic study, which had demonstrated a possible dominant gene influence on dyslexia, and were studying genetic linkage in extended families with dyslexia to find such genes. In 1983, we published an article in *Science* that presented evidence for a gene influencing dyslexia located near the centromere of chromosome 15. That same year, Shelley Smith and I published in *Child Development* a review of what was then known about genetic influences on learning disabilities and speech and language disorders. Subsequently, I published a number of articles on the cognitive phenotype in familial dyslexia, finding that it was characterized by dysphonetic spelling errors and an underlying deficit in phoneme awareness.

It eventually became clear that a large proportion of the children who present clinically with dyslexia have affected relatives, and that the recurrence rate among first-degree relatives is quite high, about 35% to 45%. This means that if a parent is dyslexic, the risk for having a dyslexic child is about eight times greater than the risk in the general population. Thus, genetic influences on learning disabilities are not rare, but instead account for a substantial portion of the etiology of the most common learning disability, dyslexia.

The search for genes that influence dyslexia has continued. Shelley and I soon joined forces with John DeFries and colleagues at the Institute for Behavioral Genetics in Boulder, Colorado, who had independently conducted important family and twin studies of dyslexia. Together, we eventually identified the approximate location of a second gene that influences dyslexia, this time on the short arm of chromosome 6. Cardon and colleagues reported this discovery in *Science* in 1994. Three years later, a separate team at Yale and Bowman Gray medical schools essentially replicated both our linkage results, those on 15 and 6, in an independent sample of families with dyslexia (Grigorenko et al., 1997). Taken together, these findings are essentially the first replicated genetic linkage results for a complex behavioral disorder.

Therefore, some, but not all, of the questions I began with have been answered. Learning disabilities exist in much the same way that other complex medical phenotypes (such as obesity or heart disease) exist. There are genetic influences on them and a substantial portion (about 50% according to twin studies) of the variance in the most common learning disability, dyslexia, is attributable to genes. The approximate locations of two of these genes influencing dyslexia are now known. Other disorders have shown us that understanding genetic mechanisms can illuminate the brain mechanisms underlying learning disabilities. The challenge for the future (and for future developmental neuropsychologists) is to better understand both genetic and brain mechanisms in dyslexia and other learning disorders.

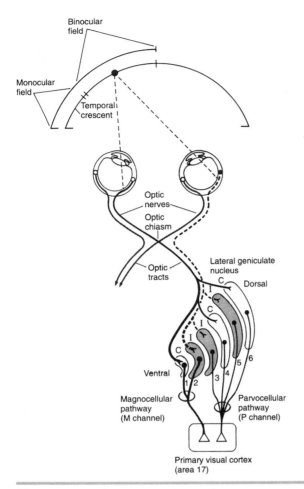

Figure 11.1 Magnocellular and parvocellular visual systems. The ventral magnocellular pathways are designated 1–2, and the dorsal parvocellular pathways are indicated by 3–6. (Adapted from Mason, C., & Kandel, E. [1991]. Central visual pathways. In E. Kandel, J. Schwartz, & T. Jessell [Eds.], *Principles of neural science* [3rd ed., p. 425, Figure 29-6]. New York: Elsevier Science, by permission of the McGraw-Hill Companies.)

Initial support for anomalies of the magnocellular system in dyslexic persons stems from investigations (Galaburda & Livingstone, 1993) of the lateral geniculate bodies of normal-reading and reading-disabled adults. Brain autopsies revealed that the parvocellular cells of the two groups were similar, but the magnocellular cell bodies were generally smaller and more variable in size and shape in the dyslexic group. The investigators propose that the structural differences in magnocellular cells are consistent with slower visual processing.

In a more recent study (Demb, Boynton, Best, & Heeger, 1998) of young adults with a history of dyslexia, tasks were presented that required the visual detection of moving stimuli. Dyslexic and healthy adults underwent functional magnetic resonance imaging (fMRI) while performing the tasks. The fMRI showed less activation in the magnocellular pathway of the individuals with dyslexia relative to control participants. Furthermore, magnocellular-occipital areas of activation correlated significantly with reading speed, which is supportive of a relation between magnocellular deficits and reading performance. Although dyslexia may be causally related to the disruption of magnocellular-parvocellular visual processing, it may also represent a more generalized deficit in rapid temporal processing.

Phonologic Model of Dyslexia

Although dyslexia as a consequence of underlying deficits in visual processing has received attention, impairment in phonologic processing as the central feature of the disorder has received greater support (Swanson, Mink, & Bocian, 1999). The term *phonologic processing* refers to the application of rules for translating letters and letter sequences into their corresponding speech–sound equivalents. This processing is supported by **phonologic awareness,** the awareness of and ability to differentiate between individual phonemes, or speech sounds (Rumsey, 1996a). Children with dyslexia exhibit deficits in translating letter strings into word sounds, also called *word decoding.* Deficits in this process cause reading to be slow and nonautomatic, disrupting efforts to identify and comprehend presented words (Pennington, 1991). The word recognition deficits of the child with dyslexia are most evident when he or she must read novel or unfamiliar words, that is, when the determination of letter–sound associations is most critical. Moreover, children with dyslexia often have problems spelling because they are unable to efficiently translate the phonologic representation of a word to its visual configuration, a process that is the converse of reading. Despite these deficits, children with dyslexia frequently demonstrate preserved "listening comprehension" when someone reads material to them. Furthermore, higher order cognitive functions such as general intelligence and reasoning, vocabulary, and syntax are typically unimpaired (Shaywitz & Shaywitz, 2005).

Early deficits in phonologic processing are predictive of later reading achievement, and interventions to remediate phonologic skill weaknesses facilitate the acquisition of reading skills (Shaywitz & Shaywitz, 1999). Individuals with severe phonologic deficits continue to show reading deficits into adolescence and adulthood, suggesting that reading deficits are often a lifelong problem. Interestingly, adults who were dyslexic as children, but who show good reading outcomes in adulthood, continue to exhibit phonologic deficits and a slow reading rate. For example, they continue to experience significant decoding deficits when required to read or spell nonwords, such as *yite*. Researchers believe their improvement in reading reflects a compensatory expansion of their sight vocabulary.

Deficits in phonologic processing are often accompanied by a second deficit, naming speed. Reduced naming speed is commonly evident in dyslexic populations. Naming speed refers to the rate of retrieval of names for letters, digits, colors, and objects (Catts, Gillispie, Leonard, Kail, & Miller, 2002). Although debate continues as to whether naming speed is independent of phonologic awareness or a generalized deficit of cognitive processing, there are indications that naming speed is a precursor to reading fluency. The identification of two primary deficits associated with disabled reading has led to the double-deficit hypothesis. The **double-deficit hypothesis** poses that reading disabilities can result from deficits in either phonologic processing or naming speed. However, children with both deficits are at the greatest risk for reading impairment (Schatschneider, Carlson, Francis, Foorman, & Fletcher, 2002; Waber, Forbes, Wolff, & Weiler, 2004).

In addition to phonologic and naming speed deficits, some children with dyslexia also demonstrate limitations in working memory (a form of short-term memory in which information is both maintained and manipulated). As discussed earlier (see Chapter 9), working memory can be conceptualized as a higher order *central executive system* that interacts with and regulates two "slave systems," the articulatory phonologic loop and the visuospatial sketchpad (Baddeley & Hitch, 1994). The articulatory phonologic loop is a temporary buffer for maintaining and manipulating auditory and verbal information, whereas the visuospatial sketchpad provides the same functions for visual and visuospatial information.

All three working memory components support reading performance, but disruption of the central executive system and phonologic loop are more strongly related to reading disabilities. Support for the involvement of the executive system is provided by studies of the memory performance of children with dyslexia. When performing measures of auditory and verbal working memory (subserved by the phonologic loop), children with dyslexia show significantly poorer performance than unimpaired readers (Kibby, Marks, Morgan, & Long, 2004). They also demonstrate deficits when performing tasks that assess temporal order memory (memory for the sequence of events across time). Temporal order memory involves higher order cognitive processes supported by the executive system (Howes, Bigler, Burlingame, & Lawson,

2003). Further support for the involvement of the executive system includes the finding that under conditions of high-processing demands, such as attempting to recall and manipulate complex information, children with dyslexia demonstrate poorer memory for *both* verbal and visual information than unimpaired readers (Swanson & Sachse-Lee, 2001). That is, the executive system fails to effectively allot attentional resources to coordinate the two slave systems when confronted with high-processing demands. Despite these findings, it remains unclear whether working memory deficits are central or contributory to the etiology of dyslexia.

Neuropathogenesis of Dyslexia

The genetics of dyslexia is an area of significant study. Twin studies demonstrate that reading deficits are highly heritable ($h^2 = 0.81$), with a concordance rate of 83% for identical twins (Alarcón, Pennington, Filipek, & DeFries, 2000). Genetic studies have identified a linkage between reading disorders and genes on chromosomes 6 and 15. The heritability rate of phonologic processing is higher than that of sight-reading, suggesting a greater genetic basis for the former (Grigorenko et al., 1997). Although other genes are the focus of study, research investigations have most consistently replicated the link between chromosome 6 and reading disabilities (Wood & Grigorenko, 2001).

The primary emphasis of neuropsychological research concerning dyslexia has focused on the language cortex of the left hemisphere of right-handed individuals. The **planum temporale** of the left posterior temporal lobe (Figure 11.2) is one of the neural regions specifically implicated in phonologic processing (Hynd & Hiemenz, 1997; Morgan & Hynd, 1998). For most people, the planum temporales of the left and right hemispheres are asymmetric, with the left planum temporale being larger than the right (L > R). Neuroimaging shows that individuals with dyslexia often exhibit left-right planum temporale symmetry (L = R), or reversed normal asymmetry (R > L). However, the precise relation of atypical symmetry to dyslexia awaits clarification.

Regional anomalies of the brains of dyslexic individuals are also associated with differences in brain activation as revealed by cerebral blood flow. For example, a positron emission tomography (PET) study by Rumsey and colleagues (1992) reported less activation of the left posterior temporal and temporoparietal cortices of individuals with dyslexia relative to normal-reading control individuals when performing a task sensitive to phonologic awareness, namely, rhyme detection. A related PET study (Flowers, Wood, & Naylor, 1991) of dyslexic and normally

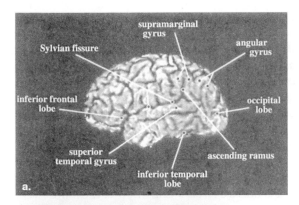

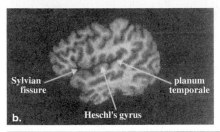

Figure 11.2 Brain regions implicated in dyslexia: (a) lateral view of the left hemisphere of the brain; (b) parasagittal slice through the left hemisphere. (Reproduced from Rumsey, J. M. [1996]. Neuroimaging in developmental dyslexia. In G. R. Lyon, & J. M. Rumsey [Eds.], *Neuroimaging: A window to the neurological foundations of learning and behavior in children* [p. 61]. Baltimore: Paul H. Brookes, by permission of Brookes Publishing Company.)

reading children found that the rate of cerebral blood flow to both the Wernicke's area (region surrounding the planum temporale) and angular gyrus related to reading performance.

Further evidence for disruption of the temporal and temporoparietal regions is provided by postmortem investigations of the brains of dyslexic individuals. Postmortem studies revealed **neuronal ectopias** (small loci of abnormally placed neurons, sometimes referred to as "brain warts") and **cytoarchitectonic dysplasia** (focal pathologic changes of cortical architecture) of the left plenum temporale, suggesting abnormal neural development, most likely between the 5th and 7th month of fetal gestation (Hynd & Hiemenz, 1997). During this period, the gyri are rapidly forming, suggesting that the origin of developmental dyslexia, whether genetically determined or a consequence of an insult, can be traced to a specific period of fetal development. However, not all studies have replicated the finding of atypical planum temporale development (Filipek, 1996; Rumsey, 1998), suggesting that other neural regions/systems may be involved in the etiology of dyslexia.

Greater specification of the neural substrates that support phonologic processing is emerging (Horwitz, Rumsey, & Donohue, 1998; Pugh et al., 2000). PET studies of regional cerebral blood flow activation demonstrate that regions of the left angular gyrus, superior and middle temporal gyri (part of Wernicke's area), inferior frontal cortex (near Broca's area), and extrastriate and striate cortex (occipital) activate when individuals without dyslexia read irregular words (reading that requires orthographic familiarity) and pseudowords (reading that requires the use of phonologic rules). The activation of these regions significantly correlates, suggesting a functional network supportive of reading. In contrast, individuals with dyslexia demonstrate reduced activation across the functional network, and the left angular gyrus fails to significantly correlate with the activation patterns of the other reading-related regions. The latter finding prompted the investigators to conclude that the left angular gyrus of individuals with dyslexia is functionally disconnected from the other regions of the network. Insofar as the angular gyrus is involved in the cross-modal transformation of visual (written) information into linguistic representations, the disconnection would limit or distort input to the other regions of the left hemisphere necessary for reading-related processing. Whether the functional disconnect is the result of anomalies in the white matter interconnecting pathways that link the left angular gyrus with the other reading-related regions of the left hemisphere, functional anomalies specific to the angular gyrus, or some other unknown set of factors remains to be determined.

In a particularly well-designed study, Shaywitz and colleagues (1998) endeavored to identify the neural substrates that correlated with reading performance. Hierarchically arranged orthographic and phonologic tasks, progressing from simple to complex, were presented to adolescents and adults with dyslexia and participants without dyslexia while undergoing fMRI. The progression and type of tasks presented were as follows: (1) judgment of line orientation (visuospatial processing without orthographic demands); (2) lowercase and uppercase letter discrimination (orthographic processing without phonologic demands); (3) single-letter rhyming (orthographic to phonologic coding and analysis); (4) nonword rhyming (complex orthographic to phonologic coding and analysis); and (5) semantic categorization (orthographic, phonologic, and semantic analysis). As the presented tasks progressed from lowercase and uppercase discrimination through nonword rhyming, unimpaired readers manifested increasing and systematic activation of the *left* posterior superior temporal gyrus, angular gyrus (parietal), and extrastriate and striate cortices (occipital), whereas individuals with dyslexia did not demonstrate this progressive activation. The dyslexic group showed greater activation of the right inferior frontal gyrus as phonologic demands became more complex. This increased activation of the right anterior regions suggests that individuals with dyslexia rely on alternative or "spared" circuitry to process reading contents. Thus, individuals with dyslexia demonstrated decreased activation of posterior brain regions that encompassed *both* visual and language areas, and an increased activation of anterior brain regions. This activation profile may provide a neural "marker" for identifying individuals with dyslexia.

Shaywitz and associates (2002) extended their study to dyslexic and non–reading-impaired children and adolescents. The participants underwent fMRI while performing the previously discussed hierarchically arranged orthographic and phonologic tasks. The regional activation patterns of the children and adolescents with dyslexia differed from those of the nonimpaired readers. Furthermore, the regional activation patterns paralleled those identified in Shaywitz and colleagues' (1998) earlier study. Based on the findings of these two studies and subsequent investigations (Shaywitz et al., 2003; Shaywitz & Shaywitz, 2005), three reading-related systems were posed. Two of these systems involve the left posterior region, and the third involves the left anterior region of the brain. The first system, located in the left dorsal parietotemporal area (angular gyrus and posterior portions of the superior temporal gyrus), is believed to support the mapping of visual print to its phonologic representation. This word analysis system operates on individual units of words (for example, phonemes), requires attentional allocation, and processes information slowly. The second system encompasses the left ventral occipitotemporal region (portions of the middle occipital and middle temporal gyrus) and operates on the whole word (visual word recognition). This visual word system requires minimal attentional allocation and serves the automatic and rapid recognition of words. The final system is localized in the left inferior frontal region of the brain (Broca's area) and is implicated in articulation, silent reading, and naming. Disruptions of the two posterior systems are the primary determinants of dyslexia.

Two other neural regions, the corpus callosum and frontal cortex, have received attention in the study of dyslexia. Investigative studies of the structural integrity of the corpus callosum of dyslexic groups have produced contradictory findings. Specifically, studies of the anterior (genu) and posterior (splenium) areas of the corpus callosum of individuals with dyslexia and individuals with preserved reading skills have not shown consistent structural differences in these regions (Hynd et al., 1995; Larsen, Hoien, & Odegaard, 1992). Causal explanations for the relation of the corpus callosum to dyslexia, when structural differences are identified, center on increased or decreased interhemispheric communication or inappropriate inhibition of one hemisphere by the other. Neuroscientist believe that these conditions disrupt the flow and integration of information between the two hemispheres that is necessary for reading.

The frontal cortex has also received attention, with researchers observing tentative differences between proficient and disabled readers. Children with either dyslexia or ADHD presented bilaterally smaller frontal cortices than a group of healthy children (Hynd, Semrud-Clikeman, Lorys, Novey, & Eliopulos, 1990). Moreover, the children with dyslexia differed from the other two comparison groups by exhibiting greater symmetry of the anterior region because of the smaller width of the right frontal lobe (R = L). Similarly, in a more recent pilot study (Semrud-Clikeman, Hooper, Hynd, Hern, Presley, & Watson, 1996), the smaller width of the right anterior frontal cortex was one of several anatomic variables that discriminated among dyslexic, ADHD, and healthy control children. The functional relation of the anatomic difference of the frontal lobe to dyslexia is unclear. However, the frontal lobes mediate a number of executive functions, such as mental shifting, allocation of attention, and working memory, that are crucial to reading (James & Selz, 1997). Support for a relation between executive dysfunction and dyslexia is emerging. For instance, in one study (Helland & Asbjørnsen, 2000), children with dyslexia showed deficits on measures of attentional flexibility and shifting relative to the performance of healthy control children.

In summary, reading is an exceptionally complex process that requires letter identification, phonologic and orthographic skills, naming speed, sequencing skills, attention, mental flexibility, and working memory. Furthermore, the **lexicon stores** (our "internal dictionaries") must be accessed to determine the meaning of words and to comprehend what is being read. These myriad functions require the support of multiple brain systems, with the left posterior regions serving a central role in skilled reading.

The next section explores NVLD. Children exhibiting NVLD potentially manifest distinctly different neuropsychological profiles from those with verbal learning disabilities. Whereas verbal learning disabilities are generally attributed to left hemisphere dysfunction and are implicated in reading disturbances, NVLD is attributed to right hemisphere dysfunction and is associated with deficits in mathematics (dyscalculia).

NONVERBAL LEARNING DISABILITY SYNDROME

Clinical Presentation and Prevalence

The concept of NVLD as a neuropsychological disorder has emerged from the ongoing investigations of Byron Rourke, who has attempted to identify the neurocognitive, psychosocial, and adaptive characteristics of children with learning disabilities. His investigative efforts revealed two basic subtypes of learning disability: one labeled R-S, for reading and spelling disability, and the other NVLD, for nonverbal learning disability syndrome. R-S children demonstrate weak psycholinguistic skills with relatively preserved skills in visual-perceptual, tactile-perceptual, psychomotor, and nonverbal/novel problem solving (Table 11.1). Reading and spelling skills are poor, with greater competency evident in mechanical arithmetic, although their performance is still below age expectancy. Rourke (1993) hypothesizes that the neuropsychological deficits of the R-S group are associated with left hemisphere dysfunctions.

In contrast, children in the NVLD group present essentially the opposite pattern of strengths and deficits as the R-S group (Table 11.2). That is, the NVLD group show relatively poor skills in visual-perceptual, tactile-perceptual, psychomotor, and nonverbal/novel problem-solving skills coupled with strengths in the psycholinguistic domain. They manifest major academic weaknesses in basic arithmetic but demonstrate preserved linguistic skills such as sight word reading (Harnadek & Rourke, 1994). Both groups exhibit comparable deficits in actual arithmetic achievement; however, Rourke (1993) attributes the poor performance of the R-S group to verbal deficits, and the low performance of the children with NVLD to weaknesses in visual-perceptual and nonverbal reasoning.

Researchers estimate the prevalence rate of NVLD within clinic populations at 5% to 10% (Rourke, 1989). Furthermore, NVLD represents between 0.1% and 1.0% of the entire learning disability population, with an overall male-to-female ratio of approximately 1.2 to 1.0 (Pennington, 1991).

Neuropsychological Pathogenesis

Rourke (1993) considers that NVLD reflects right hemisphere (particularly posterior) damage, or dysfunction, whereas R-S deficits more closely reflect problems in the left, language-dominant, hemisphere system. Rourke has adopted Goldberg and Costa's (1981) theorization of

Table 11.1 Core and Clinical Features of the Reading and Spelling Group

Neuropsychological Assets	Neuropsychological Deficits
Primary assets	*Primary deficits*
Motor and psychomotor	Auditory perception
Novel material	
Tactile perception	
Visual perception	
Secondary assets	*Secondary deficits*
Tactile attention	Auditory attention
Visual attention	Verbal attention
Tertiary assets	*Tertiary deficits*
Concept formation	Auditory memory
Problem solving	Verbal memory
Tactile memory	
Visual memory	
Verbal assets	*Verbal deficits*
Pragmatics	Phonology
Prosody	Verbal association
Semantic > phonology content	Verbal output (volume)
Verbal associations function	Verbal reception
	Verbal repetition
	Verbal storage
Academic assets	*Academic deficits*
Reading comprehension (late)	Comprehension (early)
Mathematics	Graphomotor
Reading	Mechanical arithmetic
Science	Reading
	Spelling
	Verbatim memory
	Word decoding
Socioemotional/adaptive assets	*Socioemotional/ adaptive deficits*
Activity level	Undetermined
Adaptive to novelty	
Emotional stability	
Social competence	

Source: Rourke, B., & Fuerst, D. (1996). Psychosocial dimensions learning disabilities subtypes. *Assessment, 3,* p. 281, by permission.

Table 11.2 *Core and Clinical Features of Nonverbal Learning Disability Syndrome*

Neuropsychological Assets	Neuropsychological Deficits
Primary assets	*Primary deficits*
Auditory perception	Complex psychomotor
Rote material	Novel material
Simple motor	Tactile perception
	Visual perception
Secondary assets	*Secondary deficits*
Auditory attention	Exploratory behavior
Verbal attention	Tactile attention
	Visual attention
Tertiary assets	*Tertiary deficits*
Auditory memory	Concept formation
Verbal memory	Problem solving
	Tactile memory
	Visual memory
Verbal assets	*Verbal deficits*
Phonology	Oral-motor praxis
Verbal association	Phonology > semantics content
Verbal output	Pragmatics function
Verbal reception	Prosody
Verbal repetition	
Verbal storage	
Academic assets	*Academic deficits*
Graphomotor (late)	Graphomotor (early)
Spelling	Mechanical arithmetic
Verbatim memory	Reading comprehension
Word decoding	Science
Socioemotional/adaptive assets	*Socioemotional/adaptive deficits*
Undetermined	Activity level
	Adaptive to novelty
	Emotional stability
	Social competence

Source: Rourke, B., & Fuerst, D. (1996). Psychosocial dimensions learning disabilities subtypes. *Assessment, 3,* p. 281, by permission.

brain functioning in conceptualizing the neuropathogenesis of NVLD. Goldberg and Costa propose that the right hemisphere, relative to the left, is more diffusely organized, has more association regions, and shows greater specialization for *inter-regional* integration of information. Because of its capacity to integrate input from multiple brain regions, the right hemisphere is more adept at processing complex, novel, or ambiguous information. In contrast, the left hemisphere is more focally organized, presents greater modality-specific cortical regions, and shows greater specialization for *intraregional* integration of input. The specialization of the left hemisphere is hypothesized to relate to the routine application of previously acquired cognitive strategies. The two hemispheres complement each other, with the right hemisphere showing prominence in establishing new rules, routines, or strategies, and the left storing and applying these newly established computations in similar situations or with comparable tasks in the future (Fisher, DeLuca, & Rourke, 1997).

Rourke (1995) maintains that the primary deficits of tactile-perceptual, visual-perceptual, and psychomotor abilities of NVLD are consistent with damage or dysfunction of right hemisphere inter-regional integration, whereas assets of auditory-perceptual and verbal skills suggest a relatively intact left hemisphere. He also views deficits such as poor problem solving in novel situations, or in the face of complexity, weaknesses in conceptual thinking, and impaired socioemotional skills as emanating from right hemisphere involvement.

Rourke suggests that, although right hemisphere damage is *sufficient* to produce NVLD, it is the destruction of the white matter (myelinated circuitry) required for inter-regional integration that is *necessary* for producing the disorder. That is, the development of NVLD can be caused by damage to white fibers (1) accessing the right hemisphere, (2) connecting cortical regions within the right hemisphere, or (3) linking cortical to subcortical regions within the right hemisphere (Rourke, 1995). Interestingly, Rourke hypothesizes that damage to these different communicating fibers accompanies diverse disorders in association with NVLD. For example, early damage to the association fibers of the right and left hemispheres could potentially cause both the primary features of NVLD and the global linguistic deficiencies that characterize autism.

Although Rourke emphasizes the posterior right hemisphere as playing an important role in the pathogenesis of NVLD, he proposes that the anterior brain regions may also be involved. For example, children with NVLD performed in a less efficient manner than children with

Table 11.3 *Brain Disorders and Insults Associated with Nonverbal Learning Disability Syndrome*

Asperger's syndrome

Autism

Callosal agenesis (absence of the corpus callosum)

Congenital hypothyroidism

Cranial irradiation

Fetal alcohol syndrome

Hydrocephalus

Insulin-dependent diabetes mellitus

Intracranial tumors

Metachromatic leukodystrophy (genetic metabolic disorder)

Myelomeningocele (neural tube defect)

Sotos syndrome (growth disorder)

Traumatic brain injury

Triple X syndrome (genetic neurodevelopmental disorder)

Turner's syndrome

Williams syndrome (genetic neurodevelopmental disorder)

Source: Adapted from Tsatsanis, K., & Rourke, B. (1995). Conclusions and future directions. In B. Rourke (Ed.), *Syndrome of nonverbal learning disabilities: Neurodevelopmental manifestations* (p. 486), New York: The Guilford Press, by permission.

verbal learning disabilities when presented tasks requiring higher order mental operations such as conceptual thinking and mental flexibility (Fisher, DeLuca, & Rourke, 1997). Moreover, Rourke (1995) indicates that the frontal system is necessary for (1) integrating lower level systems (such as sensorimotor) to formulate higher order levels of abstraction; (2) responding to novelty and complexity; and (3) **metacognition,** that is, the ability to understand the operation of one's own cognitive processes. Rourke believes that damage to the interconnecting white matter tracks between the frontal lobes and the posterior regions of the right hemisphere contributes to the deficits of higher order cognition evident in NVLD.

Many disorders and brain insults accompany NVLD, spanning genetic, chromosomal, structural, and environmental anomalies. Table 11.3 presents a partial list of implicated disorders. Although these disorders and insults represent a varied and seemingly dissimilar set of causative factors, clinical presentations, and developmental courses, Rourke and Del Dotto (1994) suggest that each shares a common pathway to NVLD, namely, dysfunction of the

white matter of the brain. These disorders represent a spectrum of neurodevelopmental conditions that vary in the severity of expression of NVLD, ranging from disorders that present virtually all the assets and deficits of NVLD (such as hydrocephalus and Asperger's syndrome), to those that display a majority of the assets and deficits (such as fetal alcohol syndrome and Turner's syndrome), and finally, to those that exhibit only a subset of the assets and deficits of the NVLD (such as autism). Thus, varying numbers of assets and deficits of NVLD are comorbid manifestations of these disorders caused by damage to the white matter (Rourke, 1995).

Neuropsychological Assessment

Harnadek and Rourke (1994) attempted to identify the primary neuropsychological deficits of the NVLD and R-S groups. The neuropsychological test data of three groups, NVLD, R-S, and healthy control children, was subjected to statistical analysis to determine the most discriminating measures for classifying the children into their respective groups. Two sets of tests statistically differentiated the NVLD, R-S, and healthy control groups. The first set of measures assessed visuospatial organization, tactile-perceptual, and psychomotor skills, and the second, academic (reading) and auditory-perceptual skills. The measures of visuospatial-tactile-psychomotor skills contributed significantly to the discrimination of the NVLD group from the R-S and healthy control groups, whereas the academic-auditory skill measures differentiated the R-S from the NVLD and healthy control groups. These two sets of measures accurately classified the children in their respective groups at an overall classification rate of 98%. Recently, using a larger sample of children with NVLD or reading/spelling deficits, the two sets of measures once again accurately classified children with R-S and NVLD into their respective groups (Pelletier, Ahmad, & Rourke, 2001).

As noted earlier, children with NVLD frequently exhibit arithmetic deficits. Rourke and Conway (1997) hypothesize that during the initial learning of arithmetic skills in childhood, the novel, visuospatial, and conceptual nature of the content recruit mainly right hemispheric systems. Once these skills are learned, however, they shift to the left hemisphere because of its greater facility in processing and retrieving automatic information (Dool, Stelmack, & Rourke, 1993).

Examining the mathematics performance of children with NVLD, researchers have identified seven overlapping errors (Rourke, 1993): (1) errors in spatial organization, (2) misreading or omitting required mathematic symbols, (3) failure to apply or misapplication of mathematic procedures, (4) poorly formed or spaced numbers, (5) failure to remember number facts or arithmetic rules, (6) difficulties shifting from one set of arithmetic operations to another, and (7) poor arithmetic judgment and reasoning. The latter error involves production of unreasonable solutions, or failure to generalize solutions, strategies, or plans for new or different arithmetic problems. Although children with other forms of learning and neuropsychological deficits can show errors involving spatial and retrieval deficits, several of the errors, particularly those due to poor judgment and reasoning, discriminate children with NVLD from other learning-disabled children. Errors in cognitive shifting, judgment, and reasoning potentially implicate deficits in executive function.

Socioemotional Characteristics

A broad set of adaptive and socioemotional disturbances accompany NVLD. Rourke believes these deficits are a direct consequence of the core deficits of the disorder (see Table 11.2). Of these deficits, the most prominent lie in the communication and interactional domains. The communication deficits appear in both verbal and nonverbal behaviors. At the verbal level, children and adolescents with NVLD tend to talk excessively, present tangential contents, and show a poor understanding of the **pragmatics of language,** that is, the emotional and social content of a message. Moreover, they find it difficult to understand the nonverbal behavior of others and to convey information through their own nonverbal behaviors (Rourke, Bakker, Fisk, & Strang, 1983).

Regarding social behavior, deficits in social sensitivity, interactional skills, social problem solving, and judgment seriously hinder the efforts of individuals with NVLD to relate to others. They are prone to misread or fail to appreciate the social intents, perspectives, or feelings of others. In addition, they do not accurately assess social cause-and-effect relations (Rourke & Fuerst, 1996). Social problem solving of children with NVLD is particularly compromised in new, changing, or complex social situations, often resulting in rigid or stereotypic responses that are inappropriate to the demands of the situation. Because of poor social judgment, caretakers and peers view the individual with NVLD as lacking in common sense. Frequently, the child or adolescent encounters difficulties generalizing social skills learned in one situation to another, even though the new situation is similar to the original learning context. Social conventions, such as maintaining eye contact and appropriate social distance, are often violated. Finally, the poor psychomotor skills and clumsiness of children with NVLD can elicit teasing and taunting from peers.

Although prone to acting-out behaviors and symptoms of ADHD while young (Voeller, 1996), children with NVLD tend to become shy and withdrawn with increasing age. Assessment by their mothers reveals that children with NVLD often present internalizing symptoms such as anxiety, depression, withdrawal, and poor social skills. Whether this is a direct response to their failures within the social sphere is unclear, although it is likely that social failings contribute to the emotional distress of children and adolescents with NVLD. The finding that children with NVLD exhibit increasing and more severe internalizing psychopathology (anxiety, depression, emotional lability, social isolation, and withdrawal) with age is of concern (Pelletier et al., 2001). In contrast, children with R-S deficits are less likely to demonstrate increased internalizing or externalizing (acting-out patterns) with advancing age.

Neuropsychological Model

Rourke's model of learning disability, with regard to subtypes such as NVLD and R-S, is summarized as follows:

Subtypes of LD [learning disabilities] are manifestations of distinct profiles of neuropsychological assets and deficits; the subtypes of LD may lead to specific problems in academic functioning, psychosocial functioning, or both; and, the relationship between profiles of neuropsychological assets and deficits, LD, and academic and social learning deficits can be understood fully only within a neurodevelopmental framework that takes into consideration the changing nature of the academic, psychosocial, and vocational demands that humans in a particular society confront. (Rourke & Fuerst, 1996, p. 278)

A hierarchical organization is evident, with primary neurocognitive assets and deficits leading to predictable and differential patterns of neuropsychological functioning (secondary, tertiary, and linguistic) that, in turn, directly affect academic, socioemotional, and adaptive functioning (see Tables 11.1 and 11.2). Thus, the adequacy of the child's sensorimotor development sets the stage for subsequent levels of cognitive development. The young child experiences the world through touch, movement, and vision. Contacting and exploring the environment through the basic sensory modalities fosters the development of increasingly complex and higher level mental structures. The early deficits of the child with NVLD in the tactile-perceptual, visual-perceptual, and psychomotor domains limit sensorimotor learning; and thus, hinder the formation of the basic building blocks necessary for the development of more advanced mental structures. Rourke and others believe these early limitations bias the later development of conceptual thinking, creative problem solving, communication skills, and socioemotional interactions. As the child moves into adolescence and developmental tasks become increasingly complex, the functional deficits become more apparent. Unfortunately, the impairments of the adult are even more pronounced, as evident in the common finding of marginal adaptive success across behavioral domains.

Little (1993) indicates that the primary deficits and assets of NVLD are a robust finding in the studies of learning disabilities. However, support for the socioemotional aspects of the disorder is less compelling. For example, Guy (1996) failed to find a greater prevalence of internalizing psychopathology in children with NVLD relative to healthy control children and children with verbal learning disabilities.

Developmental Course

The developmental course of NVLD is somewhat similar to the natural history reported for Turner's syndrome and higher functioning autistic/Asperger's syndrome children (see Pervasive Developmental Disorders section later in this chapter). For the NVLD infant/toddler, exploratory behavior and motor skills lag behind language development. With increasing age, delays hinder the development of self-help skills, and the child tends to depend too much on caretakers. Increasingly, the child encounters difficulties in the social domain, with playmates being either younger or older than the child with NVLD.

In the elementary years, children with NVLD are prone to act out, respond impulsively, exhibit hyperactivity, and encounter problems in sustaining attention (Rourke, Fisk, & Strang, 1986). Despite relatively advanced verbal skills, their communication patterns (both verbal and nonverbal) are often inappropriate. Misperceptions of social situations impair social problem solving and judgment, and poor social skills compromise efforts to relate successfully with peers. The child develops few, if any, close friendships, and during adolescence, peers often avoid teenagers with NVLD. Increasingly, teenagers with NVLD become socially withdrawn and isolated and show internalizing symptoms of anxiety and depression. Developmental patterns for adults with NVLD await clarification. Unfortunately, NVLD adults show elevated rates of psychopathology, and their risk for depression and suicidal behavior appears to be great.

Treatment

Because of the communication and social deficits often associated with NVLD, the child needs help developing verbal and nonverbal communication skills, basic social skills (such as greeting), and more advanced social skills (social awareness, friendship skills, and social problem solving). Early and ongoing interventions focused on the development of communication and social skills may improve the child's acceptance by peers. The young child with NVLD who exhibits ADHD symptoms may benefit from increased structuring of home and school activities, and the introduction of psychostimulant or related medications. Furthermore, parents can profit from learning management techniques to foster greater self-help skills and independence by the child.

Children with NVLD are at risk for development of psychological difficulties. Parents and professionals should be aware of this risk and prepare to provide early interventions if psychological problems arise. They should pay particular attention to the NVLD youngster with depressive symptoms that might signal an increased risk for suicide.

Rourke and Del Dotto (1994) have developed a comprehensive intervention program for children and adolescents with NVLD. The program actively involves the caretakers from its inception. A set of general principles organizes and guides treatment, with each program requiring individualization to accommodate the strengths and deficits of each child. Initially, the program provides the caretakers with information that helps them understand the nature and extent of the child's disorder and develop realistic expectations. Then the program provides interventions that will help the child (1) understand, learn, and generalize cognitive and social problem-solving strategies; (2) develop necessary communication skills; (3) engage and interact appropriately with others; (4) explore and experience his or her environment; (5) use available aids (such as a digital watch for learning time concepts); and (6) gain a realistic view of his or her strengths and weaknesses.

School-age children with NVLD are at risk for academic difficulties, particularly if spatial reasoning or executive deficits are severe. Academic subjects that can be particularly challenging to children with NVLD include handwriting and mathematics. Since it is highly unlikely that children with NVLD will outgrow these deficits, programs should be directed toward helping them develop compensatory skills and strategies. For example, children with NVLD often struggle with writing because of spatial and motor deficits. Accordingly, parents and professionals should encourage them, at an early age, to develop word-processing skills. Similarly, adolescents with NVLD need help in developing realistic academic and career goals in light of their individual strengths and visuospatial and mathematic weaknesses.

Evolution

NVLD, similar to other syndromes, is an evolving disorder. That is, the validity and clinical utility of the disorder is being evaluated based upon ongoing clinical investigations and research. This process is clarifying the major tenets, as well as prompting the modification of defining features, diagnostic criteria, and specification of differences from other disorders. For example, research is suggesting that children with NVLD do not necessarily exhibit deficits in the area of math calculation but rather in the visuospatial aspects of calculation. Venneri, Cornoldi, & Caruit (2003) determined that children with NVLD show knowledge of math facts and an understanding of calculations similar to that of healthy control children. In contrast, they made significantly more errors in the execution of written calculations, particularly when regrouping ("borrowing" or "carrying") was involved. In addition, children with NVLD demonstrated significantly poorer performance on measures of visuospatial skills and visuospatial working memory than healthy control children. The authors hypothesize that the poorer performance of the children with NVLD relates to visuospatial skill deficits, including visuospatial working memory weaknesses. Forrest (2004) has recently determined that children with NVLD were proficient in math operations (concepts and application) that allowed for the application of verbal abilities, but they faltered when confronted with mechanical arithmetic. The latter involved solving written calculations (for example, $3 + 9 = 12$), that is, problems that place greater demands on visual perceptual processing. Likewise, the author determined that visual-perceptual deficits were not generalized across all forms of visual and visuomotor tasks; rather, they appeared specific to the location of objects in space (spatial). Interestingly, children with NVLD did not demonstrate a greater prevalence of internalizing psychopathology (namely, depression or anxiety) than children with verbal disabilities and healthy control youngsters. This finding conflicts with an earlier study (Carey, Barakat, Foley, Gyato, & Phillips, 2001) of children treated for brain tumors who, upon assessment, demonstrated a profile consistent with NVLD including internalizing behavioral problems and social deficits. The children that participated in these two studies (Forrest, 2004; Carey et al., 2001) represent significantly different clinical populations, and further investigations are needed to determine under what conditions children with NVLD do or do not exhibit internalizing psychopathology.

Pervasive Developmental Disorders

Pervasive developmental disorders encompass a set of severe neuropsychological deficits that are evident early in childhood and have a poor prognosis for achieving normal adaptive functioning. To varying degrees, each of the pervasive developmental disorders involves impairment in one or more of the following domains of development: social interactions, verbal and nonverbal language, range of interests and activities, and flexibility of behavior. The behaviors manifested in these domains are age inappropriate and are disproportionate to the child's intelligence and age, even though mental retardation is frequently a correlate of the disorders. Researchers hypothesize that a myriad of central nervous system abnormalities play roles in the etiology of the pervasive developmental disorders. However, in many cases, the origin of the disorder remains unknown. Table 11.4 summarizes the primary pervasive developmental disorders and their associated behavioral features.

Table 11.4 *Distinguishing Features of Pervasive Developmental Disorders*

Autistic Disorder

Impairment or delays in the domains of social interactions and communications (including symbolic and imitative play), and repetitive and stereotyped patterns of behavior, interests, and activities, with age of onset evident before age 3.

Asperger's Disorder

Symptom presentation similar to autism with regard to delays in developing age-appropriate social interactions and repetitive and stereotyped patterns of behavior, interests, and activities. Unlike autism, few significant developmental delays in language, cognitive, adaptive (other than social), self-help, and exploratory behaviors are evident.

Rett's Disorder

Initial normal psychomotor development with normal head circumference. Between 5 and 48 months, head growth decelerates, accompanied by the loss of acquired hand motor movements, diminished social interest, emergence of poorly coordinated gait or trunk movements, and severely impaired language development with psychomotor retardation. Present only in female children.

Childhood Disintegrative Disorder

Normal development across behavioral domains is evident until 2 years of age or later. Previously acquired skills deteriorate in two or more of the following domains: language, social or adaptive behaviors, elimination control, play, or motor skills. The emergence of autistic-like symptoms in social relatedness, communication, and repetitive and stereotypic behavior is evident. The loss of skills can plateau or continue to decline if accompanied by a degenerative neurologic disorder. Present in male and female children, with greater prevalence in male children.

AUTISM

Background and Clinical Presentation

Leo Kanner and Hans Asperger are credited with the identification, first theoretical conceptualizations, and labeling of the developmental disorder **autism** (Frith, 1989). Autism entails severe impairments in social relatedness and language development, and the presentation of unusual, repetitive, and/or stereotypic patterns of behavior. Kanner, working in Baltimore, and Asperger, working in Vienna, each studied a group of disturbed children for whom there was little recognition, much less understanding. Independently, each published their classic articles (Asperger, 1944/1991; Kanner, 1943) without consultation or reported awareness of the other. Remarkably, both used the term *autistic* in characterizing the disorder. Asperger's work, largely ignored until recent years, is often associated with a higher functioning level or subtype of autism, **Asperger's syndrome,** in which near-normal to normal functioning is evident in several behavioral domains (Frith, 1991).

The first area of disturbance in autism, impairment in the ability to relate to others, particularly with regard to understanding and entering into reciprocal social relationships, is the cardinal symptom of the disorder. Kanner (1943) referred to this dramatic aspect of behavior as **"autistic aloneness,"** a psychological state of profound separation and disconnection from other people. At a behavioral level, the child with autism exhibits this social disconnection by displaying the following characteristics: (1) a limited awareness of, or interest in, the desires, needs, distress, or presence of others; (2) an emotional remoteness or aloofness; (3) a failure to share activities, pleasures, and achievements with others; (4) a lack of understanding of social convention; (5) an impairment in social perspective and empathetic role taking; (6) a restricted repertoire of social skills, such as greeting behavior; and (7) awkward or stereotypic responses to others (Bailey, Phillips, & Rutter, 1996). Moreover, children with autism often show deficits in **joint attention** (reciprocal attention between the child and another), poor conversational skills, lack of eye contact, unusual body postures or gestures, and inappropriate facial expressions (Charman, 1997; Tanguay, 2000).

The second core characteristic of autistic behavior, deficits in communication, appears as impairments of language expression and comprehension. Spoken language may be delayed in onset or fail to develop altogether, and the child makes little effort to compensate through nonverbal behaviors such as gestures or facial expressions. When language is used, the child may restrict it to the repetitive use of stereotypic or idiosyncratic content. Caretakers see deficits in the understanding and use of pragmatics of language (Rumsey, 1996b) and deviant forms of language such as **echolalia** (repeating the words or phrases of others), pronoun reversal, and **neologisms** (invention of words). The ability to understand language is often impaired and is limited to the comprehension of simple, literal contents.

The ability to initiate and enter into symbolic, pretend, or imitative play is minimally developed (McDonough, Stahmer, Schreibman, & Thompson, 1997). Initially, the child shows little interest in toys, suggesting delayed or poor comprehension of the symbolic meaning of toys (Rutherford & Rogers, 2003). As interest develops, the child manipulates toys repetitively as objects without symbolic or imaginative connotations. Insofar as pretend play is considered necessary for the development of social and communication skills, it is diagnostically significant that the child with autism rarely partakes in complex, imaginative, or cooperative play.

The third core feature of autism relates to one or more of the following unusual behavioral patterns: (1) preoccupation with specific areas of interest, objects, or qualities of objects; (2) demands for environmental or behavioral sameness; and (3) stereotypic body movements or abnormalities of posture (American Psychiatric Association [APA], 1994).

A fascination with and abnormal focus on areas of interest (such as geography), objects (fans, vacuum cleaners, and so on), parts of objects (such as buttons), movement of objects (such as spinning toys), or activities (such as drawing) can dominate the child's daily pursuits. Moreover, the child may demand the maintenance of constancy (for example, the child's room cannot be altered), order (toys must be lined up in a certain manner), or routine (the child must always walk the same route to the playground). Interference or disturbance of the child's involvement in areas of interest or the child's efforts to maintain constancy can prompt a range of responses from irritation, to overwhelming anxiety, to thunderous rage. Finally, disturbances of motility can encompass a wide range of movements such as rocking, spinning, twisting, or hand flapping. A variety of unusual postural movements may also be evident, such as a tendency to walk on tiptoe, holding the hands in an awkward manner, and walking without moving the arms.

Demographic and Comorbid Conditions

Researchers estimate the prevalence rate of autism at 10 affected children per 10,000, whereas the prevalence rate for Asperger's syndrome is 2 to 2.5 per 10,000 (Fombonne, 2001, 2003a). Males outnumber females with autism by a 2:1 to 6:1 ratio.

Concern exists that the prevalence of pervasive developmental disorders, particularly autism, is increasing at an alarming rate. A review of relevant epidemiologic studies reports an increase in prevalence from 4.4 per 10,000 for the years 1966 through 1991 to 12.7 per 10,000 for the years 1992 through 2001 (Fombonne, 2003a). An examination of the studies suggests that the increase may be spurious. Specifically, the increase may relate to the following factors: (1) changes and broadening of the diagnostic criteria for autism (for example, APA, 1994); (2) different methods used to identify individuals with autism; (3) increased focus and emphasis on identification, especially for the very young; (4) increased referrals for services and interventions; and (5) diagnostic substitution (Fombonne, 2003a,b; Volkmar, Lord, Bailey, Schultz, & Klin, 2004). Concerning diagnostic substitution, a study (Fombonne, 2003b) of the prevalence rate of autism in the state of California showed an increase from 5.8 to14.9 per 10,000 for the years 1987 to 1994, whereas the number of children diagnosed as mentally retarded during this same period decreased from 28.8 to 19.5 per 10,000. The change in the two prevalence rates suggests that greater numbers of individuals who, in earlier years, would have been classified as mentally retarded were being identified as autistic. There is a dearth of well-developed and comprehensive epidemiologic studies concerning the incidence and prevalence rates for autism, and we await the development and results of future studies to determine whether the rates of autism are actually increasing.

Many children with autism (approximately 70%) function within the retarded range of intelligence, as evident in intelligence quotient (IQ) scores below 70 (Fombonne, 2003a). Interestingly, the ratio of male to female individuals with autism is largest for those of normal intelligence, but is approximately 2 : 1 (male/female) for those individuals with autism who are mentally retarded. An inverse relation exists between IQ and severity of autistic symptoms. That is, the higher the level of intelligence, the less severe the autistic symptoms. Circumscribed abilities and skills of exceptional levels (such as **hyperlexia,** or early acquisition of reading skills without comprehension) may appear within the context of severe mental retardation. The rate of **savant skills**—that is, extraordinarily developed skills within the context of limited cognitive capability—in autism is estimated to be 10 times that of the normal population (Waterhouse, Fein, & Modahl, 1996). The risk for seizure disorders is high in

autistic groups, with a mean rate across studies of 16.8% and even higher for autistic children with IQs less than 50 (Fombonne, 2001; Fein, Joy, Green, & Waterhouse, 1996).

High-Functioning Autism or Asperger's Syndrome?

Currently, controversy exists over whether the two primary representatives of pervasive developmental disorders, autism and Asperger's syndrome, are separate disorders, overlapping subtypes, or one disorder with Asperger's syndrome representing individuals with autism who are higher functioning, both cognitively and adaptively. Before considering this controversy, we review the symptom presentation of Asperger's syndrome.

The term *Asperger's syndrome* refers to a group of children, adolescents, or adults who exhibit autistic-like symptoms but do not strictly fulfill the autism criteria. The criteria for autism and Asperger's syndrome of the American Psychiatric Association (1994) show a significant overlap in symptoms related to impairments in social interactions and preoccupations with narrow, repetitive, and stereotypic patterns of behavior, interests, and activities. Despite this overlap, the APA proposes several differences. Specifically, children with autistic-like behavior are *not* to receive the diagnosis of Asperger's syndrome if they exhibit the following characteristics: (1) significant impairment in verbal and nonverbal communication skills, (2) a lack of developmentally appropriate symbolic or imaginative play, (3) delayed language development or absence of language, (4) cognitive deficits, (5) impairment in self-help and adaptive skills (excluding those involving social interactions), and (6) limited or absent exploratory curiosity (Bailey et al., 1996). These exclusionary criteria are consistent with Asperger's original behavioral description of children exhibiting the disorder. That is, these children display poor social skills, odd and eccentric behaviors, and restrictive patterns of interests and activities, without significant delays in cognitive or language abilities.

Research studies (Eisenmajer et al., 1996; Volkmar et al., 2004) have sought to further clarify the differences between Asperger's syndrome and autism. Children diagnosed as exhibiting Asperger's syndrome, as contrasted with autism, show a greater (1) desire for social contact and friendship; (2) willingness to participate in play with other children centered on their special interest, such as dinosaurs; (3) likelihood of normal onset of language development and an absence of echolalia and pronoun reversal; (4) use of odd words of speech, pedantic speech, and one-sided, repetitive conversations; (5) tendency to pursue narrow and limited areas of interest, such as preoccupation with clocks; and (6) likelihood of being inattentive, impulsive, and overactive. However, these differential characteristics have been challenged in recent studies (Macintosh & Dissanayake, 2004; Mayes & Calhoun, 2001).

The separation of the two disorders poses several challenges. First, varied definitions and differential selection criteria artificially blur the boundaries between the two disorders, hindering efforts to identify commonalities and differences in cognition and behavior, etiology, and responsiveness to differential treatments. In addition to the major diagnostic criteria of the DSM-IV (APA, 1994) and International Classification of Diseases (ICD-10; World Health Organization, 1992), no less than five other widely publicized definitions of Asperger's syndrome exist (Volkmar & Klin, 2000). Each definition leads to differences in selection criteria, areas of study, and research results, thus hindering efforts to determine whether the two disorders are independent of one another.

Second, the reported difference between autism and Asperger's syndrome may reflect the level of intellectual or language development of the two disorders. By definition, one criterion for differentiating Asperger's syndrome from autism is the relative absence of language and cognitive impairment in Asperger's syndrome. Thus, children with Asperger's syndrome may simply be brighter children with autism who show fewer language deficits.

Third, a number of studies are flawed by the failure of the investigators to use outcome measures that are independent of those used for the selection of the participants. For instance, it is certainly appropriate for researchers who are interested in identifying the differential characteristics of Asperger's syndrome and high-functioning autism to use a measure of motor functioning to form the two groups. As a result of this selection criterion, one group would consist of children who exhibit motor deficits and the other group would include children who did not. However, in the formal study of the two groups, it would then be inappropriate to assess them with motor measures in an effort to determine whether motor deficits differentiated between the groups. The circularity of this approach is evident, because the groups were originally selected based on their differences in motor functioning.

Fourth, young, higher functioning children with autism frequently exhibit behaviors consistent with Kanner's characterization of autism. However, with maturity, they often show fewer differences in symptom presentation from individuals with Asperger's syndrome (Howlin, 2003; Volkmar et al., 2004). Accordingly, Asperger's syndrome may merely reflect the changing presentation, over time, of higher functioning individuals with autism.

The case study of Tom Z. familiarizes the student with Asperger's syndrome (Neuropsychology in Action 11.2). The study details the symptoms, evaluative data, and family history of Tom Z., as well as some rather surprising neuroimaging findings.

Neuropsychological Pathogenesis

Various researchers attribute the development of autism to a host of causative factors. There are indications that the disorder is either familial or genetic in origin; however, the finding of high rates of perinatal complications in the history of children with autism also implicates environmental factors. Some evidence exists for an autistic diathesis, that is, a genetically mediated vulnerability for autism that interacts with an early environmental insult to produce the disorder (Pennington, 2002). However, a definitive number of environmental risk factors for the development of autism have not been identified. For instances, there is public concern that the combined measles-mumps-rubella (MMR) immunization (or substances used as a preservative of the active immune agents) places children at risk for autism. Empirical studies, to date, have not supported a relation between autism and immunizations (Fombonne, 2003b). For instance, in Yokohama, Japan, the combined MMR immunization was withdrawn beginning in 1988 with no child receiving the vaccine as of 1993 or thereafter. Single immunizations for each of these diseases continued to be administered. The cumulative incidence of autism increased significantly between 1988 and 1993, with the highest increase evident in 1993 (Honda, Shimizu, & Rutter, 2005). The findings indicate that the increased incidence of autism was unrelated to the MMR vaccination. Unfortunately, the public concern over a possible relation between the MMR immunization and autism has prompted some parents to withhold MMR inoculations from their children. Clearly, such a decision increases the risk for the children to contract one or more of these diseases.

Support for a familial/genetic component of autism is the finding of relatively high rates of the disorder in the siblings of children with autism. The rate is approximately 3% to 6%, which is 25 to 50 times greater than the incidence in the normal population (Fombonne, Bolton, Prior, Jordon, & Rutter, 1997; Sutcliffe & Nurmi, 2003). Heritability studies of identical twins reveal co-occurrence rates of 60% to 92%, whereas rates for fraternal twins range from 0% to 10% (Tanguay, 2000). The substantial

Tom Z. is a tall, stocky 15-year-old male adolescent. He was born after an uncomplicated pregnancy, and subsequent developmental milestones were achieved within normal limits. Tom talked before he walked. He taught himself to read by age 3 and was reading adult-level books by age 4. By the age of 2.5 years, he had atypical interests that were pursued to the exclusion of other activities. Over the years, these interests have included stop signs, arrows, storm drains, windmills, clocks, mathematics, and computers.

In nursery school, he had poor peer relations, talked incessantly about topics of interest only to himself, failed to listen to the comments of others, and was often oppositional and impulsive. A clumsy and poorly coordinated child, he often seemed markedly odd. A preschool psychological assessment recommended special education placement, and the parents tried various programs with limited success. They finally moved him to homebound education. Despite precocious academic achievements, Tom continued to have significant problems with social interaction and in controlling his behavior.

At his first formal evaluation, when he was 9.5 years old, Tom had no friends, poor interpersonal skills, and signs of depression. His fascination with clocks pervaded all conversation. His poor social judgment was clearly evident, particularly in his description of interactions with peers. He showed limited nonverbal social behaviors, such as gestures, facial grimaces, emphasis of voice, and nonliteral communications. Interestingly, Tom's father had a history of similar problems. For example, Mr. Z. carried a small notebook to write down the names of important people he met because, "I can never remember people's faces; I can only remember names when I write them down."

Tom was evaluated again when he was 12 years old. He continued to show a markedly eccentric social style and engaged in one-sided conversations about computers

and mathematic concepts in a loud, poorly modulated voice. His limited awareness of social conventions was evident in his one-sided conversational style, his tendency to belch and pass gas in public, and his use of graphic expletives without apparent intention to shock others. He was preoccupied with the subject of girlfriends and his sexual needs.

Tom's clinical presentation and assessment results were extreme in many respects. There was a significant discrepancy between his Wechsler Intelligence Scale for Children–Third Edition (WISC-III; Wechsler, 1991) verbal and performance abilities (Verbal IQ = 139; Performance IQ = 127). He had superior scores in verbal reasoning, except for tasks involving social comprehension. Although able to describe social demands, he could not translate this knowledge into appropriate conduct. He also exhibited significant deficits in visuomotor skills, speed of processing, and motor functioning. Moreover, a large difference existed between his superior intelligence score and his ratings on a measure of adaptive skills. His adaptive rating score was significantly below average, indicating severe deficits in meeting the demands of everyday life.

Neuroimaging

Father and son underwent magnetic resonance imaging (MRI) of the brain. The father's sagittal brain images showed a large V-shaped wedge of missing tissue in the dorsolateral frontal region of the brain (Figure 11.3a). This region of tissue loss appeared in the same location of both hemispheres, but was somewhat larger in the left. Given the absence of a history of trauma, the tissue loss likely represented an area of focal dysmorphology of unknown origin.

Tom showed a similar but noticeably smaller region of structural anomalies in exactly the same area of both hemispheres. His abnormality, however, was somewhat

larger on the right, the reverse of the father's (see Figure 11.3b). In addition, he showed decreased tissue in the anteromesial region of the left temporal lobe (see Figure 11.3c). The similarity of abnormalities in Mr. Z. and Tom indicated potential familial transmission.

Discussion of Magnetic Resonance Imaging and Psychological Testing

A three-dimensional rendering of the father's brain showed his neurodevelopmental abnormality to be in the region of the middle frontal gyrus (see Figure 11.3d). The deficit was a recessed area of absent tissue. Furthermore, the three-dimensional image showed an abnormality that did not appear on the two-dimensional images: both right and left frontal lobes showed an abnormal pattern of gyri and sulci. Normally, the frontal lobe consists of three prominent horizontal gyri (the superior, middle, and inferior gyri) that run in parallel from anterior to posterior. Although the father's superior frontal gyrus appeared normal, the middle frontal gyri were vertical in both hemispheres. This aberrant pattern of surface structure may have originated from an abnormal prenatal developmental process.

Because of movement artifacts, a clear three-dimensional representation of Tom's brain was not possible. However, researchers reconstructed coronal images by computer methods to evaluate his left temporal lobe abnormality. The images showed a large region of missing tissue and also an asymmetry of the lateral ventricles.

Any single case report must be interpreted with caution, yet it is of interest that Tom's neuropsychological deficits are understandable in light of his brain abnormalities and other studies of individuals with autism, Asperger's syndrome, and similar disorders (for example, see Piven et al., 1990). As described earlier, Tom's psychological testing demonstrated significantly higher WISC-III Verbal IQ relative to Performance IQ. Consistent with his greater nonverbal difficulties, Tom's frontal lobe abnormalities were

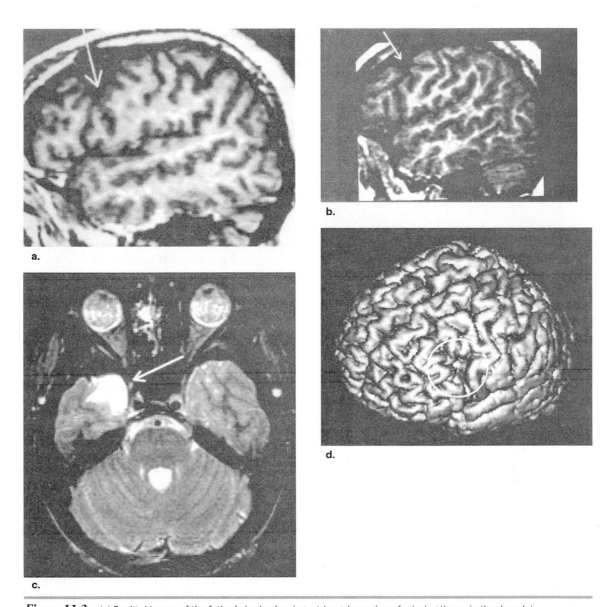

Figure 11.3 (a) Sagittal image of the father's brain showing a triangular region of missing tissue in the dorsolateral aspects of the left frontal lobe. (b) Sagittal image of the son's brain showing a similar but smaller abnormality in exactly the same location as the father's brain. (c) Axial view of the son's brain. The arrow points to the anterior mesial aspects of the left temporal lobe, where a pocket of cerebrospinal fluid fills a region of decreased brain tissue. (d) Three-dimensional reconstruction of the father's brain images. The circle encompasses the region of missing tissue first seen in two dimensions in (a). (Reproduced from Volkmar, F. R., Klin, A., Schultz, R., Bronen, R., Marans, W. D., Sparrow, S., & Cohen, D. J. [1996]. Asperger's syndrome. *Journal of the American Academy of Clinical and Adolescent Psychiatry, 35,* 121–122, by permission.)

more prominent on the right than the left side. The right hemisphere is also more prominently involved than the left hemisphere in regulating language prosody and pragmatics (Kolb & Whishaw, 1990), two areas in which Tom performed poorly. Moreover, the volume of his left hemisphere was somewhat larger than that of the right. In a study published several years ago, Willerman, Schultz, Rutledge, & Bigler (1992) found that a larger left than right hemisphere predicted a higher Verbal IQ than Performance IQ in male individuals.

(continued)

(*continued*)
The frontal lobe findings may clarify Tom's motor difficulties and conceptual inflexibility. The structural abnormality was at the juncture of the primary motor strip, premotor area, and dorsolateral convexity, thus potentially affect-ing the functions mediated by each of these regions. The dorsolateral prefrontal cortex is known to be involved in the executive functions of working memory and shielding of cognitive operations from disruption by unwanted distractions (Goldman-Rakic, 1987a).

Source: Adapted from Volkmar, F. R., Klin, A., Schultz, R., Bronen, R., Marans, W. D., Sparrow, S., et al. (1996). Asperger's syndrome. Journal of the American Academy of Child and Adolescent Psychiatry, 35, 118–123.

co-occurrence rates for identical twins suggest that genetic factors play a significant role in the etiology of autism. Genetic research has implicated at least 20 genes as contributing to autism risk. Of these implicated genes, anomalies of chromosome 15q11-q13 have been frequently replicated across studies (Nurmi et al., 2003; Sutcliff & Nurmi, 2003).

The neural substrates considered to produce autism are numerous, but none has received unanimous support. Anatomic abnormalities, hypothesized or identified in autistic samples, have included most cortical and subcortical regions of the brain. In addition, empirical studies reveal differences in neurochemical systems, brain volume, proportion of white-to-gray matter, neuronal metabolism, and cellular migratory patterns of the cortex, prefrontal cortex, cerebellum, and limbic system (hippocampus, amygdala, and other limbic nuclei).

Studies have implicated abnormalities involving neurotransmitters as pathogenic of autism, with serotonin receiving the most attention. Serotonin (5-HT) is involved in regulating a number of brain functions, including learning, memory, sleep, pain responsiveness, mood, and inhibitory processes. In addition, there are indications that excessive 5-HT can disrupt social affiliation and attachment. Children with autism show 25% to 50% increase in serotonin (**hyperserotonemia),** although the precise role of 5-HT in the production of autistic symptoms is unclear. Even more troublesome are studies showing that elevated levels of serotonin are not specific to autism, with other disorders such as mental retardation also exhibiting hyperserotonemia (Anderson, 2002; Fein et al., 1996).

Converging evidence indicates that a large proportion of children with autism (14–30%) have a greater head circumference than healthy control children. Brain size is also larger (approximately 10%) in autistic populations (Volkmar et al., 2004). Of importance is the finding of small brain size at birth, followed by two periods of accelerated growth occurring at 1 to 2 months and 6 to 14 months of age. Subsequently, brain size in autism reaches its maximum growth by ages 4 to 5 years and thereafter begins to gradually decline. By adolescence and adulthood, brain size is similar to that of healthy adults (Courchesne, Carper, & Akshoomoff, 2003). Although the underlying neurobiological factors accounting for this developmental pattern are unknown, this growth profile may provide an early warning signal for the risk for autism. However, head or brain size enlargement may not have a direct causative role in autism insofar as there is little relation between head/brain size and specific autistic symptoms. In addition, other clinical populations show increased head/brain size, specifically **fragile X** syndrome and tuberous sclerosis (Tanquay, 2000).

A second area of convergence relates to the finding of atypical white-to-gray brain matter ratios in autistic populations (Schultz, Romanksi, & Tsatsanis, 2000). Although the pathogenic relation of disproportionate white-to-gray matter to autism remains to be clarified, it is hypothesized that it represents a disruption of the brain's interconnectivity (Volkmar et al., 2004). In turn, integrative brain functions are impaired. Interestingly, there is also speculation that the atypical white-to-gray matter may result in modularity of brain functions. Modularity relates to brain functions that are specific to relatively separate and independent brain regions or circuits. The high rate of savant capabilities in cognitively impaired autistic groups is consistent with a modular organization—that is, a set of neurally distinct, preserved, and self-contained mental functions.

Historically, the cerebellum has been thought to mediate motor behavior. Increasingly, clinical and research studies are reporting that the cerebellum is involved in a number of cognitive operations including attentional behavior, classical conditioning, and executive functions. Structural and functional abnormalities of the cerebellum in autistic populations are evident. For instance, studies have identified hyperplasia or hypoplasia of the cerebellar vermis lobules (Courchesne, Townsend, & Saitoh, 1994; Filipek, 1995). Malformation of the cerebellar vermis lobules is believed to cause a disruption of attentional shifting and possibly other cognitive processes often evident in autism. However, subsequent studies of cerebellar structure have produced negative results (Schultz et al., 2000). Furthermore, cerebellar anomalies are not specific to autism, as evident in similar malformations in the brains of mentally retarded populations.

The temporal and limbic system structures, including the amygdala, hippocampus, and entorhinal cortex, appear to play a major role in mediating human socioemotional behavior. Studies of the temporal lobe-limbic system of autistic populations reveal volumetric reductions, hypofunctional activity, and abnormalities in neuronal size and density (Schultz et al., 2000). The important findings of atypical facial processing in autistic groups are of particular interest. Orienting to and focusing on the faces of others initially occurs in early infancy and is an important precursor of healthy emotional and social development. Children with autism show a lack of interest in human faces and, in contrast, a preferential interest in objects as early as the first year of life.

The medial temporal-limbic system is intimately involved in facial and emotional processing. The fusiform and inferior temporal gyri (and possibly the lateral occipital gyrus and parahippocampal gyrus) are preferentially involved in facial and object processing, respectively. Because of its activation in facial processing, an area in the middle region of the fusiform gyrus is referred to as the fusiform face area (FFA). At least seven different studies of children, adolescents, and adults with autism (Piggot et al., 2004; Schultz et al., 2003; Wang, Dapretto, Hariri, Sigman, & Bookheimer, 2004) show reduced activation of the FFA to images of human faces. For instance, Schultz and associates (2000) have investigated the fMRI activation patterns of autistic (autistic and Asperger's syndrome) and healthy young adults of normal intelligence when performing facial and object discrimination tasks. The study revealed that subjects with autism demonstrated decreased activation in the FFA and increased activation of the inferior temporal gyrus when performing the facial discrimination task. In contrast, the healthy control participants showed significant activation of the FFA and decreased activation of the inferior temporal lobe. Both healthy control participants and those with autism activated the inferior temporal gyrus when viewing objects. Likewise, autistic groups have been found to show reduced activation in the FFA when required to match emotional facial expressions or identify mental states based on facial details (Piggot et al., 2004; Schultz et al., 2003). Overall, these studies indicate that autism is associated with atypical activation of a brain region related to a basic building block of socioemotional behavior, namely, facial processing. A failure to attend to the faces of significant others, and people in general, disrupts normal socioemotional learning during development and potentially contributes to the significant social disinterest and atypical interaction patterns that characterize autistic groups.

There are indications that the FFA may have an even broader role in the mediation of socioemotional behavior. In an ingenious experiment, Klin (2000) used a task, the Social Attribution Task, to assess the social cognitions of young adults with autism. The Social Attribution Task involves the presentation of systematic movements of geometric shapes that, when viewed by healthy individuals, are imbued with social meaning. In contrast, individuals with autism do not impose social meaning on these movements; instead, they describe the physical features of the stimuli. In a recent fMRI study (Schultz et al., 2003), healthy control participants were presented the Social Attribution Task, a face perception task, and control tasks. Of importance to our discussion is the finding of marked activation of the FFA for both the Social Attribution Task and face perception tasks, but not for the control tasks. The authors conclude that the FFA appears to have an important role in social attribution and judgment. However, the FFA is but one functional component of the limbic system, and attention by neuroscientists has also focused on other limbic structures, such as the amygdala.

The amygdala is richly interconnected with the temporal cortex and other cortical and subcortical regions. It is involved in emotional arousal, appraising the behavioral significance of environmental stimuli, attributing emotional valence to stimuli, and emotional learning (Schultz et al., 2003). Animal research demonstrates that damage to the limbic system, including the amygdala, can produce autistic-like behaviors (Bachevalier, 1994). In addition, atypical neuroactivation of the amygdala is apparent in autistic groups when processing facial (Wang et al., 2004; Sparks et al., 2002) and theory of mind tasks (Baron-Cohen, O'Riordan, Stone, Jones, & Plaisted, 1999).

Evidence also exists of anomalies in frontal lobe functioning associated with autism. Neuroimaging studies show atypical activation of the orbital and medial prefrontal cortices and anterior cingulate in individuals with autism (Schultz et al., 2000). Because of the rich interconnections of the frontal regions with limbic and other brain structures, the frontal cortices are in a position to integrate and regulate the internal and external inputs necessary for socioemotional behavior.

Increasingly, research and clinical work with autism and other populations has led to the theorization of a social brain network. Interconnected orbital and medial prefrontal cortices, anterior cingulate, amygdala, superior temporal sulcus, and FFA are believed to underpin the social brain. It is hypothesized that the orbital and medial prefrontal cortices play a role in integrating and regulating affective and cognitive processes, whereas the dorsomedial prefrontal cortex and cingulate support social cognition (thinking about the thoughts, feelings, and intentions of others and social judgment). The amygdala appears to be involved in modulating and interpreting the emotional significance of stimuli and in assisting the cortex with the integration of emotion and cognition for evaluation and action by the frontal lobes. The superior temporal sulcus supports facial expressions, social gestures, eye gaze, and facial recognition, while the FFA assists in facial discrimination and social attribution. Together, the latter two structures support the perception of social behavior (Schultz et al., 2000, 2003). Damage to different aspects of this distributed social brain network may account for the heterogeneity of cognitive, emotional, and social deficits of autistic populations. Obviously, the social brain network warrants additional empirical verification and possible expansion to include other limbic structures.

Neuropsychological Assessment

The diagnosis of autism requires a careful review of the child's developmental history and observations of the child with family members, teachers, and peers. In addition, a complete medical evaluation and review of pertinent medical records should be standard practice because of the potential presence of genetic and chromosomal abnormalities, the high likelihood of co-occurring medical conditions (such as seizures), and the association of autism with other neurodevelopmental disorders. Moreover, assessments by other disciplines (such as speech and language) are often needed to augment the evaluation.

The neuropsychological evaluation of the child with autism should involve a comprehensive assessment of cognitive and related behaviors. The selection of measures depends heavily on the unique presentation of the child. For example, the evaluation and selection of measures may be quite different for the child who has not developed language than for the child who has rudimentary language. Currently, the Autism Diagnostic Interview-Revised (Rutter, Le Couteur, & Lord, 2003) and Autism Diagnostic Observation Schedule (Lord et al., 2000) are two well-standardized measures that are considered the "gold standards" for the assessment of autism.

Cognitive Profiles—It was initially proposed that children with Asperger's syndrome and autism demonstrated differential cognitive patterns (Ehlers et al., 1997; Minshew,

1997). The Asperger's syndrome profile involves greater facility in verbal relative to visuospatial or visuomotor problem solving. This cognitive profile is consistent with that demonstrated by children with NVLD (Rourke & Conway, 1997; see Nonverbal Learning Disability section earlier in this chapter). The autism cognitive profile is the converse of the Asperger's syndrome profile. That is, children with autism demonstrate relative strengths in visual-perceptual and visuospatial as contrasted with verbal problem solving. The majority of subsequent studies (Macintosh & Dissanayake, 2004) are not supportive of these differential cognitive profiles. In fact, several of these studies have found no differences between the two groups, whereas others have shown the opposite cognitive profiles, with autistic groups showing relatively advanced verbal relative to visuospatial and visual-perceptual abilities.

Although differential profiles for autism and Asperger's syndrome are not fully supported, they do highlight the variability of performance that may be encountered in the neuropsychological assessment of this group, particularly as contrasted with mentally retarded populations where a more uniform suppression of cognitive abilities is often evident. However, individuals with autism often demonstrate poor performance on tasks that require higher level conceptual processes such as reasoning, inferring, integrating, and abstracting (Minshew, 1997). This deficit cuts across the domains of cognition involving language, memory, executive functions, and academic performance. In addition, individuals with autism tend to be more detail oriented and have difficulty with (1) integrating parts into wholes, (2) identifying central elements or themes, (3) differentiating between relevant and irrelevant information, and (4) determining meaning (Ozonoff, 2001). Their thinking is often literal and concrete. The high rate of hyperlexia in autism exemplifies this disparity. The autistic child with hyperlexia learns to read (decode) early but is impaired in comprehending the reading material. Interestingly, the cognitive and learning profile of autism is the converse of learning disabilities such as dyslexia. The dyslexic child cannot decode words but shows preserved listening comprehension when another person reads the material aloud. In summary, deficits in higher order thinking processes are evident across the autistic spectrum, including those individuals who are higher-functioning.

Executive Function—Similarities in the behaviors of individuals with autism and patients with prefrontal damage have prompted speculation that executive dysfunction may be of causative significance in autism. Empirical efforts to determine the validity of this speculation, and to identify differential patterns of executive performance, are growing.

Consistent with this line of investigation, Hughes, Russell, and Robbins (1994) have determined that children with autism perform in an inferior and differential manner on executive measures compared with healthy control children. Specifically, the autistic group exhibited poorer complex planning and mental shifting performance and also a unique type of executive deficit termed **"stuck in set" perseveration.** The researchers interpreted the concept of "stuck in set" perseveration as a failure to disengage the current attentional focus from ongoing cognitive operations (Ciesielski & Harris, 1997). Such disengagement is necessary if the person is to shift attentional focus to a new set of demands, activities, or goals.

The most robust executive deficit associated with autism is that of higher order planning (Ozonoff, 2001). **Executive planning** involves complex, means–end problem solving to achieve a behavioral goal and is supported by a number of component processes to include working memory, mental flexibility, **response inhibition** (the ability to delay a response), and the ability to project ahead in time. Research using tower tasks (Tower of London/Hanoi) to assess executive planning consistently shows poorer performance by autistic groups (both high- and low-functioning) relative to healthy and other clinical groups (Pennington & Ozonoff, 1996). A set of studies by Ozonoff and others (Ozonoff & Jensen, 1999; Ozonoff & Strayer, 2001) revealed distinct executive profiles for autistic, Gilles de la Tourette's syndrome, and ADHD groups. Specifically, autistic groups showed impaired planning and mental flexibility, whereas ADHD groups exhibited deficiencies in response inhibition. The Gilles de la Tourette's syndrome and healthy control groups did not differ in their performance across executive function tasks.

Ozonoff (2001) calls attention to the importance of subtle or overlooked factors that may affect the performance of individuals with autism. For instance, when examining studies of executive performance, particularly those that involved tower tasks, the performance of autistic groups varied from impaired to unimpaired. She discovered that most of the studies reporting unimpaired or improved executive performance involved computerized administration of the executive measures. In contrast, impaired performance was more likely to be evident when the measures were presented in a face-to-face format. Subsequent investigations indicated that the issue is much more subtle than type of test administration. The important variable appears to be the mode of feedback, human versus nonhuman. Individuals with autism appear to show poorer performance when feedback is presented within a verbal, social-interactive, as contrasted to an impersonal, computer-generated context.

Social Cognition—Converging evidence is revealing that autism is associated with deficits in social cognition. Social cognition encompasses a diverse set of processes such as facial perception, social orientation, joint attention, imitation, and **theory of mind** (TOM). We have reviewed facial processing in autism (see Neuropathogenesis earlier in this chapter). Deficits in social orientation (interest in and preference for human contact over objects) and joint attention (sharing a common focus of attention with another) are evident in autistic children. Likewise, imitation of others is a key component of social learning. Research reports that children with autism often do not imitate the actions of significant others and peers (Pennington, 2002).

TOM has received considerable empirical and theoretical attention. TOM, or "mentalism," refers to the ability to represent or infer mental states such as the beliefs, motives, and intentions of others. This ability enables people to make attributions, to reason about mental states, and to understand and predict the behavior of others (Rowe, Bullock, Polkey, & Morris, 2001). It is posed to be involved in or support the social behaviors of perspective-taking, "mind-reading," empathy, and the detection of deception, irony, humor, and faux pas (Baron-Cohen et al., 1999; Lawson, Baron-Cohen, & Wheelwright, 2004). An example of TOM would be observing a person and inferring what the person is "thinking" or predicting how the person would respond. This example portrays a first-order TOM. Higher levels of TOM are also evident. A second-order TOM would involve representing or inferring one person's mental state about another person's mental state ("Bill thinks that Mary believes that Joe believes . . ."). Young children are capable of performing first-order tasks, whereas success with second-order TOM tasks is not achieved until a later age, depending on the complexity and difficulty of the task presented. Unimpaired TOM processing is viewed as central to the development of appropriate interpersonal and communication patterns.

Investigations reveal deficits in TOM for autistic groups relative to healthy control participants (Jarrold, Butler, Cottington, & Jimenez, 2000; Ozonoff & Griffith, 2000; Rutherford & Rogers, 2003). Suggestions have been made that TOM performance is supported, in part, by the orbital prefrontal cortex (Baron-Cohen, Ring, Bullmore, Wheelwright, Ashwin, & Williams, 2000), a region implicated in higher order socioemotional regulation. A number of imaging studies have also demonstrated a relation between TOM performance and the medial prefrontal cortex activation (Shallice, 2001). In a relatively recent investigation (Stuss, Gallup, & Alexander, 2001), patients with lesions of the frontal and nonfrontal cortices were presented with measures of TOM. In contrasting the performance of the different lesion groups, significantly poorer TOM performance was associated right and bilateral frontal lesions, particularly lesions of the right medial prefrontal cortex.

Although TOM has enhanced our understanding of autism, it has received its share of criticism. For example, TOM deficits are evident in other clinical groups, indicating a lack of specificity to autism (Pennington, 2002). Furthermore, TOM performance is related to verbal ability and general cognitive level which undermines its utility as a specific index of social cognition. Finally, TOM has been variously defined as a cognitive, language, emotional, or social construct, leading to confusion as to what processes are actually encompassed by the theory. Therefore, we await further theoretical developments and research to clarify the meaning, boundaries, and utility of TOM.

Although psychological constructs such as executive function and social cognition have enabled us to characterize and predict certain autistic behaviors, they lack the theoretical breadth necessary to account for the diverse communication, language, and social behaviors associated with the disorder. We next turn to a theoretical model that endeavors to provide a comprehensive neurofunctional model of autism.

Comprehensive Neurofunctional Model

Multiple theories and models are available to account for the behavioral manifestations, core deficits, and cause of autism. These conceptualizations focus on impairments of attention (shifting and selective), TOM, social attachment, socioemotional perception, memory, language, and executive function (Fein et al., 1996). The majority of these theoretical efforts are rather narrow with regard to the specific autistic behavior that is interpreted or predicted. Accordingly, most fail to account for the multiple behavioral manifestations and proposed neural impairments of autism.

Waterhouse and coworkers (1996) propose a comprehensive model to account for the heterogeneity of symptoms and causes of autism. The comprehensive model rests on a series of assumptions relating human social behavior to brain functioning. It proposes four neurofunctional impairments that, in interaction, account for the social and related behavioral disruptions of autism:

1. **Canalesthesia** involves the fragmented processing of incoming information from the different sensory modalities. Because of this fragmentation, sensory information in consciousness, working memory, and declarative memory fails to integrate properly, resulting in distorted representations of the information.
2. **Impaired affective assignment** is the disrupted linking of appropriate emotional meaning or significance to novel and social stimuli. This disruption impairs appropriate responses to new situations and the social actions of others.
3. **Asociality** is a profound disturbance of normal social attachment and interdependence with others. Social interest and bonding motivation are minimal or lacking altogether.
4. **Extended selective attention** is an overextended attentional focus and inordinate delay in shifting attention, resulting in a variety of inappropriate responses such as hypersensitivity to sensory input and perseverative behaviors.

Waterhouse and coworkers (1996) link each of the aforementioned neurofunctional impairments to relatively distinct neural regions and circuitry. That is, dysfunction of the hippocampus and amygdala of the temporal lobes produces canalesthesia and the impaired assignment of affective significance, respectively. Asociality relates to the aberrant functioning of three interrelated neurochemical systems: oxytocin and vasopressin neuropeptide, endogenous opiate, and serotonin. Finally, the researchers consider extended selective attention to relate to a disruption of the temporal and parietal association areas. Although each of these supporting neural regions and circuitry links to specific broad functions, they interact and overlap to produce the deficits that the child with autism displays. Interestingly, Waterhouse and coworkers view brainstem, cerebellum, and frontal lobe damage—all of which other researchers and theorists have considered of etiologic significance in autism—as only secondary causes or by-products of aberrant input from other neural systems.

An impressive body of supporting research based on neuroimaging, electrophysiology, neuropathology, and animal studies supports the four neurofunctional impairments as pathogenic of autism. An individual with autism can present all four of these impairments. However, some individuals present three or fewer impaired neurofunctional systems. In such cases, the number and form of the symptoms exhibited relate to damage to the individual system or group of systems. For example, if damage is restricted to the oxytocin-opiate system, the model predicts that most of the autistic symptoms will be absent, except for those behaviors associated with disrupted social attachment and lack of affiliation with others. Although the validity and utility of the comprehensive model requires further empirical verification, it represents a bold effort to integrate the theories and empirical findings of autism.

Developmental Course

Autism is a chronic, lifelong disorder that parents and professionals generally detect before the child reaches age 3. A number of distinguishing characteristics appear as the child with autism develops, although individual differences are evident. In infancy, the baby with autism may be passive and unresponsive to being held and cuddled. Social or interactive behaviors directed to the infant by caretakers often fail to elicit recognition or interest.

As the child with autism moves into the toddler and preschool years, the onset of speech and language is often delayed or may fail to develop altogether. Moreover, as language develops, echolalia, reversed pronouns, and neologisms may emerge. Self-help skills lag in development. The child with autism is less likely than healthy children to imitate the gestures or vocalizations of adults (Sigman, 1994; Tanguay, 2000) and has only a limited desire or ability to communicate with others.

The play of the child with autism lacks sophistication in both structured and unstructured situations. The developmental stages of parallel and cooperative play are delayed or not attained at all. Stereotypic motor behaviors, unusual interests or preoccupations, demands for order and sameness, and other peculiar behaviors may dominate the child's daily activities. Unusual reactions, such as hypersensitivity to specific environmental stimuli (such as noise) or advanced abilities or skills (such as hyperlexia), may also be apparent.

During the toddler and early preschool years, the parents begin to realize their child is not developing appropriately. Professional services are typically sought, and the child is involved in a series of medical, psychological, speech, language, and related evaluations. At this point, there is a rendering of the diagnosis of autism for the first time, and comorbid conditions, such as mental retardation, are identified. Subsequently, the parents often enter the child into a preschool special education or treatment program with supportive services.

Autistic behavioral excesses and deficits continue to be evident during the child's elementary school years. However, as discussed earlier, improvement across behavioral domains begin to be evident with increasing age, particularly for the higher functioning child with autism. Despite this improvement, the child remains developmentally delayed and continues to exhibit unusual behavioral patterns. Many of these children cannot enter a normal educational program. Academic achievement is variable and poor, particularly if cognitive or intellectual deficits are pronounced. Peer interactions are minimal, and most children with autism never develop a close friendship.

Continued improvement may be evident with the advent of adolescence, particularly for the higher functioning child with autism. However, most individuals with autism continue to exhibit deficits in one or more of the core impairment areas, and unfortunately, some teenagers with autism regress (Piven, Harper, Palmer, & Arndt, 1996). Low-functioning adolescents with autism often need continued training in the more basic life skills and placement in a program, such as a sheltered workshop, that emphasizes the development of rudimentary vocational skills. Higher functioning teenagers with autism, despite relative success in academics, lack social acceptance by peers because of their ongoing deficits in socialization and communication and their unusual interests and patterns of behavior.

Approximately 80% of individuals with autism are unable to move fully into the workforce, and up to half require lifelong residential care (Pennington, 1991). Others can function effectively in a sheltered workshop or higher level of employment if the work environment is supportive. Higher functioning individuals may be capable of life in a group home or other assisted living program in the community. Only about one-third are able to live independently.

Treatment

Currently, the most significant treatments for autism and other pervasive developmental disorders include behavioral interventions, special education, and occasionally, pharmacotherapy. Despite early intervention and application of currently available treatment options, autistic and related disorders generally do not fully resolve.

Caretakers generally use behavior modification as an intervention in an autistic child's comprehensive treatment program. Several investigators consider behavior modification one of the more effective treatment options for children with autism. Generally, the use of behavioral interventions involves a functional analysis of targeted behaviors to determine the relation of environmental antecedents and consequences to the child's behavior. Using this analysis, psychologists develop a behavioral plan to generate behaviors (such as social skills), strengthen appropriate actions (such as increased eye contact), and reduce or eliminate maladaptive behaviors (such as aggression or self-injury). Caretakers use both rewarding and aversive behavior interventions to bring about desired change. Positive reinforcement and token systems are two examples of rewarding interventions used to produce or strengthen target behaviors. Aversive behavioral techniques incorporate the use of corrective feedback, time-out, response cost, and overcorrection to reduce inappropriate behaviors. **Response cost** involves the loss of a reinforcer contingent on the child demonstrating an inappropriate behavior, whereas **overcorrection** involves having the child practice a positive response that is incompatible with an inappropriate behavior. Overcorrection is particularly effective in reducing self-stimulating behaviors, such as repetitive mouthing of objects.

Insofar as deficits in language and communication skills are often dramatic, initial treatment efforts focused on increasing language acquisition and production. That is, the interventions centered on prompting speech and reinforcing the child's verbalizations. Although verbalizations increased, the child's actual ability to communicate did not necessarily improve. The realization that verbal production does not equate with communication has prompted a shift in treatment focus to increasing the child's spontaneous, communicative language. Moreover, social skills training is receiving increased attention as a treatment modality. These interventions target one of the central deficits of autism, the impaired ability to relate to others. Finally, some children with autism benefit from pharmacologic interventions to reduce self-injurious behaviors, hyperactivity, ritualistic behaviors, and aggressiveness. However, a number of the medications (such as haloperidol [Haldol]) require careful monitoring for potentially serious side effects. The advent of atypical antipsychotic medications (for example, risperidone [Risperdal]) is receiving support for treating severe behavioral disturbances, significant agitation, and self-injurious or stereotypic behaviors (McDougle et al., 2000). Similarly, selective serotonin reuptake inhibitors (for example, fluoxetine hydrochloride [Prozac]) are efficacious in treating compulsive, stereotypic behaviors and aggression.

In summary, children with autism frequently require special educational services tailored to their individual learning, social, and adaptive needs. In addition to academic and daily living skills, many require ancillary services such as speech, language, and physical therapy. Vocational training and supervised job placement, often in a sheltered workshop environment, provide meaningful employment and the opportunity for social and recreational activities for individuals with autism.

 # Disruptive Behavioral Disorders

The APA (1994) currently classifies disruptive or externalizing behavioral disorders as psychiatric disorders. These disorders feature a variety of poorly controlled or acting-out behaviors that are developmentally inappropriate or violate societal dictates for acceptable behavior. The three primary representatives of this category are ADHD, oppositional defiant disorder (ODD), and conduct disorder (CD). As a developmental disorder, ADHD has generated an enormous number of theoretical and empirical studies since the mid-1980s. It is to this disorder, the most prevalent of childhood disruptive disorders, that we turn our attention next.

ATTENTION-DEFICIT/HYPERACTIVITY DISORDER

Clinical Background and Presentation

The clinical manifestations of children exhibiting an **attention-deficit/hyperactivity disorder (ADHD)** are variable, although clinicians generally agree that the core symptom patterns include age-inappropriate inattention, impulsivity, and hyperactivity. These symptom patterns are chronic, cross situational in presentation, and developmental in origin (APA, 1994). Thus, the behavioral symptoms of ADHD are not transient in presentation and generally continue into adolescence and adulthood. Furthermore, these symptoms are typically observed before school age and across multiple contexts such as home, school, and the community.

Since its inception in 1980, the diagnosis of ADHD has undergone several revisions (Table 11.5). These revisions involve introducing different diagnostic models, changing exclusionary criteria, and delineating specific subtypes. Despite these modifications, the diagnosis retains the core symptoms of inattention, impulsivity, and hyperactivity, although the combinations, relations, and definitions of these symptom patterns have altered.

Demographic and Comorbid Conditions

Currently, ADHD accounts for a third to half of all childhood referrals for psychological services (Richters et al., 1995). Prevalence rates of 3% to 9% for childhood populations are commonly cited (Spencer, 2002). The breakdown of ADHD figures by sex reveals that boys, compared with girls, are more frequently diagnosed as exhibiting ADHD, with cited ratios ranging from 3:1 to 9:1 (Pennington, 1997a). However, some researchers suggest that girls are

Table 11.5 *Changing Attention-Deficit/ Hyperactivity Disorder Criteria*

DSM	Symptom Presentation
DSM-III (1980)	
Attention-deficit with hyperactivity	Inattention, impulsivity, and hyperactivity
Attention-deficit without hyperactivity	Inattention and impulsivity
DSM-III-R (1987)	
Attention-deficit/ hyperactivity disorder	Inattention, impulsivity, and hyperactivity
Undifferentiated attention deficit disorder	Inattention
DSM-IV (1994)	
Attention-deficit/hyperactivity disorder—combined type	Inattention, impulsivity, and hyperactivity
Attention-deficit/hyperactivity disorder—inattentive type	Inattention
Attention-deficit/hyperactivity disorder—impulsive-hyperactive type	Impulsivity and hyperactivity

DSM-III = *Diagnostic and Statistical Manual of Mental Disorders, Third Edition;* DSM-III-R = *Diagnostic and Statistical Manual of Mental Disorders, Third Edition, Revised;* DSM-IV = *Diagnostic and Statistical Manual of Mental Disorders, Fourth Edition.* Reprinted with permission from the *Diagnostic and Statistical Manual of Mental Disorders,* Fourth Edition. Text Revision, Copyright 2000, American Psychiatric Association.

under-represented, partly because of the greater likelihood that boys will present with higher levels of overactivity and aggressive behaviors that quickly draw the attention of caretakers. Although a childhood disorder, 30% to 60% of diagnosed children continue to exhibit symptoms of ADHD in adulthood (Sheppard, Bradshaw, Purcell, & Pantelis, 1999). Currently, increased focus has been on the identification and treatment of adults with ADHD.

There is a growing recognition that ADHD frequently coexists with other psychiatric and psychological disorders. ODD and CD are the most prevalent comorbid conditions of ADHD, with reported rates of occurrence ranging from 40% to 65% (Barkley, 1990; Wilens et al., 2002). ODD is characterized by chronic, age-inappropriate, angry mood and resistant, stubborn behaviors, and CD involves the repeated violations of the rights of others or of societal norms. Assaultive behaviors and illicit drug use are examples of the types of violations CD children exhibit. The basis for the high rates of comorbidity of ODD/CD with ADHD is unclear. However, evidence suggests that social factors such as family sociopathy,

rather than genetic determinants, are contributors to the pathogenesis of these disorders.

ADHD also covaries with anxiety and depressive disorders at rates ranging from 18% to 51%, depending on the childhood population sampled for study (Eiraldi, Power, & Nezu, 1997; Jensen, Martin, & Cantwell, 1997; Wilens et al., 2002). Estimates of the rate of comorbidity of ADHD and Gilles de la Tourette disorder range from 25% to 50% (Cirino, Chapieski, & Massman, 2000). Finally, from 15% to 20% of children with ADHD also exhibit learning disabilities (Richters et al., 1995). The high rates of comorbidity have led to speculation that ADHD is one disorder within a spectrum of related disorders.

Neuropsychological Pathogenesis

Neuropsychologists consider ADHD a neurobiologically based developmental disorder that responds to specific types of environmental and pharmacologic interventions. However, the etiology of ADHD is currently unknown. We review areas of investigation that are expanding our knowledge of the pathogenesis and symptoms of ADHD.

Familial and Genetic Influence—Accumulating evidence suggests that ADHD is a familial disorder, possibly inheritable. The familial nature of the disorder is clear from the elevated rates of ADHD in first- and second-degree relatives. The presence of familial ADHD does not necessarily signal that the disorder is genetically determined because little is known of the psychosocial environmental transmission of ADHD across generations. The finding of significant parental discord and psychopathology in families of children with ADHD suggests that environmental factors may be of causative significance. However, the high rate of concordance of ADHD for identical twins and the discovery of a potential linkage between ADHD and genetic markers tips the balance in the direction of a genetic component as the primary determinant of the disorder. Regarding the latter, researchers have linked a thyroid gene to a narrow subgroup of children with ADHD (Hauser et al., 1993) and have also identified a relation between ADHD and a number of gene variants.

The *D4* receptor gene on chromosome 11 has been implicated in the etiology of ADHD (Holmes et al., 2000; Smalley et al., 1998). One variant of the *D4* gene, the 7-repeat allele (a segment of the DNA is repeated seven times), has been associated with the personality trait of "novelty seeking" or "thrill seeking," a characteristic often evident in children with ADHD. Several studies have found that children with ADHD are more likely to have the 7-repeat allele than healthy children. However, only 25% to 30% of children with ADHD carry the 7-repeat allele, indicating that the gene is neither necessary nor sufficient to produce the disorder (Barr, 2001; Pliszka, 2003).

The dopamine transporter gene (*DAT1*), located on chromosome 5, governs the reuptake of dopamine into the neuron. The presence of one variant of the *DAT1*, 10-repeat (segment of DNA repeated 10 times) allele, is associated with greater risk for ADHD (Daly, Hawi, Fitzgerald, & Gill, 1999; Waldman et al., 1998). The genetic research with "knockout" mice that examines the relation of the *DAT1* gene to behavior is of interest. Knockout mice are bred without selected genes to study the effects of mutations and other genetic alterations. Investigations of knockout mice without the (*DAT1*) gene reveal that the animals demonstrate hyperactivity, poor spatial performance, and other behaviors suggestive of disrupted inhibitory control. When administered a psychostimulant medication (for example, methylphenidate [Ritalin]), the mice showed a calming response, similar to that evident with medicated children with ADHD (Gainetdinov & Caron, 2001).

Other genes implicated in ADHD are the dopamine receptor *D5*, catechol *O*-methyltransferase (*COMT*; codes for the enzyme that catalyzes the breakdown of dopamine and norepinephrine), and monoamine oxidase (*MAO*; codes for the enzyme that breaks down dopamine and norepinephrine after reuptake into the neuron). However, there are both confirmatory and contradictory studies regarding the association of the dopamine receptor (*D5*), *COMT, MAO,* and other genes with ADHD (Pliszka, 2003), indicating the need for further research to clarify and expand our knowledge of the role of genetics in the pathogenesis of ADHD.

Neural Substrates—Numerous neural substrates have been implicated in the etiology and neuropsychological manifestations of ADHD, including most major cortical and subcortical systems, regions, and axes of the brain. Currently, four cortical-subcortical brain regions are the focus of study. The first relates to possible abnormalities in the structure of the corpus callosum. Such anomalies are believed to disrupt the transmission of impulses between the cerebral hemispheres, thereby interfering with the communication necessary for integrated behavioral control. However, neuroimaging studies of the genu (anterior portion) and splenium (posterior portion) of the corpus callosum of children with ADHD have produced inconsistent results, with subjects displaying anatomic differences in both regions, in only one region, or in neither region, relative to healthy control children (Hynd, Semrud-Clikeman, Lorys, Novey, & Eliopulos, 1991; Giedd et al., 1994; Semrud-Clikeman et al., 1994).

The second neural substrate considered of pathologic significance for ADHD is the frontal lobes. The parallel between the symptom patterns of patients with acquired frontal lobe damage and those of children with ADHD has fostered speculation that disruption of the frontal lobes may contribute to the etiology of the latter disorder (Bensen, 1991). Neuroimaging investigations have provided some support for this speculation. The majority of these investigations (Castellanos et al., 1994; Filipek, Semrud-Clikeman, Steingard, Renshaw, Kennedy, & Biederman, 1997; Hynd et al., 1990) have found a lack of normal asymmetry (R > L) in the frontal lobes of children exhibiting ADHD, with the right prefrontal region being anatomically smaller and, therefore, symmetric with the left prefrontal lobe (R = L). In addition, there are indications that both left and right frontal lobes may be smaller for groups with ADHD relative to those without the disorder (Sowell et al., 2004). The frontal lobes contribute to the control of attentional functioning, and the finding of atypical symmetry and volume suggests a relation to ADHD. However, studies have not always replicated these findings of structural differences, nor have they determined that differences in symmetry of the prefrontal lobes are specific to ADHD. For example, Hynd and colleagues (1990) have also identified atypical symmetry (R = L) of the prefrontal lobes in children exhibiting dyslexia.

Studies of cerebral blood flow within the frontal lobes have revealed differences between individuals with ADHD and healthy volunteers. Zametkin and coworkers (1990), in a PET study of adults with ADHD, discovered that the participants exhibited hypofrontality in glucose use/cerebral blood flow. Hypofrontality can reflect a disruption in executive inhibitory control of behavior. However, subsequent studies of children and adolescents with ADHD have not consistently replicated these findings, particularly when contrasting male and female adolescents (Ernst, Cohen, Liebenauer, Jons, & Zametkin, 1997; Ernst, Liebenauer, Jons, & Zametkin, 1994; Zametkin et al., 1993).

Recently, a preliminary proton magnetic resonance spectroscopy (^{1}H-MRS) and MRI study (Yeo et al., 2003) of children with ADHD and healthy control children examined the relation of neurometabolite concentration, frontal volume, and attentional performance. For healthy control children, a significant relation between neurometabolite concentration, frontal volume, and attentional performance was not evident; however, a significant relation was evident for those children with ADHD. Specifically, concentration levels of Cre (sum of intracellular creatine and phosphocreatine indexing cellular energy metabolism) and *N*-acetylaspartate (a marker of neuronal

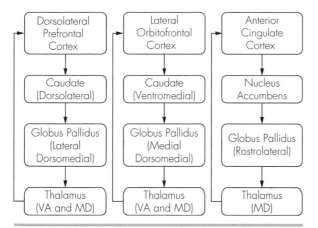

Figure 11.4 Three of the frontal-basal ganglia circuits involved in the mediation of higher order behavior. MD = mediodorsal; VA = ventral anterior. (From D. G. Lichter and J. L. Cummings, "Introduction and Overview," in D. G. Lichter and J. L. Cummings, eds., *Frontal-subcortical Circuits in Psychiatric and Neurological Disorders,* New York: The Guilford Press, 2001, p. 6, Figure 1. 2. Reprinted by permission of the American Medical Association.)

viability) correlated with right dorsolateral volume and poorer performance on a measure of sustained attention for children with ADHD. These findings contribute to the growing body of evidence that ADHD is associated with atypical neurobiology at the cellular level. Clearly, further investigations are needed to verify the findings of this study and to clarify the relation of atypical metabolic activity to attentional functioning, and possibly other cognitive processes associated with ADHD.

The third focus of study asks, "How significant is disruption of the frontal-basal ganglia circuitry to the cause of ADHD?" The basal ganglia are subcortical nuclei embedded below the frontal lobes. The prefrontal lobes send projections to the basal ganglia (caudate, putamen, globus pallidus, and nucleus accumbens) that, in turn, direct projections back to the prefrontal lobes via thalamic nuclei, forming neural circuits. Figure 11.4 portrays the frontal-basal ganglia circuitry involved in mediating higher order behavior. These frontostriatal pathways have been the focus of attention in the study of ADHD.

Early investigations suggest that the basal ganglia are primarily involved in motor control (Denckla & Reiss, 1997). Increasingly, investigators are realizing that the basal ganglia may play a role in cognitive functioning, although the precise nature of this role remains unclear. Neuroscientists have posed many and varied speculations as to the cognitive role of the basal ganglia, with most suggesting an inhibitory function that parallels or serves to augment executive control of the frontal lobes.

Neuroimaging of the frontostriatal circuitry of children with ADHD has identified decreased cerebral blood flow or other abnormalities of metabolism in several of the basal ganglia nuclei (Castellanos, 1997; Zang et al., 2005). For instance, adolescent boys with ADHD were scanned (fMRI) while performing a measure of response inhibition. Relative to healthy control participants, the ADHD group showed less brain activation of the right inferior frontal lobe and left caudate nucleus in performing the inhibitory measure (Rubia et al., 1999). Different striatal nuclei have been associated with decreased activation, with most being specific to the right hemisphere. Similarly, there is evidence of a reduction in the size of basal ganglia nuclei in individuals with ADHD (Aylward, Reiss, Reader, Singer, Brown, & Denckla, 1996; Faraone & Biederman, 2004). Unfortunately, inconsistent findings exist regarding whether volumetric differences are specific to the right or left hemisphere (Casey et al., 1997; Castellanos et al., 1994, 1996; Hynd et al., 1993) or whether hypoactivation or hyperactivation of frontostriatal structures characterize children with ADHD (Schultz et al., 2005). Finally, psychostimulant medication known to significantly reduce the core symptoms of ADHD can increase, or normalize the blood perfusion of the basal ganglia (Teicher, Polcari, Anderson, Andersen, Glod, & Renshaw, 1996), providing additional evidence for the involvement of these nuclei in the etiology of ADHD.

Finally, morphologic differences in the cerebellum are implicated in the pathogenesis of ADHD. Structural neuroimaging reveals smaller volume of the cerebellar hemispheres, particularly the posterior vermis lobules, for children with ADHD (Hill, Yeo, Campbell, Blaine, Vigil, & Brooks, 2003). However, the specific lobules or the proportion of volume found to be reduced differs across studies (Castellanos et al., 2001; Mostofsky, Reiss, Lockhart, & Denckla, 1998). It has been speculated that the cerebellum supports motor control, inhibition, temporal processing, attention, and executive functions (Giedd, Blumenthal, Mollowy, & Castellanos, 2001; Halpern & Schulz, 2006).

Overall, support is growing for anomalies in the frontal-striatal-cerebellar regions and circuitry in the pathogenesis of ADHD. Although the frontostriatal circuits are implicated in the inhibition, selection, initiation, and execution of complex motor and cognitive responses, and cerebellar circuits provide ongoing guidance of activated programs (Giedd et al., 2001), the precise role of these neurosubstrates in ADHD remains to be specified.

Neuropsychological Assessment

The heterogeneity of children diagnosed with ADHD; the failure to delineate sensitive, specific, and verifiable neuropsychological markers of the disorder; and the inability to identify the underlying pathogenesis of the disorder have hampered assessment. This state of affairs has resulted in a diagnosis by exclusion. That is, clinicians must first rule out all other disorders that could account for the child's inattentive, impulsive, and overactive behaviors before they can diagnose ADHD. This process becomes even more muddled when the child identified as ADHD exhibits comorbid psychological disorders such as ODD.

An assessment to determine whether a child is displaying ADHD warrants the integration of information drawn from developmental data and school records; systematic interviews with the parent, child, and other significant adults; behavioral observations and rating scales completed by the parent, teacher, and child; and a comprehensive battery of neuropsychological measures. Often, a team approach enables professionals from a variety of disciplines (for example, neuropsychologist, physician, social worker, and educators) to answer specific questions concerning the child's functioning.

Executive Function—The current focus on frontostriatal dysfunction as a cause of ADHD has prompted efforts to assess the executive functions attributable to these neural circuits. Investigators have found that children with ADHD perform in a differential manner on measures of executive function (see Chapter 9). Pennington and Ozonoff (1996) have reviewed 18 studies that sought to assess the executive functions of children with ADHD. Table 11.6 lists the executive measures that most markedly and consistently differentiated children exhibiting ADHD from healthy control children. Of these measures, the Tower of Hanoi (TOH) was the most sensitive to ADHD. The TOH is a complex measure that assesses executive planning, working memory, and inhibitory control.

Researchers report executive deficits for a variety of disorders, including Turner's syndrome, fragile X, autism, phenylketonuria (PKU, a genetic metabolic disorder), and Gilles de la Tourette's syndrome. Thus, impairment of executive performance may be a common impairment of developmental disorders. This does not, however, rule out the possibility that a specific executive function (such as cognitive flexibility) or set of executive functions (such as planning and working memory) may be unique to ADHD. Several investigators (Barkley, 1998; Pennington, 1997b) have proposed that a deficit of inhibitory control may be central to ADHD.

Table 11.6 Consistency of Differences and Average Effect Size of Executive Measures in Attention-Deficit/Hyperactivity Disorder

Measures	Consistency[†]	Average d
WCST perseverations	4/10	0.45
TMT B time	4/6	0.75
MFFT		
_Time	4/6	0.44
_Errors	5/5	0.87
Stroop Test time	4/5	0.69
Mazes	3/4	0.43
TOH	3/3	1.08
Motor inhibition tasks	6/6	0.85

[†]Number of studies finding a significant group difference divided by the number of studies using the measure.

WCST = Wisconsin Card Sorting Test (Heaton, 1981); TMT B = Trail Making Test B (Reitan & Davison, 1974); MFFT = Matching Familiar Figure Test (Kagan, 1964); Stroop Test (Golden, 1978); TOH = Tower of Hanoi (Welsh, 1991).

Source: Pennington, B., & Ozonoff, S. (1996). Executive functions and developmental psychopathology. *Journal of Child Psychology & Psychiatry, 37,* 63, by permission of Cambridge University Press.

To familiarize the student with the neuropsychological assessment of ADHD, Neuropsychology in Action 11.3 provides a case study. As will soon become evident, the case study demonstrates significant impairments in several executive functions that have been implicated in ADHD.

Neuropsychological Models

Several neuropsychological models of attentional functioning have evolved that are relevant to the understanding and treatment of ADHD. The following sections provide brief reviews of the representative models of Allan Mirsky (1995, 1996), Michael Posner (1992; Fernandez-Duque & Posner, 2001), and Russell Barkley (1997a, 1997b, 1997c).

Mirsky's Model and Attention-Deficit/Hyperactivity Disorder—As discussed in Chapter 9, Allen Mirsky (National Institute of Mental Health, Bethesda, MD) provides an empirically derived neuropsychological model that identifies five elements of attention, and he relates these elements to neuropsychological measures and underlying neural systems. The five elements of attention are *focus-execute* (selective attention and rapid perceptual-motor output),

Neuropsychology in Action 11.3

Case Study of a Child with an Attention-Deficit/Hyperactivity Disorder

by William C. Culbertson

B.C. is a 10-year-old boy with a history of school and home difficulties. His parents and regular class teacher were concerned about his inconsistent academic performance and poor behavioral control. The teacher reported that B.C. frequently failed to complete his assignments, appeared distracted, failed to follow directions, and rarely checked his work. Furthermore, he was prone to call out in class, leave his seat, walk about the room, and squirm when required to remain seated. Despite his classroom difficulties, his group achievement test scores demonstrated average to above-average skill development.

At home, he was "always on the go," could not sit quietly unless playing with building blocks, and rushed when completing chores or homework. It was difficult for B.C. to initiate or focus on his homework unless a parent sat with him to guide his efforts. His ability to plan and organize activities (for example, picking up his toys, organizing game activities with friends, and so forth) was described as very poor. Despite his behavioral difficulties, he was characterized as a gentle child who was rarely aggressive or noncompliant.

Neuropsychological Findings

Behavioral rating scales were completed by the teacher and parents regarding B.C.'s behavior. These ratings showed very high rates of inattention, impulsivity, and hyperactivity. Formal neuropsychological results revealed that B.C. was functioning within the average range of intelligence. Verbal and performance intelligence were both comparably developed in the average range. Relative weaknesses were evident on subtests sensitive to attentional weaknesses. His memory performance was age appropriate. However, he demonstrated very poor sustained attention and high rates of impulsivity on auditory and visual measures of continuous performance. Relatedly, he performed poorly on measures sensitive to selective attention and response inhibition, goal persistence and impulse control, and cognitive flexibility.

B.C. manifested very poor executive planning on the Tower of London-Drexel University test (TOL^{DX}) (Culbertson & Zillmer, 1998a, 1998b, 2005) relative to the performance of his peers. His planning attempts were quick, without adequate forethought or reflection. From a qualitative perspective, his problem-solving approach was impulsive, rigid, and comparable with that of a much younger child.

The integration of the developmental, rating, and neuropsychological findings supported the diagnosis of an attention-deficit/hyperactivity disorder–combined type. The neuropsychologist developed behavioral interventions with B.C.'s teacher and family. These interventions focused on B.C.'s inattention, impulsivity, hyperactivity, and planning deficits. Although he was responsive to behavioral interventions, his behavioral disinhibition remained high. Accordingly, the neuropsychologist sought a medical consultation to determine the feasibility of stimulant therapy. Stimulant medication was introduced and gradually titrated to therapeutic levels. A significant additive effect (behavioral interventions and medication) was evident, with attention, impulse, and activity control showing marked improvement.

---

shift (attentional flexibility), *sustain* (vigilance and persistence of attention), *encode* (working memory), and *stable* (consistence of attentional effort). The five components constitute an attentional system that is widely distributed throughout the brain. Accordingly, the system is quite vulnerable to disruption after brain injury; yet, it is also resilient. A specific attentional function may be compromised by injury, but undamaged neural regions may provide some degree of compensation.

Support for the utility of the model for identifying and understanding the attentional processing of children with ADHD is emerging. In an early study (Lowther & Wasserman, 1994), a battery of attentional measures selected to represent each element of attention was administered to children with ADHD and healthy control children. Each element of attention differentiated ADHD and healthy children and correctly predicted group membership with 91% accuracy. Recently, Kunin-Batson and associates (2002), in a double-blind, placebo–control study of children, determined that the introduction of psychostimulant medication significantly augmented the "sustain" and "stable" components of attentional functioning, but not the "focus-execute" or "encode" elements of attention. Measures of the "shift" attentional component were not included for study in the investigation. Finally, as reviewed later, clinical childhood groups demonstrate differential patterns of performance on measures sensitive to Mirsky's components of attention and the attentional processes that Michael Posner poses.

Posner's Model and Attention-Deficit/Hyperactivity Disorder—As discussed in Chapter 9, Michael Posner has developed a model of attention from the perspective of cognitive psychology and neuroscience. He hypothesizes that ADHD may result from disruption of the *vigilance attention system,* insofar as children with ADHD are impaired in their ability to maintain attention over time. The study revealed that children with ADHD showed deficits, relative to healthy control children, on measures sensitive to the functioning of the vigilance and *anterior attention system* (Pearson, Yaffee, Loveland, & Norton, 1995; Swanson et al., 1991). Thus, disruption of both the vigilance *and* anterior attentional systems may play a key role in the etiology of ADHD.

The utility of Posner's model was recently examined in a study (Brewer, Fletcher, Hiscock, & Davidson, 2001) of three groups of children (ADHD, congenital hydrocephalus, and healthy control children). The children were presented with measures sensitive to attentional focus, maintenance, and shifting. Furthermore, the measures allowed for the separation of the **disengage, move,** and **engage** processes of Posner's model of attention. Relative to the control group, the children with hydrocephalus demonstrated deficits in focusing and shifting attention, whereas the children with ADHD were impaired in sustaining and shifting attention. The difficulties of the hydrocephalus groups with focusing and shifting attention were related to impairments of disengaging and moving the focus of their attention. These impairments are consistent with disruption of the *posterior attention system.* In contrast, the shifting difficulties of the ADHD group reflected preservative errors consistent with anterior system involvement. Likewise, poor sustained attention implicates impairment of the vigilance and anterior systems. The findings of greater posterior versus anterior attentional dysfunction in the congenital hydrocephalus and ADHD groups correlate with the neuroanatomic and neurofunctional differences identified for the two groups.

Recently, Swanson and colleagues (2000) have proposed a tentative model linking the symptoms of ADHD delineated in the DSM-IV (APA, 1994) to the cognitive processes and neural circuits that Posner proposed (Table 11.7). Different symptoms of inattention reflect disruptions to the alerting and orienting processes supported primarily by the right frontal and posterior parietal neural networks. Alerting symptoms relate to deficits in persistence of attention (sustained) and vigilance, whereas orienting symptoms define deficits of selective attention. The hyperactivity-impulsive symptoms are linked to perturbations of the executive control processes underpinned by the anterior cingulate region of the brain. Although the neural circuits are relatively distinct, they interact and overlap in their support of the complex behavioral manifestations associated with ADHD. When considering the distribution of the neural

Table 11.7 *Diagnostic and Statistical Manual of Mental Disorders, Fourth Edition,* **Attention-Deficit/ Hyperactivity Disorder Symptoms, Cognitive Processes, and Neural Networks**

Symptom Domains	Cognitive Processes	Neural Networks
Inattentive	Alerting	Frontal
Difficulty sustaining attention		Right frontal cortex
Fails to finish		Right posterior parietal
Avoids sustained efforts		Locus ceruleus
Inattentive	Orienting	Posterior Parietal
Distracted by stimuli		Bilateral parietal
Does not appear to listen		Superior colliculus
Fails to pay close attention		Thalamus
Hyperactive-Impulsive	Executive control	Anterior cingulate
Blurts out answers		Anterior cingulate
Interrupts or intrudes		Left lateral frontal
Cannot wait		Basal ganglia

Source: Adapted from Swanson, J., Posner, M., Cantwell, D., Wigal, S., Crinella, F., Filipek, P., Emerson, J., Tuciker, D., & Nalcioglu, O. (2000). Attention-deficit/ hyperactivity disorder: Symptom domains, cognitive processes and neural networks. In R. Parasuraman (Ed.), *The attentive brain* (p. 455, Table 20.2). Cambridge, MA: The MIT Press, by permission.

networks implicated in ADHD, damage within or between networks could produce variability in the symptom presentation of children with the disorder. In fact, significant variability exists in the symptoms demonstrated by children with ADHD, and the proposed model may help clarify and further specify the behavioral manifestations of this disorder. We await the clinical and empirical application of the model.

Barkley's Model of Attention-Deficit/Hyperactivity Disorder— Russell Barkley (1997a,b,c) proposes a three-tiered executive model of ADHD (Figure 11.5). The first tier, behavioral inhibition, is central to the model. Behavioral inhibition involves three inter-related processes: (1) the inhibition of a **prepotent response,** (2) stopping an ongoing response, and (3) protecting an ongoing mental operation from disruption by competing external or internal events **(interference control).** These inhibitory processes are necessary for the effective operation of the four executive functions of tier 2: working memory; internalization of speech; regulation of arousal, emotions, and motivation; and reconstitution (recombining behavioral elements to create

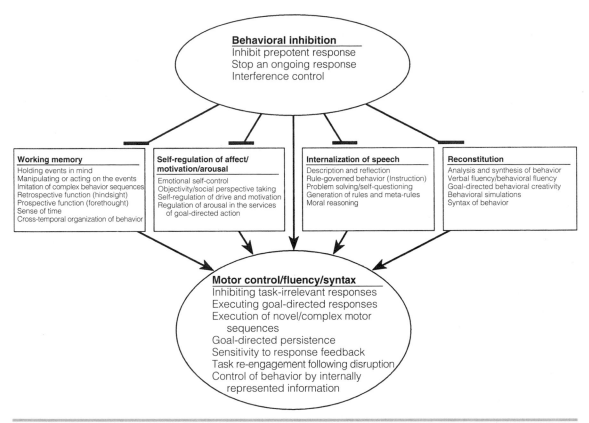

Figure 11.5 Schematic configuration of a conceptual model linking behavioral inhibition with the performance of the four executive functions that bring motor control, fluency, and syntax under the control of internally represented information. (Reproduced from Barkley, R. A. [1997]. Behavioral inhibition, sustained attention, and executive functions: Constructing a unifying theory of ADHD. *Psychological Bulletin, 121,* 73, by permission of the American Psychological Association.)

new behaviors). Tier 2 functions, in turn, affect the control, organization, and flexibility of the behavioral output of tier 3. Although the brain as a whole supports these processes, the prefrontal and frontal cortices are primarily responsible for the inhibitory and executive processes.

When inhibitory and executive processes are intact, the child develops the capacity to regulate behavior by using internal representations of events in thought and image. These internal representations enable the child to link past learning and experience with both present demands and future consequences of actions. Furthermore, the capacity to internally manipulate and guide behavior via internal representations allows for the regulation of emotion and motivation and the generation of new behavioral patterns to augment goal-oriented behavior, particularly when something thwarts intended actions. In ADHD, impaired inhibitory control processes disrupt the operation of the executive processes. The cascading effect of this impairment results in a host of behavioral excesses

and deficits, including poor impulse control, inattention, and hyperactivity.

Barkley's model continues to spawn studies of inhibitory control and executive function as they relate to ADHD. Support is amply evident for poor inhibitory control and executive functions deficits in ADHD populations (Nigg, 2001; Purvis & Tannock, 2000), although the verification is stronger for inhibitory weaknesses than executive dysfunctions. Varieties of methodologic issues cloud recent efforts to determine the factors that account for differences in findings. A primary problem is the selection of developmentally appropriate tasks to assess executive functions. Executive functions emerge at different points in childhood, continue to develop in a multistep manner, and reach final maturity in adolescence or early adulthood. Thus, the assessment of a specific executive skill requires a measure sensitive to the stage/level of maturation of that particular skill. For example, the ability to inhibit a motor response is more fully developed than interference control (shielding a cognitive operation from distracting, nonrelevant intrusions) during the early childhood years. Interference control has a more contracted developmental trajectory that continues through the upper elementary years. Accordingly, comparing the performance of healthy preschool children with a group of children with ADHD on a measure of interference control will likely show minimal differences, because neither group fully possesses the executive skills to perform the measure.

Recently, Berlin, Bohlin, Nyberg, and Janols (2004) presented children with ADHD and healthy control children (age 7–10 years) with a battery of developmentally appropriate measures of inhibitory control and executive function. The measures were selected to target the executive domains articulated in Barkley's model. The results revealed that the children with ADHD performed significantly poorer across the measures of inhibitory control and executive function, except for one, reconstitution. More importantly, when the measures that differentiated the two groups were combined for prediction (logistic regression), 86% of the children were correctly classified into their diagnostic groups. The sensitivity (probability that a child with ADHD would be correctly classified) and specificity (probability that a healthy child would be correctly classified) rates were 81% and 88%, respectively. In addition, inhibition, working memory, and self-regulation were determined to be distinct predictors of group membership. The latter finding indicates that the three executive functions were each assessing a relatively unique set of abilities. Overall, the findings of the study are supportive of Barkley's model, but suggest that it be reduced to three major components: inhibition, working memory, and self-regulation.

Developmental Course

As a developmental disorder, ADHD is evident early in childhood and, with maturation, shows changing symptom manifestations. In infancy, children displaying ADHD tend to be highly active, overly responsive to stimulation, quick to anger, and show low adaptability to change. During the toddler and preschooler years, children with ADHD are constantly "on the go," seem "driven by a motor," continually manipulate objects, and shift across activities. Moreover, they constantly run and climb, often without apparent consideration for the consequences of their actions. Preschoolers exhibiting ADHD are at risk for accidental injury due to their inattention, impulsivity, and high activity levels. One 3-year-old, for example, was so inattentive and hyperactive that he ran into walls, doors, and other stationary objects on a daily basis!

In a preschool setting, children with ADHD often find it difficult to remain seated, fail to listen to or follow directions, become too excited when stimulated, and talk loudly and incessantly. Peers describe classmates with ADHD as bossy, uncooperative, and intrusive into their activities and games. The parents may be asked to remove their child from the preschool program if the child is also highly oppositional or aggressive. The traditional elementary school environment is referred to as the "showplace" for ADHD. The demands of school highlight the regulatory deficits of children with ADHD. Specifically, the following school requirements all tax the controlling efforts of children displaying ADHD: (1) attention to work that can be boring, tedious, and effortful; (2) organization of assignments and belongings; (3) completion of work without rushing; (4) remaining seated for long periods; (5) adherence to multiple classroom rules; (6) reflection before responding; (7) refraining from talking unless permitted; and (8) cooperation with others. It is during the elementary school years that children with ADHD begin to avoid homework assignments, which inevitably leads to significant conflict with teachers and parents. Furthermore, peers often begin to move away from these children, finding their impulsivity, hyperactivity, and inattention to rules of behavior difficult to tolerate.

As children with ADHD enter middle and high school, their inability to meet the expectations for greater independence in managing the academic demands of multiple teachers leads to an ever-increasing sense of failure and frustration. Perplexed, if not angry, teachers and parents continually confront these adolescents over their failure to live up to expected levels of academic performance. The normal adolescent strivings for independence and self-direction fuel resistance to parental offers of assistance or attempts to provide structure to the teenager's studying and homework habits. Ongoing rejection by peers, particularly if the adolescent is aggressive, often results in the teenager gravitating toward peers who are experiencing similar difficulties. Cumulatively, these negative experiences diminish the adolescent's self-esteem and contribute to a growing realization that future educational and vocational aspirations may be unattainable.

As adolescents who exhibit ADHD move into adulthood, some show greater regulatory control and a related reduction or resolution of core symptoms of inattention, impulsivity, and hyperactivity. Unfortunately, a significant number of the adolescents (Weiss & Hechtman, 1993) continue to manifest the core or residual symptoms as they enter adulthood. Early failings in school, rejection by peers, and disappointed family members evolve into problems related to achieving success in work, marriage, and family life. Not surprisingly, investigators report high rates of mood disorders, alcoholism, substance abuse, and antisocial personality disorders among adults with ADHD (Barkley, 1998). Adults with ADHD are generally gainfully employed and self-sufficient, although they tend to have poorer work records and lower vocational status than their adult peers without ADHD. Clearly, many children and adolescents manifesting ADHD continue to encounter adjustment difficulties in adulthood.

Treatment

The treatment of children with ADHD warrants a comprehensive, multimodal approach due to the multiplicity of deficits and difficulties that these children present. Each child presents a unique set of strengths and weaknesses and, accordingly, warrants an individual treatment plan tailored to his or her individual needs. When targeting the ADHD child's needs, the core symptoms of inattention, impulsivity, and hyperactivity serve as the primary point of intervention. These core symptoms, as they are manifested across contexts (family, educational, and social), expand and alter the specific treatment components. The presence of comorbid conditions (such as depression) further modifies the treatment interventions appropriate for the child. Typically, caretakers and teachers are involved in the process of implementing treatment interventions because of their key roles in engendering, exacerbating, or attenuating the child's presenting symptoms.

The two primary and most successful interventions with ADHD are behavioral management and psychopharmacology. Behavioral management involves using learning principles to develop interventions to facilitate or inhibit behavior. Externally imposed interventions, such as token systems or response costs, appear more effective for managing the child's impulsivity, inattention, or overactivity than cognitive-behavioral interventions that focus on the child developing internal verbal self-control (Barkley, 1998).

Psychologists mold behavioral interventions to the specific needs of the child in the home, school, and community. Such interventions frequently lead to significant positive change in targeted ADHD core symptoms and coexisting emotional-behavioral difficulties. Unfortunately, this improvement in behavioral control does not often generalize beyond the specific context for which the interventions were developed. For example, the improvement in impulse control brought about by behavioral interventions in a classroom may not transfer to the home and community unless psychologists develop additional behavioral interventions for these contexts. A serious limitation of behavioral management interventions is the rapid reappearance of the child's core ADHD symptoms when the behavioral systems are faded out. In addition, it is difficult to implement behavioral management systems for older children and adolescents because they naturally resist external structuring and control.

Various psychopharmacologic interventions currently are available for treating ADHD. The psychostimulant medications (namely, methylphenidate [Ritalin], methylphenidate hydrochloride [Concerta], amphetamine [Adderall], and dextroamphetamine sulfate [Dexedrine] are the most frequently prescribed medications for ADHD. If the child is presenting other comorbid disorders, the physician may introduce additional medications in combination with the psychostimulants. For example, a depressed child with ADHD may need an antidepressant medication in conjunction with a psychostimulant medication. A relatively recent addition to the medication armamentarium of the physician is atomoxetine (Strattera). Atomoxetine is a nonstimulant medication (norepinephrine reuptake inhibitor) that has been determined to significantly reduce the symptoms of ADHD (Weiss et al., 2005). It is a viable treatment option for children who are nonresponsive to or unable to tolerate psychostimulant medications.

Several factors prompt the use of medication. As noted earlier, behavioral improvement often does not generalize beyond the setting in which the training occurs. Moreover, behavioral interventions may not fully manage the more seriously involved children who exhibit moderate to high levels of core symptoms. Finally, parents and educators often find it difficult to use and maintain behavioral interventions unless the psychologist who develops the interventions closely supervises and supports them.

The behavioral improvements exhibited by children treated with psychostimulant medications can range from slight to dramatic. Psychostimulant medications have enabled children with ADHD to remain in the regular classroom due to the substantial improvement in their behavioral control and academic achievement. Negative parent–child interactions frequently decline as a consequence of the child's new ability to complete homework, follow home rules, and behave appropriately in public settings. Peers can often identify when a child is medicated because of noticeably improved behavioral control, although it is unclear whether the medications actually contribute to increased peer acceptance. Interestingly, despite the widespread use and effectiveness of psychostimulant medications, neuroscientists do not completely understand the neurochemical actions of the drugs. Researchers have proposed a number of hypothesized actions, most implicating the impact of psychostimulant medication on the brain's neurotransmitters, specifically dopamine and norepinephrine, resulting in increased inhibitory control across cognitive and behavioral systems.

Despite the positive effects of psychostimulant medications, these drugs also have several limitations: (1) side effects are common, such as temporary appetite suppression and sleep disruption; (2) the therapeutic effectiveness of the medications vary from child to child; (3) the child may show a brief intensification of core symptoms at the end of the last daily dose ("rebound effect"); (4) children often resist compliance with the medication regimen; (5) the medications have minimal effect on certain problems (such as learning disabilities); and (6) the medications do not "cure" the disorder. Regarding the latter limitation, the core symptoms re-emerge when the child is not medicated.

We now discuss Gilles de la Tourette's disorder, a tic disorder that can be baffling to observers and distressing to the affected child or adolescent. Unfortunately, Gilles de la Tourette's disorder frequently co-occurs with ADHD and obsessive-compulsive disorder.

Tic Disorders

Motor and/or vocal tics can be transient, episodic, or chronic. Tics are particularly intriguing to neuroscientists insofar as they appear to represent a type of behavior that is both voluntary and involuntary with regard to expression. Whether a tic condition constitutes a "disorder" depends on a number of factors such as chronicity; disturbance to academic, social, or work performance; or degree of subjective distress. The most serious tic disorder is that of Gilles de la Tourette's syndrome, which involves the presentation of both motor and vocal tics.

GILLES DE LA TOURETTE'S SYNDROME

Background and Clinical Presentation

Gilles de la Tourette was a brilliant neurologist who studied with Charcot at the Parisian Hôpital de la Saltpêtrière during the latter part of the seventeenth century. Because of his work, the disorder of multiple motor and vocal tics, **Gilles de la Tourette's syndrome (GTS),** bears his name. Unfortunately, Gilles de la Tourette's professional contributions were overshadowed by a series of tragedies during his life. He suffered gunshot wounds inflicted by a

psychiatric patient, struggled with bouts of depression and mania in later life, and is believed to have died of syphilis (Bradshaw, 2001).

GTS is a developmental disorder that exemplifies the hazy boundary between neurology and psychiatry. Initially, GTS was viewed as a psychiatric disorder and, consistent with the early development of psychiatry, considered amendable to psychoanalytic interpretation and therapeutic interventions (Cohen & Leckman, 1994). The APA (DSM IV, 1994) lists it as a "mental disorder," despite advances in the neurosciences and related fields elucidating the neuropathogenesis of the disorder. More accurately, GTS appears to be a product of a complex and only partially understood interplay of genetic, neurophysiologic, and psychological factors.

Tics refer to repetitive, stereotypic, nonrhythmic, and reoccurring motor movements or vocal responses of brief duration (≤ 1 second). Tics are fragments of normal motor/vocal behavior that are semivoluntary in expression. They occupy an intermediate point on the continuum of motor behavior, with one end represented by involuntary movements (for example, resting tremor associated with Parkinson's disease) and the other end characterized by volitional, deliberate, and purposeful actions. The semivoluntary nature of tics relates to the fact that they can be temporarily either suppressed or expressed in an altered or concealed manner (for example, integrating the tic into a series of voluntary movements). An example of a semivoluntary behavior that we all experience is yawning. The urge to yawn can be temporarily suppressed or concealed (namely, covering one's mouth), but if we are truly tired, it will ultimately emerge. Similarly, the tic is often preceded by an urge or sensation (premonitory urge/sensation) that can be suppressed, but this produces tension and discomfort that, in turn, compels the release of the movement or vocalization. Furthermore, the release of the movement/vocalization provides short-term relief from the tension and discomfort. Unfortunately, the relief is followed by renewed tension and discomfort, producing a cycle of repeated tic behaviors.

Tics are classified as simple or complex. Table 11.8 presents examples of each. Simple tics appear more reflexive, whereas complex tics appear more purposeful and coordinated. In extreme cases, motor or speech actions are performed compulsively.

Developmentally, tics are evident in healthy developing children, but resolve over time. Tic disorders are classified as transient, chronic, and GTS. A transient tic disorder refers to motor and/or vocal tics that are exhibited from 1 to 12 months. A chronic disorder relates to the presentation of motor *or* vocal tics for a period greater than 12 months.

Table 11.8 *Simple and Complex Motor and Vocal Tics*

Simple Motor	Complex Motor	Simple Vocal	Complex Vocal
Blinking	Jumping	Throat clearing	Repeating others' speech
Facial twitches	Touching others	Sniffing	Repeating one's own words
Head or arm jerk	Smelling	Snorting	Obscene words
Shoulder shrugs	Facial expressions	Yelping	
Foot stomping	Hand or head gestures	Barking	
	Squatting	Clicks	
	Twirling	Grunts	
	Spinning in a circle	Speech fragments	
	Imitating others' behaviors	Phrases	
	Obscene gestures	Humming	

Finally, GTS encompasses the expression of motor *and* vocal tics for a period exceeding 12 months. The tics associated with GTS are also required to cause significant distress or interfere with the child's or adolescent's adjustment to home, school, or community.

The onset of GTS can be gradual or rapid, with initial motor tics involving the head and face, and later showing a caudal progression. The motor and vocal tics of GTS fluctuate ("wax and wane") in their nature, location, frequency, severity, and duration of presentation. Thus, it is a condition that tends to be intermittent in its expression—periods of tic behaviors that abate, only to reoccur at another point in time—through childhood and adolescence. The average age of onset is 7 years of age, although cases are known to occur both earlier and later than this age.

Tics tend to exacerbate with the onset of adolescence, but generally lessen or resolve by adulthood (Figure 11.6). Unfortunately, the public media often presents *copropraxia* (obscene gestures) and *coprolalia* (obscene or inappropriate speech) as representative of GTS. In fact, these extreme behaviors are relatively rare, occurring in less than 10% of the cases (APA, 1994).

Tic behaviors are exacerbated by stress, boredom, and excitement. Conversely, they tend to diminish when the child is relaxed, intensely focused on an activity, or emotionally calm. Interestingly, tics significantly abate when the child is asleep.

Prevalence

The prevalence of GTS for school-age children is estimated to be 1 to 8 per 1000 children (Costello et al., 1996;

Hornsey, Banerjee, Zeitlin, & Robertson, 2001). Boys are affected at a higher rate than girls, with estimated ratios ranging from 1.8 to 8 boys to 0 to 6.6 girls (Leckman, Peterson, Anderson, Arsten, Pauls, & Cohen, 1997). A generally accepted estimate is a 4:1 ratio of boys to girls. GTS does not appear to have a disproportional affect on any specific racial or ethnic group.

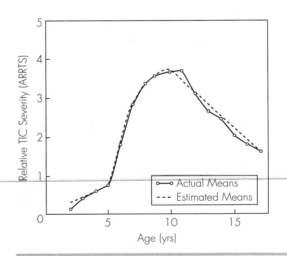

Figure 11.6 Plot of mean tic severity for ages 2 to 18 years. Tic severity reaches its highest point between 10 and 12 years of age and begins to decline thereafter. (Reproduced from Leckman, J., Peterson, B., Schultz, R., & Cohen, D. [2001]. Tics: When habit-forming neural systems form habits of their own. In C. Nelson & M. Luciana [Eds.], *Handbook of developmental cognitive neuroscience* [p. 557, Figure 35.5]. Cambridge, MA: The MIT Press, by permission.)

Comorbid Conditions

Individuals with GTS often experience anxiety, depression, and aggression. Aggression can range from oppositional responses to overt acting-out behavior. However, the two major conditions most likely to co-occur with GTS are **obsessive-compulsive disorder** (OCD) and ADHD. OCD is estimated to occur in approximately 30% to 60% of individuals with GTS, whereas 25% to 50% of children and adolescents with GTS exhibit a co-occurring ADHD (Cirino, Chapieski, & Massman, 2000; Leckman et al., 1997).

Obsessions are repetitive, intrusive, unwanted, and often inappropriate thoughts or images. Obsessive thoughts/images typically relate to themes of aggression, sexuality, contamination, cataclysmic events, symmetry, and exactness. Often, obsessions prompt compulsions that are thoughts or actions to resist, suppress, or neutralize the obsessions. Compulsive behaviors are many and varied, frequently involving checking, counting, ordering, washing, seeking reassurance, and ritualistic behaviors (Bradshaw, 2001). Unfortunately, the anxiety reduction produced by compulsions is short-lived. Obsessive thoughts/images reoccur and prompt, once again, the compulsive behaviors.

When GTS and OCD co-occur, it can be difficult to differentiate complex motor tics from compulsive behaviors. The two disorders can sometimes be differentiated by the dynamics of the two conditions. The sequence of events in GTS is as follows: a premonitory urge or sensation (sensorimotor prompting), followed by the release of the tic behavior and momentary relief of the tension and press associated with the premonitory urge/sensation. In contrast, OCD involves an unwanted image or thought (cognitive prompting) that engenders anxiety and distress. The compulsive behavior serves to alleviate the anxiety associated with the obsessive thought/image.

As we have discussed, ADHD relates to the manifestation of age-inappropriate inattention, impulsivity, and hyperactivity. The comorbidity of ADHD, OCD, and GTS is highly disruptive to the child or adolescent's academic performance, social acceptance, and self-valuing. A number of interpretations have been posed to account for the comorbidity of OCD and ADHD with GTS. Of significance, however, are research findings indicating that all three disorders appear to relate to perturbations of the frontostriatal brain systems.

Neuropsychological Pathogenesis

GTS is one of the most familial of the neuropsychiatric disorders and appears to be transmitted via autosomal dominant genes with incomplete penetrance (incomplete expression in affected individuals) (Bradshaw, 2001; Pennington, 2002). With monozygotic twins, the rate of concordance for GTS is 50% to 56%, and it increases to 77% to 94% when GTS and chronic tic disorders are combined. The concordance rate for dizygotic twins is 8% to 18%, but increases to only 23% when combined with chronic tic disorder (Leckman et al., 1997; Leckman & Cohen, 1996; Pennington, 2002). The dopamine D2 A1 allele and dopamine *D3* and *D4* receptor genes and chromosomal abnormalities (8, 18, and 22) have also been implicated (Alsobrook & Pauls, 1999; Bradshaw, 2001; Casey, Tottenham, & Fossella, 2002).

Alterations of neurotransmitters intrinsic to the frontostriatal pathways have been posed as pathogenic to GTS (Bradshaw, 2001; Sheppard et al., 1999). The catecholamines (dopaminergic, serotonergic, and noradrenergic systems) have received the greatest attention. Of these transmitters, dopamine appears to play the crucial role in GTS. In part, this is based on the effects of medications that either inhibit or facilitate dopamine activity. Dopamine (D2) receptor antagonists such as haloperidol (Haldol) reduce motor and vocal tics. In contrast, dopamine agonists such as central nervous system stimulants (for example, methylphenidate [Ritalin]) can exacerbate motor and vocal tics. It is unclear whether striatal D2 receptors are hypersensitive to dopamine or whether there is a dopaminergic hyperinnervation of the striatum (Leckman et al., 1997). The effectiveness of clonidine (Catapres) and guanfacine (Tenex) (α_2 noradrenergic receptor agonists) in the treatment of the symptoms of both GTS and ADHD further suggests a role of noradrenalin in the modulating cortico-striatal-thalamo-cortical pathways. Support for the role of serotonin in the cause of GTS is limited, although there is significant evidence for its role in OCD (Pennington, 2002). Currently, the role of other central neurotransmitters in the pathogenesis of GTS awaits clarification.

Since the mid-1990s, ongoing research has focused on the role of environmental factors that place a child at risk for the development of tic disorders. Extensive research has been directed toward determining whether there is a risk for the development of tic disorders as part of an autoimmune response. Clinical findings of a temporal relation between β-hemolytic streptococci and the onset or exacerbation of tic disorders and/or OCD provided the impetus for this research. The National Institute of Mental Health labeled this disorder *pediatric autoimmune neuropsychiatric disorders associated with streptococcal infections* (PANDAS). Pathogenically, it is hypothesized that the human body's antibodies targeting the streptococci also cross-react with the basal ganglia, with resulting damage and production of tics and OCD behaviors. A number of studies have supported differences between increased levels of antistreptococcal antibodies for GTS relative to control groups; however, others have not (Hoekstra, Kallenber, Korf, & Minderaa, 2002). Moreover, the mechanism of action of antistreptococcal antibodies with regard to the development or exacerbation of tics remains to be elucidated. Insofar as streptococcal infections are common among children and most do not develop tics and/or OCD, additional investigations are needed to determine what factors account for the development of tics and/or compulsions in a select few individuals.

Structural and functional neuroimaging studies have reported alterations of brain structure and metabolic activation patterns associated with GTS. A consistent finding across studies is reduced volume or atypical asymmetries of the caudate, putamen, and globus pallidus of the basal ganglia (Peterson et al., 2003; Sheppard et al., 1999). Altered activations of the prefrontal cortex (lateral orbitofrontal and anterior cingulate), motor cortex, somatosensory association areas, and thalamus have also been reported (Jeffries, Schooler, Schoenbach, Herscovitch, Chase, & Braun, 2002). Jointly, the neuroimaging studies provide growing evidence for the role of the frontostriatal pathways in the pathogenesis of GTS (Singer & Minzer, 2003). The motor and vocal tics of GTS are hypothesized to relate to disinhibition (possibly because of hypersensitivity of dopamine receptors or hyperinnervation of the striatum) of the frontal motor-striatal circuit, particularly at the level of the caudate, resulting in the release of motor programs. Notably, the frontal motor circuit includes projections from the somatosensory cortex, implicating its potential role in the generation of premonitory urges. Hypoactivation at the level of the lateral orbitofrontal and anterior cingulated cortex suggests a disruption of top-down voluntary control.

While there are indications of hyperactivation and hypoactivation of different frontostriatal circuits in OCD and ADHD, the interactive pathogenic role of the circuits in co-occurring GTS, OCD, and ADHD is not well understood. The comorbidity of the three disorders implicates some level or degree of dysfunction across the major frontostriatal circuits; however, we await research findings explicating the nature and cause of this dysfunction.

Neuropsychological Assessment

Because of the putative role of disinhibition in the expression of motor and vocal tics, studies of inhibitory control have been undertaken. The evidence from these studies has been inconsistent in supporting inhibitory weaknesses as specific to GTS (Channon, Pratt, & Robertson, 2003). Similarly, little evidence exists of deficits in executive functions supported by the dorsolateral prefrontal cortex, such as planning, rule finding, and set shifting (Ozonoff & Jensen, 1999). Lateral frontal regions are believed to contribute to strategic, working, and procedural memory

processes, and at least one study (Stebbins, Singh, Weiner, Wilson, Goetz, & Gabrieli, 1995) has identified weaknesses in this domain for adults with GTS participants.

Deficits related to visual-construction, visuomotor integration, and motor performance are frequently evident in children and adults with GTS, possibly reflecting disruption of the motor-striatal pathway (Leckman, Peterson, Schultz, & Cohen, 2001). Unfortunately, many of these studies have not controlled for the high frequency of comorbid conditions that accompany GTS, potentially contributing to conflicting and equivocal results. However, selected studies controlling for comorbidity and GTS are available. For example, Silverstein, Como, Palumbo, West, and Osborn (1995) found that the poor attentional performance of adults with GTS is related to the presence of ADHD and OCD, and not a unique deficit associated with GTS. In a more recent study, Channon and colleagues (2003) compared GTS, GTS + ADHD, GTS + OCD, and healthy control children and adolescents on measures of executive functioning, memory, and learning. Children and adolescents with only GTS differed from the healthy control youngsters on one measure of response initiation, whereas the GTS + ADHD group demonstrated deficits on several measures of executive function assessing response inhibition, strategy generation, and multitasking. Furthermore, the GTS + OCD group did not differ in their executive performance from the healthy control group. Finally, none of the clinical groups differed from healthy control individuals in memory or learning performance.

Casey and colleagues (2002) have extensively studied the frontostriatal regions and circuitry of children with developmental disorders and healthy children. Reflecting this ongoing research has been the development of a model of cognitive control. One critical aspect of cognitive control is the ability to suppress or override competing attentional and behavioral responses to resolve conflict. The inhibition of three forms of cognitive-motor processing (stimulus selection, response selection, and response execution) was studied with healthy control and clinic groups (children with GTS, ADHD, childhood onset schizophrenia, and **Sydenham's chorea**). The Sydenham's chorea group was selected because of the high rate of OCD (75%) associated with the disorder. The intent of the studies was to determine whether the separate disorders demonstrated different cognitive control deficits.

The children were administered a battery of tasks that assessed the three cognitive control processes. The stimulus selection task requires the inhibition of attention to visual features previously viewed in order to attend to a new feature. The response selection task involved the learning of a series of responses to specific stimuli, and then the production of a different (incompatible) set of responses to the same stimuli. In the latter condition, the child was faced with inhibiting the first learned response set in order to select and generate the second response set. In contrast, the third task, response execution, involved the creation of a prepotent response through the frequent association of the response with a specific stimuli and then periodically requiring the inhibition of the response to a different stimuli. Relative to healthy children, the GTS group demonstrated significantly poorer performance in response-execution, whereas the ADHD group showed deficits in stimulus selection and response-execution. Furthermore, the childhood schizophrenic group was impaired in stimulus-selection, and the Sydenham's chorea (OCD) group showed deficits in response-selection. Mapping of these cognitive processes to the neural circuits is incomplete, although there are indications that the right prefrontal cortex is primarily involved in stimulus-selection, the right orbital/anterior cingulate circuits are related to response execution, and the basal ganglia-thalamocortical circuits, at the level of the caudate, underpin response selection. Confirmation of these findings should increase our neuropsychological understanding of GTS and other disorders and provide differential information to aid diagnosis and treatment.

Treatment and Developmental Course

The two primary treatment interventions for GTS are behavioral modification and pharmacologic therapy. A wide range of behavioral interventions has been applied to GTS with varying degrees of success. The techniques that have been introduced in the treatment of GTS include: (1) massed practice (rapid and repeated voluntary production of a tic); (2) operant conditioning (providing reinforcement for tic-free periods); (3) anxiety management training (for example, training in muscle relaxation for use in anxiety-engendering situations); (4) exposure plus response prevention (stimuli or conditions are presented that increase the likelihood of premonitory urge, and the child is not allowed to release the tic); and (5) habit reversal (performing a competing and incompatible physical response contingent on the urge to perform the tic). Of these techniques, habit reversal has received the greatest support as an efficacious treatment (Piacentini & Chang, 2001). Although each of these techniques can lead to tic reduction, the treatment effects often fail to generalize to other situations and are frequently short-lived.

The medications used for GTS treatment are generally dopamine antagonists, such as the neuroleptic haloperidol (Haldol), which are effective in the treatment of the disorder. Unfortunately, the use of typical neuroleptics can result in a number of undesirable and sometimes se-

vere side effects. These side effects range from cognitive slowing to Parkinsonian-like motor disturbances. The use of the newer atypical antipsychotic medications such as risperidone (Risperdal) reduces the likelihood of side effects, but their efficacy has not been fully established. Recently, there has been interest in the dopamine antagonist metoclopramide, which has been found to be effective in tic reduction without significant neuroleptic-like adverse side effects (Nicolson, Craven-Thuss, Smith, McKinlay, & Castellanos, 2005). However, further studies are warranted to assess its efficacy and safety over long periods of use. Clonidine (Catapres) and guanfacine (Tenex) are α_2 agonists and have been used with varying success in reducing tic behaviors. The precise mechanism of action of α_2 agonists is unknown, although there are indications that dopamine utilization is increased in the frontal regions of the brain (Pennington, 2002).

The child or adolescent with GTS and comorbid OCD often requires the introduction of behavioral and cognitive behavioral interventions that target tic behaviors and disruptive obsessions and compulsions. Often, these techniques are insufficient, and medication is introduced. Clomipramine (Anafranil), a tricyclic antidepressant, is efficacious for the treatment of OCD. However, because of the potential for significant side effects associated with Anafranil, selective serotonin reuptake inhibitors (SSRIs) are currently the first line of pharmacologic intervention. Paroxetine (Paxil) is an SSRI that has been determined to be helpful in reducing intrusive ideations and compulsive behaviors for both children and adults. Importantly, SSRIs do not typically exacerbate motor or vocal tics.

A particularly difficult presentation is the child with GTS and ADHD. The psychostimulants, although effective for treating ADHD, can exacerbate the motor and vocal tics associated with GTS. However, not all children who receive a psychostimulant medication experience acceleration of tic behaviors. For the child who is unable to tolerate a psychostimulant, clonidine or guanfacine may be introduced to reduce tics, as well as the hyperactivity and impulsivity associated with ADHD. However, the α_2 agonists are not always effective in the treatment of GTS or ADHD. In addition, the child medicated with a α_2 agonist warrants careful monitoring because of the potential for adverse cardiac effects. Recently, atomoxetine (Strattera) was approved for the treatment of ADHD. Atomoxetine is a noradrenaline reuptake inhibitor that, in addition to reducing ADHD symptoms, does not appear to exacerbate co-occurring motor and vocal tics. In more severe cases of GTS with co-occurring OCD and/or ADHD, a combination of medications is often needed to reduce disruptive symptoms.

Neuropsychological strengths and weaknesses warrant consideration when mapping out the child's educational curriculum. The teacher and classmates of the child with GTS can profit from a discussion with the neuropsychologist or other informed person concerning what tic behaviors are and are not, the intermittent expression and possible increasing severity of tic behaviors, and what they are to do or not to do when the child is exhibiting tic behaviors. This information is important for increasing their understanding of GTS, disabusing misinterpretations, and reducing negative responses to the afflicted child. Interventions to help the teacher and child to cope with tics within the classroom are important. For example, the teacher may need to allow the child to leave the classroom and go to the nurse's office if a significant exacerbation of tic behavior occurs. While in the nurse's office, the child can be helped to initiate any techniques that have been found to be effective in reducing his or her tics. Seating the child in the front row of the class can reduce the detection of tics by classmates, because the majority of them

will be seated behind the child. Most important, the teacher and educational staff need to be alert and intervene quickly if they observe teasing or taunting of the child by peers.

Adolescence can be a difficult period of development for a healthy teenager. The motor and vocal tics of GTS, coupled with ADHD and/or OCD comorbidity, can be disruptive to the adolescent's efforts to affiliate with peers, initiate dating relationships, develop a positive body image, and establish a healthy self-identity. Fortunately, as discussed earlier, motor and vocal tics of GTS begin to attenuate or resolve during adolescence and early adulthood. Most adolescents with GTS graduate from high school and demonstrate appropriate adaptation to their disorder. In cases when GTS symptoms do not reduce, or even exacerbate, social, vocational, and emotional adjustment in adulthood may be compromised (Brown & Ivers, 1999). Hopefully, future pharmacological advances and refinements will identify medications that will effectively address vocal and motor tics at all age levels while producing fewer negative side effects.

Summary

Several developmental disorders currently are the focus of extensive research by neuropsychology and other disciplines. The neuropsychological identification of the potential brain and behavior correlates of dyslexia and NVLD have enhanced our understanding of learning disabilities. Although most theorization and research has focused on disorders of reading and mathematics, other forms of learning disabilities, such as dysgraphia, await investigation. Autism has a profound and often global impact on the cognitive and behavioral development of a child. Advances have been made in the understanding of the neuropathogenesis, neuropsychological assessment, neuropsychological models, developmental course, and treatment of autism. However, the cause of autism remains elusive, and treatment interventions often fail to significantly alter the symptoms of the disorder. ADHD is one of the most studied childhood disorders of our time. Researchers have redefined and relabeled the disorder, spawned numerous hypotheses and theories, and generated multiple interventions. Unfortunately, the etiology of ADHD remains unknown; the interplay of mediating variables such as the child's personality, environmental effects, and presence of comorbid disorders is also poorly understood; and the current treatment options are limited and often ineffective. Although the entrance of neuropsychology into the study of ADHD is relatively recent, optimism remains high that its contribution will provide new and much needed direction to the study and understanding of the disorder. Finally, GTS is a significantly disruptive and potentially embarrassing disorder that falls on the boundary of voluntary-involuntary behavior. The high frequency of comorbidity of other disorders with GTS highlights the diverse effects of frontostriatal dysfunction.

Critical Thinking Questions

- Why are the symptoms of NVLD and ADHD so often displayed by children exhibiting a wide range of developmental disorders?
- Can a child with autism or Asperger's syndrome develop normal social awareness and attachment? If so, how would this be accomplished?
- How would you respond to the comment, "ADHD does not exist, it is merely a diagnosis to excuse lazy and undisciplined children?"

■ As our understanding of the neural correlates of learning and neuropsychiatric disorders expands, what impact will this have on traditional psychological and educational treatment?

■ Does the finding that the symptoms of GTS often attenuate or resolve in later adolescences or early adulthood support a conceptualization of the disorder as a developmental lag? How do you account for individuals who do not show such improvement and struggle with GTS as a lifelong disorder?

Key Terms

Dyslexia
Dyscalculia
Dysgraphia
Surface dyslexia
Deep dyslexia
Flicker fusion rate
Magnocellular visual system
Parvocellular visual system
Saccadic eye movements
Phonologic awareness
Double-deficit hypothesis
Planum temporale
Neuronal Ectopias

Cytoarchitectonic
    dysplasia
Lexicon store
Metacognition
Pragmatics of language
Autism
Asperger's syndrome
Autistic aloneness
Joint attention
Echolalia
Neologism
Hyperlexia
Savant skills

Hyperserotonemia
Fragile X
"Stuck in set" perseveration
Executive planning
Response inhibition
Theory of mind
Canalesthesia
Impaired affective
    assignment
Asociality
Extended selective
    attention
Response cost

Overcorrection
Attention-deficit/hyperactivity
    disorder (ADHD)
Disengage attention
Move attention
Engage attention
Prepotent response
Interference control
Gilles de la Tourette's syndrome
    (GTS)
Obsessive-compulsive
    disorder (OCD)
Sydenham's chorea

Web Connections

http://www.bda-dyslexia.org.uk
Dyslexia—provides a large collection of references on dyslexia.

http://www.cognitivedesigns.com
Cognitive Designs—provides educational and clinical tools to teach and treat children with autism or other developmental learning disorders.

http://www.mentalhealth.com/dis/p20-ch06.html
Autistic Disorder—comprehensive site that provides descriptions, treatments, research references, books, magazine articles, and various links concerning autism.

http://www.mentalhealth.com/fr20.html
Attention-Deficit Hyperactivity Disorder—provides a comprehensive overview of ADHD: a review of descriptions, treatment options, books, and magazine articles.

http://www.mentalhealth.com/dis/p20-ch02.html
Conduct Disorder—provides a complete listing of materials on CD; links are provided and reviews of treatments, books, and magazine articles.

http://www.mentalhealth.com/dis/p20-ch05.html
Oppositional Defiant Disorder—provides a complete listing of materials on oppositional defiant disorder; links are provided and reviews of treatments, books, and magazine articles.

http://www.tsa-usa.org
Tourette Syndrome Association—provides parents and professions with information related to the identification, treatment, and education of individuals with Tourette's syndrome.

Chapter 12

CEREBROVASCULAR DISORDERS AND TUMORS

In whatsoever house I enter, I will enter to help the sick.
—*Hippocrates (460–377 B.C.)*

Overview

The normal functioning central nervous system (CNS) can be affected by a number of neurologic disorders and diseases. Some will result in similar types of damage, and some will be vastly different. Some result in focal effects, others result in diffuse damage. Physicians expect some, if not complete, recovery after many types of brain damage, such as mild head injuries. Other types of brain diseases are more severe and may result in lasting impairment, as is often the case in stroke, or may be even fatal, as is Alzheimer's disease, with which there is an inevitable decline in health culminating in death. Thus, brain disorders may have a wide-ranging impact on a person's well-being. Often, significant neuropsychological deficits exist that result in marked disabilities, alterations in personality, and a decline in quality of life.

This chapter discusses the most common neurologic problems and neuropsychological sequelae that are associated with cerebrovascular accidents (CVAs) and tumors. Chapter 13 discusses the impact on the brain and its recovery related to head injury. Chapters 14 and 15 present degenerative disorders, which are good examples of diffuse and generalized involvement of brain pathology. Chapter 16 reviews disorders of consciousness, in which the typical clinical picture is also more generalized, with many behavioral adaptive skills possibly affected.

For each disorder, we examine neuropathology, neuropsychological sequelae, appropriate treatments, and case examples of patients we have treated. We present the information within a neuropsychological perspective; that is, we describe the disorders with particular relevance to the relations among brain anatomy, biological processes of the brain, and their behavioral product.

Pathologic Process of Brain Damage

This section reviews examples of brain damage and their mechanisms of action within the brain. These examples are not necessarily mutually exclusive, and many conditions may result in more than one problem. They also are not totally inclusive, but are meant to provide an overview of some of the more common terms and conditions you will encounter as you read about various pathologies throughout this book. Although some examples result in specific behavioral effects, many terms, such as "lesion," are more generic, and their behavioral effects often depend on the specific location and extent of damage within the brain.

BRAIN LESIONS

What are lesions, and what effects do they have on the brain? Brain **lesions** (derived from Latin *laesio,* meaning "to hurt") are any pathologic or traumatic discontinuity of brain tissue. Lesions result in "holes" or "cavities" in the brain and almost always entail loss of function. Depending on their size and location, lesions result in minor or major behavioral effects. Lesions may be caused by traumas, such as punctures from bullet wounds, fragments of skull fractures, or other foreign objects entering the brain. Other events that cause lesions include CVAs, surgical removal of tumors, or diseases such as multiple sclerosis or Creutzfeldt–Jacob disease.

Neurons that are completely severed often degenerate. The tissue that surrounds the lesion shrinks and dies

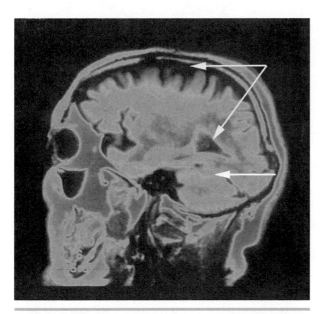

Figure 12.1 Sagittal magnetic resonance imaging of brain with small stroke in the superior portion of the cerebellum (bottom). Significant atrophy is associated with increased size of the lateral ventricles and intracranial space (top). See inside covers for color image. (Courtesy Eric Zillmer.)

within hours. Cerebrospinal fluid (CSF) then fills the cavity. With time, surrounding brain tissue may collapse the cavity, which may concomitantly distort other areas of the brain or ventricles, depending on the size of the lesion (Figure 12.1). Any dead neuronal debris is engulfed by the brain's micro "cleaning machines," the phagocytes, which are forms of glial cells (see Chapter 4). As a result, glial cells may be all that remains in the cavity of the lesion where neurons were once active. This obviously results in a blockage or interruption of neural transmission.

ANOXIA AND HYPOXIA: OXYGEN DEPRIVATION TO THE BRAIN

Most readers will know that reduced flow of oxygen to the brain is dangerous. CVAs or strokes imply by definition a disruption or stoppage of blood to the brain. Strokes almost always result in neuronal loss or degeneration. Neurons need oxygen to break down glucose into carbon dioxide and water. Furthermore, the brain has no reservoir of glucose or oxygen. Thus, the brain depends on a constant and immediate supply. An elaborate blood system carries oxygen and important nutrients to the brain. Although weighing less than 3 pounds, the brain is

rather demanding, requiring more than 20% of the body's oxygen to keep functioning effectively. As a result, the brain is particularly vulnerable to oxygen depletion.

If a neuron lacks oxygen for some time, the neuron will die. This **necrosis,** or *neuronal cell death,* is a direct result of a crucial interference with the cellular metabolism of the neuron. A complete absence of oxygen supply to the brain is **anoxia.** The most common causes of anoxia are cardiopulmonary failures associated with heart attacks, complications of anesthesia, accidents such as near-drowning episodes, or other severe traumas to the brain, such as are often seen in gunshot wounds to the head. In these cases, where there may be respiratory or cardiac arrest, permanent brain damage follows unless oxygen is restored quickly. Most anoxic episodes appear to result in damage to subcortical and limbic areas, the frontal lobes, and the cerebellum.

In contrast, **hypoxia** describes a reduced, but not complete, oxygenation of brain. Hypoxia typically entails not cell death, but some possible interference in the functioning of the neuron. In general, 4 to 6 minutes of anoxia may cause necrosis, although this is highly variable and depends on individual and environmental characteristics. Hypoxia can occur at high altitude, during acute cardiac crisis, during the aftermath of open-heart surgery, and during exertion in deep-sea divers. It may also be seen in carbon monoxide poisoning, may accompany sleep in the aging brain, and is present in people with chronic obstructive pulmonary disease related to chronic, intermittent lowered oxygen saturation in the blood.

A growing body of literature suggests that individuals who are otherwise healthy and who experience mild-to-moderate hypoxia may demonstrate significant difficulties in concentration, short-term memory, new learning, and judgment. At extreme altitude—that is, more than 22,000 feet—hypoxia can impair a human's cognitive function, including motor speed, judgment, verbal fluency, learning, and short-term memory. Severe hypoxia produces more dramatic deficits, often resulting in irreversible brain damage. However, under specific environmental conditions (such as cold water submersion), children may recover completely from acute hypoxia, even if it has lasted as long as 20 minutes. The reasons for this are unclear, but are probably related to young age and the poorly understood effects of cold-water submersion on brain metabolism.

Hypoxia can occur at high altitudes. For example, climbers refer to elevations above 25,000 feet as the "death zone," because of the low oxygen level in the air (Krakauer, 1997). The air is so thin that even conditioned climbers may become hypoxic. In fact, if one were to "pluck" a person from sea level and drop him or her on Mount Everest, which has an elevation of 29,028 feet, death by anoxia would occur within minutes. Even when adapted to extreme elevations, many climbers must use supplemental oxygen. Nevertheless, at such high altitudes, one becomes careless, sluggish, and fatigued. To conserve oxygen, the brain may diminish oxygen supply to more distal parts of the body, increasing the risk for frostbite and hypothermia, and sometimes edema of the brain and death. Recent neuropsychological studies conducted on the ascent and the summit of Mount Everest clearly indicate hypoxia in climbers and a related dysfunction in memory and concentration (for example, see Virues-Ortega, Buela-Casal, Garrido, & Alcazar, 2004).

Medical conditions can also affect oxygen uptake. For example, chronic obstructive pulmonary disease is a disorder in which the lung has lost its capacity to efficiently exchange oxygen with white blood cells. **Sleep apnea** (derived from Greek *apnoia,* meaning "negative breathing") is a good example of chronic hypoxia during sleep. Breathing is disturbed throughout the night and often completely stops for periods as long as a minute. These hypoxic episodes often occur with more severity during rapid eye movement (REM) sleep, because the voluntary muscles that assist in breathing are paralyzed during dream sleep. Under normal circumstances, blood is 95% oxygenated, but in sleep apnea patients, this can decrease to 50% and less. Consequently, people with sleep apnea often report morning headaches, poor attention and concentration and, of course, sleepiness during the day (Zillmer, Ware, Rose, & Maximin, 1988). It is unclear whether the effects of hypoxia reverse with increased oxygen saturation in the blood. To some extent, they appear to, because patients often completely recover. Reversibility is likely related to the length of deprivation.

HYDROCEPHALUS

Hydrocephalus is a condition in which the ventricles enlarge abnormally, because of increased CSF production, decreased CSF absorption, or a blockage of CSF flow through the ventricles. There are several medical reasons why this occurs. You may recall from Chapter 5 that the ventricles produce and circulate CSF through and around the brain and spinal cord. Spinal fluid and waste products are then reabsorbed, in part by the ventricles. The presence of blood or blood products mixing with the CSF,

perhaps as a result of hemorrhage or infection, may interfere with reabsorption. This condition is called **communicating hydrocephalus.** Finally, blockage of the circulation of CSF is termed **obstructive hydrocephalus.** In young children, obstructive hydrocephalus is often caused by a congenital narrowing or stenosis of the aqueduct of Sylvius between the third and fourth ventricles. In adults, obstructive hydrocephalus is most likely caused by brain tumors protruding into the ventricles.

Damage to the brain caused by hydrocephalus results from the pressure of squeezing parts of the brain against an immovable skull. If not corrected quickly, intense pressure can cut off the blood supply and result in cell death. Behaviorally, hydrocephalus results in symptoms of increased cranial pressure, such as sleepiness, severe headache, and nausea. Hydrocephalus is usually an acute condition, but physicians can reverse it by releasing the pressure; they surgically insert a tube to shunt the CSF into the peritoneal cavity of the body—the potential space around the lining of the abdominal and pelvic walls. If not treated quickly, progressive hydrocephalus can be life threatening, because it impinges on vital brainstem functions such as respiration and arousal.

Overview of Cerebrovascular Disorders

Bubbeh had to die, as you and I will one day have to die. Just as I had witnessed the decline of my grandmother's life force, I was present when it gave the first signal of its finality. It was early on an ordinary morning; Bubbeh and I were doing ordinary things. Having finished breakfast a few minutes before, I was still hunched over the sports section of the *Daily News* when I became aware that there was something very strange in the way Bubbeh was trying to wipe clean the surface of the kitchen table. Even though we had long since realized that such household tasks were beyond her, she had never quite given up trying, and seemed oblivious to the fact that one or another of us always repeated the work after she laboriously shuffled out of the room. But when I looked up from the tabloid, I saw that her wide circular strokes were even more ineffectual than usual. Her sweeping hand had become aimless, as though acting on its own with no plan or direction. The circles ceased to be circles and soon became mere languid, useless drags of the moist cloth that was barely held in her flaccid hand, adrift on the table without purpose or weight. Her face was turned straight ahead. She seemed to be looking at something outside the window behind my chair instead of at the table in front of her. Her unseeing eyes had the dullness of oblivion; her face was expressionless. Even the most impassive of faces betrays something, but I knew at that instant of absolute blankness that I had lost my grandmother. I shouted, "Bubbeh, Bubbeh!" but it made no difference. She was beyond hearing me. The cloth slipped from her hand and she crumpled soundlessly to the floor.

I bounded to her side and called her name again, but my shouting was as futile as my attempts to comprehend what was happening. Somehow, and I remember not a moment of it, I gathered her up and staggered to the room we shared. I laid her down in my bed. Her breathing was stertorous and loud. It blew in long, forceful blasts from only one corner of her mouth, and it flapped her cheek out like a buffeted wet sail each time she exhaled from that noisy bellows somewhere down deep in her throat. I can't recall which side it was, but one entire half of her face seemed toneless and flaccid. I rushed to the phone and called a doctor whose office was not far away. Then I contacted my aunt Rose at the Seventh Avenue dress factory where she worked. Rose got there before the doctor could free himself from a waiting room filled with early-morning patients, but we knew there was nothing he could do anyway. When he arrived, he told us Bubbeh had suffered a stroke, and wouldn't live more than a few days. She outsmarted the doctor and hung on for the next 14 nights. (Nuland, 1993, p. 58–59)

Cerebrovascular disease is reported to be the most common cause of neurologic disability in the Western world, the second leading cause of death among the oldest old (age >85), and the third most common cause of death in the developed countries of the world. Only cancer and heart attacks affect more people. Strokes are a major health concern in the United States, and they can significantly affect the quality of life of those afflicted, as well as their families.

In the United States, stroke affects approximately 500,000 people each year, and it is the major cause of disability among adults. The death rate associated with strokes is approximately 5%, corresponding to approximately 150,000 deaths each year in the United States. Another 150,000 people are left with permanent severe disability. Individuals suffering from a cerebrovascular disorder place a significant financial and emotional burden on the families who take care of their loved ones. The estimated public health costs related to stroke amount to billions of dollars per year and are expected to accelerate steadily as advances in emergency medicine allow more stroke victims to survive.

The average age of a stroke victim is approximately 70 years (see Zillmer, Fowler, Waechtler, Harris, & Khan, 1992). As the population of the United States is growing, life expectancy is likewise increasing. Today, people are living longer and into the age-groups that are more at risk for CVAs. In fact, gerontologists have called the over 65 age-group the fastest-growing segment of the U.S. population. This increase in the elderly population greatly swells the number of those at risk for strokes, creating a situation in which more people in the population will actually be suffering from CVAs.

STROKE DEFINITION

The term *stroke* itself is not clearly defined and is not a precise medical term. A more technical term for stroke is **cerebrovascular accident (CVA),** which describes a heterogeneous group of vascular disorders that result in brain injury. The brain's blood vessels are damaged, which can decrease blood flow within and to the brain. In simple terms, stroke "suffocates" brain tissue and often produces an area of dead or dying brain tissue. A stroke always occurs in the brain and is the most common type of cerebrovascular disease. Thus, CVA or stroke is a common label assigned to clinical syndromes that are caused by blockage in blood supply or by bleeding in the brain. Stroke can result from a wide variety of different vascular diseases, but not all vascular disorders produce stroke. Although the onset of symptoms is rapid (hence the term *stroke*), the full development of the clinical picture may take an appreciable time, sometimes hours, depending on the rate of the bleed and its final cessation (Bannister, 1992).

In the past, people have conceptualized stroke as a "fait accompli"; That is, once it occurred, little could be done. Recent medical technology, however, has made advances in treating the stroke patient immediately; therefore, early diagnosis and intervention have become a high priority. Physicians now treat stroke as a "brain attack," a medical emergency similar to a heart attack. Stroke can produce an array of disorders of great complexity. Most strokes occur, or are localized, in only one of the cerebral hemispheres, although in some instances, multiple strokes or one major subcortical stroke affects the entire brain. In general, the deficits directly relate to the location or the hemisphere where the stroke occurs.

Neuropsychologists play a crucial role in CVA diagnosis and rehabilitation. They are at the forefront in many significant advances in long-term treatment and rehabilitation of stroke patients. In addition, neuropsychologists conduct research on CVA survivors because it provides them with clinical data by which to examine localized lesions, propose strategies for intervention and rehabilitation, and indirectly develop knowledge of the functioning intact brain (Naugle, Cullum, & Bigler, 1998).

IMPAIRMENT OF BLOOD SUPPLY TO THE BRAIN

The clinical presentation of a patient after stroke reflects the damage to the anatomic structures of the brain. Disruption of major arteries can cause characteristic symptoms according to the area of the brain that artery serves (the vascular system of the brain is reviewed in Chapter 5). For example, the symptoms of a right hemisphere stroke are quite different from those of a left hemisphere CVA. Almost always behavior is disrupted, and thus physicians often consult neuropsychologists to evaluate stroke patients. The following three related neuropsychological events often occur after a stroke, all of which interfere with normal brain functioning. Victims may have to contend with these three serious consequences of stroke:

1. Disrupted blood supply decreases oxygenation, as in hypoxia or anoxia, of the involved brain tissue.
2. Related to bleeding (or hemorrhage), a space-occupying mass or pocket of blood often develops, which may press on nearby brain structures, affecting their integrity. As a result, **intracranial pressure (ICP)** may suddenly increase.
3. When blood spills out of the artery and into brain plasma, many toxins in the blood can interfere with normal brain metabolism. In an intact vascular system, the blood–brain barrier (BBB) protects the surrounding tissue from any toxic properties contained in blood, but exposed blood outside of the artery irritates brain tissue.

Types of Cerebrovascular Disorders

To effectively rehabilitate the patient and provide appropriate guidance to the family and patient, neuropsychologists differentiate among three different types and mechanisms of stroke:

1. "Temporary" strokes arise from insufficient blood supply to an area of the brain. These events, collectively called ischemia, often manifest in short-lasting attacks that cause only transient deficits.
2. Blockage of an artery causes a more severe loss of blood supply. This **infarction** often results in more lasting neuropsychological deficits.
3. The third type of stroke is related to bleeding and to displacement of the brain that arises from a hemorrhage. **Hemorrhages** are the most severe form of stroke and often cause permanent brain damage or death.

Each cerebrovascular event is described in more detail in the following paragraphs.

TRANSIENT ISCHEMIC ATTACKS

Neuropsychologists call an acute, focal (localized) neurologic deficit, evidenced by a transient loss of function, a **transient ischemic attack (TIA).** Recovery should occur within 24 hours, but is often complete within a much shorter time, often minutes. The attacks vary from infrequent (that is, less than one a month) to very frequent (that is, several times a day).

Rudolf Virchow, a German physician and the founder of German medicine, coined the term *ischemia* (derived from Greek *ischein,* meaning "to hold in check," and *haima,* meaning "blood"); literally, ischemia means "a holding in check of the flow of blood" to refer to the temporary disruption of blood flow. Deficits from TIAs heal gradually, and the patient most often returns to normal neurologic and neuropsychological functioning. An important assumption in a TIA is that no actual damage to any neurons has occurred, just a temporary insufficiency of oxygen supply (Powers, 1990).

TIAs most commonly involve the internal carotid, middle cerebral, or the vertebral-basilar arteries. Clinically, neuropsychologists divide the deficits into the anterior circulation involving the carotid system and those affecting the posterior circulation involving the vertebral-basilar system. If the ischemic attack affects anterior circulation, the deficits manifested will most likely relate to brief clumsiness or weakness of a limb, dysarthria, or aphasia. If the attack affects the posterior circulation, deficits may include dizziness, neglect, double vision, and numbness or weakness of the extremities. Individuals suffering from TIAs rarely lose consciousness completely, and as mentioned earlier, cognitive and physical functioning usually return to normal once the attack has ceased.

Because one of the first "signs" of stroke is TIAs, their occurrence should be taken seriously. People suffering from TIAs have a 20% to 35% greater risk for stroke than do unaffected individuals, and they go on to suffer obvious infarction (see later). Little research has been conducted, however, to determine which individuals suffering from TIAs go on to experience development of the more severe infarctions. Another third continue to have TIAs without any permanent disability, and the remainder

Table 12.1 *Symptoms of a Transient Ischemic Attack*

- Sudden tingling or numbness on one side of the face

- Confusion as to time, place, or person

- Loss or impairment of speech for understanding and/or communicating

- Sudden slurring of speech, dizziness

- Visual disturbances such as blurring or double vision

- Other cognitive changes such as difficulty reading, writing, or thinking

- Weakness on one side of the body (arm or leg)

have attacks that cease spontaneously. Two-thirds of those suffering from TIAs are male or hypertensive, or both (Powers, 1990). A neurologist or neuropsychologist easily recognizes symptoms of a TIA (Table 12.1). Unfortunately, the person suffering the TIA, because of confusion or an impaired capacity to use judgment, often does not recognize the symptoms resulting from a TIA. In other cases, the TIA symptoms are so peculiar and vague that clinicians find them difficult to establish, because of their waxing-and-waning, transient nature. This is particularly frustrating to the patient, who may be inadvertently referred to a psychiatrist or psychologist because his or her presentation does not appear to fit any established medical categories or because physicians can find nothing physically wrong.

INFARCTIONS

When ischemia is severe enough to kill the nerve cell, neurologists consider the neuron infarcted. Infarctions result from an inadequate blood supply to an area of the brain, causing tissue death or necrosis from the lack of oxygen. This event most often relates to obstruction of the local vascular circulation by blockage or occlusion of a vessel, stopping blood flow. Occlusions are typically caused by either a blood clot or a fatty deposit lodged in a vessel. The area of the brain in which this occlusion occurs depends on clot size. Occlusion can happen to the brain as a whole, as in severe heart failure; in one of the major arteries or their branches supplying blood to the brain; or in a small capillary. Cerebral infarction is most likely the result of a thrombotic or an embolic vascular occlusion in blood flow. We discuss both ischemic events in more detail in the following paragraphs.

Thrombosis

Thrombosis is the formation of a blood clot or *thrombus* (derived from Greek meaning "clot") within the blood vessel. A thrombosis at the heart is a heart attack. A thrombosis in the brain is a stroke. The most common basic neuropathologic process in infarction is that of **atherosclerosis.** In atherosclerosis, irregularly distributed yellow fatty plaques are present in large- and medium-size arteries. Fat deposits build up along blood vessel walls, reducing the size of the cerebral artery. In atherosclerosis, the blood clot lodging in the vessel reduces or completely blocks blood flow through the vessel. Thus, atherosclerosis often precipitates infarction due to occlusion. Atherosclerosis is not a uniform process throughout the cardiovascular system; it can affect certain parts of the arterial system more than others. The most common location for atherosclerosis is at the bifurcation of arteries (the point where the division occurs), specifically at the common carotid artery. This condition is progressive, variable, and difficult to predict, although it tends to become worse as a person grows older. Atherosclerosis restricts blood supply to the brain and results in inadequate oxygenation of brain tissue. This produces a general decline in neuropsychological abilities of a diffuse nature. TIAs often, but not always, precede stroke that results from cerebral thrombosis.

The pathologic process underlying a thrombosis involves **platelets.** Platelets are disk-shaped cells found in the blood of all mammals. They are important for their role in blood coagulation and are produced in large numbers in the bone marrow. From there, they are released into the bloodstream, where they circulate for approximately 10 days. While circulating, these cells do not adhere to each other or to the wall of a blood vessel. When the **endothelium,** the layer of epithelial cells that line the blood vessels, is breached, however, the blood-clotting properties of the platelets activate. That is, they change shape and stick to the vessel wall, each other, and red blood cells. If this occurs pathologically—that is, in a normal vessel—it leads to a thrombosis, ultimately occluding the vessel. Aspirin is an important antithrombotic agent.

The middle cerebral artery on the left side is the most commonly reported site for an occlusion. Research has shown that blood clot formation most frequently stems from abnormality within the vessel wall and less frequently from an abnormality of the blood itself (Brown, Baird, & Shatz, 1986). If a thrombus forms and blocks the flow of blood to the brain, a cerebral infarction occurs. The area of the brain in which this occlusion occurs depends on the size of the blood clot. If it is large, it may lodge in one of the major arteries; if smaller, it will lodge

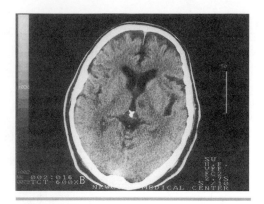

Figure 12.2 Lacunar infarcts of the thalamus as seen on computed transaxial tomography scan. (Courtesy Eric Zillmer.)

in a branch of the major arteries. The effects of occlusions in small and large vessels differ. People with long-standing hypertension and diabetes often have occlusions of small vessels, called *lacunar infarctions* (derived from Latin *lacuna,* meaning "hole"), because the infarctions are generally small and round. Patients with lacunar infarctions frequently have multiple small lesions. Because the lesions are small and typically deep in the brain (Figure 12.2), they produce not disturbed alertness, headache, or electroencephalographic changes, but usually pure motor and sensory deficits. The disease course is often fluctuating or stepwise.

Embolism

The term ***embolism*** (derived from Greek *embolos,* meaning "plug" or "wedge") refers to a blood clot that has traveled from one part of the body to another. Sometimes a piece of plaque originally formed in the heart can "break" off into the blood circulation and travel to the brain. If the blockage is not relieved rapidly, the brain area served by that artery dies of infarction. Embolism are often (up to 33%) associated with a condition known as **atrial fibrillation,** an arrhythmia of the heart. Research has recently established that cardiac surgery (such as valve replacement) may potentially contribute to cerebral emboli. When a traveling blood clot or embolism lodges in a distal intracranial branch of a blood vessel, it may block blood flow to specific parts of the brain, so a cerebral infarction occurs. At younger ages, embolic strokes are more prevalent than thrombotic strokes and are more likely to involve the anterior areas of the brain. Embolisms develop suddenly, often without immediate warning. Most often the patient is awake and active (Toole, 1990).

HEMORRHAGE

Hemorrhage (derived from Greek *haima,* meaning "blood," and *regnynai,* meaning "to burst forth") results from rupture of a blood vessel causing heavy spilling of blood into cerebral tissue. The large accumulation of blood within tissue is called a **hematoma.** Onset of cerebral hemorrhage is abrupt and usually occurs during waking hours, presumably because the person is more active and thus has a higher blood pressure. Although the severity may vary from a small, symptomless bleed to massive hemorrhage leading to sudden death, prognosis for cerebral hemorrhage is usually poor, especially if the patient is unconscious for more than 48 hours. A hemorrhage usually occurs when a weak spot in a blood vessel, called an *aneurysm,* ruptures. Such hemorrhages are usually massive, cause the most severe damage structurally, and often result in death. A large, space-occupying bleed may discharge itself through the ventricles and can be detected using a spinal tap. Often alterations in consciousness accompany hemorrhages, ranging from disorientation to coma. Severe motor and sensory deficits are also usually present, although the degree of deficits depends on the speed and extent of the bleed. Hemorrhages occur most commonly in brain regions that are susceptible to the presence of aneurysms. Those include the putamen (50%), cerebral white matter (16%), thalamus (12%), pons (8%), cerebellum (8%), and caudate nucleus (6%) (Barnett, Mohr, Stein, Yatsu, 1986). There are two kinds of hemorrhagic strokes: intracerebral and subarachnoid.

Intracerebral Hemorrhage

Intracerebral means "within the cerebrum," or within the brain. In this type of hemorrhage, a defective artery bursts and floods the surrounding brain tissue with blood. Intracerebral hemorrhages most often accompany hypertension and result in deficits localized to either the left or right hemisphere. Medical and neuropsychological problems resulting from an intracerebral hemorrhage occur not only because of the disruption of blood flow that would normally reach the brain tissue from the intact artery, but also because of increased ICP on the brain tissue from the increased amount of blood flow into the skull. Large hemorrhages not only destroy brain tissue, particularly if the bleed continues, but also displace vital brain centers, which may prove fatal. Less serious hemorrhages may disrupt the integrity of adjacent brain tissue without destroying it and produce highly localized symptoms. When the bleeding does cease, there is usually no recurrence from the same site, a situation unlike that of a bleed resulting from an aneurysm.

Subarachnoid Hemorrhage

A **subarachnoid hemorrhage** occurs when a blood vessel on the surface of the brain bursts and blood flows into the subarachnoid space, the small cavity that surrounds the brain. As with intracerebral hemorrhages, a major problem that can occur from this type of stroke is increased pressure on the brain. The extent of dysfunction seen with subarachnoid hemorrhages depends, in part, on how much pressure is exerted on the brain. Acute symptoms include sudden headache, vomiting, and a possible interruption of consciousness. Because of the diffuse effects on the brain, localized symptoms, such as paralysis, typically are not present during a subarachnoid hemorrhage.

Aneurysms

Aneurysms represent weak areas in the walls of an artery that cause the vessel to balloon. These localized dilations of blood vessels may be of congenital origin, but are also present after trauma, infection, and arteriosclerosis. Aneurysms can produce more significant disorders when they begin to hemorrhage and are a major cause of stroke-related mortality and disability. Aneurysm bleeds range from minor to a complete rupture resulting in a hemorrhage, as described earlier. Approximately 50% of aneurysms occur in the middle cerebral artery and are most likely inherited or related to a pathologic process that weakens arterial walls. Many vascular anomalies remain undetected only to begin causing problems when they rupture because of such factors as high blood pressure. The base rate for adults is 4%; and among those who have aneurysms, 20% have multiple ones. Aneurysms, which expand with time, are most often less than 6 to 7 mm in diameter, with giant aneurysms expanding to 2.5 cm. It is relatively rare that small aneurysms rupture (Bannister, 1992).

Arteriovenous Malformations

Arteriovenous malformations (AVMs) represent direct and essentially useless communications between arteries and veins without an intervening capillary network. AVMs are typically congenital collections of abnormal vessels that result in abnormal blood flow. Because they are inherently weak, AVMs may lead to stroke or to inadequate distribution of blood in the regions surrounding the vessels. Rupture of AVMs may produce intracerebral and subarachnoid bleeding. Like aneurysms, AVMs have a tendency for recurrent bleeding. The clinical symptoms of AVMs can include headache, which is similar to migraine in that it is related to the dilation of vessels, or other more vague cognitive complaints (Neuropsychology in Action 12.1). Often, AVMs have no identifiable clinical consequence and many individuals are not aware

they have the condition. The most serious complication of AVMs is bleeding, typically at a very slow rate. Table 12.2 summarizes the various types of cerebrovascular disorders reviewed in this chapter.

Diagnosing Cerebrovascular Disease

Because of their sudden onset, infarctions are relatively easy to differentiate from other focal neurologic disorders such as tumors. Gradual obstruction of one vessel, however, may not produce an infarction at all. Because the occlusion develops over a long period, its eventual course into full occlusion may have few or mild effects, because alternative blood sources for the affected brain tissues may have formed over time. The major diagnostic task in differentiating stroke from other neurologic conditions is to exclude other causes of lesions that produce similar clinical pictures or cause a bleed. A precise diagnosis

---

Table 12.2 *Summary of Different Types of Vascular Disorders*

Arteriovenous malformation—arteriovenous malformations (AVMs) represent abnormal, often redundant vessels that cause abnormal blood flow. Because they have inherently weak vessel walls, AVMs may lead to slow bleeding or inadequate distribution of blood in the regions surrounding the vessels.

Embolism—a type of artery occlusion in which the clot forms in one area of the body and travels through the arterial system to another area, in this case, the brain, where the clot becomes lodged and obstructs cranial blood flow. Approximately 14% of all CVAs are caused by an embolus.

Hemorrhage—means bleeding, or literally, the escape of blood from the vessels. It is the most severe form of cerebrovascular accident (CVA), characterized by the rupturing of a blood vessel. Hemorrhages account for approximately 10% of all strokes. Most hemorrhages stem from increased blood pressure and the presence of abnormal formations of blood vessels, including aneurysms.

Migraine stroke—a rare type of stroke caused by severe transient ischemic attacks (TIAs), typically associated with classic migraine.

Thrombosis—a type of occlusion in which a clot or thrombus forms in an artery and obstructs blood flow at the site of its formation. This is the most common form of stroke and accounts for approximately 65% of all CVAs.

Transient ischemic attack—a temporary (transient) lack of oxygen (ischemia) to the brain. This temporary lack of oxygen can cause a time-limited set of neuropsychological deficits. TIAs technically are not considered a stroke, because neuronal death does not occur.

Neuropsychology in Action 12.1

Migraine Headache: A Vascular Disorder of the Brain

by Eric A. Zillmer

Although the primary symptom of migraine is a seemingly subjective and excruciating headache, migraine is, in fact, a neurologic disorder of the brain's vascular structure. Symptoms consist of a moderate to severe lateralized, "throbbing" headache, typically behind the eye, associated nausea, and an increased sensitivity to light, odors, and sounds. Often, a family history shows similar headaches, but the diagnosis is indicated only if no evidence of other organic disease, such as tumor or stroke, could account for the symptoms. Migraines are common: 24 million or 1 of every 11 people in the United States suffer from migraine (Lezak, Howieson, & Loring, 2004). Migraines are more prevalent among women than men (by a 3:1 ratio) and occur most often between ages 30 and 45. The typical frequency of migraine is intermittent (about 2–5 per month), and an attack lasts between 4 and 72 hours. A migraine attack can incapacitate the victim, so high labor costs arise from decreased work productivity and increased absenteeism. About 20% of migraine sufferers experience an **aura,** a neurologic event that occurs before the onset of pain and is most likely caused by a TIA. The aura presents usually as a visual symptom including flashing lights, zigzag lines, or blurred or partial loss of vision. Other neurologic symptoms may also be present during an aura, including increased numbness of the skin (especially in the arms), difficulties in motor coordination, and symptoms of aphasia.

The trigeminal nerve, a large cranial nerve with three branches, has been implicated in migraine. The trigeminal nerve conveys sensory information including pain, touch, and temperature from most of the face and the scalp. A proposed mechanism for migraine implicates the sensory "pain" fibers of the trigeminal nerve that surround the cranial arteries that supply blood to the

meninges. In people with migraine, these nerve fibers sometimes release chemicals known as *peptides*. As a result, blood vessels become inflamed, and cranial blood flow changes, first abnormally constricting and then dilating.

Migraine auras occur during the constriction phase. This is such a common event among migraine sufferers that many patients notice this as a first sign of the oncoming migraine. During the subsequent dilation, patients experience the symptoms of the migraine attack. Swollen blood vessels stimulate surrounding nerve fibers to relay impulses to the brain, where they are perceived as pain. The accompanying severe nausea perhaps relates to a compromise in the blood–brain barrier, which, in turn, allows toxins naturally present in the blood to enter into brain tissue. The neurotransmitter serotonin plays a major role in migraine (Figure 12.3). During migraine attacks,

serotonin levels decrease and medications or substances that deplete serotonin (such as chocolate or the food additive MSG) often trigger a migraine. Conversely, administering a serotonin agonist (such as sumatriptan succinate [Imitrex]) often relieves the headache.

Although many individuals with migraines experience development of transient ischemic attacks (TIAs), few go on to suffer from a cerebrovascular accident (CVA). Although rare, **migraine strokes** do occur and seem to account for a small proportion of CVAs in people younger than 40 years, particularly female individuals. Medical research has demonstrated that individuals suffering from migraines are actually at less risk for stroke than the general population (Bannister, 1992). This is because the migraine patient's cardiovascular system is inherently flexible, which allows the constriction and dilation of arteries in the first place (Walton, 1994).

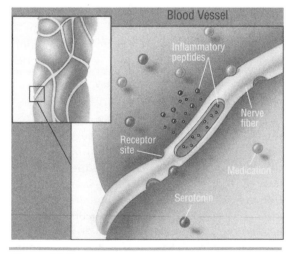

Figure 12.3 The role of serotonin in migraine.
(Courtesy Beth Willert © 2000. Reprinted by permission of the artist. From packaging display for GlaxoWellcome, Inc.)

is important to the medical team, as well as the neuropsychologist, to plan an appropriate rehabilitation program for the stroke patient. The following sections review diagnostic procedures that are used to document stroke.

COMPUTED TRANSAXIAL TOMOGRAPHY

Computed transaxial tomography (CT) is a powerful, almost risk-free technique for imaging the structure of the brain (see Chapter 2). The CT scan often provides the first evaluation in diagnosing stroke, particularly in differentiating between hemorrhagic and nonhemorrhagic stroke. On CT scans, hemorrhages appear initially as round, well-circumscribed lesions of uniform high density. Over time, the circumference of the lesions becomes more irregular and the lesion less dense. CT scans provide information not only about the location of a hemorrhage, but also size, possible edema (swelling), displacement of other brain structures, and presence of blood in the ventricular system. Tumors, which appear on CT with a different density, are easily differentiated. Contrast-enhanced CT typically does not increase detection of hemorrhages. TIAs are less easily monitored on CT because of their small size.

ANGIOGRAPHY

Angiography represents the most accurate diagnostic procedure for vascular disorders. Angiography can also provide an evaluation of collateral vessel potential and a diagnosis of coexisting neurologic problems. Angiography is an invasive diagnostic procedure that entails some risk (see Chapter 2). Therefore, it is usually reserved as the final diagnostic test for stroke, and CT typically precedes angiography. The two most common routes for angiography are via the venous and arterial systems (see review in Chapter 2). Arterial angiography is more popular in diagnosing stroke, because it provides precise images of cerebral arteries. This is because the specialist can pass the catheter, which injects the contrast medium, up the aortic arch and selectively place it into the carotid or vertebral arteries. Angiography can also show whether the obstructing lesion is significantly impairing carotid blood flow and whether the lesion can be removed surgically. Precise diagnosis of cerebral aneurysms, AVM, artery occlusion, and **stenosis** (narrowing of an artery) are all possible using angiography.

OTHER TESTS

An alternative to angiography and imaging are noninvasive tests, typically targeted at detecting anatomic and physiologic information of the common and internal arteries. These devices, which use ultrasonic waves, function on the principle that extensive lesions to the carotid arteries may produce distorted sound-wave feedback. In addition, pulse-wave Doppler imaging systems may be sensitive to blood flow velocity. In most cases, a conclusive diagnosis is not made; rather, noninvasive devices for carotid blood flow serve to screen for subsequent referral to the more invasive angiogram. CSF analysis using a lumbar puncture is also of value in ruling out or confirming a subarachnoid hemorrhage not seen on CT.

Treatment and Prognosis of Vascular Disorders

FACTORS INVOLVED IN STROKE RECOVERY

Once an individual has had a stroke, the type of damage or lesion and associated neuropsychological symptoms depend on a number of medical and neuroanatomic factors. These include the extent of the lesion, the general health of the cerebrovascular system, the presence of collateral circulation in the brain, and the location of the lesion. These factors influence the extent and nature of associated cognitive symptoms, as well as the possibility and prognosis for recovery and extent of rehabilitation.

Size of Blood Vessel

If a small blood vessel (such as a capillary) is interrupted, the effects are more limited than the often devastating consequences of damage to a large vessel, such as the internal carotid artery or other cerebral arteries. Strokes of these large arteries can result in lesions that include large portions of the brain and produce serious behavioral deficits, coma, and even death.

Remaining Intact Vessels

If a CVA occurs in one restricted portion of the brain, the prognosis may be rather good, because healthy blood vessels in surrounding brain tissue often can supply blood to at least some of the deprived areas. In addition, the presence of **collateral blood vessels** allows redundant blood supply to take more than one route to a given region. The term *collateral* is used to describe redundant blood flow present in the vascular network after occlusion of an artery. If one vessel is blocked, a given region may be spared an infarct because the blood has an alternative route to the affected brain area. Conversely, if a stroke occurs in a region surrounded by weak or diseased vessels (as in arteriosclerosis), the effects may be much more serious, because there is no possibility of compensating. The surrounding weak zones may also be at an increased risk for stroke.

This communication between blood vessels by collateral channels is also known as **anastomosis** and provides an important defense against stroke. The properties of collateral communication that provides a sufficient blood supply to obstructed areas vary considerably among individuals. Thus, damage to the same vessel in different people can produce symptoms that vary considerably. Anastomosis can provide some relief to blood-depleted brain areas, particularly if the primary vessel affected is gradually blocked, rather than rapidly occluded.

Premorbid Factors

The presence of previous strokes is a strong predictor of disability. A small stroke in an otherwise healthy brain will, in the long run, have a good prognosis for substantial recovery of function. However, the effects of an additional lesion most often are cumulative. As a result, destruction of a functional zone of brain tissue may produce serious consequences for the patient.

Location

The location of brain tissue involved in a vascular disorder has neuropsychological significance. A lesion in the temporal lobe can produce a deficit in understanding speech; a stroke in the hippocampus can cause memory deficits; and a lesion in the brainstem can trigger heart failure, resulting in death. Thus, behavioral symptoms of vascular disorder are important clues to the neuropsychologist for locating the area of brain damage and assessing the extent of damage.

MEDICAL TREATMENT

The initial treatment of the stroke patient involves medical stabilization and control of bleeding, if necessary through surgery. Common medications include anticoagulants to dissolve blood clots or prevent clotting, vasodilators to dilate or expand vessels, and blood pressure medication and steroids to control cerebral edema. Surgeons have developed interventions to reduce the risk for bleeding for some aneurysms by "clipping" them (Figure 12.4). Other surgical procedures are used in the case of hemorrhages when it may be necessary to operate to relieve the pressure of the blood from the ruptured vessel on the rest of the brain. Small hemorrhages typically are not treated surgically, but rather are controlled by altering the patient's blood pressure.

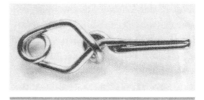

Figure 12.4 Aneurysm clip
(approximate size = 6 mm).
(Courtesy Eric Zillmer.)

Physicians typically treat infarctions by intravenously administering heparin (a potent anticoagulant agent), but only if diagnosis rules out a mass lesion from a trauma or hemorrhage (either intracerebral or subarachnoid). Administering an anticoagulant agent to a patient with a hemorrhage can be fatal; therefore, establishing a precise differential diagnosis is important. In medium-size bleeds, surgical draining is often effective, although this technique may leave a surgical hole in the brain that may later entail neuropsychological deficits. Other ways to decompress the brain include artificial hyperventilation, corticosteroids, and diuretics. In most cases, physicians artificially lower the blood pressure. Treatment for TIA symptoms, which is more difficult because the symptoms are ambiguous, is often restricted to pharmacologic intervention with anticoagulants. An obvious danger in using anticoagulants is the inherent risk for an uncontrolled bleed.

AVMs are often surgically removed or are embolized artificially. In the latter technique, the surgeon delivers an agent that blocks the blood vessel close to the lesion, in some cases permanently. The embolization agent is a sponge, ball, coil, or balloon and entails certain risks. This delicate technique uses highly selective catheterization procedures and close radiographic monitoring. The reason for this care is that the delivery system must advance as close to the lesion as is possible; otherwise, healthy arteries may be embolized, or the embolus may migrate to the lung or heart.

PREVENTING STROKE

Many people who have had a stroke say that it "struck out of nowhere"—there seemed to be no obvious warning. Typically, a stroke that occurs spontaneously results from an embolism or a hemorrhage. That one can have a stroke with little or no warning testifies to the importance of identifying the many risk factors associated with stroke. The most prominent risk factor is a history of stroke. In fact, as mentioned earlier, stroke recurrence is an important contributor to disability. In addition, common demographic factors predispose an individual to cerebrovascular disease, including:

Heredity (cardiovascular disease in one's family)

Sex (men are at greater risk for stroke than women, a risk related to their higher incidence of heart disease and hypertension)

Ethnicity (African Americans have one of the highest stroke rates, 40% greater among women and 10% greater among men)

Lifestyle indices also affect the probability of cardiovascular disease. A well-known risk factor of CVA is hypertension. Elevated blood pressure means that the force of the blood against the walls of the arteries is too high. As a result, over time the arteries become weakened and can burst. If this happens in the brain, it results in a cerebral hemorrhage. High blood pressure can also increase the force of the blood against the artery walls and break off some plaque along those walls, which then travels as an embolus through the bloodstream until it clogs a narrower vessel. The dangerous part of hypertension is that most people do not feel it, and thus do not seek medical help.

Other risk factors for stroke are diabetes and high cholesterol. Individuals with diabetes run a greater risk for stroke. Vascular diseases are most often related to problems in artery linings, which become hardened by deposits of cholesterol, fat, calcium, and other materials such as fibrin, a substance that encourages clot formation. Fat causes plaque to build up along the lining of blood vessels, which can break off and lead to embolic stroke or can become so built up that thrombotic stroke can occur. Because smoking is a vasoconstrictor, it is an additional risk factor for stroke. Smoking a cigarette constricts an already too-narrow blood vessel.

Small amounts of alcohol may actually thin blood and can serve the same purpose as one aspirin per day. Also, some evidence suggests that a glass of wine with dinner reduced cholesterol. Alcohol becomes a risk factor when consumed in large quantities. Excessive consumption contributes to high blood pressure and may result in ataxia (poor balance), which is often already a problem after a stroke. Also, alcohol is a sedating drug and may not interact well with other drugs. Finally, obesity contributes to the onset and maintenance of diabetes, hypertension, heart disease, and high cholesterol. Obesity is medically defined as being 25% over your ideal weight. Approximately 26% of men and 30% of women in the United States are overweight. Cardiovascular complications in obesity are related to the high correlation between being overweight and hypertension, a precursor of coronary heart disease.

Neuropsychological Deficits Associated with Stroke

Significant functional and cognitive impairments are often the result of stroke. These deficits can seriously impair the patient's ability to function independently and are often incapacitating and serious enough to lead to hospitalization in a rehabilitation facility. Typically, long-term hospitalization occurs because the patient is exhibiting symptoms of inattentiveness, apraxia, communication difficulties, apathy, or general intellectual impairment.

Many factors influence cognitive changes as a result of stroke. These factors include the patient's age, interval between the stroke onset and time of rehabilitation, nature of the stroke (infarction or hemorrhage), and size and location of lesion (such as right or left brain, anterior or posterior). The patient's medical history is important, particularly as it relates to the presence of previous strokes (such as lacunar strokes), prior CNS trauma or disease, and premorbid level of functioning. Many stroke-related cognitive deficits may resolve over time, sometimes immediately after the stroke. For example, the more localized the effects, the more positive the prognosis. But residual deficits may remain that require an evaluation of cognitive abilities and subsequent rehabilitation (Brown, Baird, & Shatz, 1986).

Because of their complexity and variability from patient to patient, the cognitive deficits associated with stroke are not easily classified into simple categories. For didactic purposes, neuropsychologists correlate cognitive deficits with the specific type of stroke. Correlating the location of an anatomic lesion with the stroke patient's cognitive impairments has been only modestly successful. Thus, the neuropsychology student should be careful not to rigidly adhere to specific patterns of deficits and recovery, but instead should realize that the disease course in individual patients varies greatly (Weimar et al., 2002).

NEUROPSYCHOLOGICAL RISK FACTORS

Several important principles govern the properties of neuronal processes that are particularly relevant to understanding the neuropsychology of cerebrovascular disorders. These principes are explained in the following paragraphs.

Necrosis

Neurons that have died as a result of necrosis do not spontaneously regenerate. In most instances, lost neurons in the CNS are incapable of healing after the developmental period (see Chapter 4). Thus, no cellular regeneration of the neuron or regrowth of damaged neurons to their normal target occurs. Neurons lost as a result of stroke are not replaced. Fortunately, functional losses entailed by these structural losses are not necessarily permanent, because the brain has redundant pathways for supplying blood to various areas. Specifically, redundant blood supply in the brain may minimize neuronal death because there is sufficient blood supply to brain areas that have been damaged. Also, the process of rehabilitation allows some compensation of functional losses with behaviors that have been left relatively intact. Rehabilitation may alleviate enough disruption caused by stroke that the victim regains some or nearly all of his or her premorbid level of functioning. In fact, neuropsychologists have made significant headway recently in developing assessment, prosthesis, and cognitive rehabilitation techniques to compensate for disrupted functional brain systems. In addition, neuroscientists are making some progress in designing drugs that facilitate the regrowth of injured neurons.

Disinhibition

An important principle of neuronal processes relevant to understanding the neuropathology of stroke relates to the capacity for inhibiting behavior after a stroke. As discussed in previous chapters, many of the neuronal collections, particularly in the frontal lobe, serve to inhibit rather than initiate behavior. This is important because losing inhibitory neurons to stroke may actually result in an inappropriate increase in behavior or disinhibition, and often causes striking behavioral and personality changes in stroke victims. Damage to an excitatory collection of fibers, of course, results in losing some function. This is why many traumas to the brain, including stroke, often show both loss of function (such as aphasia and the inability to speak) and disinhibition (increased likelihood of inappropriate behavior) including impulsiveness, hypersexuality, and inappropriate feelings. This was made painfully clear when a colleague of ours was leading a stroke support group. All members of the support group had sustained a stroke, and many had significant related cognitive deficits. Almost all members demonstrated poor judgment and disinhibition when it came to operating an automobile, and they spent much time in the group discussing this. Nevertheless, they insisted on continuing to drive and drive poorly; in fact, many accidents happened in the parking lot before and after group meetings. When group participants returned from trips, they would discuss and bring along pictures of their recent accidents. They described these crashes with

some bravado, reflecting poor insight and a general lack of awareness of the dangers. This is a typical example of disinhibition because victims do not inhibit high-risk behavior, as they may have done premorbidly, that is, before the stroke. The incapacity to drive after a stroke is one of the most sensitive issues facing health care workers, stroke victims, and their families.

Disconnection Syndrome

Because the substructures of the brain connect so intricately, observed deficits in a stroke patient may not necessarily correspond to the lobe or site where the stroke occurred. For example, a stroke in the visual area of the cortex (occipital lobe) ordinarily results in some form of visual impairment. In addition, however, these visual deficits may also disturb motor behavior or gait. Furthermore, a stroke may disrupt important pathways of neurons that project to other centers of the brain. This is a common problem when strokes occur near subcortical structures such as the striatum, a common stroke site. Such a stroke commonly results in higher order cognitive deficits, because injury has severed projections to the cortex. This problem is called *disconnection syndrome,* because important pathways in the brain have been "disconnected."

ATTENTION DEFICITS

Many types of brain dysfunction typically reduce efficiency of the brain in processing information. This is certainly true for CVA. In milder cases, stroke victims cannot sustain their attention to one particular stimulus for long periods or select information from competing sources (selective attention). This impairment may be minimally present and detectable only with formal neuropsychological testing, or it may be profound and easily noticeable by any observer. Sometimes cognitive changes in stroke patients are so pervasive that the patient is considerably confused and disoriented as to time, place, and person. Deficits of arousal typically relate to damage of the patient's frontal lobe circuitry or the brainstem region. In contrast, deficits in attention may relate to local or global brain damage.

Motor and Sensory Impairment

General behavioral slowing and a reduction of psychomotor activity can be dominant characteristics of stroke. Both the right and left hemispheres are associated with changes in motor and sensory functioning from stroke. Such changes can be as benign as mild motor slowing or as debilitating as complete paralysis, particularly if the lesions are in the thalamic area or the motor and premotor areas of the frontal lobes. Motor deficits of the right brain resemble those of the left brain. Right hemisphere stroke motor deficiencies, however, are generally less severe, because the nondominant left hand is not as important for skilled tasks.

Severe motor deficits are often apparent without formal testing and may involve impairment in motor speed, strength, steadiness, and fine-motor coordination. Even mild deficits may significantly reduce the efficiency on highly demanding manual tasks, interfere with self-care or light housework, deteriorate handwriting skills, and slow reaction times, which may require the victim to give up driving. Diminished sensory functioning is most likely in areas of visual acuity, visual field perception, and hearing.

MEMORY PROBLEMS

Stroke survivors commonly report that their memory is not as good as it was before the stroke, and on occasion, they may not recall a person's name, even when they know that person well. Many stroke patients exhibit intact memory for old learning, but not always for new learning. That is, they can remember events that happened years ago, but may be unable to remember what they had for lunch today. Unless the lesion is extensive, CVAs do not typically cause loss of primary, immediate, or long-term memory, but are most pronounced in the area of short-term memory. This most likely relates to the stroke patient's decreased capacity to organize and process large amounts of information ("chunking") in a fashion that lends itself to easier memory storage or retrieval. Not uncommonly, these patients recall only a small amount of new material 30 minutes after it is presented to them.

Patients that have stroke-related hippocampal damage experience significant memory difficulties, may require repetition of new information, and may show significant problems with forgetfulness associated with a variety of everyday tasks. Such patients have frequent difficulty recalling details of recent experiences, tend to misplace things, fail to follow through on new obligations, and tend to get lost more easily in unfamiliar areas.

Stroke patients with the most severe memory deficits are virtually unable to retain any information, particularly if their attention has been directed elsewhere. Such individuals also cannot profit from repeated exposures to stimuli. They need substantial assistance in daily living and characteristically cannot take care of themselves, because they may create fire hazards at home and cannot manage financial affairs or keep track of scheduled activities. For such patients, it helps to create an environment where important objects are kept in the same place, the same daily routines are maintained, and instructions are verbalized in the same sequence. A major concern related to memory impairment is the stroke patient's ability to manage his or her own medication schedule.

DEFICITS IN ABSTRACT REASONING

Impaired judgment, loss of insight, and diminished capacity for abstract and complex thinking are common cognitive changes among stroke victims, particularly if anterior aspects of cortical areas are involved. People with mildly impaired abstract reasoning and new concept formation can often use their past accumulated knowledge to exercise reasonable judgment for routine daily activities. Those who show more serious cognitive decline often encounter difficulties with tasks that require complex planning or organization and with novel situations. Such patients cannot assess new situations accurately and demonstrate poor judgment, with serious consequences to themselves or others.

COGNITIVE DEFICITS ASSOCIATED WITH RIGHT BRAIN STROKES

Researchers have directed much research attention toward distinguishing the cognitive deficits between left versus right hemisphere brain damage. In general, patients with left-sided brain damaged show markedly impaired language comprehension and communication, and stroke patients with damage to the right hemisphere exhibit significantly more impairment in ability to process and execute behaviors that require visual-perceptual ability (Lezak, Howieson, & Loring, 2004; Reitan & Wolfson, 1993).

Deficits that affect the right cerebral artery involve areas responsible for spatial, rhythmic, and nonverbal processing. Right hemisphere symptoms, although serious in the patient's overall functioning, can be less striking in the acute phase, particularly if they do not involve motor dysfunction. Right brain damage occurs as a consequence of right-sided CVAs and is often associated with contralateral motor and sensory impairment. Patients with right-sided brain injury present a variety of symptoms that pose a particular challenge to the neuropsychologist. First, the deficits often found among patients with right hemisphere brain damage are not as striking initially as the deficits observed among patients with left hemisphere brain damage, in which case the patient is often aphasic. Second, many patients with right-sided brain damage display a range of emotions from indifference to euphoria. This is in contrast with the depression often observed among patients with left hemisphere brain damage.

Neuropsychology in Action 12.2

Case Example of a Left Stroke

by Eric A. Zillmer

The patient is a 32-year-old, married, right-handed woman with 12 years of education. She worked as a manager for a fast food restaurant and lived with her husband and two young children in a two-story house. One month before my evaluation, she sustained a sudden onset of aphasia, right-sided weakness, and headache. Computed transaxial tomography (CT) scan showed an infarction in the area of the left cerebral hemisphere. A carotid angiogram showed an occluded internal carotid artery. Medical history was unremarkable.

I tested her neuropsychologically 1 month after the stroke. In my clinical interview with the patient, her speech was marked by paraphasias (the substitution of wrong words or phrases) and verbal perseverative tendencies (unnecessary repeating), which are signature symptoms for a left hemisphere stroke. She was oriented to person and could state her name, age, and date of birth. She was somewhat oriented to place; that is, she knew she was in a rehabilitation hospital but could not give its name or location. She could write the correct date, but could not recall the current or last president. She showed a significant sensory and motor deficit on her dominant right side. She could not feel light touch on her right hand with single or double simultaneous stimulation. On verbal tasks, she was able to perform automatic tasks such as counting from 1 to 20 and reciting the alphabet, but she could not perform any other tasks that required voluntary and purposeful speech. The patient's gross- and fine-motor ability and speed were intact on her nonaffected left side. However, on her dominant right side, she showed a marked hemiparalysis and could not voluntarily move her right shoulder, arm, hand, or fingers. She did not show any evidence of motor apraxia and could copy simple designs adequately with her nondominant hand, suggesting intact right hemisphere functioning.

As expected, her verbal functions were severely impaired, consistent with the location of her cerebrovascular accident (CVA) in the distribution of the left middle cerebral artery. Receptive language skills were moderately impaired, as she could follow only one-step commands without difficulty. She became easily confused with two-step commands. Expressive speech was severely impaired. On the word fluency item, which requires the individual to name as many animals as possible in 30 seconds, she was able to name only one and perseverated with the word *baseball,* which was an incorrect response to a previous item. She was able to correctly repeat words and phrases after the examiner, but was unable to initiate a correct response on her own. She also demonstrated alexia and agraphia for written language.

Therefore, it is easy to assume that the deficits from right brain damage are not as serious as those from left brain damage. However, this is not true, because both types of problems can be highly disruptive to patient and family alike, often even exceeding the problems associated with left hemisphere CVAs.

For example, research has shown consistently that patients with right hemisphere stroke remain longer in rehabilitation facilities than do patients with left hemisphere strokes (Zillmer et al., 1992). This difference is related to the pervasive deficits that patients with right hemisphere damage present in visuospatial abilities and the extended rehabilitation required for dressing, ambulating, and other self-care behaviors.

Right hemisphere stroke patients are not diagnosed as rapidly as are left hemisphere stroke patients. This is probably related to the difficulty that left hemisphere stroke patients display in using language—an obvious symptom that helps a family member identify that something is "wrong" with their loved one. In contrast, patients with right-sided brain damage often use language fluently. Thus, on the surface, they "sound" okay. Furthermore, patients with right-sided brain damage tend to be unaware of their problems. Such patients often deny that there is anything wrong with them. As a result, patients may be blamed for being "rude," "disruptive," or "inappropriate," when they are actually exhibiting symptoms of right brain injury, including impulsivity, verbosity, inattention, and poor judgment. Thus, although neuropsychological deficits in patients with right hemisphere stroke may be more subtle, they are equally and sometimes more functionally disabling than the more obvious language impairments typically associated with left hemisphere stroke.

Visuospatial Deficits

Deficits in right hemisphere stroke patients almost always include visuospatial deficits—that is, the patient's capacity to accurately perceive his or her surrounding world in its completeness. Neuropsychologists report that visuospatial deficits occur particularly after right hemisphere stroke and include both visual-perceptual and visual-constructional abilities. Patients with problems in spatial relations have difficulty estimating the distance between different objects, as well as between themselves and other

The patient's visuospatial functions were basically intact. Figure–ground distinctions, spatial manipulation, visual sequencing, facial recognition, and spatial orientation all tested within normal limits. Her visual memory appeared to be within normal limits for both immediate and delayed recall procedures. However, verbal memory was severely impaired secondary to her receptive and expressive aphasia. She was able to correctly repeat a list of five words for four separate trials. However, on the recognition task (2 minutes later), she could identify only two words and made five false positive responses.

Her judgment/problem solving appeared moderately impaired secondary to her receptive and expressive aphasia. Yet, she did demonstrate some reasoning skills on the purely visual problem-solving items such as the visual analogies. She showed a moderate degree of psychological distress.

Overall, she showed a moderate degree of cognitive impairment for left hemisphere functions, which was consistent with the site of her CVA. Interestingly, on casual observation, she looked more impaired than she was on testing, given that laypeople almost always evaluate a person's cognitive status based on the vocabulary they use.

I retested the client 1 month later after she had completed her inpatient rehabilitation program. Overall, she showed significant improvement in orientation, verbal functions, memory, judgment/problem solving, psychological distress, and activities of daily living skills. The client correctly responded verbally to all the orientation questions except for one, which asked what town the hospital was located in. Verbal functions improved dramatically. The client showed good receptive speech in that she was now able to follow two-step commands easily. Verbal fluency remained limited but still showed a dramatic improvement. On the animal fluency item, she went from zero to five words and could now read and write sentences to dictation. Memory functions showed a significant improvement in her verbal memory, because she could now encode verbal information and retrieve it spontaneously. Judgment/problem solving showed some problems with concrete thinking, but generally good common sense, reasoning, and judgment. The reported amount of psychological distress experienced by this young woman decreased significantly, and she showed remarkable increase in her level of independent functioning in her activities of daily living.

In summary, neuropsychological testing proved a valuable technique in tracking this young woman's recovery from stroke during the acute stage of recovery. It was also effective in demonstrating the breadth of improvement this client made in cognitive, psychological, and physical skills, as well as documenting the residual areas of impairment in verbal functioning and verbal memory. A follow-up evaluation as an outpatient 12 months after stroke was recommended. The neuropsychology student should note that the precise extent of this patient's deficits and partial recovery is not obvious even to health care workers and the immediate family. That is why neuropsychological testing can be so important, not only in quantifying cognitive abilities but also in setting realistic expectations for recovery and rehabilitation. In this case, the family was focusing primarily on the patient's residual impairment in memory and language. In charting the patient's remarkable recovery, I was able to help the family reframe their perceptions of the perceived strengths and weaknesses, thus helping them also cope with this potentially devastating disease.

---

people or things. Common examples of mistakes that patients make with this kind of disturbance include knocking items off a table when dusting, misplacing items on tables so that they are no longer centered or are in danger of falling off, and misjudging steps or thresholds, which puts them in danger of falling.

Obviously, patients with spatial relations disturbance may have difficulty driving a car, and they may often need help in other areas of their lives such as stair climbing and activities of daily life such as dressing, bathing, toileting, and eating. It is in unfamiliar environments and in novel situations that driving is difficult for these patients. In case of marginal impairment, it may be helpful to limit patients to driving only in their own neighborhoods. In difficult cases, a neuropsychological evaluation can aid in making this decision. Motor impersistence is also a common sign—the stroke patient cannot persist with a motor response for any length of time (such as keeping eyes closed or holding arms over the head). Often, others may perceive the patient as being oppositional or stubborn, when, in fact, he or she is not in control of the skills required to perform the action.

COGNITIVE DEFICITS ASSOCIATED WITH LEFT BRAIN DAMAGE

In general, cognitive profiles are most robust when associated with damage of the left versus the right brain hemisphere. For example, the middle cerebral arteries serve major sensory and motor areas; thus, significant motor and sensory deficits often affect the side contralateral to the stroke. One of the most common infarctions is that of the left middle cerebral artery, in which deposits have traveled up from the heart and then blocked the middle cerebral artery. Disorders of the left middle cerebral artery most often involve cortical areas of the brain responsible for both expressive and receptive speech. Thus, one of the most dramatic symptoms of a left middle cerebral artery stroke is the impairment in speaking or understanding speech, or both. Deficits also include severe motor and tactile symptoms on the contralateral right body side in addition to expressive aphasia (Neuropsychology in Action 12.2).

Understanding and being understood by others is the goal of most human interactions. When a stroke damages that part of the brain that controls language and communication, the effects can devastate both patient and family. Several types of communication problems can occur with stroke, and neuropsychologists play an important role in diagnosing and rehabilitating specific forms of communication problems in stroke survivors. Many patients also have apraxia, a loss of voluntary movement that makes it difficult or impossible for patients to use gestures to communicate their needs. The presence of apraxia is the main reason why speech pathologists do not routinely attempt to teach aphasic patients sign language to compensate for spoken language difficulties.

Often, patients lose not only spoken language but written language as well. Writing is one of the most complex of language abilities. If writing is disturbed by impairment to the limb that produces letters and words, neuropsychologists do not consider that a disorder of language. Rather, in written language deficits, words, letters, or numbers may appear foreign or incomprehensible because the person cannot recall the form of letters. His or her attempts to write may be filled with real or imagined letters that make no sense to others. With time and training, the person may be able to understand simple written language—for example, single words such as bath or food—but still be unable to comprehend more complex written language such as sentences or paragraphs.

Many so-called behavioral problems seen with stroke patients with aphasia occur because of receptive aphasia. In moderate cases, the patient can understand part but not all of the communication. Sometimes patients' apparent noncompliance is actually caused by their misunderstanding the communication. Thus, a patient may act as though he or she had not heard a word at all (so-called word deafness) or as though he or she had heard only fragments of the word. The most common defect lies not in failing to recognize that someone spoke a word, but in failing to attach meaning to the word. Some patients with aphasia comprehend individual words, but not certain grammatical constructions.

Often, stroke patients with visual disorders have considerable difficulty reading because they are blind to certain visual fields. This problem is not related to receptive aphasia; rather, the patients cannot see the word—if they could, they would read it correctly—or are unaware of additional words that need to be read, as in unilateral inattention. The classification of aphasias into receptive and expressive is a useful didactic tool, but in reality, most left hemisphere stroke patients have a combination of both aphasia types, because the left middle cerebral artery serves both expressive and receptive areas.

ANTERIOR VERSUS POSTERIOR STROKES

Disorders of the anterior cerebral artery may cause motor or sensory impairment involving the leg. Because the anterior cerebral arteries serve the prefrontal lobes, deficits consistent with a prefrontal syndrome, including disinhibition and dysfunction of executive skills, are also characteristic. Strokes in the posterior cerebral artery are less common and typically cause visual field loss and sensory loss of one side. Basilar artery disorders may have a similar effect as posterior cerebral arteries stroke if the posterior communicating artery provides insufficient blood supply. Those include blood flow disruption of the brainstem, including cranial nerve involvement, the cerebellum (see Figure 12.1 for an example of a cerebellar stroke), and the occipital lobes.

EMOTIONAL AND BEHAVIORAL CHANGES AFTER A STROKE

After a stroke, it is common for patients to respond differently to people and events in terms of their emotional reactions. This relates, in part, to the experience of significant stress in the patient's life, but also to that the integrity of the brain has been compromised.

Depression

Depression is a common and not surprising reaction to stroke. Depression may be indicated if patients feel overwhelmed with sadness, believe they have failed completely, blame themselves for their problems, and often feel like crying. Poor sleep, decreased appetite, low self-esteem, and reduced efficiency are present as well. Whenever people experience loss, depression is a natural response. Depression is most likely to occur among patients with right-sided weakness and corresponding left hemisphere stroke. Often, a patient does not show signs of depression until 6 to 12 months after a stroke, when the scope of the loss has sunk in and there is time to think about how life has changed. Research and experience tells us that depression is best treated with a combination of psychotherapy and antidepressant medication.

Apathy

Apathy, or indifference, involves lack of emotions. The person is not sad or happy. In fact, the person may not appear to have any emotions. The voice sounds monotone, the face lacks expression, and if you ask the patient what he or she feels, the answer will be neutral, or without affective tone. On occasion, patients who lack vocal and facial expression nevertheless report that they feel depressed, afraid, or angry. Both depression and apathy are quite common after a stroke, especially after anterior medial damage. This is related, in part, to the loss of function that can accompany stroke, but also to reduced brain efficiency after such trauma. Thus, part of the depression or apathy in a stroke patient is related to the stroke itself. In this sense, the depression is more biological than psychological.

Euphoria

Euphoria is an overriding positive emotional response that is "too happy" given the circumstances. Euphoric people are not sad, indifferent, or apathetic; in fact, they are full of ideas and energy. Patients with euphoria seem positively happy about or despite their condition. Euphoria goes beyond a capacity to overcome obstacles—it is as if no obstacles existed. Apathy and euphoria are especially common among patients with left-sided weakness—that is, those suffering from right hemisphere stroke.

Impulsive Emotional and Behavioral Displays

An impulsive emotional response is one that appears to come without warning. Patients who have labile emotions will cry or laugh in response to events or phrases that others around them might find only mildly arousing. For example, most people respond to the National Anthem before a baseball game with a smile. The stroke patient may respond with seemingly uncontrolled tearfulness or laughter. Labile emotional responses usually embarrass the patient and upset the family members. As a consequence, family members often avoid talking about important family topics, lest the discussion "upset" the patient. It is important to remember that labile emotional responses are a physiological and not an emotional response to a stroke. In fact, patients often cry in response to happy events—as when a therapist compliments them.

Impulsivity of behavior also affects a person's ability to stop motor actions. For example, a stroke survivor may automatically stand up and begin to walk on legs that cannot support him or her. This is dangerous to the well-being of the stroke patient, and therapists spend much time in rehabilitation helping the patient to inhibit dangerous or inappropriate behaviors.

Lack of Initiation

On the other end of the spectrum, strokes can also impair a person's ability to initiate (or start) a behavior (akinesia). For example, the person may be hungry, and food may be sitting there ready to be consumed, but the person fails to bring the food to his or her mouth. In the extreme, the person may fail to chew once food has been placed in his or her mouth. The inability to initiate behavior may appear in the person's verbal responses. For example, it may take a long time to answer questions. A difficulty related to problems initiating actions is the perseveration of behavior. Perseveration is the inability to stop behaviors once they have started. A patient may perform a motor movement over and over again, unable to stop it. Motor rigidity, perseveration, motor impersistence, and disinhibition are common problems in stroke patients and generally improve with rehabilitation.

Poor Judgment

Many stroke victims demonstrate poor judgment, especially with prefrontal cortical damage. Ironically, many such patients often can verbalize the appropriate actions they "should take," but cannot follow through with those actions. For example, individuals with a spatial problem may be able to verbalize the steps in preparing a cup of coffee, but nevertheless continue to let coffee overflow when pouring a cup. It is as if their words and actions were not related. The brain trauma has impaired their ability to monitor their own behaviors and to understand the consequences of their own actions.

Tumors of the Brain

When I was in graduate school my aunt (EAZ) was diagnosed with a brain tumor. The MRI suggested that it was consistent in size and appearance with a malignant tumor. A decision was made to operate and remove as much of the tumor as was possible. Because the tumor was the size of a baseball it had already displaced and invaded healthy brain tissue. As a result, my aunt's speech was severely impaired and she complained of headaches and dizziness. The brain surgery would immediately relieve many of my aunt's symptoms and would allow for a biopsy to classify the exact type of tumor cell.

To reach such a tumor, a team of specialists first drill a series of holes into the patient's skull, not unlike the burr holes used in the ancient procedure of trephination (reviewed in Chapter 1). Then the surgeon connects the holes with a surgical jigsaw. After he or she lifts the oval-shaped piece of skull the dura mater is exposed, a thick membrane that protects the brain and spinal cord. My aunt's tumor was inside of the brain tissue and thus the neurosurgeon had to proceed through healthy brain tissue to reach the tumor. The neurosurgeon had to navigate carefully, dividing the tumor from the normal brain, cauterizing severed blood vessels along the way. Gradually the tumor was cut, actually siphoned, away from my aunt's brain and extracted. A lab autopsy verified the initial diagnosis: a malignant glioma, a fast-growing and dangerous tumor (discussed later). By the following day, she would be walking the halls and feeling much better. Her long-term prognosis was poor, however, since research clearly demonstrated that similar patients only live 6 to 12 months, even after a successful operation. No matter how careful the surgeon cuts out the malignant tumor, the few stray cancer cells that are inevitably left behind will begin to grow again. My aunt's death sentence had been postponed, perhaps by a year.

The term *tumor* refers to a morbid enlargement or new growth of tissue in which cell multiplication is uncontrolled and progressive. Tumors are also called **neoplasms,** which means "new tissue." The new cell growth resembles cells already normally present in the body. This growth is, however, often arranged in disorganized ways, does not serve any functional purpose, and often grows at the expense of surrounding intact tissue. Brain tumors make up approximately 5% of all cancers and appear in approximately 2% of all autopsies. Because cancer is the second most frequent cause of death, the actual number of victims with brain tumors is actually quite high. Brain tumors can occur at any age, but are most common in early and middle adulthood (Golden, Zillmer, & Spiers, 1992).

Brain tumors can be conceptualized according to two principal forms:

1. **Infiltrative tumors**—take over (or infiltrate) neighboring areas of the brain and destroy its tissue
2. **Noninfiltrative tumors**—are encapsulated and differentiated (easily distinguished from brain tissue), but cause dysfunction by compressing surrounding brain tissue

Tumors can be further classified according to two additional descriptors:

1. **Malignant**—indicates that the properties of the tumor cells invade other tissue and are likely to regrow or spread
2. **Benign**—describes cell growth that is usually surrounded by a fibrous capsule, is typically noninfiltrative (noninvasive), and will not spread

The primary feature of malignant tumors is that they are much more likely to reappear after surgical intervention. Because they are infiltrative, it is difficult to completely remove malignant tumors surgically. Malignant tumors may also "travel" to other organs in the body through the bloodstream. This form of spreading is called **metastasis.**

Metastatic brain tumors typically originate from primary sites other than the brain, most frequently the lung or the breast. Even benign tumors, however, are troublesome if they occur in the brain. This is because the skull completely encloses the brain, and any mass-producing lesion displaces healthy brain tissue. You may already realize that nerve cells are not likely to cause brain tumors, because neurons do not grow or heal spontaneously. This is correct. Tumors of the brain arise mostly from the supporting cells of the brain. As a result, neurons are only indirectly affected. **Neuromas** are tumors or new growths that are largely made up of nerve cells and nerve fibers.

One method of evaluating the malignant features of a brain tumor is to **grade** them from slow-growing neoplasms to rapidly growing tumors. The grade of a tumor is determined by its malignancy, the tendency of a tumor to grow at a fast rate, causing severe destruction of brain tissue and eventually death. Grading is from 1 to 4, with a Grade 1 tumor representing a slow-growing tumor accompanied by few neuropsychological deficits. Grades 2 and 3 represent intermediate rates of growth and neuropsychological dysfunction. Grade 4 tumors grow fast and typically have a poor prognosis for recovery. Table 12.3 reviews the different characteristics of brain tumors. Neurological and neuropsychological dysfunction results from the invasion and destruction of brain tissue by the tumor. Secondary effects include increased ICP and cerebral swelling (edema), which displace and compress brain

---

Table 12.3 Characteristics of Intracranial Tumors

1. Characteristics of brain tumors
   - Atypical, uncontrolled growth of cells
   - Cells do not serve functional purpose
   - Tumor grows at the expense of healthy cells

2. Infiltrating tumors
   - Take over and "invade" neighboring areas of the brain and destroy surrounding tissue

3. Noninfiltrating tumors
   - Encapsulated, well differentiated, and noninvasive

4. Malignant
   - Indicates that the properties of the tumor cells invade other tissue and that there is a propensity for regrowth

5. Benign
   - Describes abnormal cell growth that is usually surrounded by a fibrous capsule and is noninfiltrative; a much smaller probability for regrowth

6. Grading
   - A classification system of tumor growth; grading is in order of increasing malignancy from Grades 1 to 4, depending on cell type.

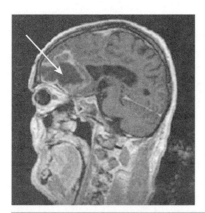

Figure 12.5 Magnetic resonance imaging (MRI) examination of a patient with a cerebral glioma. The patient had suffered from increasing headaches for 6 weeks, memory impairment, and increasing paresis of the left side. Walking remained undamaged. MRI examination indicated a tumor 65 × 56 × 69 mm in size in the right frontal lobe. The tumor displaced the anterior part of the right lateral ventricle and moved a part of the corpus callosum to the left. (Courtesy Dorota Kozinska, University of Warsaw, Warsaw, Poland.)

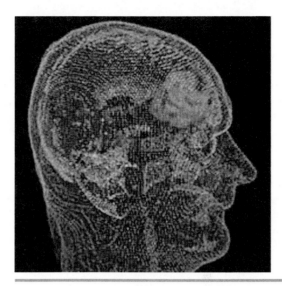

Figure 12.6 Injected magnetic resonance imaging–visible dye amplifies boundaries of right frontal tumor, a glioma, in relation to cortex and scalp surfaces. See inside covers for color image. (Courtesy Dorota Kozinska, University of Warsaw, Warsaw, Poland.)

tissue, cranial nerves, the cerebral vascular structure, and the CSF system.

Types of Intracranial Tumors

INFILTRATING TUMORS

As mentioned earlier, infiltrative tumors are not clearly differentiated from surrounding brain tissue. The most common infiltrative tumors are **gliomas,** which make up approximately 40% to 50% of all brain tumors. Gliomas are relatively fast-growing tumors that arise from supporting glial cells (Figures 12.5 and 12.6). Any type of glial cells can form a tumor, including gliomas (arising from neuroglial cells), astrocytomas (which are formed from astrocyte cells), and oligodendrogliomas (composed of oligodendrocyte cells). A particularly destructive and fatal glioma is the **glioblastoma multiforme (GBM),** which generally arises after middle age and is most often confined to one hemisphere. A GBM is typically a large, Grade 4 tumor that grows rapidly, with symptoms arising within several weeks. Surgical removal is often incomplete because of the highly infiltrative and malignant characteristics of these tumors. Thus, regrowth and eventual death are common within 6 to 12 months after surgery, even after aggressive radiation therapy. **Astrocytomas** are infiltrative tumors of astrocytes, a type of glial cell. Astrocytomas grow

more slowly than GBMs; thus, they have a somewhat better prognosis. Gliomas of the brainstem are typically astrocytomas and often affect cranial nerves V, VI, VII, and X. Finally, an **oligodendroglioma** is a rare, slowly growing tumor that affects primarily young adults.

NONINFILTRATING TUMORS

Meningiomas

The most common noninfiltrative tumors are the **meningiomas,** which represent approximately 15% of all brain tumors. Meningiomas are highly encapsulated benign tumors that arise from the arachnoid layer of the meninges. Their incidence increases with age, and they are more frequent in women than in men (by a 2:1 ratio). Meningiomas grow slowly and can become rather large before the gradually increasing pressure on the brain and displacement of surrounding healthy brain tissue cause symptoms. Technically, a meningioma is not a brain tumor, because the growth is in the brain's covering, outside the brain. This is why we refer to all tumors discussed in this chapter as *intracranial* (within the skull) rather than as *brain* tumors. With meningiomas, brain tissue is not destroyed, but neuropsychological impairments may appear because the space-occupying mass puts physical pressure on the cortex, especially in large meningiomas. Because meningiomas grow over many years, the brain can often accommodate the size of the tumor. Thus, focal or severe deficits usually do not accompany this type of tumor. Because the brain adapts to the slowly growing meningiomas, tumors in the frontal area may grow relatively large before ICP produces behavioral symptoms. Therefore, meningiomas often cause no symptoms and remain undiagnosed, only to be discovered later on autopsy.

The neurosurgeon finds meningiomas relatively easy to remove because they are encapsulated outside the brain. Removal can, however, become complicated if the tumor is difficult to access, as when the lesion is in the intrahemispheric fissure or the inferior parts of the brain. Meningiomas arising from the optic nerve sheath may be particularly difficult or impossible to remove, because they almost envelop the optic nerve. Nevertheless, because they are encapsulated and benign, meningiomas offer the best prognosis for complete recovery of any of the brain tumors.

M e t a s t a t i c   T u m o r

A malignant but encapsulated tumor is a **metastatic tumor.** *Metastasis* is a medical term for the transfer of disease from one organ or part not directly connected with it. The capacity to metastasize is a characteristic of all malignant tumors. Metastatic tumors arise secondarily to cancerous tumors, which have their primary site in other parts of the body, such as the lungs, breasts, or lymph system. The secondary growths arise because cancer cells from the primary neoplasm detach. The bloodstream can carry the cells to the brain, where they multiply. This is why early diagnosis in cancer is so important: to keep tumor tissue from "metastasizing." Metastatic brain tumors typically have multiple sites and represent up to 40% of all brain tumors seen in elderly adults. They generally grow fast and typically occur at the junction of gray and white matter, close to the cortex surface, although they can grow at any location in the brain. Metastatic brain tumors in adults arise most frequently from bronchogenic carcinoma (lung cancer), adenocarcinoma of the breast (breast cancer), and malignant melanoma (skin cancer).

A typical clinical picture in metastatic tumor is the diagnosis of an elderly man with lung cancer related to a long history of cigarette smoking. Examination of the patient's lymph nodes shows evidence of a tumor. Twelve weeks later, the patient develops a gait disturbance. Neuropsychological evaluation shows that the patient is cognitively intact but has motor slowing on the left side, an intention tremor, and difficulty walking in a straight line. Diagnostic imaging shows a metastatic tumor in the left

hemisphere of the cerebellum (recall that cerebellar deficits involve the ipsilateral arm and leg). Despite intensive chemotherapy and radiation therapy, the patient dies. The prognosis in metastatic brain cancer is typically poor because cancer invades multiple organs and produces multiple growths in the brain. Neurosurgeons usually do not consider extracting metastatic tumors if multiple sites are present. But as with any disease, there are exceptions, and disease progress is often difficult to predict. For example, U.S. cyclist Lance Armstrong was diagnosed with testicular cancer. His cancer metastasized to his lungs and his brain, spawning multiple tumors. After surgery, Armstrong made a remarkable recovery and has not only stayed cancer free, but went on to win the month-long Tour de France, the most grueling bicycle race in the world, a record seven times.

A c o u s t i c   N e u r o m a

Acoustic neuromas are progressively enlarging, benign tumors within the auditory canal arising from Schwann cells of cranial nerve VIII, the auditory vestibular nerve, which sends sensory hearing and equilibrium information to the brain. Initial symptoms include ringing in the ears (tinnitus), followed by partial deafness, such as in distinguishing speech sounds and rhythmic patterns. Acoustic neuromas typically begin to grow in the internal auditory canal and then grow medially. They affect the cranial nerves V (the trigeminal nerve, which provides sensory information of the face and motor control for chewing and swallowing) and VII (the facial nerve, which provides sensory information from the tongue and motor control of facial expressions and crying). As a result, the patient may lose his or her sense of hearing, followed by reports of a loss of taste on one side. Physicians often consult audiologists in diagnosing acoustic neuromas.

P i t u i t a r y   T u m o r s

The classification and neuropathology of **pituitary tumors** is complex because of the relation of the pituitary gland to the chemistry of the nervous and endocrine systems. Scientists traditionally divide pituitary tumors into **functioning** and **nonfunctioning adenomas. Pituitary adenomas** are benign neoplasms of the pituitary gland. Nonfunctioning adenomas produce symptoms caused by pressure on the pituitary and adjacent structures. As the tumor grows out of the sella—the bony capsule that holds the pituitary—headaches are common. Visual field deficits may also occur due to compression of the optic chiasm (bitemporal hemianopsia). Hypothalamic compression usually causes diabetes insipidus.

Functioning pituitary tumors play an "uninvited" role in the operation of the pituitary gland, often affecting the release of the gland's hormones. Functioning tumors of the pituitary gland include the **acidophilic adenoma,** a tumor usually found in the anterior lobe of the gland. The acidophilic adenoma provokes excessive secretion of growth hormones, often resulting in giantism, a condition featuring enlarged jaw, nose, tongue, hands, and feet. The **chromophobic adenoma** also appears in the anterior aspects of the pituitary gland and often produces hyperpituitarism or hypopituitarism. **Basophilic adenomas** also occur in the anterior lobe of the pituitary gland, but cause excessive secretion of adrenocorticotropic hormone (ACTH), which can cause **Cushing's syndrome.** This syndrome, named after Boston surgeon Harvey Cushing (1869–1939), is a severe systemic illness most often seen in female individuals that includes neurologic symptoms and changes in bone structure, hypertension, and diabetes. The ACTH-secreting tumor is the most serious condition encountered by any of the pituitary tumors and can necessitate complete removal of the tumor, including the pituitary gland.

CHILDHOOD TUMORS

Childhood tumors are less frequent than brain tumors in adults. The most frequent is the **medulloblastoma,** a rapidly growing and malignant tumor located in the inferior vermis close to the exit of CSF from the fourth ventricle. This type of tumor accounts for about two thirds of all tumors in children and causes increased ICP due to obstructive hydrocephalus. Early symptoms include vomiting and headache. Other common childhood tumors are cerebellar astrocytomas, gliomas of the brainstem and optic nerve, and **pinealomas.** Pineal tumors are most common in prepubescent boys. The tumor often compresses the aqueduct of Sylvius, causing hydrocephalus, papilledema, and other signs of ICP. Table 12.4 summarizes the different types and features of brain tumors.

DIAGNOSIS OF BRAIN TUMORS

The overall incidence of brain tumors for male and female individuals is about equal, but cerebellar medulloblastomas and GBM are more common in male individuals, and meningiomas are more frequent in female individuals. The overall frequency of various types of intracranial tumors is approximately 45% for gliomas, 15%

Table 12.4 *Types of Brain Tumors*

Acoustic neuroma—a benign tumor growing from the sheath of the acoustic nerve at the cerebellopontine angle

Gliomas—a tumor composed of tissue representing neuroglia; the term *glioma* is often used to describe all primary, intrinsic neoplasms of the brain and the spinal cord

Glioblastoma—Malignant forms of astrocytoma

Glioblastoma multiforme—an astrocytoma of Grade 3 or 4, a rapidly growing tumor usually confined to one cerebral hemisphere and composed of a mixture of spongioblasts, astroblasts, and astrocytes

Astrocytoma—a malignant tumor composed primarily of astrocytes

Ependymal glioma—a bulky, solid, firm vascular tumor of the fourth ventricle

Oligodendroglioma—a neoplasm derived from and composed of oligodendrocytes

Optic glioma—a slowly growing glioma of the optic nerve or optic chiasm, associated with visual loss and loss of ocular movement

Meningioma—a typically benign tumor arising from arachnoid cells; produces neuropsychological deficits by exerting pressure on surrounding brain substances or cranial nerves

Metastatic tumor—a growth of a tumor, often multiple, distant from the site primarily involved in the morbid process

Pituitary adenoma—a tumor of the pituitary gland; pituitary adenomas are often classified as functioning (changing the secretion of the pituitary gland) and nonfunctioning (benign)

Pinealoma—a tumor of the pineal body

for pituitary adenomas, 15% for meningiomas, 15% for metastatic brain tumors, and 10% for other types.

Early behavioral symptoms in the diagnosis of tumor include a sudden onset of headaches, nausea, loss of cognitive function, or seizures. The ICP triad often accompanies the growth of brain tumors and includes:

1. Headache
2. Nausea and vomiting
3. A positive papilledema, a swelling of the optic disk in the eye

Of course, not every patient reporting a headache has a brain tumor, but headache often accompanies brain tumor because of the enlarging tumor mass.

The introduction of the CT scan and the more recent magnetic resonance imaging (MRI) has literally revolutionized diagnosis of tumors. High-resolution CT can visualize even tiny tumors. Three-dimensional reconstruction can often demonstrate the intimate relations of the tumor to its surrounding brain structure, facilitating precise removal of the tumor by surgeons. Today, neurologists most efficiently diagnose brain tumor using CT or MRI, which often provides the definitive diagnosis (see Chapter 2 for a comprehensive review of medical diagnostic procedures). Neurologists have used functional MRI (fMRI) to differentiate brain tissue from tumor tissue, as well as to identify areas of the brain that are particularly vital for cognitive functions. This is often important, because using fMRI neurologists can identify a safe corridor through the brain into the tumor, which the surgeon can then use. In addition, fMRI can help differentiate whether the cancer itself contains vital brain tissue. Somatosensory-evoked responses and direct stimulation of the brain can also help separate important brain tissue from brain tumor tissue. Neurologists often use plain X-ray films in diagnosing and planning surgery to remove meningiomas, because this type of tumor can erode the skull in a high percentage of patients, as shown in radiographic changes on skull X-ray films.

Angiography occasionally can be useful in tumor diagnosis to identify which primary branches of the cardiovascular system supply the tumor with its blood supply. Modern imaging is most effective in diagnosing the presence of a tumor, but not in diagnosing its type. Histologic examination via brain biopsy is necessary to precisely diagnose the type of tumor and to select the most appropriate intervention. Neurologists most frequently do this using CT-guided stereotaxic biopsy, which interfaces stereotactic frames that fasten to the patient's head with steel pins. A biopsy needle is affixed to the frame, which the neurosurgeon can move with precision in all three dimensions. Using this procedure and with the patient under local anesthesia, the neurosurgeon can take a brain specimen through a burr hole. Subsequent laboratory examination can then provide the exact diagnosis of the tumor.

TREATMENT OF BRAIN TUMORS

The preferred treatment for brain tumors is total surgical excision of the tumor whenever possible. The prognosis for recovery after removing a brain tumor depends on two primary factors, the location and type of tumor. For example, a relatively simple surgical excision may involve a well-differentiated tumor, such as a meningioma, particularly if the tumor is in an easily accessible location (as in superior aspects of the cortex). If the tumor is malignant, local radiation therapy typically follows surgical removal to prevent regrowth. If the tumor is inaccessible, for example, in the region of the thalamus or brainstem, radiation therapy is the primary intervention. A fast-growing glioblastoma in a nonresectable location is often fatal within 12 months. Thus, the prognosis for GBMs is not good, but combined treatments have a small success rate. For tumors that are difficult to access, located at the base of the skull or covering the superior sagittal sinus, the neurosurgeon often uses a sophisticated operating microscope or a laser.

Chemotherapy for brain tumors is playing an increasingly important role in the battle against cancer. Chemotherapy is most effective in tumors that have a high growth fraction; that is, tumors that are actively dividing and producing DNA. When a tumor is young, most of its cells are making DNA. When antitumor drugs reach tumor cells in the phases of cell cycling, the cells die. As the tumor ages, growth fraction decreases and drug sensitivity declines. Thus, the most effective form of chemotherapy is when the tumor is young and 100% of its cells are in the growth fraction—this again emphasizes the importance of early diagnosis. However, the BBB, which protects the brain from foreign substances, complicates chemotherapy for brain tumors. The BBB prevents cancer-killing drugs from entering brain tissue via the bloodstream. Thus, antitumor drugs targeting brain tumors are limited to agents easily transported across the BBB—typically, very lipid-soluble substances. In recent years, however, researchers have discovered that some chemicals (such as the bradykinin agonist, RMP-7) are highly effective in opening the BBB by making capillary walls "leaky." As a result, chemotherapy drugs can act directly on the tumors, increasing their effectiveness as much as 10-fold.

Medicine will only achieve a cure in the fight against brain tumors, however, when it can enlist the patient's own immune system to attack the cancer. Tumors produce a chemical that tricks the immune system into ignoring them. Recent genetic engineering research in animals has shown some promise in discovering substances that turn off the ability of the tumor cells to produce their own vaccine. The tumor cells then become immediate targets of the immune system, which destroys them.

Treating brain tumors is not only complicated from a scientific perspective, it also takes a psychological toll on the patient, as well as the patient's family. As a result, psychologists also play an important role in counseling patients undergoing cancer treatment or in hospice centers—health care centers that provide medical and emotional support for the terminally ill and their families.

Brain Tumors and Neuropsychology

The neuropsychological manifestations of brain tumors depend on the location, size, and grade of the tumor, rather than on its histologic type. Smaller tumors near primary motor areas may cause seizures and loss of motor function, whereas deeper intracranial tumors may grow rather large before focal clinical symptoms appear. Evaluations also find a general decline in adaptive areas, as well as in overall cognitive functioning, because the tumor displaces neighboring areas. The neuropsychological deficits of a GBM are profound. The destruction of whichever cerebral hemisphere is involved is severe and nearly complete. In the acute stages of GBM, neuropsychological evaluation typically is not undertaken, because the deficits are so severe and the overall medical condition of the patient is of foremost concern. Patients with astrocytomas may have longer histories of increasing problems, because of the slow growth of these neoplasms. Oligodendrogliomas typically produce few neuropsychological effects because they grow so slowly.

Focal neuropsychological symptoms of brain tumors stem from localized destruction, compression of nervous tissue, or altered endocrine function. Tumors in the frontal lobes are most commonly meningiomas and gliomas. They can produce both localized and generalized cognitive deficits, including expressive aphasia (if located in the dominant hemisphere) or difficulties smelling (anosmia) related to a meningioma at the base of the frontal lobe. Inattention and changes in motivation commonly accompany tumors that affect both frontal hemispheres. Parietal lobe tumors may contralaterally impair sensory modalities, stereognosis, contralateral homonymous hemianopsia, and apraxia. Speech disturbances, agraphia, and finger agnosia may appear if the left hemisphere is involved, and neglect is characteristic of patents whose right hemisphere is affected.

Temporal lobe tumors may produce mixed expressive and receptive aphasia of the dominant temporal lobe. Nondominant temporal tumors often do not have "obvious" cognitive signs. Tumors deep in the temporal lobe may cause contralateral hemianopsia. Occipital lobe tumors most often entail visual deficits, typically a contralateral quadrant defect in the visual field or a hemianopia with sparing of the macula. Subcortical tumors that involve the internal capsule produce contralateral hemiplegia. Thalamic tumors produce contralateral sensory impairment. Basal ganglionic tumors often result in tremors. All brain tumors may produce seizures, which may be preceded by an aura that may indicate the location of the tumor.

Metastatic tumors are often associated with neuropsychological test results indicating focal areas of deficits. Skills that the tumor does not affect may be relatively intact. Later stages of metastatic tumors with numerous sites and sizes may produce a diffuse loss of most neuropsychological abilities. Acoustic neuromas typically do not entail severe cognitive loss, but rather a hearing impairment. A meningioma produces its behavioral effects by compressing the brain. Meningiomas near the optic nerve result in visual disturbances and are difficult to remove because of their location. Pituitary tumors also produce visual field defects because of the close relation between the optic chiasm and the pituitary gland.

Neuropsychological evaluations have proved most useful in establishing a cognitive baseline before neurosurgery and in evaluating outcomes of patients after surgery. As mentioned earlier, neuropsychologists also provide counseling and education to patients with brain tumor and their families. More recent research has focused on the neuropsychological implications of radiation therapy (Neuropsychology in Action 12.3).

Other Neurologic Disorders

BRAIN ABSCESS

Brain abscesses are similar to tumors, both in appearance and on visualization using imaging. Compared with a tumor, however, a brain abscess arises from an infection spreading to the brain or originating in the brain. Abscesses begin as an area of generalized inflammation and progress to a "walled off," localized pocket of pus within the brain. The abscess can gradually expand, destroying and compressing brain tissue as it grows. Compared with brain tumors, however, imaging typically shows an empty center within the abscess, differentiating it from a tumor, which appears more "solid." In addition, the patient typically presents with a history of prior infection.

INFECTIONS

Infections and infectious diseases tend to attack specific brain structures depending on the type. At least 20 different types of infections affect the brain. Many are obscure and rare. Among the well studied are **meningitis, herpes encephalitis,** and **human immunodeficiency virus (HIV).**

Neuropsychology in Action 12.3

Neuropsychology of Treatments for Individuals with Brain Tumors

by Carol L. Armstrong Ph.D., Department of Neurology, University of Pennsylvania and the Joseph Stokes Research Institute, Children's Hospital of Philadelphia, Philadelphia, PA

Effective brain tumor treatment is always a compromise, involving the protection of healthy cells and the destruction of aggressive cancer cells that have infiltrated healthy tissue. Treatment choices are complex and should involve input from a team of oncologic professionals, including neurosurgeon, oncologist–hematologist, radiation therapist, neuroradiologist, neurologist, and neuropsychologist. Surgical interventions range from biopsy, or the removal of enough tissue for microscopic determination of histologic type and pathologic grade of tumor cells, to the resection of 100% of tumor tissue as a method of preventing tumor regrowth. Brain surgery may also involve Wada testing or functional magnetic resonance imaging (see Chapter 2), with the aid of the neuropsychologist in determining hemispheric dominance of movement and language, and help from the neuroradiologist in outlining blood flow patterns in the brain. Specialists also may use brain mapping to localize function and preclude resection of brain tissue crucial for language or memory.

Besides surgical treatments for brain tumors, medical professionals often give radiation therapy and chemotherapy, either alone or in combination. The most common method of radiotherapy involves external photon beam radiation; with this method,

technicians administer a total dose of radiation in fractions over a period of about 6 weeks, 5 days a week. If the treatment is to prevent metastasis or the seeding of tumor cells by blood- or lymph-based cancer, then radiation may include the whole brain. However, to shrink or prevent the spread of a primary tumor, radiation is focused on just parts of the brain. The best current alternative therapies include conformal and stereotactic radiotherapy, surgical placement of chemotherapy wafers in the tumor bed, and gene therapy.

The natural history of radiotherapy effects is not well understood. Experimental animal studies demonstrate brain damage or decreased cell density from radiotherapy. Several studies in humans have associated damage to the brain's white matter with delayed radiation effects (Corn et al., 1994). In addition, chemotherapy interacts with radiotherapy to exacerbate radiation damage. Although studies of children and several retrospective studies have found alarming effects of radiation injury, some studies of adults have not. The methodology used is often the source of the discrepancies. For example, retrospective studies find abnormally high rates of white matter damage, low IQ, memory impairment, and even dementia in both adults and children from 3 months to

many years after irradiation (DeAngelis, Delattre, & Posner, 1989). A late effect, up to 20 years after treatment, may result in an atherosclerotic-like disorder if carotid arteries were irradiated. Conclusions are confounded when patients are tested at irregular time periods, only brief neuropsychological evaluations are conducted, or no baseline neuropsychological testing (before treatment) is ordered.

Memory deficits have been implicated as the most frequent and severe delayed effect of radiation therapy. Researchers consider the early delayed effects, occurring 2 to 3 months after completion of radiation treatment, to be mild and temporary. The late delayed effects of radiation therapy are more severe, may progress, and are irreversible. We compared longitudinal research on patients who received radiation therapy with patients with similar tumor types but who did not have radiotherapy. Patients with low-grade, cortical, primary brain tumors often have long life expectancies and relatively few cognitive deficits. Neuropsychologists give these patients a repeatable, comprehensive battery of tests that includes many sensitive measures of attention and memory processes. Evaluations occur just before irradiation, and then at 3-, 6-, and 12-month intervals. Thus far we have learned

---

Meningitis is a bacterial or viral infection of the meninges that provide the protective covering of the brain. Meningitis can also be a result of brain surgery (there is an up to 5% incidence rate); physicians routinely administer antibiotics to patients who have undergone intracranial procedures to prevent such infections. Interestingly, such infections acquired during brain surgery vary, not only from hospital to hospital depending on the thoroughness of sterilization of the operating room but also among operating rooms within a single hospital. Such data are, however, not commonly published for the consumer, for

obvious reasons. Herpes encephalitis (not to be confused with genital herpes) aggressively attacks the medial temporal and orbital frontal areas. This appears to destroy much of the limbic system, especially the hippocampus. The result is a near total inability to learn new information (anterograde amnesia). The HIV/AIDS virus has wider effects on the brain, because it progressively destroys the immune system. The virus itself may have direct consequences for the brain, but it also opens the brain to opportunistic infections and other diseases that can attack the brain.

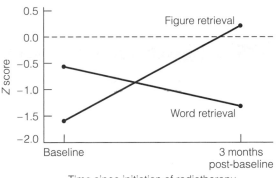

Figure 12.7 Double dissociation of patient's word and figure retrieval after delay at baseline and at point of early delayed phase of radiotherapy. (Reproduced from Armstrong, C., Corn, B., Ruffer, J., Pruitt, A., Mollman, J., & Phillips, P. [2000]. Radiotherapeutic effects on brain function: Double dissociation of memory systems. *Neuropsychiatry, Neuropsychology, and Behavioral Neurology, 13,* 100–111, by permission.)

that robust patterns of neurocognitive change appear during the first year after radiotherapy (Figure 12.7). Visual-perceptual memory learning and recall are impaired at baseline but improve steadily over 1 year. Verbal-semantic retrieval is often not affected at baseline, but declines at the early delayed phase. Researchers think the early delayed phase of radiation damage is caused by interruption of myelin synthesis, which stems from inhibition of glial mitosis. Thus, verbal-semantic retrieval appears sensitive to the damaging effects of radiotherapy and may be sensitive to the more crucial late delayed phase of irradiation. The initial impairment and improvement in visual memory may represent recovery from surgical injury to the hippocampal memory system.

We discovered that radiation selectively impairs verbal-semantic memory significantly more than motor control, visual and auditory attention, visual and auditory working memory, visual long-term memory, language, visuospatial perception, processing speed, and reasoning. Why would retrieval be so sensitive to radiation? Retrieval, the end point of remembering, depends on reconstructive processes in which the system associates the contents of current consciousness with information stored in permanent memory. Several other cognitive processes theoretically could account for the patient's failure to retrieve words from long-term memory, including failure of selective attention, working memory deficit, slowed processing speed, and failure to regenerate the attributes of the target. However, we found that none of these related cognitive processes explained the retrieval impairment. We are pursuing the questions of whether the rate of reconstruction of current memory or the recall of novel arrangements of memory attributes predicts the retrieval deficit, and how these processes correspond with regions of the brain's white matter.

Neuropsychological findings have influenced the treatment of brain tumors. Neuro-oncologists have become more selective about the doses and timing of radiotherapy. Radiation oncologists may advise patients about the early delayed effects on memory. Patients are more likely to receive referrals for rehabilitative therapies, and neuropsychologists are more cautious when recommending return to work. Neuro-oncology researchers are investigating other potential damaging effects on the brain, such as the possible association with Alzheimer's-like neural changes in gray matter. Researchers are also aiming studies at developing pharmacologic treatments to block the damaging effects of radiotherapy and at identifying chromosomal markers of beneficial sensitivity to cancer treatments. Neuropsychologists can play an important role in helping to understand the psychological (Neuropsychology in Action 12.4) and the cognitive changes associated with brain tumor treatment.

NEUROTOXINS

Neurotoxins include any substances that are poisonous to the brain (Lezak, 1995). These may include drugs, alcohol, solvents, fuels, pesticides, and metals such as lead or mercury. Many substances can be toxic to the brain in high doses, whereas they may not be toxic in low doses. Many prescription drugs fall into this category, for example, lithium, which is used to treat bipolar affective disorder (manic depression).

Many heavy metals, such as lead or mercury, can be extremely damaging to the body and the CNS, even in low dosages (Zillmer, Lucci, Barth, Peake, & Spyker, 1986; Zillmer, 1995). Although not many people come in contact with heavy metals, the general population may be exposed to some toxins routinely or by accident. For example, more than half a million accidental poisonings from pesticides are reported each year worldwide. One common group of pesticides are chlorinated hydrocarbon insecticides (for example, chlordane, heptachlor, and lindane), which people use extensively to combat household pests such as flies, cockroaches, fleas, termites, and mosquitoes, as well as agricultural crop enemies. Because chlordane maintains its effects for approximately 15 or more years after application, it offers an economically

Neuropsychology in Action 12.4

Family and Child Adjustment to Cognitive Aspects of Cancer in Children

by Lamia P. Barakat   Ph.D., Associate Professor of Psychology, Department of Psychology, Drexel University, Philadelphia, PA

Lisa, a 21-year-old woman, was referred to a consulting psychologist by her pediatric oncologist because of depressed mood, behavioral manifestations of seizures with no associated neurologic changes, and family conflict. When she was 10 years old, Lisa was treated for acute nonlymphoblastic leukemia through bone marrow transplant, which included high-dose, whole-body radiation. Sequelae of the cancer and its treatment included apparent seizures (particularly when stressed); cognitive deficits associated with cranial radiation, including limitations in general intellectual functioning; and a pattern of deficits associated with nonverbal learning disability (Carey, Barakat, Foley, Gyato, & Phillips, 2001), cataracts, and infertility. At the time of referral, Lisa lived with her parents and her younger brother. Although a high school graduate, she was not employed and spent most of her time alone at home. Although her parents were caring and protective, they did not encourage Lisa to branch out of the home, because they feared she would have a seizure in a public place, were uncertain of her capabilities, and viewed the cancer and its consequences as severe and insurmountable. Despite her current situation, Lisa hoped to go to college, get married, and have children.

The complexities of Lisa's medical condition placed a considerable burden on the family as a whole. The role of the patient's cognitive factors in family functioning is complex; some detrimental effects may appear, but some families can cope with these problems (Carlson-Green, Morris, & Krawiecki, 1995). A key to understanding the relations among cognitive aspects of childhood cancer, child adjustment, and family functioning may be child and parent perceptions or appraisals of the impact of the illness. A series of studies on childhood cancer survivors and their parents consistently relate perception of life threat associ-

ated with cancer, and its treatment in the past and present, and appraisals of treatment intensity to child, parent, and family adjustment (Barakat, Kazak, Meadows, Casey, Meeske, & Stuber, 1997; Foley, Barakat, Herman-Liu, Radcliffe, & Molloy, 2000). However, objectively rated intensity of the treatment, severity of medical late effects, and history of cranial radiation treatment are not consistently associated with adjustment in children treated for cancer.

These findings provide strong evidence for the importance of child and parent subjective appraisals or perceptions of cognitive limitations in understanding child and family functioning after cancer diagnosis and treatment. Importantly, preventive interventions can modify child and parent appraisals of cognitive limitations and the impact of the illness, to improve long-term family adaptation (Barakat & Kazak, 1999). It is essential to work with families from the point of cancer diagnosis to provide a realistic but optimistic framework for understanding children's capabilities and needs. The intervention must consider the child's ability to comprehend this information, given cognitive limitations.

Such interventions must also take into account developmental process in families. As the children grow older, families must reassess and reintegrate the meaning of cognitive limitations for their child and family. For example, as children enter formal schooling, families must balance the need to address potential learning problems with the need for children to engage in routine activities with peers. As children reach adolescence and strive for autonomy, families must be able to set realistic goals with their children while allowing them to achieve independence in functioning. On the flip side, children and adolescents should gain guidance in choosing academic, vocational, and social goals that they can attain.

In addition to addressing perceptions, it is necessary to foster positive changes in family interactions (such as interactions around homework, rules in the home, and peer relationships) to promote children's competencies and, in turn, improve functioning. In relation to this, frequent communication among other systems, such as the school, religious community, or medical treatment team, decreases conflicting information provided to families and improves coordination of support. For instance, the child, parents, and teachers may cooperatively develop and implement a plan aimed at homework completion that provides structure and builds on the child's cognitive strengths.

Finally, improving parent resources and coping helps improve the functioning of families dealing with the long-term strains and medical sequelae of cancer treatment, including cognitive changes. Family-to-family contact and support through multiple-family groups is an integral part of bolstering children's and their parents' resources. Families learn from one another which coping strategies most facilitate healthy family development as the childhood cancer survivor moves into adulthood.

After complete neurologic and psychological evaluations, Lisa was diagnosed with grand mal seizures, as well as unexplained seizure activity, and major depression with dissociative features. Treatment entailed achieving a therapeutic dose of medication for her seizures and individual and family therapy. The goal of family therapy was to help Lisa and her parents realistically assess her skills and recognize her potential. Initially, through increasing her responsibility in the home, trips to the mall (where she was free to shop on her own), and engagement in hobbies, Lisa's sense of competence improved. Her parents' perceptions of her abilities became more optimistic, and their appraisals of her illness severity lightened. Lisa and her parents began to focus on increasing Lisa's independent functioning. She successfully entered a vocational rehabilitation program and made plans for a clerical position in the future. She began to make friends and to attend social functions through her rehabilitation program. Lisa made a number of overnight visits with siblings, and her parents took a long-needed vacation without their daughter. Concurrently, counselors gently guided Lisa through cognitive interventions to understand and come to terms with her limitations, particularly those relevant to her hopes for a college education and children. Lisa's seizures and depression remitted.

appealing long-term treatment against termites. Chlordane is readily absorbed through the gastrointestinal tract, respiratory tract, or unbroken skin, and it is stored in body fat. Once absorbed, chlordane is an axon poison, which disturbs the normal action of the sodium-potassium adenosinetriphosphatase (ATPase) pump, interfering with the transmission of nerve impulses. Because of its chemical stability, chlordane can be detected in approximately 70% of U.S. homes today and ranks among the most ubiquitous neurotoxic materials being released into the ecosystem (Zillmer, Montenegro, Wiser, Barth, & Spyker, 1996).

In general, toxic effects on the brain cannot be described in simple terms, because the mechanisms of action are so varied. Most common are cognitive deficits ranging from mild to severe on tasks that require speeded processing, problem solving, and delayed memory. Somatization, hysterical features, and depression often dominate the clinical picture. Thus, the medical profession increasingly recognizes that chemicals can have significant neuropsychological effects (Hartman, 1995), and that neuropsychology offers promise in increasing knowledge of the effects of toxins on the human CNS, describing specific patterns of performance, and monitoring the course of treatment.

Summary

In general, damage to the brain may result from either primary or secondary damage and may have either acute or long-term effects. In addition to damage within the immediate area, there may also be damage to more distal areas because of disconnected neuronal pathways. The diagnosis of primary damage relates to the initial injury or insult to the brain. If axons are completely severed or destroyed, the damage is often permanent and that tissue is lost. Secondary brain damage, in contrast, may result in either permanent or temporary damage. Secondary damage is caused by the aftereffects of the primary injury. Hemorrhage or bleeding causes oxygen deprivation and can lead to cell death known as necrosis. Edema, or "brain swelling," hemorrhage, and infection may all cause increased cranial pressure. This pressure in the nonexpanding skull may effectively "cut off" areas of brain functions. If these secondary effects can be controlled quickly, the damage and functional effects may reverse in the acute stages of recovery. What is considered primary damage in one situation may be secondary damage in another. For example, a head injury (see discussion in Chapter 13) may cause primary axonal severing, destruction of brain tissue, and secondary swelling and hemorrhaging. The primary damage of a stroke may be caused by a hemorrhage, but there may still be secondary swelling and ICP. Sudden traumas such as stroke tend to have more striking and noticeable behavioral effects than slowly emerging processes. The most frequently encountered cerebrovascular disorders may, at times, produce multiple cognitive disabilities; yet, often such dysfunction is relatively localized for the anatomic area involved, as well as the corresponding neuropsychological sequelae. However, more general neuropsychological disabilities are possible when, for example, larger areas of the brain are infarcted. Brain tumors affect a significant proportion of the population and may lead to many debilitating conditions. Neuropsychologists are at the forefront in researching cerebrovascular and tumor treatment and rehabilitation. In Chapter 13, we discuss other neurologic disorders of the brain, specifically the neuropsychological consequences and rehabilitation of traumatic head injuries.

Critical Thinking Questions

- What are the neurologic, behavioral, and emotional symptoms of a stroke?
- What are the major forms of treatment for stroke?
- Why do some stroke victims downplay their illness, whereas others go into a deep depression?

- Describe the most common neuropsychological deficits associated with stroke.
- Would you want to know what type of cell a tumor arises from if one of your family members had brain cancer? Why? Should physicians routinely inform their patients of such medical details?
- What is the neuropsychologist's role in diagnosing and treating patients with brain tumors? What is his or her role with the patient's family?
- How do children who have brain tumors react differently to their disease from the way adults do? How do their families react?

Key Terms

Lesions	Atherosclerosis	Tumor	Pituitary tumors
Necrosis	Platelets	Neoplasm	Functioning adenomas
Anoxia	Endothelium	Infiltrative tumors	Nonfunctioning adenomas
Hypoxia	Embolism	Noninfiltrative tumors	Pituitary adenoma
Sleep apnea	Atrial fibrillation	Malignant tumors	Acidophilic adenoma
Hydrocephalus	Hematoma	Benign tumors	Chromophobic adenoma
Communicating hydrocephalus	Intracerebral	Metastasis	Basophilic adenoma
Obstructive hydrocephalus	Subarachnoid hemorrhage	Neuromas	Cushing's syndrome
Stroke	Aneurysms	Grade of tumor	Medulloblastoma
Cerebrovascular accident (CVA)	Arteriovenous malformations	Gliomas	Pinealoma
Intracranial pressure (ICP)	(AVMs)	Glioblastoma multiforme (GBM)	Optic glioma
Infarction	Aura	Astrocytomas	Brain abscess
Hemorrhage	Migraine stroke	Oligodendroglioma	Meningitis
Transient ischemic attack (TIA)	Stenosis	Meningiomas	Herpes encephalitis
Ischemia	Collateral blood vessel	Metastatic tumors	Human immunodeficiency virus
Thrombosis	Anastomosis	Acoustic neuromas	(HIV)

Web Connections

http://www.med.harvard.edu/AANLIB/home.html
Harvard Medical School: CVA Facts—This site for the Whole Brain Atlas has an excellent section of images demonstrating various types of CVAs discussed in our text. A great way to visualize the extent of damage different types of CVAs may manifest. Also shows MRI and single-photon emission computed tomography images of various neoplastic diseases, including glioma, metastatic tumors, and meningioma.

http://neurosurgery.mgh.harvard.edu
Brain Aneurysm and AVM Center—Links you to the Harvard Brain Aneurysm and AVM Center at Mass General, where you can find discussions of the latest treatment for these and other cerebrovascular disorders.

http://www.stanford.edu/group/neurology/stroke
Stroke Awareness—Stanford Medical Center's site for stroke awareness and treatment information.

http://www.ninds.nih.gov
National Institute on Neurological Disorders and Stroke—An excellent site for the most up-to-date information on CVAs and related disorders. Internal search engines allow you to be as specific as you would like in obtaining information.

Chapter 13

TRAUMATIC HEAD INJURY AND REHABILITATION

If you want to understand God, you study the anatomy of the brain.
—*Keith Black (neurosurgeon)*

Traumatic Head Injury
Epidemiology of Traumatic Head Injury
Mechanism of Impact: Neuronal Shearing, Stretching,
   and Tearing
Complications of Moderate and Severe Brain Injury
Mild Head Injury: "Concussions"
Treatment of Head Injuries
Recovery, Rehabilitation, and Intervention of Traumatic
   Brain Injury
Adaptation and Recovery
Overview of the Rehabilitation Process
Treatment Methods for Neuropsychological
   Rehabilitation

Neuropsychology in Action

13.1 Case Study: Penetrating Head Injury
13.2 Can a Concussion Change Your Life?
13.3 Consensual Sex after Traumatic Brain Injury:
      Sex as a Problem-Solving Task
13.4 It Is More Than a Black Box

> ## Keep in Mind
>
> ■ Do different injuries to the brain have similar effects on the brain, or should we expect a variety of effects?
>
> ■ What is the difference between a penetrating and a closed head injury?
>
> ■ What role do neuropsychologists play in the diagnosis and treatment of head injuries?
>
> ■ How do rehabilitation programs further the process of recovery and adaptation with traumatic brain injury?
>
> ■ What is the specific role of the neuropsychologist on the rehabilitation team?

Overview

Neurologists commonly differentiate neurologic disorders of the brain by whether they have a particular focus or site, or are more generalized, affecting the brain as a whole. There are, however, many exceptions to this simple classification paradigm. As discussed in Chapter 12, a stroke or a bleed in the brain is a focal disorder because the damage occurred at a specific location. In contrast, many small bleeds or very large hemorrhages often present a diffuse clinical picture. Similarly, a single brain tumor may represent a precise focal deficit, whereas a large tumor or multiple small tumors of the brain may leave the patient with more wide-reaching deficits, which typically entail diffuse neuropsychological deficits. For the most part, neuropsychologists consider tumors to be focal disorders of the brain, because most often they entail more or less circumscribed brain damage.

In contrast, diffuse disorders most often involve dysfunction of the entire brain and most frequently appear in closed head injuries (CHIs), toxic conditions, and degenerative disorders. This classification paradigm is not entirely accurate, but it helps the neuropsychologist make an overall determination of the severity and extent of possible dysfunction. In a car accident, the rotational forces on the head often result in blunt trauma to the brain, and thus cause diffuse damage. In contrast, a gunshot wound to the head may present a relatively localized but devastating trauma to the brain and may have more localized deficits. Therefore, keep in mind that this categorization is not a hard-and-fast rule. In principle, focal disorders may interrupt a small area of brain functioning, whereas other areas of the brain remain relatively intact. Sometimes the loss of brain tissue is so small that it may not be noticeable except with sophisticated neuropsychological testing or advanced imaging techniques.

This chapter discusses the more diffuse traumas of the brain related to head injury. Finally, less frequently encountered neurologic disorders are discussed, including brain abscesses, infections, and neurotoxins.

Traumatic Head Injury

The Kennedy clan (that is, President John F. Kennedy's family) engage in an annual family ritual during their skiing vacation in Aspen, Colorado. The Kennedy clan and friends gather at a mountaintop bar, waiting until the lifts shut down at about 4 P.M. Then, with few other skiers on the trails, they play football down the slope, with skis but no poles. A cross between Frisbee and touch football, "ski football" is an old Kennedy pastime. They divide into two teams and start tossing a makeshift football through the thin mountain air toward a goal, typically a trail marker. The rules of the game demand that a player must pass the ball to a teammate within 10 seconds or turn the ball over. This seems like a lot of fun, but inherent in skiing, as is true for most sports, is risk in the form of speed. Sports, in fact, account for 17% of all head injuries, second only to motor vehicle accidents (MVAs). The most dangerous sports are equestrian events, gymnastics, and cheerleading. Among intercollegiate sports, gymnastics, football, lacrosse, and ice hockey are the most likely to lead to head injuries. Skiing is actually a relatively safe sport—there is less than 1 death per 1 million skied days. But that New Year's Eve afternoon the conditions were getting worse, the slopes were slick and icy, and the sun was setting behind the mountains, making it hard to see in the shadows and flat light. On the quintessential "last run" on the last day of the year, Michael L. Kennedy, the 39-year-old son of Ethel and the late Senator Robert, turned his head to catch the ball. He hit a fir tree headfirst on the left side of the trail. Yes, it was reckless to ski while playing a daring game of mountainside football. The ski patrol had warned against it. Tossing a makeshift football back and forth may have distracted Kennedy just enough that he was not able to stop or swerve before striking the tree. According to eyewitnesses, Kennedy—a good skier—first struck the tree with a tip of his ski, which caused him to catapult slightly and slam his head directly into its trunk without slowing down. With his three youngest children watching in horror, Michael Kennedy died of a severe head injury to the back of his fractured skull. His injury must have damaged his brainstem, because his sister Rory, who was the first to his side, noticed no pulse or breathing. The medulla oblongata, a part of the lower brainstem, mediates vital functions necessary for life such as respiration, blood pressure, heart rate, and basic muscle tone. Damage to the medulla can interrupt motor and sensory pathways, as well as threaten life itself. The death, ruled accidental, adds yet another tragedy to America's most famous clan.

Would a helmet have saved his life? Those who survive head injuries often sustain significant brain damage, which can change them for a lifetime, both physically and emotionally. This can result in a markedly altered lifestyle for the survivor, those who take care of him or her, the family, and loved ones.

Epidemiology of Traumatic Head Injury

Human brains have evolved over hundreds of thousands of years, but only recently have people invented technology, both recreational and occupational, that has put brains in motion, often at high speeds. The skull and the dura mater protect the brain well, but they are no match for the physical forces unleashed on the brain during a head injury, which often can result in brain damage. Head injuries do not occur in isolation, and additional injuries are common; thus, most cases require additional medical attention to other seriously traumatized parts of the body, complicating the overall prognosis and intervention.

Accidents are the leading cause of death in people ages 1 to 30. In the 1970s, the medical profession first recognized head injuries, particularly those related to MVAs, as a national epidemic. Researchers estimate that 500,000 people suffer brain injury every year. A majority of those are in the mild range, but millions of people in the United States are surviving and living with a moderate to severe brain trauma (Zillmer, Schneider, Tinker, & Kaminaris, 2006). After MVAs, the causes of head injuries are, in order, sports injuries, falls, violence, and industrial accidents. In individuals younger than 45 years, head injuries cause more deaths and disability every year than any other neurologic illness. Those most at risk are young, under age 30, single, and male. The male/female ratio may be as high as 4:1. Young adults between ages 15 and 24, followed by children and adolescents aged 5 to 14, are at greatest risk for traumatic brain injury (TBI). But no one is immune. Studies implicate alcohol in one third to half of all traumatic head injuries. In fact, head injuries are such a significant health problem among developed countries that they play a role in approximately half of all deaths related to trauma (Rimel, Giordani, Barth, Boll, & Jane, 1981).

Most often head injuries show no visible physical "scars." However, significant changes in behavior and emotion follow head injuries, often most noticeable by people close to the victim. As recently as the mid-1980s, hospitals typically discharged survivors of head injuries, after recovering medically, without consideration of whether they had recovered cognitively or emotionally. Neuropsychologists now know that even mild head injuries may entail a variety of learning and mood disorders. Head injuries also place a financial burden on society. On average, each brain injury costs more than $100,000 in acute medical care and rehabilitation. Neuropsychologists play an important role in assessing survivors and in providing rehabilitation. Because of the complexities of brain functions and the sequelae of TBI, the neuropsychology student must understand the pathophysiologic aspects of head trauma, as well as their neuropsychological correlates.

Mechanism of Impact: Neuronal Shearing, Stretching, and Tearing

Bumps to the head are something everyone has endured. But when does a "bump" become a TBI? The pathomechanism of head injuries relates to the physical forces placed on the neuron, specifically the axon and cell body (Figure 13.1). Neurologists have described these forces as shear and straining effects at the neuron level. The axon in particular can take only a certain amount of physical

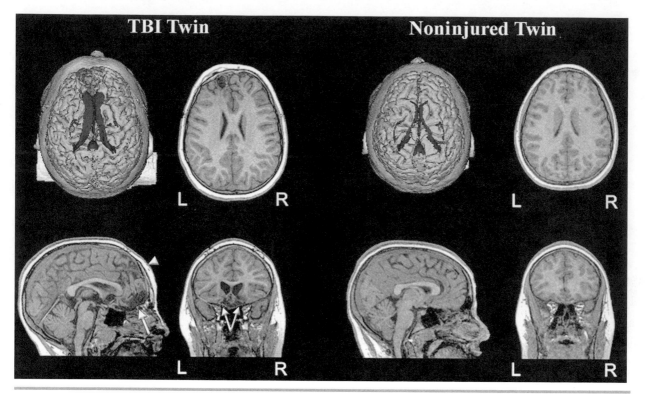

Figure 13.1 Magnetic resonance imaging (MRI) of a 12-year-old who sustained a traumatic brain injury (TBI). The MRI scans demonstrate frontal contusions and atrophy with associated enlarged ventricles, compared with the MRI of the noninjured twin. The three-dimensional representation of the brain shows the increased lateral ventricles in the TBI survivor. See inside covers for color image. (Courtesy Erin Bigler, Ph.D., Brigham Young University, Provo, UT.)

stress; the **tensile strength** of the axon is its resistance to longitudinal stress, measured by the minimal amount of stress required to rupture the axon. Brain trauma may deform, stretch, and compress the brain and its tissue, exceeding normal tissue's extendibility, particularly along the axon. These forces may tear the axon, and once damaged, the axon may degenerate back to the cell body, which may lead to cell death. This process is called **retrograde degeneration.** Conversely, the tear or rupture of a cell body can lead to the axon fiber degenerating, called **anterograde degeneration.** Because the neuron dies, the now-damaged axon is not activated by the postsynaptic axon. This may lead to a "domino effect," that is, metabolic changes in the postsynaptic neuron and possible cell death. The shearing effect on axons is most noticeable at the junction of gray and white matter regions of the brain (Naugle, Cullum, & Bigler, 1998). Recent advances in understanding of neuronal changes in the brain have improved knowledge of the microanatomic changes related to TBI. This knowledge has confirmed the long-assumed idea that during brain trauma, real physical changes at the cellular level may have associated cognitive deficits.

These types of degeneration most likely result from rapid acceleration and deceleration that shake the "Jell-O–like" brain within the cranial cavity. The types of traumas most likely to cause such shaking are CHIs, in which the head impacts another object or is suddenly thrown back in whiplash. Only neurons that are not completely severed may "resprout" axonal projections. Shearing, tearing, and stretching may result in axonal sprouting, or new growth from the damaged neurons. Perhaps these new connections will bypass damaged areas and restore function. New axonal sprouting, however, is not always beneficial. Neurons may also form unwanted connections, resulting in behavioral disturbances. Apparently, much axonal activity occurs in the area of the neuronal injury. There may be not only axonal sprouting from damaged neurons but also collateral sprouting from nearby intact neurons.

Damage to the brain itself results either from an object penetrating the skull or from rapid acceleration or deceleration of the brain. Thus, it is useful to divide the mechanisms of impact according to two major classifications of head injuries:

1. Head injuries associated with a penetrating mechanism, called **penetrating head injury**
2. **Closed head injuries** (CHIs), associated with a blow to the head, but not penetrating the skull

PENETRATING HEAD INJURY

A penetrating head injury occurs when a small object has lodged in the brain, such as a knife, scissors, or a bullet from a gun. Penetrating head injuries are extremely dangerous to the cortical integrity of the brain because of two factors. The first factor is the location and extent of the damage. For example, a gunshot wound to the brainstem is almost always fatal. Conversely, damage to a cortical association area may entail "less" damage. The second factor is the complications typically associated with penetrating head injuries, which include infection and hemorrhaging.

Although most gunshot wounds to the head result in fatal brain damage, survivors almost always receive a neuropsychological evaluation to outline the deficits and residual strengths associated with the injury. We have consulted on many cases in which patients with seemingly fatal penetrating head injuries have survived, although with neuropsychological deficits (Neuropsychology in Action 13.1).

Penetrating head injuries can greatly damage the brain, which is often incompatible with sustaining life. A large-caliber gunshot wound to the brain usually causes death, because there is significant tearing of blood vessels and destruction of brain tissue along the bullet's path through the brain. Small-caliber gunshot wounds can also be fatal, because they can "bounce" within the skull, fatally damaging a strategic area of the brain.

Self-inflicted gunshot wounds to the head are the primary way men commit suicide, followed by jumping off high buildings and hanging. There are more than 25,000 suicides in the United States every year, with a majority being from gunshot wounds.

People who survive penetrating head injuries are often disabled for life. A well-documented case is James Brady, who was President Ronald Reagan's press attaché. During an assassination attempt by John Hinckley, Jr., Brady was struck by bullets to his right frontal lobe. Hinckley used "killer bullets," which, on impact, explode into hundreds of fragments. Surgeons completely removed Brady's right frontal lobe, which was seriously damaged. Hinckley, a paranoid schizophrenic, later used the insanity defense to avoid prison; he is currently hospitalized in St. Elizabeth's Hospital in Washington, DC. Brady was left hemiplegic on the left side of his body and has many other, more subtle, neuropsychological symptoms. He and his wife have been the primary political forces behind the Brady Bill, which seeks to control handgun purchases by former mental patients and people with a criminal record. Countries that monitor gun purchases have shown dramatic success in reducing gun-related deaths and injuries. For example, in Norway, a small, northern European country of approximately 5 million people, less than 10 deaths a year are attributed to gunshot wounds to the head. The latest statistics from the U.S. Department of Justice report that of all homicides perpetrated in the United States in 1998, 52% or 14,000 were committed with handguns.

CLOSED HEAD INJURY

Closed head traumas have many different causes, but common to all is that the brain undergoes either marked acceleration or deceleration, or both. In **acceleration,** the brain experiences a significant physical force that propels it quickly from stationary to moving. Examples are the brain being hit by a moving object such as a baseball bat or a car, or a passenger in a rocket accelerating very fast. In **deceleration,** the brain is already in motion, traveling at a certain speed, and then stops abruptly, sometimes instantaneously. Examples include most MVAs and the skiing accident described earlier. The kinetic potential—that is, the physical forces acting on the brain—can be expressed mathematically for both types of injuries.

Let us first start with acceleration injuries. You can measure acceleration by noting the time elapsed from the start of acceleration and multiplying it by the acceleration of gravity, or $g = 9.8$ m/sec^2, and time, according to the following formula: velocity (v) = the product of acceleration (g) and time (t) or $v = gt$. For example, think of yourself jumping off a 3-meter-high diving board. There are two ways you could get hurt. The first is related to acceleration from the forces (in this case, from gravity) that your brain is experiencing during the period of free fall. In mathematical terms, you can calculate this using the preceding formula. Thus, maximum impact velocity (v) for a 3-meter board would be 12.94 m/sec, corresponding to approximately 29 mph maximum impact speed (depending how high you jump off the board; see Zillmer, 2003c).

The second type of injury you could receive is related to how fast your kinetic energy that you have acquired (29 miles/hour), as a result of the free-fall deceleration, is absorbed by your body and brain. For example, you may have performed a jump in which you landed flat on your stomach. In this case, you decelerate much more quickly than you would if you entered the water feetfirst. You can calculate deceleration (*a*) by dividing velocity over time

Neuropsychology in Action 13.1

Case Study: Penetrating Head Injury

by Eric A. Zillmer

This case concerns a patient I treated in a trauma intensive care unit (ICU). The client was a 25-year-old, right-handed, unemployed, single mother with a 12th-grade education. She was suffering from severe depression when she shot herself in the forehead with a small .32-caliber pistol. She was right-handed and held the pistol to her right temple, an inch above her right eye. With her two young children in the home, she then pulled the trigger. The bullet pierced her right frontal skull, sending fragments of bone into her right frontal and parietal lobe. The bullet itself, sterilized by the heat from the acceleration from the gun barrel, came to rest in the left frontal lobe (Figure 13.2). Damage to her brain was confined to her frontal lobes. She did not injure subcortical structures and motor areas of the frontal lobes, and no vital arteries or veins were severed. In a way, she lobotomized herself, and surprisingly, she was actually conscious and responsive when she arrived in the emergency department!

She underwent a right frontal craniotomy for debridement of the gunshot because the bone and skin fragments presented a risk for infection. Surgeons inserted a metal plate in her right skull to repair the damage where the bullet had entered. The bullet itself was too deeply lodged in the brain to be removed. The neurosurgeon decided not to extract the bullet, because doing so would have required cutting through intact brain tissue to reach the bullet. The bullet remained in her brain.

I conducted a neuropsychological evaluation while the client was still in the trauma ICU, 3 days after trauma. It was not possible to administer a complete neuropsychological examination of the patient because of her level of fatigue and poor endurance. The results from the screening showed that she was alert and oriented to person, place, and time. She was aware that her speed of processing was extremely slow and kept asking, "Why am I taking so long to respond to these questions?" Attention was mildly impaired. She could repeat up to 5 digits forward and could do automatism, such as counting from 1 to 20 and reciting the alphabet. On tasks requiring more sustained attention/concentration, however, she showed moderate problems, because she could repeat only up to two digits backward and made errors adding serial threes.

Her motor functions showed decreased motor speed and motor-sequencing problems on the nondominant left hand. Visuospatial functions showed mild problems in spatial orientation and a left visual neglect syndrome. Copying of designs showed a neglect of the left visual space. For example, her drawing of a clock was missing the numbers from 6 to 10 on the left side. Receptive speech was adequate: She could follow two-step commands, but her processing speed was very slow. Expressive speech showed markedly decreased fluency. Immediate visual and verbal memory were adequate. On delayed recall, however, she showed mild-to-moderate short-term memory problems. Her overall abstract reasoning and planning were significantly impaired.

I include this evaluation here to demonstrate the neuropsychologist's role in a critical care setting, as well as to document the neuropsychological functioning of a gunshot victim. In making this neuropsychological evaluation, I established some cognitive impairment and identified this client as a potential rehabilitation patient. The relatively mild degree of impairment, given the nature of the trauma, suggests that the integration centers of the brain were spared from damage. It could have been a lot worse neuropsychologically and medically, although the patient continued to struggle with depression.

Another account of penetrating gunshot wound from our clinical experience concerns a depressed man who tried to kill himself by using a shotgun. He placed the shotgun underneath his chin, pointing the gun straight up, and pulled the trigger. The blast removed his chin, nose, mouth, and most of the prefrontal cortex. The suicide attempt also left him blind. But vital areas of the brain, including the brainstem, hypothalamus, and subcortical structures, remained intact, and the patient survived. Interestingly, the patient had inadvertently given himself a prefrontal lobotomy. His depression was not present anymore, but he had many cognitive deficits and a bad temper.

In another, final example, during a prison fight, one inmate plunged a pair of scissors into another inmate's brain, straight down the parietal cortex. The scissors missed the superior sagittal sinus and must have been short enough to avoid penetrating subcortical areas. The prisoner walked into the emergency department with the scissors still implanted in the skull—only the handles showed!

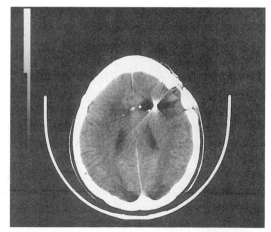

Figure 13.2   Computed transaxial tomography (CT) scan of .32-caliber bullet gunshot wound. CT scan shows that the gunshot was to the right frontal area with bone fragments in the right frontal lobe. (Courtesy Eric Zillmer.)

($a = v/t$). You have already calculated the velocity, so all you need to establish is the time it takes to decelerate. If that time period is instantaneous—if you were to hit the asphalt rather than the water—the deceleration would be high and injury likely. If, however, it takes the diver 1 or 2 seconds to decelerate, then the forces are much less. The time of deceleration is an important variable in the deceleration equation. If very short, it corresponds to higher deceleration. This is why downhill skiing or race car crashes that take a "considerable" amount of time, although horrific to the observer, are actually safer, because the brain is decelerating more slowly.

Using the preceding formula, a springboard diver experiences approximately a corresponding deceleration of 16.28 m/sec^2 or approximately 2 g when jumping off a 3-meter board. If you were to hit asphalt from the same height, the approximate deceleration expressed in mathematical terms would be more than 50 $g!$ In their cars, race car drivers at the Indy 500 carry G-meters, which can corroborate the amount of gravity forces the driver experiences during a crash. In one crash during practice, a driver hit the retaining wall almost head-on. The G-meter indicated a force of 87 g, incompatible with sustaining life. Because car racing is dangerous and drivers are at risk for CHIs, Indy race car drivers undergo preseason neuropsychological testing to establish a baseline in cognitive abilities if injuries occur during the season. This is also the case for the National Hockey League (NHL), which has started baseline neuropsychological testing for all its players to evaluate the effects of mild CHIs (also called concussions), which have cut short some of the players' careers.

In CHIs, the physical forces acting on the brain tissue may occur at the point of impact (an **impact injury**) or its opposite pole, because the brain "tears" away from the skull (**countercoup injury**). Diffuse injury is also common and most likely to occur at the frontal lobes and temporal poles, because of the uneven, "sandpaper-like" surface of the tentorial plates that hold those brain structures in place. The physical forces may shear, tear, and rupture nerves, blood vessels, and the covering of the brain. In severe head injury, those forces are so strong that they reduce the brain to a bloody, swollen pulp. As a result, there may be severe complications associated with neuronal disruption, ischemia, hemorrhaging, and edema.

ASSESSING THE SEVERITY OF BRAIN INJURY

The severity of a traumatic head injury has been most often associated with corresponding scores on the **Glasgow Coma Scale (GCS)** (Teasdale & Jennett, 1974). This mea-

sure gives the head injury trauma team a rapid, reliable measure of coma depth by assessing separate symptoms, including language, consciousness, and motor domains. Neuropsychologists generally accept the GCS as the standard measure for determining severity of injury in patients with compromised consciousness, from the mildest confusional state (scores >13) to deep coma (scores <5; Table 13.1). Medically, coma is defined as a score of 8 or less, which corresponds to a severe head injury. Thus, the standard definition of **coma** is that a patient cannot open his or her eyes, make any recognizable sounds, and follow any commands (Levin, Benton, & Grossman, 1982). Depth of coma, together with post-traumatic amnesia (PTA; described later in this chapter), is a reliable measure of the overall level of brain damage and prognosis. The GCS has proved a good outcome measure after coma, with scores greater than 8 indicating a good recovery. Greater mortality is typically associated with scores less than 7.

Coma is not the same as "being asleep." In fact, electroencephalographic (EEG) monitoring shows that a comatose patient has sleep–awake cycles even while in coma. Coma is directly associated with an injury to those areas of the brain, typically the lower brainstem and reticular activating system (RAS), that are involved in brain arousal. Although it is not clear what precisely causes coma, researchers believe it is related to RAS damage. In animal experiments, researchers found that a linear acceleration blow did not result in coma, but when the head was free to move in a rotational plane, as in injuries from MVAs, coma did appear. Coma is also not a binary phenomenon: It is incorrect to conceptualize the patient as either in a coma or not. Rather, coma falls along a continuum. That is, patients can be in a deep coma or in a light, shallow coma, or somewhere in between. Alternatively, head injury survivors may not be in a coma at all, but may be confused and disoriented. When patients recover from coma, they do not "suddenly awake" from it. Rather, they slowly progress from deeper stages to more shallow stages of coma. In this respect, the GCS has been a useful tool for monitoring recovery of comatose patients. Limitations of the GCS are twofold: First, incorrect assessment is possible because of confounding factors including eye swelling that prohibits assessment of eye opening and the presence of an endotracheal tube and the use of drugs (such as barbiturates or anticonvulsants), both of which can prevent verbal response. The second limitation relates to that a small lesion to the brainstem can cause coma, although most of the brain is not injured. In such a case, the coma, although serious and potentially life threatening, is not a good indicator of overall brain damage, because the cortex, for example, may be entirely intact.

Table 13.1 *Glasgow Coma Scale*		
Dimension	**Score**	**Description**
Eye opening (E)		
Spontaneously	4	Eyes are open; scored without reference to awareness
To speech ("Open eyes.")	3	Eyes are open to speech or shut without implying a response to a direct command
To pain	2	Eyes are open with painful stimulus to limbs or chest
Not at all	1	No eye opening, not attributed to ocular swelling
Best verbal response (V) ("What year is it?")		
Oriented	5	Aware of self, environment, time, and situation
Confused	4	Attention is adequate and patient is responsive, but responses suggest disorientation and confusion
Inappropriate	3	Understandable articulation, but speech is used in a nonconversational manner or conversation is not sustained
Incomprehensible	2	Verbal responses (moaning), but without recognizable words
None	1	
Best motor response (M) ("Show me two fingers.")		
Obeys commands	6	Follows simple verbal directions
Localizes pain (by touch)	5	Moves limbs to attempt to escape painful stimuli
Withdraws from pain	4	Normal flexor response
Abnormal flexor response	3	"Decorticate": abnormal adduction of shoulder
Extensor response	2	"Decerebrate": internal rotation of shoulder
None	1	Flaccid
Glasgow Coma Scale score (E + V + M) = 3–15		

Source: Adapted from Teasdale, G., & Jennett, B. (1974). Assessment of coma and impaired consciousness. *Lancet, 2,* 81–84.

Research has demonstrated a relation between the severity of a head injury, defined by the GCS, and neuropsychological outcome. The most severe injuries entail the most substantial neuropsychological deficits (Levin et al., 1982). Although initial severity of GCS is an important prognostic indicator for the patient's survival, other indicators, such as number of days to reach a GCS of 15, have also been associated with long-term neuropsychological outcome.

 ## Complications of Moderate and Severe Brain Injury

The major complications of moderate and severe CHIs are edema of the brain and associated brain herniation, intracranial bleeding, and skull fractures. We describe each of these processes next because they are important variables for a positive neuropsychological outcome.

EDEMA

Edema of the brain refers to swelling. Just as swelling follows a bruise to a leg, the brain swells as a result of trauma. The problem with brain edema is that there is no space for the brain to swell into. As a result, internal pressure of the brain increases, often dramatically. Therefore, the trauma team almost routinely places an intracranial monitoring catheter into the ventricles or the subarachnoid space to monitor **intracranial pressure (ICP).** ICP can cause diffuse damage to the brain. In fact, in moderate and severe head injuries, severe and uncontrollable ICP is the main cause of death.

BRAIN HERNIATION

Besides head injury, other pathologic processes occur in the brain, including hemorrhages, tumors, or infections, which may displace and deform the brain. This process, called **brain herniation,** is associated with increasing ICP often related to the presence of a large pocket of blood (also called a hematoma). In more than 75% of severe CHI cases, there is an associated ICP of greater than 20 mm Hg (or Torr; normal is 0–15 mm Hg). Such a high ICP often results from an intracranial hematoma and a generalized swelling of the brain. These displace the brain downward. This **transtentorial herniation** is characterized by downward displacement of the parahippocampal gyrus and uncus of one or both temporal lobes through the tentorial hiatus. There is only one large opening in the skull, the foramen magnum, which is the normal anatomic site of the lower brainstem. Brain herniation can place extreme pressure on the lower brainstem, typically cutting off the cranial nerve III (the oculomotor nerve) and compromising the integrity of the brainstem. The cranial nerve symptom causes initial constriction, followed by dilation of the pupil on the herniation side. Furthermore, the patient may lose motor functions on the same side as the herniation. Compression of the posterior cerebral artery may obstruct blood circulation and eventually cause necrosis. In the herniation syndrome, consciousness deteriorates to a state of deep coma within minutes to hours. If left untreated, the patient goes into a coma and dies of respiratory failure because the brain centers, among them the medulla oblongata, have been damaged and life-sustaining functions cease to operate.

Because edema thus progresses to brain herniation, controlling ICP is the main medical issue in acute CHI. Medical trauma personnel carefully monitor ICP, and if it is elevated, they treat it, often aggressively. Reducing the patient's blood pressure medically or by hyperventilation is often enough to stabilize ICP. In extreme cases, the trauma staff artificially places the patient in a coma. Of course, he or she is already in a coma related to the brain injury, but a pharmacologically induced coma additionally reduces brain metabolism, and hence swelling. A last resort in controlling ICP is evacuation (surgical removal) of a lobe, such as the right frontal lobe, to make room for the brain to swell into. This happened to one of our patients, Frank, a 22-year-old college student. One night he joined a friend to travel by car to a questionable location of the city to buy marijuana. The drug dealers mistook Frank for someone else who, the night before, either did not pay for drugs or started an altercation. His attackers were never caught. They pulled Frank from the car, beat him up with a baseball bat, and left him for dead. Miraculously, he survived, but with a severe CHI and in a coma. His ICP was so severe that he would have not lived had not the neurosurgeons removed his right frontal lobe, although there was no specific injury to that lobe. They simply removed it because Frank's brain needed the additional space to expand. Frank has now been through 10 years of rehabilitation. He has severe cognitive deficits and needs supervision 24 hours a day. His life has changed dramatically. He has had to learn all over again how to walk and talk. The rehabilitation hospital where Frank now lives has built a special room for him with soft padded walls, because of his uncontrollable temper. To his parents he is a completely different person from who he was before the assault. His parents deal with the situation as if their son had died that night and as if the new Frank were their new son.

EXTRADURAL AND SUBDURAL HEMORRHAGE

As a result of a head injury, cerebral blood vessels may tear, producing pools of blood within and between the meninges. Subdural and extradural bleeding frequently complicate head injuries and are medically significant. A **subdural hematoma,** in particular, may be associated with trivial bleeding only to cause problems weeks after the injury (Figure 13.3). Acute subdural or intracerebral bleeds most often appear in severe head injury. Together with brain edema, they are present in most fatal cases. The classic symptom in the subdural is an initial period of unconsciousness, but because the dura adheres tightly to the skull, the bleeding delays and a prolonged interval occurs during which the patient is conscious and functioning more or less normally. Once the bleed enlarges, it pushes the brain laterally and downward, causing brain herniation. As the hematoma enlarges, level of consciousness deteriorates quickly. This sequence of events is very dangerous, because the patient appears to have recovered from the trauma to the head, only to deteriorate once more quickly—and often fatally.

The frequent subdural hematoma corresponds to a bleed between the dura and the arachnoid space. A subdural hematoma is most likely caused by an acute venous hemorrhage related to rupture of a cortical vein, such as the superior sagittal sinus. Subdural bleeding typically occurs over the outward surfaces of the frontal and parietal lobes. Subdural hematomas are medical emergencies and typically develop within 1 week after the injury (if the bleed is slow) to as quickly as within 1 hour. Skull fractures (of which MVAs are the most frequent cause) cause more than half of all subdurals. Alcohol is a major catalyst, because of its anticoagulant properties in blood. Left untreated, the brain pressure increases to such a degree that the brain herniates, ultimately resulting in death. Symptoms of subdural hematoma include contralateral hemiparesis, ipsilateral pupil dilation, and changes in level of consciousness. Radiologists can easily make the diagnosis using computed transaxial tomographic (CT) imaging.

The less frequent **extradural hematoma** is a bleed that occurs between the skull and the dura. Bleeding of the large middle meningeal artery most often causes an extradural hematoma. An **epidural hematoma** represents a bleed between the meninges and the skull and is less common only occurring in 1% to 3% of major CHIs. The cause of an epidural is most often related to

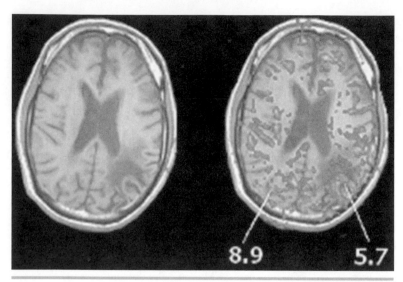

Figure 13.3 Images obtained from a 42-year-old man, 4 years status after work-related landscaping accident where a branch from a tree struck the left posterior portion of his skull. His initial Glasgow Coma Scale was 3, and his duration of loss of consciousness was greater than 2 weeks. The left image is a magnetic resonance imaging (MRI) scan showing significant neuronal loss secondary to massive subdural hematoma. Right image is an MRI scan with cerebral blood flow (CBF) superimposed. Numbers (5.7 ml/100 compared with 8.9 m/ml) reflect lower average CBF in lesioned brain area. See inside covers for color image. (Courtesy Frank Hillary, Ph.D., Pennsylvania State University.)

the rupture of an artery, but in some cases, an epidural develops as a result of injury to a meningeal vein or to the dural sinus.

Surgeons treat an epidural or subdural hematoma by drilling one or more burr holes over the parieto-occipital and temporal regions. This drains the pocket of blood and is the most rapid and effective intervention. In essence, the hematoma drains through a shunt placed within the bleed. Drainage needs to occur as quickly as possible once the hematoma has been diagnosed, and before the blood coagulates, which would have to be removed by neurosurgery. If such intervention occurs in a timely manner, the outcome of the subdural or epidural hematoma is generally good, with few, if any, cognitive deficits.

INTRACRANIAL BLEEDING

"Space-occupying clots" appear in about 15% of fatal head injuries. Most frequent are microscopic hemorrhages, commonly formed by shearing forces that tear blood vessels in subcortical white matter, the corpus callosum, and the orbital surfaces of the frontal and temporal lobes. Focal lesions do not occur as frequently, but appear as contusions and intracranial hematoma (a collection of

blood, typically clotted). Technically, epidural and subdural hematomas are not intracerebral hematomas, in which the bleed is intracranial—that is, within the brain. Epidural and subdural bleeds are actually outside the brain. Intracerebral hematomas are more difficult to treat than epidural and subdural hematomas and may require emergency neurosurgery.

SKULL FRACTURES

Examiners find skull fractures in approximately 75% to 90% of all patients with intracranial or epidural hematoma. Two different types of skull fractures exist. The first is the relatively benign linear fracture, which results in a rather distinct, straight line. The second is the more complicated depressed skull fracture, in which the impact has often driven fragments of the skull into the underlying dura and brain. Location is another important variable. Fractures to the base of the skull are difficult to detect in X-ray films and often entail more damage than do the simple linear fractures. Although the brain can be severely damaged without any skull damage, the presence of a skull fracture always creates the possibility of infection, cerebrospinal fluid leaks, and bleeding. Skull fractures may also rupture meningeal arteries or large venous sinuses, resulting in epidural and subdural hematomas.

The relation between skull fractures and neuropsychological functioning has been debated. Clearly, for the skull to fracture a significant force must have acted on the cranial plates. This force may have transferred to the brain, making actual brain damage more likely. The physics of skull fractures are complicated. In a skull fracture, the skull itself may have absorbed much, if not most, of the kinetic energy, thereby protecting the brain from damage. This is analogous to falling off a bicycle while wearing a helmet. The helmet absorbs much of the physical force, which transferred to the physical structure of the helmet (often destroying it), thereby protecting the head and the brain. For these reasons, skull fractures may not be directly related to specific levels of neuropsychological dysfunction. However, brain damage is more likely in skull fractures because the initial forces that fractured the skull must have been high, increasing the likelihood of brain damage.

POST-TRAUMATIC EPILEPSY

Seizures are a major complication after head injury. Post-traumatic epilepsy follows about 10% of severe closed head wounds and 40% of penetrating head injuries. The causes of the seizures relate to the presence of scar tissue, specifically alterations in neuronal membrane function and its structure. Neurologists consider seizures stemming from a head injury secondary, because they result from a known pathologic lesion. It is difficult to predict which head injury survivor may experience development of seizures, because onset can be delayed as much as 2 years after the trauma. Risk factors that increase the likelihood of for development of post-traumatic seizures include penetrating type head injury, severity of brain damage, prolonged periods of coma, PTA (described later in this chapter), inflammation associated with the wound, and residual neurologic symptoms. Seizures are such a frequent complication of head injury that patients receive anticonvulsant medication prophylactically (routinely) to control even the possibility of seizures.

Mild Head Injury: "Concussions"

The concept of a mild head injury is relatively recent. In the early 1980s, one of our mentors, Jeffrey T. Barth from the University of Virginia Medical School, was curious about what happens to patients who report to the emergency department for a head injury complaining of a concussion. These patients typically have had no or a short loss of consciousness, followed by prompt recovery without any localizing neurologic signs. They exhibit few immediate cognitive or physical complaints beyond a headache, feeling dizzy, and vague memory problems. Together with a team of neurosurgeons and neurologists, Barth examined hundreds of patients who were turned away from the emergency department, usually with no referral follow-up, because their injury was not thought to be severe enough to hospitalize the patient. The assumption was that there were no long-term problems. In the early 1980s, concussions were not considered a medical emergency.

Perhaps this indifference relates to how society deals with mild head trauma. For example, in athletics, concussions are often tolerated with some bravado: "I was hit in the head and didn't know the score of the football game." In fact, television football announcers recount how "amusing" it was to have someone knocked out, only to return to the opponent's sideline rather than his own. They recall with great humor how a teammate, after being knocked out, proceeded to run with the football in the wrong direction. Similarly, the symptoms of "seeing stars" has not been thought of as a neurologic symptom in this society, although it clearly is, but as a relatively benign, perhaps comic, event. In fact, many comic strips use "stars" to characterize transient confusion (Figure 13.4).

Until recently, researchers have not studied and understood the medical, neurologic, and psychological manifestations of mild head injuries. Since the early 1990s, an appreciation for milder forms of injuries to the head has appeared in the scientific literature. Mild head injuries often entail dizziness, fatigue, or headaches, with no loss or only brief loss of consciousness (Levin, Eisenberg, & Benton, 1989). The traditional literature often calls this type of head injury a "concussion." However, neuropsychologists now treat mild head injury as a significant medical event that has real, even long-term, consequences (Neuropsychology in Action 13.2). This finding is related not only to clinical evidence, in which patients have described physical and cognitive symptoms, but also to experimental evidence. Research studies have demonstrated that earlier studies using only the light microscope were incorrect in finding no reliable association between mild head injury and pathologic lesions in the brain. Recent animal research, using histologic staining techniques, shows that neurons exposed to forces consistent with a mild head injury are damaged and die (Barth et al., 1983).

Neuropsychology in Action 13.2

Can a Concussion Change Your Life?

by Ronald M. Ruff Ph.D., Director of Neurobehavioral Rehabilitation, St. Mary's Medical Center; Associate Adjunct Professor, Department of Neurosurgery and Psychiatry, University of California at San Francisco, San Francisco, CA

After attending a research meeting in Vail, Colorado, on traumatic brain injuries, my colleague, a 42-year-old neurosurgeon, decided to hit the ski slopes. While descending a modest incline, he lost his balance and fell, striking his head. He was immediately knocked unconscious for a period of only 10 to 15 seconds. On awakening, he experienced confusion that cleared within minutes, with the exception of a modest vertigo that persisted but did not interfere with his ability to ski down the mountain. Because my mentor and friend, who is a renowned specialist in brain trauma, continued to ski that day, I thought this concussion had had no effect on him. However, on returning home, he did report that he was a bit more distractible and that his memory was flawed, for example, when remembering the location of his Dictaphone, briefcase, and keys. He also noticed that when talking with colleagues and residents, he could no longer quickly recall references to articles. His speed of information processing was not affected, nor was his skill and judgment as a neurosurgeon; however, he did fatigue more quickly than before.

What exactly is a concussion? The term *concussion* refers to an injury to the brain, resulting either from a collision between the head and an object or from a rapid, forceful acceleration and deceleration. Neuropsy-chologists typically diagnose a brain injury when the consequences include one or more of the following: (1) an alteration or loss of consciousness, (2) a loss of memory for the events immediately before and after the injury, and (3) neurologic symptoms. The degree of injury can vary significantly, from a mild concussion to death. The terms *concussion* and *mild traumatic brain injury* (TBI) frequently are used as synonyms, although I focus here on mild TBI. What features separate a mild from a moderate brain injury? Medical professionals generally accept that a "mild" rating should not involve a loss of consciousness that exceeds 30 minutes; in addition, memory loss for events after the trauma should not exceed 24 hours, and the neurologic symptoms should not lead to a deterioration of the patient's Glasgow Coma Scale (GCS) score to less than 13.

How many of us have sustained a mild TBI? Neurologists classify approximately two thirds of all brain injuries as mild. In the United States alone, researchers estimate that approximately 1,300,000 people sustain a mild TBI each year. Approximately half are the result of motor vehicle accidents, and the rest involve assaults, falls, or sports-related injuries (such as in skiing, boxing, football, horseback riding, and ice hockey). What happens to the brain during mild TBI? Currently, the best data are derived from studies of concussed animals or from humans who, in addition to having concussions, died of other medical complications such as chest wounds. Particularly because of rotational forces, brain cells tear, and this shearing of axons most often occurs in subcortical and frontotemporal regions. Because impact to the brain from the outside can vary so significantly, tearing and shearing of cells can also vary among individuals. However, postmortem examinations of concussed brains have provided evidence of microscopic changes, which can no doubt lead to neurophysiological and neurochemical alterations.

What typical difficulties do patients encounter? By evaluating patients in the first phases after a mild TBI, researchers have documented frequent impairments on neuropsychological tests of sustained attention, memory, and learning, and measures that capture speed of information processing. Most mild TBI survivors enjoy a favorable recovery in the 3 to 6 months after the injury. That is, these patients improve up to a level that is not statistically below that of a control group. One study even found a way to test patients before and after a mild TBI. Before the playing season, researchers tested college football players who had never sustained a brain injury and did follow-up testing on those who later sustained a mild TBI. This retesting showed an initial decline

Three important findings have emerged from this body of research that are important to mild head injuries:

1. Mild head injuries usually go medically unnoticed. The medical community does not widely recognize the often debilitating sequelae of such injuries.
2. During mild head injury, the physical energy transferred to the brain is related to linear and rotational mechanical forces associated with the sudden acceleration, deceleration, or both. These forces can result in shearing or stretching, and even in necrosis (cell death) of neurons, which are the central building blocks of the central nervous system (for example, see Levin et al., 1982).
3. Head injuries, including the mild variety, are cumulative in effect. For example, Gronwall and Wrightson (1975) conducted one of the first investigations to establish that after a second concussion the capacity of adults to process information declined significantly. Thus, repeated blows to the head, such as those occurring in boxing and football, are especially dangerous to the athlete's health.

on neuropsychological testing, with a positive recovery in the subsequent weeks. However, a large body of literature has unequivocally demonstrated that not all mild TBI patients enjoy a favorable recovery. A minority continue to have not only persistent cognitive problems but also physical problems, which typically include headache, vertigo, dizziness, energy loss, and in some cases, a heightened sensitivity to noise, light, alcohol, or medications. Emotional reactions commonly include irritability, elevated anxiety, or depressive symptoms. These cognitive and physical problems can, in turn, lead to emotional, psychosocial, and vocational changes. Neuropsychologists use the term *postconcussive disorder* for such cases. In the literature, researchers have estimated that postconcussive disorders occur in 10% to 20% of all mild TBI cases (130,000–260,000 cases each year in the United States). Over the years, the importance of a careful neuropsychological evaluation of patients with mild TBI has become more and more recognized.

What is the neuropsychologist's role in evaluating mild TBI? The objective tools that physicians tend to rely on for diagnosing brain injuries include computed transaxial tomography (CT) and magnetic resonance imaging (MRI). However, for mild TBI, these neuroimaging techniques lack sufficient sensitivity to visualize microscopic changes. Thus, CT and MRI scans are, as a rule, "normal" in most mild TBI cases. Although the newer dynamic neuroimaging techniques such as positron emission tomography (PET) and single-photon emission computed tomography (SPECT) scans have demonstrated greater sensitivity in case studies,

more research is required to determine whether these newer techniques can objectify mild TBI conclusively. Because objective tools cannot yet reliably evaluate the potential brain damage involved in mild TBI, medical teams frequently assign to neuropsychologists, using subjective tools, the task of providing answers. Using psychometric tests, neuropsychologists are uniquely qualified to delineate the upper thresholds of cognitive functioning. Based on a pattern analysis across a neurocognitive test battery together with a psychodiagnostic evaluation, neuropsychologists can reach a diagnosis to determine the extent to which brain damage has contributed to the postconcussive disorder. The three key challenges for making a differential diagnosis are: (1) estimating preinjury functioning levels, (2) evaluating comorbid factors, and (3) exploring interactions among the postinjury problems. Estimating preinjury functioning is paramount for capturing not only "deficits" but also any decline in functioning.

To illustrate, let us return to the earlier-mentioned neurosurgeon who struck his head while skiing. Many neuropsychologists use an impairment index that largely represents a common notion that a deficit is defined by a score that falls two standard deviations below the mean. However, this notion may lead to false negatives. For example, a 50% decrease in performance in an individual whose preinjury functioning levels were at the 95th percentile will result in a postinjury performance at the 45th percentile. This neurosurgeon commented, with respect to the challenges neuropsychologists face:

Perceptions of a disease by one who has not had the disease as a patient tend to be

modestly inaccurate. Recovery from a head injury appears to be a long process, one requiring innumerable strategies for compensation. Neurocognitive testing will indicate part of the story, only if the results are abnormal; it leaves something to be desired in predicting levels of performance for those who are adequate competitors in a modern society. (Marshall & Ruff, 1989, p. 278).

In addition to capturing a relative loss based on a comparison with the patient's estimated preinjury functioning levels, it is also crucial that the neuropsychologist become aware of preexisting medical risk factors (history of alcohol or substance abuse; prior concussion), as well as cognitive risk factors (preexisting learning disabilities) and emotional risk factors (such as hysteria, somatization, and secondary gain). Concurrent medical injuries are common in mild TBI cases, including neck, shoulder, and rib fractures, which can result in a pain syndrome. Excessive pain can interfere with sleep, and it always results in emotional reactions that can, in turn, affect neurocognitive functioning. More systematic research is called for to evaluate mild TBI cases with and without comorbid medical injuries. Finally, the interactions among postinjury problems require careful analysis. Postconcussive syndromes derail some patients from their vocations as a result of a combination of factors (such as headaches, vertigo, attentional difficulties, and mood changes). All of us who work in this field believe that we must stress prevention. The mandatory introduction of helmets, safety belts, and airbags has reduced TBI rates. Be careful: A concussion has the potential to change your life!

SPORTS-RELATED CONCUSSIONS: A NEUROPSYCHOLOGICAL PERSPECTIVE

Competitive sports participation has increased worldwide. Sports-related concussions represent a significant potential health concern to those who participate in contact sports. In the United States alone, it is estimated that approximately 1.3 million individuals sustain a mild TBI each year, approximately half of which result from MVAs. After MVAs, the causes of head injuries are, in order, sports injuries, falls, violence, and industrial accidents. Thus, a high number of athletes are at risk for concussion, approximately 2% to 10% (Ruchinskas, Francis, & Barth, 1997), representing more than 300,000 sports-related head injuries annually (Moser & Schatz, 2002).

It has been recognized only recently that concussive injuries present a significant neuropsychological event (Zillmer, 2003b). As a result, increasing emphasis has been in providing protection to athletes. Those forms of protection include rule changes to minimize concussion-type

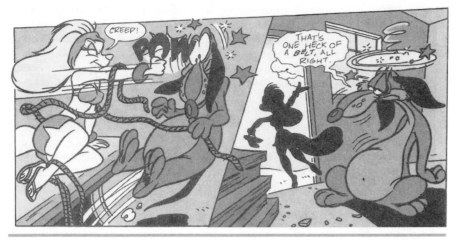

Figure 13.4   Animaniacs. (Reproduced from DC Comics, *Animaniacs,* September 17, 1996, by permission. Copyright © 1996–2000 by Warner Bros. All rights reserved.)

injuries, as well as equipment changes, including improved helmets, mouth guards, and other face and head protection to reduce the transfer of kinetic energy to the head during an athletic contest (Figure 13.5). In the area of brain-behavior research, a concomitant focus has been on understanding the neuropsychological manifestations of sports-related concussions. Neuropsychologists have directed their

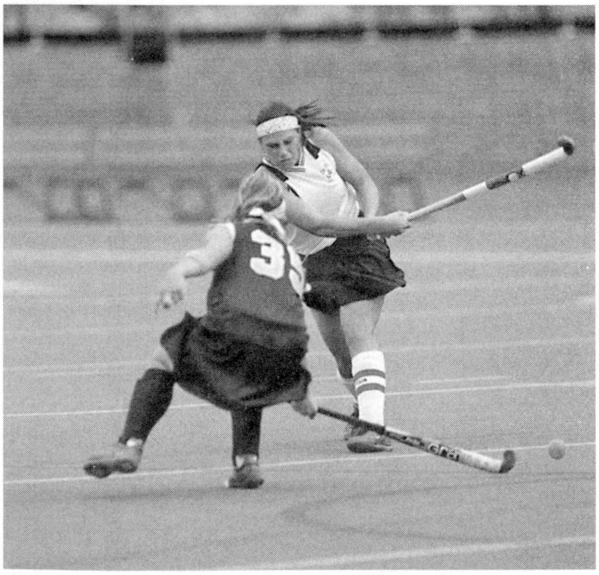

Figure 13.5   Many sports have the potential for physical contact and collision. Sport is clearly a breeding ground for physical injury. (Courtesy Drexel University, Philadelphia, PA, 2003, by permission.)

attention to defining and grading concussions, as well as to understanding the neurometabolic changes associated with concussions. In the area of clinical neuropsychology, advancements have been made for concussion assessment and diagnosis, as well as concussion management, rehabilitation, and return to play decisions. Accordingly, neuropsychologists have become an integral part of the sports medicine team involved in the care of athletes with sports-related concussions. Today, neuropsychologists are playing a leading role in the clinical and scientific aspects of sports-related concussions.

The Twentieth Century: A Revolution of Science and Sports

The history of sports-related concussions is long, but its past has been short. In the early part of the twentieth century, the frequent nature of collisions between football players called into question the safety of the sport and highlighted an awareness of head injuries in sports. Football helmets were not available until 1896, and because of the physical properties of the helmets themselves, as well as the nature of play, they were not effective in the protection of athletes (Cantu & Mueller, 2003). In fact, the 1905 college season ended with much protest over the brutality of football. On October 9, 1905, midseason, President Roosevelt met with representatives from Harvard, Yale, and Princeton to discuss making football less dangerous, in an effort to ultimately save the sport. Football was being publicly denounced as brutal and inappropriate for young men after the *Chicago Tribune* published an injury report

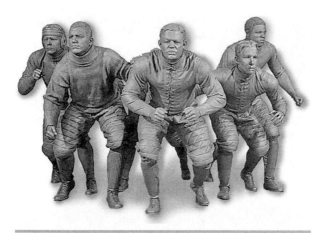

Figure 13.6 A bronze statue of the flying football wedge as seen at the NCAA museum in Indianapolis. The flying wedge revolutionized the game but also led to numerous injuries and even deaths on the field. (Courtesy NCAA Hall of Champions, Indianapolis, IN.)

listing 18 deaths and 159 serious injuries (Stewart, 1995). Led by Henry M. MacCracken, the chancellor of New York University, the parties responsible for football rules agreed to change the game. As a result, the Intercollegiate Athletic Association was established, which would later become the National Collegiate Athletic Association (NCAA), the current governing body for intercollegiate sports. The rule changes included outlawing the "flying wedge" (Figure 13.6), one of football's most violent offensive formations, during which a group of lead offensive tacklers would provide protection for the ball carrier. Overall, the consequences of head injuries in football were the primary force underlying the creation of the NCAA, which was established initially to ensure the welfare of the student–athlete.

The 1980s Virginia Football Studies

Clinical and epidemiologic studies of mild head injury in the 1980s reported neuropsychological deficits in new and rapid problem solving, attention and concentration, and memory, which lasted up to 3 months after trauma (Barth, Macciocchi, Boll, Giordani, Jane, & Rimel, 1983; Rimel et al., 1981). At about the same time, Gennarelli (1983) and Ommaya (Ommaya & Gennarelli, 1974) were performing primate studies to evaluate the histologic effects of mild acceleration/deceleration during head trauma. They documented visible axonal shearing and straining in the brainstem in experimentally induced mild

head injury. By the 1980s, there appeared to be a growing consensus that mild head injury was not as innocuous as previously thought. Still, recovery curves lacked definition and individual vulnerability of mild head injuries were not well understood. Research was needed that would control preexisting factors and assess neurocognitive functions in a laboratory setting before and after the administration of a controlled mild head injury to a human subject. In this way, the individual would act as his or her own control.

Within this context, Jeff Barth and his colleague at the University of Virginia (UVA) designed one of the most creative experiments in neuropsychology. They approached college football players as the practical solution to this research problem. Football players were at risk to experience an acceleration/deceleration mild head injury similar to the type of linear of rotational brain trauma experienced in MVAs within a natural yet controlled environment. The first landmark sports-related concussion study therefore focused on the UVA football team. These early football studies suggested that young, bright, healthy, and well-motivated student–athletes, who experience mild, uncomplicated head trauma without loss of consciousness did demonstrate neuropsychological decline in areas of information problem solving and attention, but would likely follow a rapid recovery curve and have no lasting disability (Barth et al, 1989).

Interestingly, these investigators at UVA also consulted with professional football teams hoping to extend these findings beyond the college arena. But they found little interest in allowing scientists to study the potentially negative effects of concussion, which were presumed to occur (Jeffrey Barth, personal communication, January 10, 2004). A decade later, however, Mark Lovell and his colleagues again spearheaded a movement aimed at implementing a program designed to educate and protect professional athletes. The Pittsburgh Sports Concussion Program initiated pilot baseline and postconcussive neuropsychological testing of the Pittsburgh Steelers players in the late 1980s through early 1990s. This program successfully broke down many of the barriers regarding professional football players' acknowledgment and acceptance of concussive injuries, and in combination with the NFL Players Association's growing concerns over career-ending injuries related to multiple concussions (for example, Troy Aikman and Steve Young), has now led to league-wide programs in both the National Football League (NFL; 1993) and NHL (1996) (Mark Lovell, personal communication, November 23, 2004; Pellman, Lovell, Viano, et al., 2004).

Twenty-First Century and the Refinement of Sports Neuropsychology

Besides the advances that have been made in the neuroscientific and neuropsychological community, experts on the psychology of sports injuries have made significant advances in how concussion injuries can be treated and conceptualized. Even though an injury is essentially a negative experience, some unexpected benefits have been noted; for example, the challenge in response to injury to reorder one's life and lifestyle, to develop creative solutions in overcoming physical and mental deficits, and to forge new and meaningful relationships with others (Pargman, 1999). Thus, a renewed focus on the concept of injury prevention and a multidisciplinary approach to the rehabilitation of injured athletes has been made, which includes psychological intervention, as well as medical, mechanical, and social factors. This newly conceptualized multimodal approach appears especially appropriate in the context of making return-to-play decisions with concussed athletes in view of the emergence of neuropsychology in sports medicine (Echemendia & Cantu, 2003). In addition, neuropsychological profiles of athletes may help us understand their specific strengths and weaknesses and how they may cope with sports-related concussions. As scientists and researchers provided increasing evidence for an organic basis to the clinical symptoms of concussion, it became evident that the clinical picture reflects a dynamic state of affairs in which physical, personal, social, competitive, and economic factors contributed in varying degrees (Zillmer 2003b).

Contemporary sports-related concussion research is akin to putting a complex puzzle together: What is the effect of age and sex in concussions? What is the epidemiology of the sports-related concussion injuries and how they differ by sport and sex (Figure 13.7). What neuropsychological tests are best suited to assess concussions? What is the gold standard for grading concussions? Who is most susceptible to sports-related concussion? What return-to-play guidelines are most practical?

We believe neuropsychologists play, and will continue to play, an important role in assembling this complex puzzle. In the absence of any detectable abnormalities on traditional magnetic resonance imaging (MRI) scans for cases with concussion (Bigler & Snyder, 1995), the objective nature of neuropsychological testing has become a reliable and valid approach to measuring cognitive impairment and symptom resolution for mild TBI. The future of sports-related mild head injury research is expanding and will be best served by prospective neuropsychological study of athletes at high risk for multiple concussions. Bet-

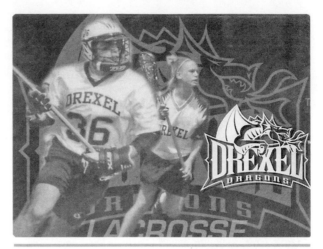

Figure 13.7 Female athletes are consistently found to be at higher risk for sustaining concussions than male athletes across all sports and all ages (Covassin, Swanik, & Sachs, 2003). Pictured are two college lacrosse players. In collegiate lacrosse men wear helmets, whereas women do not, which has initiated a debate regarding the use of head protection in the sport. (Courtesy Drexel University, Philadelphia, PA.)

ter protective equipment and devises, rule changes, and pooling of information into a comprehensive concussion data bank to better define safe return-to-play criteria should be the focus of sports medicine in the new millennium.

Future directions in the assessment and management of sports-related concussion include: increased research on prevalence rates and effects of concussions for female and young athletes, educating parents of youth athletes and family physicians on the importance of baseline and postconcussion cognitive assessments, and further validation of computerized assessment measures. Despite a paucity of research on female and youth athletes, there is evidence that female athletes are at greater risk for injury than male athletes, and that concussions may affect children and young adolescents differently than older adolescents and adults. Sideline, baseline, and postconcussion assessments have become prevalent in documenting preinjury and postinjury performance, recovery rates, and return-to-play decisions. New computerized assessment procedures are growing in popularity and are used in the NFL, NHL, NASCAR, and Formula 1.

The role of the neuropsychologist in the assessment of concussions for purposes of diagnosis and symptom resolution is one that our profession should embrace. Moreover, for those neuropsychologists who love sports, it provides a unique opportunity to merge one's professional skills with one's affinity for sports. Most often the role of the neuropsychologist in the area of sports-related concussions will be that of a consultant and a researcher. In addition to being an expert in the neuropsychological assessment of concussions, the neuropsychologist must understand the culture and epidemiology of the injuries of the athletic arena and of various sports they may be asked to cover. We believe that the neuropsychologists' training and expertise uniquely prepares him or her to play an important and rewarding role in this growing field in the future (Zillmer, Schneider, Tinker, & Kaminaris, 2006).

POSTCONCUSSIONAL SYNDROME

Medical personnel often call the behavioral and cognitive sequelae of mild head injury "postconcussional syndrome." These sequelae range over a variety of somatic and neuropsychological symptoms, including headache, irritability, dizziness, lack of concentration, and impaired memory. Researchers have documented the symptoms of mild head injury most frequently with MVAs. However, analogous situations with acceleration/deceleration of the head arise in the context of competitive sports. Many sports involve speed and the potential for collision. In fact, as mentioned earlier, 17% of all head injuries are sports related.

For example, research with football players suggests that many effects of sports-related collisions (such as tackling) that were originally thought to be relatively benign, actually have measurable neuropsychological consequences in college athletes. These collisions may not only diminish the performance of players on the field but can also compromise their health off the field. Full appreciation of impact injuries has only recently developed as many NFL quarterbacks have reported the negative effects of repeatedly being hit in the head. Frequent head impact places them at risk for losing consciousness even when experiencing relatively minor concussive forces to the head. In some cases, this has resulted in cognitive changes, including excessive dizziness and difficulty in concentrating. Several players were forced to retire, and rules were changed, disallowing tackling with the helmet or "spearing" to the opposing player's head.

Researchers have studied the neurologic aspects of professional boxing in more detail; these aspects are easily appreciated by the public because of the knockout (KO), which is a neurologic event synonymous with cerebral contusion. Only recently have researchers examined the neurologic aspects of amateur boxing, where duration of fights, rules, and protective devices differ from professional boxing. Other less obvious sports-related neurologic effects appear in soccer players who frequently head the ball. Findings indicate more EEG abnormalities among professional players (Tysvaer, Storli, & Bachen, 1989) and the presence of neuropsychological deficits among college players (Witol & Webbe, 1993). That football and soccer can involve potential mechanical forces to the head that can cause injury seems disturbing, particularly at the non-professional, "recreational" level. At that level, many elementary school, high school, and college players are particularly vulnerable to the developmental delays related to such head injuries (Levin et al., 1982).

 # Treatment of Head Injuries

An acute TBI often entails severe neurologic impairment. In severe head injuries, the patient is comatose when the medical emergency unit arrives. The initial management of severe head injury follows the ABC assessment (airway, breathing, and circulatory status); the medics establish a respiratory *airway,* often freeing the pharynx from blood and other obstructions. If they do not establish an airway, anoxia will result, adding to the physical injuries of the brain. After a clear airway has been established, medics assess the patient's *breathing.* Then the team establishes regular breathing, if necessary, artificially, with sufficient oxygen, because hypoxia is common in head injuries. Alterations in breathing may be related to brainstem dysfunction. Medics then evaluate *circulatory status* by examining blood gases and blood pressure. They initiate intravenous infusion, including blood replacement. Then, once the patient has been medically stabilized, they obtain diagnostic imaging using CT and MRI. Next, a neurologist conducts an evaluation to ascertain the level of consciousness and presence of neurologic symptoms. If the patient remains in a coma, the team may hospitalize him or her in a neuro-intensive care unit, which has a specialized environment that facilitates care of comatose patients.

As mentioned earlier, intracranial monitoring is the cornerstone of medical therapy. If ICP remains normal, the patient undergoes intensive supportive care. If ICP is elevated, medical personnel use aggressive measures to reduce it. These include controlled ventilation, which decreases cerebral blood volume and constricts cerebral vessels, thus reducing ICP. Steroid therapy may prevent intracerebral edema. Patients are typically temperature controlled with heating/cooling blankets, because elevated body temperature increases metabolic rate and hypothermia leads to other medical complications. Sometimes medical personnel administer diuretics to reduce

Neuropsychology in Action 13.3

Consensual Sex after Traumatic Brain Injury: Sex as a Problem-Solving Task

by Carrie H. Kennedy Ph.D., Lieutenant Commander, Navy Neuropsychology Fellow, University of Virginia, Charlottesville, VA

John, age 24, and Theresa, age 22, are two adults with traumatic brain injuries (TBIs). John suffered a head injury at age 17 in a motorcycle accident. At age 20, Theresa suffered a head injury when a drunk driver struck her car as she waited at a red light. As a result of their injuries, John and Theresa currently live in a community-based rehabilitation facility.

John experiences hemiplegia, difficulty in planning for future events, and memory and attention deficits. Theresa experiences seizures, as well as severe speech and memory deficits. John and Theresa enjoy each other's company and often attend community events together. More recently, John and Theresa have become interested in a physically intimate relationship.

The last issue is a concern for the agency that provides their rehabilitative services. With their specific cognitive deficits, can John and Theresa consent to have sex? Can

they each make an informed decision using information on sexual conduct, diseases, and pregnancy? Is either at a high risk for being victimized because of an inability to adequately protect himself or herself from unwanted sexual advances? To explore the answers to these questions, the issues of TBI and sexuality must be considered.

After a head injury, the often-ambiguous rules and rituals pertaining to sex can become even more difficult. Adverse effects of TBI on sexuality range from sensorimotor deficits and bowel and bladder dysfunction, to changes in sex drive and various male and female genital sexual dysfunctions. In addition to the neurologic, physical, and emotional effects on sexuality are cognitive changes associated with TBI. Cognitive changes can affect sexuality in a variety of ways, including impairment of the ability to make safe choices regarding sexual behavior. The individual can be physically able to

engage in a sexual relationship, and even be interested in pursuing one, but at the same time be cognitively incapable of consenting. An inability to make decisions can result in victimization, unwanted pregnancies, and diseases.

One hallmark of a moderate-to-severe TBI can be the loss of the ability to make complex decisions requiring judgment, insight, preplanning, reasoning, organization, and impulse control. Clearly, such cognitive deficits can impair the ability to consent to sex. When this issue arises, the neuropsychologist serves two main roles. First, the neuropsychologist, together with formal testing of cognitive and functional strengths and weaknesses, can assess an individual's capacity to consent to sex. Second, the neuropsychologist can recommend rehabilitative and educational strategies that are specially geared to a person's functioning level and cognitive abilities and

---

the ICP. If these measures do not control ICP, the prognosis is typically poor, and more aggressive measures are taken, such as inducing barbiturate coma and surgery. Administering a large dosage of barbiturates decreases the cerebral metabolic rate and constricts cerebral vessels. Inducing barbiturate coma is controversial, because it may contribute to additional neuropsychological sequelae. A final measure is to remove part of the brain to make space available.

NEUROPSYCHOLOGICAL MANIFESTATIONS

Neuropsychological sequelae, of course, are prominently associated with TBI. They range from patient reports of memory difficulty to problems with attention and concentration, as well as alterations in mood. Neuropsychologists play an important role in objectively assessing residual ability after mild, moderate, and even severe head injuries, once the patient has been medically stabilized and is no longer in a coma or in acute medical care.

In addition to the cognitive effects of brain injury, personality changes from frontal lobe damage may affect the patient's well-being and quality of life (Neuropsychology in Action 13.3). Neuropsychologists routinely test head injury survivors, because unless tested, cognitive deficits, especially memory, may at first go unnoticed, but cause problems later when the patient returns home or to work. Most recovery after severe head injury occurs within the first 6 months, with smaller adjustments continuing for perhaps as long as 2 years. In the past, rehabilitation experts have waited until the "natural" healing cycle has finished before initiating rehabilitation. More recent thinking has proved that rehabilitation is most effective when started as early as medically possible (Levin et al., 1989).

Anterograde and Retrograde Amnesia

Memory problems constitute a major deficit for people who have sustained traumatic head injuries and are of

strengths. In this way, neuropsychologists can optimize the decision making and safety of TBI survivors, whereas facilitating the return of an important aspect of quality of life, that of sexual intimacy.

Using an instrument such as the Sexual Consent and Education Assessment (SCEA; see Kennedy, 1999), neuropsychologists make a capacity determination based on prescribed legal criteria for consent. Legal criteria for sexual consent vary from state to state, but a consensus of psychologists is that individuals must have knowledge of sexual conduct, knowledge of the consequences of sexual activity, and basic safety skills to be deemed capable of consenting (Kennedy & Niederbuhl, 2001). Although, taken together, these criteria determine the capacity of any given individual, each criterion is also a separate entity directly related to cognitive abilities that neuropsychologists can measure.

The first two criteria for capacity for sexual consent, regarding the nature of sexual conduct and consequences of sexual activity, are a function of crystallized intelligence (knowledge that has been acquired over the years) in most adults. That is, individuals who have had previous sexuality education, sexual experience, or both are more likely to retain general knowledge and information regarding sexuality. Later, such adults who have experienced a TBI typically have little difficulty communicating their understanding of the nature of sexual conduct and the various consequences of sexual activity. However, individuals who have not yet obtained general knowledge about sexuality must learn it for the first time. After TBI, attentional, memory, and executive function deficits significantly hinder new learning and can make a task such as learning basic sexual knowledge daunting.

The third criterion, however, basic safety skills, appears to be the most significant hurdle for individuals with moderate to severe head injuries. This particular neuropsychological task appears to be an executive decision that involves a complex string of decision making, reasoning, judgment, and planning. Preliminary findings suggest that neuropsychological tasks that assess those abilities, such as the Tower of London–Drexel University (Culbertson & Zillmer, 2005), the Modified Wisconsin Card Sorting Test, and word fluency are able to correctly classify cognitively impaired individuals who are and are not capable of consent-ing to sexual activity (Kennedy, 2003). Additional research will provide further information regarding sexual consent and related neuropsychological requirements. In turn, investigation of these questions will also provide the basis for developing more effective rehabilitative strategies to help people with neurologic damage in regaining important parts of their lives, not least of which will be sexual intimacy. This leads us back to our original questions about John and Theresa.

John and Theresa were both tested using the SCEA and a neuropsychological battery. Theresa easily passed all aspects of the assessment, whereas John showed significant difficulty with the concepts of sexually transmitted diseases and protection against them. John was declared not capable of giving consent until he could successfully complete an educational program dealing specifically with diseases and methods of protection. The educational program, which John completed, included methods of learning that were optimal for John given his neuropsychological test findings. Subsequently, the rehabilitation facility worked with John and Theresa about establishing privacy, and their subjective quality of life is vastly improved.

---

special interest to neuropsychologists. In fact, head injury experts grade the severity of a head injury partly on the patient's memory surrounding the accident. Such memory problems are called **post-traumatic amnesia (PTA). Retrograde amnesia** is the loss of memory for the interval preceding the injury. Conversely, **antero-grade amnesia** is the loss of memory for events after trauma or disease onset. Although the patient may have residual short-term memory impairment from the head injury, as well as other cognitive deficits, neuropsychologists have established retrograde and anterograde amnesia as a relatively robust measure of the severity of trauma and its associated cognitive symptoms. Because cortical and subcortical structures mediate memory, PTA has proved a better overall indicator of brain damage than length and depth of coma, which may relate to isolated damage of the brainstem. Neuropsychologists consider these types of amnesia to relate mostly to anterior temporal lesions, an anatomic area particularly vulnerable to head injuries, because of the bony features surrounding this area of the brain.

Neuropsychological Evaluation

Often other medical personnel ask neuropsychologists to evaluate head-injured patients at their bedside, close to the time of their accident, while they are still hospitalized (see Neuropsychology in Action 13.1). This examination is typically brief and serves to assess whether the patient can tolerate more formal, longer testing. It also establishes a baseline of overall cognitive abilities for future comparisons. An example of such a neuropsychology consult is as follows:

Neuropsychology Note. Results from brief neuropsychological procedure, post-MVA with LOC (loss of consciousness) 30 min, revealed a 33 yowm (year-old white male) who was oriented × 3 (to self, time, and place) and attentive/cooperative with the exam. The patient was able to follow simple commands involving two-step learning. Memory appeared within normal limits (WNL) for immediate and short-term verbal/visual material. Expressive/receptive speech were also WNL. No sensory deficits including astereognosis, finger agnosia, neglect, right–left confusion, or hemianopsia, were observed. The patient did manifest a bilateral resting hand tremor as well as motor incoordination, and difficulty in initiating specific motor movements. Perseveration of motor behavior was also apparent. Additional frontal lobe signs included poor reasoning ability and judgment.

Results are consistent with mild to moderate head injury and bilateral frontal lesions as seen on MRI from revealing contusions in the inferior frontal regions. Psychologically, the patient appears very distressed and depressed about his hospitalization and MVA, with suicidal thoughts present (but no specific plan). No other psychiatric symptoms were noted (hallucinations, delusions). Patient should be placed on suicide watch. Psychiatric consult should be ordered, and relocation to psychiatric ward should be considered to better manage suicide threats when the patient is medically stable. Other recommendations include comprehensive neuropsychological and psychological evaluation within the next four weeks to identify functional strengths and weaknesses. Cognitive residual effects that may hinder this patient's ability to return to his previous employment as a manager include his ability to function independently in life, and his need for outpatient psychotherapy. This testing can be done on an inpatient or outpatient basis and should be repeated over a 6- to 9-month period to monitor his recovery. Once he is discharged I also recommend that he join our head injury group meetings, designed for individuals and families with histories of head injuries.

Signed: *Dr. Eric A. Zillmer, Neuropsychologist*

In general, the long-term neuropsychological effects of head trauma may vary considerably and depend on the strength of the trauma and the medical condition of the patient with the head injury. Not all head traumas produce significant neuropsychological deficits. Others cause permanent and severe deficits. In general, neuropsychologists consider CHIs a diffuse disorder of the brain, because they may affect many different areas of the brain. Thus, differences in neuropsychological presentation in a head-injured protocol typically relate to the patient's level of overall deficits.

Recovery, Rehabilitation, and Intervention of Traumatic Brain Injury

What is the potential for the human brain to recover or adapt after brain injury? First, insult to the brain can result in different effects depending on the site and mechanism of damage. What is remarkable, however, is the brain's amazing ability to try to adapt to damage. If damage does not totally destroy neurons, the brain attempts to restore functioning. If the injury was caused by shock or some other temporary mechanism, diaschisis may serve to "unmask" functioning neuronal systems. When neurons are damaged through processes such as tearing and shearing, they may reorganize through axonal resprouting, collateral sprouting, or developing supersensitivities to neurotransmitters. When neuronal damage is complete, depending to a large degree on plasticity, the brain may sometimes be able to substitute other functioning neurons or neuronal systems or rely on some redundancy to take over. The neuropsychologist should consider the following factors when evaluating influences on recovery:

1. Location and extent of damage
2. Duration of time since injury
3. Age (brain plasticity)
4. Premorbid intellectual level
5. Premorbid personality characteristics
6. Premorbid functional level
7. Medical health
8. Emotional health
9. Support system
10. Type of treatment

Behind most theories of neuropsychological recovery and rehabilitation lies the premise that if functions are not completely ablated, there is a chance that they can be restored through the ability of the brain to heal and adapt. To what degree functions may spontaneously recover versus needing aid via neuropsychological rehabilitation techniques remains unresolved. There is no doubt that some spontaneous recovery can occur, but how much does targeted training also help to restore function? What if a function is completely lost? In this case, most neurobehavioral rehabilitation focuses on **substitution,** or the use of other behavioral strategies or devices to "work around" the problem or serve as an external prosthetic device to help take the place of the lost function.

Adaptation and Recovery

DIASCHISIS

Diaschisis (first described by von Monakow, 1911) refers to an unmasking of function after temporary neuronal disruption. Monakow's theory of diaschisis (derived from Greek *schizein,* meaning "to split") described the loss of function caused by cerebral lesions in areas that are remote from the lesion, but that are neuronally connected to it. A depression in neuronal functioning can occur due to neuronal shock, intercranial pressure, edema, metabolic changes, or any condition that reduces blood flow. This transience of function inhibition implies that the neuronal systems have not been permanently damaged. Therefore, diaschisis differs from **restitution** in that it is a passive process of uncovering working systems rather than an active process of repairing damaged systems. As the condition causing the dysfunction is removed, the behavioral function re-emerges.

Researchers have proposed that diaschisis represents an imbalance between excitatory and inhibitory mechanisms (Poppel & von Steinbuchel, 1992). An interesting demonstration in animals (Poppel & Richards, 1974) provides an example. If the right occipital lobe is damaged, blindness in the left visual field results; however, if the left superior colliculus is destroyed, sight is restored. How is this so? Apparently, the colliculi of each hemisphere serve to inhibit each other while each occipital lobe excites its ipsilateral colliculus. Thus, in the normal brain, all is balanced. However, when the right occipital lobe is damaged, the right superior colliculus, which no longer is receiving input from its occipital lobe, cannot moderate the left superior colliculus. In fact, the right becomes overinhibited by the relative overactivity of the left. If the inhibitory input of the left is removed, the right becomes functional again and some sight is restored. This complicated interplay between excitatory and inhibitory functions repeats itself over and over again with different functional systems of the brain. According to the theory of diaschisis, this imbalance between excitation and inhibition resolves spontaneously.

BRAIN REORGANIZATION

Reorganization of brain function after injury has much to do with the plasticity of the brain. **Plasticity,** the behavioral or neural ability to reorganize after brain injury, appears to be one of the more important factors contributing to the speed and level of final recovery. Most research on plasticity has tested animals, leaving the relation between neuronal reorganization and behavioral organization unclear in humans. Immature nervous systems are much more plastic than those of adults; children show less behavioral effect and recover faster from brain injury. Some have suggested that recovery from aphasia in prepubescent children may be caused by the adaptability of the short-axon Golgi type II cells (Hirsch & Jacobson, 1974; Kertesz & Gold, 2003). Whereas the long axon neurons of the brain appear to be preprogrammed genetically

for certain functions, the more flexible Golgi type II cells appear to maintain flexibility until the onset of hormonal changes associated with puberty.

Axonal and Collateral Sprouting

One way in which the brain reorganizes is through the regrowth of neurons that have been only partially damaged. As mentioned in Chapter 4, unlike axons in the peripheral nervous system, those in the central nervous system are not known to regenerate after total severing. However, axons that have been sheared may resprout, and collateral sprouting can occur from nearby intact neurons. Younger organisms appear to have the greatest potential for axonal regrowth. Theoretically, sprouting could replace the lost function. Although researchers have documented that axonal and collateral sprouting does occur, they do not yet know whether the "reconnections" rebuild the previous function. Excessive sprouting may even hinder behavioral functioning.

Denervation Supersensitivity

If an area of the brain is lesioned, any remaining neurons in that area may become hypersensitive to the neurotransmitters that act on them. The mechanism appears to act via a proliferation of postsynaptic receptor sites. This may result in a greater excitatory or inhibitory potential, depending on the type of neuron.

Overview of the Rehabilitation Process

Rehabilitation seeks to retrain and re-educate people with disabling injuries, to improve level of daily functioning. The philosophy of a rehabilitation center is very different from that of an acute care hospital. In the early stages after an injury or trauma, the hospital's goal is to medically stabilize the patient. The hospital provides care for the patient and does not require the patient to be active in treatment. Rehabilitation centers expect the patient and family to take a more active role in retraining, and to become partners in treatment planning. Rehabilitation settings also use rehabilitation teams of specialists who work together in setting goals and implementing treatment. This section considers the various specialties in more detail. Traditionally, rehabilitation treatment was set up over a period of weeks to months on an inpatient unit, then followed periodically on an outpatient unit. With the advent of managed care, inpatient rehabilitation has shortened, outpatient rehabilitation has lengthened, and the role of the neuropsychologist has evolved to meet new demands for services. The final goal of rehabilitation is to reintegrate people back into the community at the highest level of functioning possible.

Rehabilitation psychology, like neuropsychology, is a distinct specialty area within psychology. Practicing rehabilitation psychologists may treat people who have suffered non-neurologic problems such as burns, chronic pain, amputation, or blindness, as well as neurologic brain and spinal cord injuries and trauma. The focus is on applying psychological principles to recovery and adjustment to disability. More specifically, for the psychologist working with brain disorders, neuropsychological rehabilitation—or brain injury rehabilitation, as it is more commonly known—represents the intersection of neuropsychology and rehabilitation. As such, the focus is on the process of recovery, adjustment, and rehabilitation of brain disorders. The conditions most often seen on brain injury units of rehabilitation hospitals include TBI caused by head injuries from accidents and falls and cerebrovascular accidents (CVAs). Less often, rehabilitation units treat patients recovering from brain tumor or brain disease. With the increasing survival rate of heart attack victims, rehabilitation centers are experiencing a greater influx of anoxic/hypoxic injuries resulting from loss of oxygen to the brain before resuscitation.

Rehabilitation hospitals are specialty hospitals, which admit patients who fit a restricted group of diagnoses, such as TBI. Length of inpatient stay varies but has shortened dramatically since the advent of managed care. As inpatient stays shortened, the focus of treatment evolved to include a greater emphasis on outpatient treatment within a person's home, social, and occupational settings.

There are about 1600 TBI treatment programs in the United States (National Directory of Head Injury Services, 1992). A large proportion of neuropsychologists work in rehabilitation settings where they apply knowledge of brain–behavior relations and neuropsychological evaluation to the process of recovery and community reintegration. A challenge for neuropsychologists working in these settings is to translate the patient's level of functioning to appropriate treatments regarding daily life, since rehabilitation neuropsychologists spend the majority of their time treating the patient and family. Those involved in research constantly wrestle with the issue of ecologic validity—that is, with developing means of evaluation and treatment specific to common issues of rehabilitation such as driving, cooking, and return to work.

ADMISSION TO REHABILITATION PROGRAMS

Although most neuropsychologists in rehabilitation work in specialty rehabilitation hospitals or treatment programs that focus primarily on treatment, others work in large, acute-care hospitals that have rehabilitation units and focus on early evaluation before transfer to a specialized facility. Brain injury specialists working in acute-care hospitals get the earliest view of a person's functioning, perhaps while emerging from coma or recovering from brain surgery. They conduct the first evaluations of alertness, attention, sensorimotor, and cognitive skills over the course of the first few days and weeks of recovery before being transferred to a longer term rehabilitation hospital. The GCS (see earlier) is a good example of a measure used early in the process of recovery from head injury. Also, acute care rehabilitation neuropsychologists conduct preoperative and postoperative assessments to document the level of change in cognitive functioning. These first neuropsychological evaluations can serve as a valuable baseline and predictor of future level of recovery. Therefore, neuropsychological evaluation becomes a valuable part of the prescreening process. Neuropsychologists design the prescreening process for entry into a rehabilitation program to select patients whom they consider to have potential for treatment success and enough social support for postrehabilitative care. In fact, admission to a rehabilitation program in itself suggests the absence of a medical life-threatening crisis and the potential for further recovery.

The rehabilitation hospital is the primary setting for learning the skills to return to a home setting. If rehabilitation facilities did not exist, a large proportion of patients with brain-damage would go directly from the acute-care hospital to a skilled nursing facility. This is because most patients admitted to rehabilitation hospitals cannot care for themselves and may still be in a state of significant cognitive confusion, and their families do not yet understand the condition and the caretaking responsibilities. The rehabilitation hospital is an opportunity to take advantage of the skills of others and to practice practical skills with professional supervision. Therefore, it is quite normal for patients to spend some time getting used to the functioning and philosophy of a rehabilitation unit. The "team" approach is also a new concept for most people accustomed to acute-care hospitals.

As patients move from the acute-care hospital to a rehabilitation program, they must make the transition from the hospital environment to the rehabilitation environment. Rehabilitation patients need time to orient to the philosophy of empowerment that rehabilitation programs advocate. The team teaches the means to maximize independence both for survivor and family caretaker. The goal for a patient is not to live in the rehabilitation hospital, but to get back to community life. Thus, patients in a rehabilitation hospital are not relegated to the traditional "sick" role or to a self-perception that earlier experiences in other acute-care medical units might have shaped.

A newly admitted patient must adapt to many factors in the rehabilitation environment, such as structured rehabilitation programs and new expectations. In addition, the sheer variety of patients of different ages recovering from myriad disorders can be overwhelming. Depending on the size of the facility and the extent of services, there are often separate units for orthopedic and brain injury patients, although sometimes the patients are mixed together. Where brain injury is involved, there is usually a preponderance of young men in their teens and 20s recovering from head injuries, gunshot wounds, or spinal cord injury. Elderly heart attack and stroke victims are also present, as well as tumor surgery patients. The patients with brain injury can be expected to have significant cognitive compromise, often still involving confusion and PTA, as they arrive at a rehabilitation facility.

The Rehabilitation Team: Goal Setting, Treatment, and Evaluation

Once a patient is accepted for admission, the typical protocol assigns him or her to a rehabilitation team. Teams usually consist of specialists in rehabilitation nursing, social services, psychology/neuropsychology, physiatry, speech therapy, occupational therapy, physical therapy, and therapeutic recreation. Treatment teams are often directed by the physiatrist, but may also be directed by psychologists or speech therapists. A "physiatrist" is a physician who specializes in physical medicine and rehabilitation. Other related specialists may also become involved, including specialists in audiology, nutrition, orthotics, optometrics, and dentistry. A variety of medical specialists are also available to patients, such as internists, urologists, cardiologists, ophthalmologists, and pediatricians. These teams generally follow a multidisciplinary or transdisciplinary approach in which each discipline works together in a coordinated fashion to achieve specific treatment goals. More and more patients and their families are becoming integral members of their own treatment teams. This approach includes them in all areas of treatment planning and evaluation of progress.

Initial treatment planning routinely puts patients on a schedule of daily "therapies"; for example, 1 hour each of physical therapy, occupational therapy, and speech therapy. As noted earlier, patients who cannot endure this daily training are generally not considered ready for comprehensive rehabilitation and may be sent to a continuing care center until they are more able. Beyond the minimum rehabilitation requirement, many rehabilitation hospitals provide additional rehabilitation hours, which consist of whatever the patient needs most. Next, we explore the individual contributions of neuropsychology, physical therapy, occupational therapy, speech therapy, and recreational therapy in greater detail. Although we discuss these as separate disciplines, as a treatment team works together over a period of time, a degree of "cross-training" often occurs. In some rehabilitation hospitals, the lines between disciplines become totally blurred as each person is referred to as a "brain injury therapist," although their individual contributions may be somewhat different.

Neuropsychology

Neuropsychologists are active in the rehabilitation process from admission to discharge. As mentioned earlier, neuropsychologists on rehabilitation units of acute-care or comprehensive hospitals may provide baseline evaluations that help determine an individual's capability to participate in a rehabilitation program. On a patient's admission to a rehabilitation unit, a neuropsychologist may conduct a formal evaluation. He or she may also evaluate functional neuropsychological skills such as meal planning and preparation, ability to plan and self-administer medication, driving, or work-related tasks. The recommendations generated specifically aim at helping the treatment team form workable goals and objectives given an individual's pattern of cognitive and emotional strengths and weaknesses. These evaluations necessarily focus on the functional level of the individual and serve as a baseline to document impairment. Notice that the focus of this evaluation is not only on the pattern of deficits exhibited but on the strengths that may aid the person in compensating for losses in other areas. During treatment planning, it is the neuropsychologist's role to discuss specific recommendations with the team regarding potential remediation strategies. For example, would memory log training be likely to be successful? How will the person's level of frustration tolerance impact his or her ability to participate in various therapies? How feasible is this training, given the cognitive demands of the patient's home environment?

During the treatment process, the neuropsychologist continues to assess progress toward goals of daily living in conjunction with other team members. Neuropsychologists take part in individual patient counseling surrounding issues of loss and cognitive readjustment. Family education and counseling regarding the effects of brain damage on behavior and strategies to cope with cognitive and behavioral deficits are also quite important to support the patient in return to the community. Finally, the neuropsychologist often coordinates compensatory strategies across settings from rehabilitation, home, community, work, and school. We discuss the neuropsychologist's assessment and rehabilitation methods in greater depth later in this chapter.

Physical Therapy

Physical therapists (PTs) focus on motor control with the aim of improving physical functioning to the highest degree possible. PTs evaluate each patient on admission to assess performance of functional activities related to strength, balance, coordination, physical endurance, and range of motion. The evaluation also considers the neurologic status of the motor systems. For example, PTs evaluate activities such as rolling, standing, sitting, transferring, using a wheelchair, and walking. PTs develop and individualize treatment programs for each patient according to specific strengths and weaknesses. For example, treatment programs for those with motor disability, weakness, or paralysis may consist of the following activities: mat activities, developmental sequences, balance training, hydro/pool therapy, strengthening exercises, transfer and wheelchair training, walking, and use of adaptive equipment. PTs accomplish goals by teaching such activities as wheelchair management and wheelchair propulsion. They instruct patients how to transfer from their wheelchairs, bed, toilet, and car. To walk again may be a major goal. PTs determine when a patient has sufficient strength, muscle control, and balance to attempt walking, and they assess the need for assistive devices such as walkers, canes, crutches, braces, or splints.

Occupational Therapy

The term *occupational therapy* is confusing to some people who think that the training is specific to individuals who have an "occupation" and want to go back to work. This is not the only goal of occupational therapy. Occupational therapy is concerned with self-care activities such as grooming, bathing, dressing, and feeding, commonly called activities of daily living (ADLs). Occupational therapists (OTs) also focus on work activities ranging from home management, meal preparation, money management, household chores, and activities involved with occupations as well as avocations (that is, hobbies).

The OT evaluates and treats the performance components that are necessary for functioning in ADLs, work, and leisure. The performance components include many aspects of human functioning. Of great importance to the OT is an assessment of sensory and perceptual-motor functioning. The use of muscles to bend, move, and perform purposive action (praxis) lies within the domain of occupational

therapy. Finally, issues of thinking, remembering, and problem solving for daily life hold special importance for the OT.

Several ways exist to distinguish the difference in specialization between PT and OT. Both are concerned with muscle strength and coordination. However, in many hospitals, PTs work primarily on the lower extremities (all muscles below the waist), and OTs work primarily on the upper extremities (everything above the waist). In those hospitals that do not distinguish between upper and lower extremity strength, the difference between PTs and OTs is usually broadly defined by strength (PT) and function (OT). In regard to the latter definition, for example, a stroke survivor may be able to walk with strength and endurance. That same patient, however, may not be able to judge distances, determine left from right, or near from far. As a consequence, walking per se adds little to the patient's independence, because walking is not safe. The OT takes on the job of applying strength gained from PT to using that strength within everyday types of activities. For example, an occupational therapy session may focus on teaching the patient to discriminate between things that are close and things that are far away (as in depth perception training) or things seen to the right versus things seen to the left (as in left neglect training). This therapy is referred to as perceptual retraining, or perceptual remediation.

Another area of occupational therapy concerns among brain injury survivors is apraxia. Stroke victims often show this lack of purposive action. In practical terms, the OT will refer to, for instance, "dressing apraxia," indicating that the patient cannot dress on command, or "on purpose." This form differs somewhat from stroke patients who fail to dress one side of their bodies because of neglect. If you say to a stroke victim, "Let's go outside," she may automatically put on the sweater that is nearby. However, if you say, "Put on your sweater so we can go outside," she may either simply go outside without regard for the sweater or may sit there and fumble with the sweater because she can no longer put it on. OTs try to use activities to meet goals; thus, in this case, the actions chosen will have the purpose or function of overcoming dressing apraxia.

Speech Therapy

Speech therapists provide therapy for patients experiencing a range of communication difficulties. These may include mechanical speech difficulties involving speech production, expressive language, hearing and understanding speech, reading, writing, and the social use of language. Speech therapists specifically trace communication problems from the basic level of auditory acuity and speech production to higher level skills of communication and linguistic integration.

The ultimate goal is to design interventions to aid in speech production and understanding and to facilitate communication. This may be accomplished through practice and retraining or with prosthetics aimed at assisting communication through artificial means.

The speech problems most commonly treated deal with articulatory difficulties, or **dysarthrias,** caused by improper muscle control of tongue, lips, or cheeks for pronouncing words. If either the left or right hemisphere is damaged, people with damage to the section of the motor strip controlling speech production will have contralateral impairment. Thus, half of the lips, cheeks, and tongue muscles used to articulate words may be weakened. Although it is not caused by a similar mechanism, if you have ever experienced slurred speech after a visit to a dentist who used Novocain, you will readily sympathize with the problems stroke survivors face in articulating speech. In the extreme case, such speech may sound garbled or unintelligible.

Neuropsychologists often design higher order language and communicative evaluations to assess the presence and degree of aphasia, alexia, or agraphia. Speech therapists may specialize in evaluations to categorize aphasias (such as expressive, receptive, transcortical, and global), and to understand the nature of reading and writing difficulties such as alexia and agraphia. At this level the interest is in cognitive-linguistic integration.

Therapeutic Recreation

Therapeutic recreation emphasizes the importance of recreational and leisure time activities. These activities serve a purpose beyond being just fun. For instance, patients are encouraged to use skills learned in physical or occupational therapy in completing craft projects. This helps in the "transfer" of learning. Therapeutic recreation also allows patients to begin socializing with each other in a structured but less formal atmosphere than that afforded in other therapy settings.

At some facilities, the therapeutic recreational specialist takes patients on community outings. Community outings allow patients to practice their skills in real-life settings, among nonhospital people. This can help patients on the first important step in their transition from the hospital setting back to their home, friends, and family. The skills addressed in community outings may include:

1. Mobility: ramps, elevators, curbs, doorways, obstacles, transfers, and so on
2. Daily living skills: money management, safety awareness, personal energy pacing, nutritional awareness, and problem solving

EVALUATION OF GOALS AND DISCHARGE PLANNING

The rehabilitation team begins planning discharge from the hospital and outpatient rehabilitation from day 1. This idea sometimes confuses patients and families, who believe they cannot make discharge plans until they absolutely know the final functioning level of the brain injury survivor. It is often difficult to realize that no one can guarantee the exact level of functioning a person will attain by the end of a rehabilitation program. However, rehabilitation teams are in the business of estimating reasonable goals and can give a solid ballpark estimate of function level. Once this expected level of functioning is determined, then everyone can make appropriate plans for what will happen after the hospital stay.

Many brain injury survivors living at home before the injury choose to consider returning home after rehabilitation. As they contemplate this option, everyone must consider the feasibility of living at home safely and happily. The treatment team, patient, and family must consider the functional requirements of a person's current living situation and his or her resources to cope with that environment.

Increasingly, rehabilitation programs are incorporating shorter inpatient stays and longer outpatient treatment into their programs. Some impetus for this, of course, is due to the financial pressures of managed care. However, there is also a move to integrate people into the community as soon as possible. We return to a discussion of community integration programs, with the example of job coaching, later in this chapter. Next, we turn to an in-depth look at the methods that neuropsychologists use in rehabilitation settings.

In summary, the philosophy of treatment in a rehabilitation hospital requires that patients and families be active in rehabilitation. They are "trained" by multidisciplinary teams, which typically consist of specialists in areas of neuropsychology, as well as physical therapy, occupational therapy, speech therapy, and therapeutic recreation. Each area contributes a unique expertise related to brain-behavior functioning. PTs focus on the motor system, OTs are concerned with applying motor functioning to daily life tasks and with other functional tasks of daily living, speech therapists evaluate and facilitate improvement in all aspects of communication, and therapeutic recreation specialists focus on leisure activities and on practicing skills in the community. Neuropsychologists provide initial and ongoing evaluation, as well as treatment for cognition, mood, and behavior disorders. The training done by each team member necessarily focuses on parallel tracks: The first is to work directly with the patient to try to restore function or compensate for lost function, and the second is to work with caregivers and family to ensure that treatment will continue after rehabilitation ends. During outpatient treatment, where community reentry is the focus, the focus of the team turns to providing bridges to employment or other vocational endeavors. The next sections take an in-depth look at the role of neuropsychologists in rehabilitation settings—first the role in assessment, then the role in treatment.

TREATMENT PLANNING

Successful treatment rests on appropriate evaluation. Assessments need to answer questions related to the possibilities of success in treatment and in returning to the "real world." What is the pattern of strengths and weaknesses according to the functional areas of verbal processing, visuospatial processing, and so forth? Will the person be able to absorb the purpose of therapy and remember instructions? Does the patient appreciate the need for therapy? When deficits appear, what exactly is the nature of the problem? For example, in language, are there more expressive or receptive difficulties? How severe is the problem? Are there residual abilities that indicate the deficit can be strengthened through practice? Are there other areas of strength that can be trained to compensate or substitute for the problem? What is the likelihood that this person will be able to return home, return to work, return to independent functioning? These questions, in addition to describing patterns of neuropsychological functioning, definitely require predictions. This forces the neuropsychologist to consider not only current level of functioning but also the accumulated research and clinical knowledge regarding the probability and time course of recovery for the particular problem. Recovery depends on numerous factors: pattern of impairment, treatment program, degree of spontaneous recovery, physical and emotional state of the person, family support, and several other factors. Prediction becomes quite a challenging task.

ASSESSMENT OF EVERYDAY ACTIVITIES

Real-world tasks such as driving, cooking, balancing a checkbook, taking medication, or navigating an unfamiliar route require numerous cognitive components. Neuropsychological assessment often attempts to isolate the effects of functional areas such as divided attention, receptive language, or memory encoding. Although this is helpful in understanding the pattern of neuropsychological strengths and weaknesses, the "whole" of a process such as preparing a meal may be more than the sum of its generic cognitive "parts." Cooking certainly requires sustained attention, the ability to read and follow recipes, the ability to organize preparation of different dishes so they are finished at the same time, the necessity to monitor time so the cake will not burn, and of course, basic visuospatial abilities. A problem in any one of these areas may lead to a dining disaster. But does the presence of basic skills ensure competence in cooking? A neuropsychological assessment that measures attention, reading, organization, and time monitoring may reveal deficits that pose problems for independent meal preparation. But if no problems are found, does this mean the person can prepare meals independently? Not necessarily. First of all, tests of general functional areas such as attention and memory may be too nonspecific to shed light on the exact neuropsychological requirements that make up successful meal preparation. Does a general test of organizational ability adequately predict organization of meals? This is a question of ecologic validity. Second, even if we can identify the basic cognitive components involved, do the demands of combining and integrating these components into fluid action somehow change the nature of the task?

To deal with these issues, neuropsychologists who develop "ecologically valid" measures can take one of two approaches, and may take both. First, they may attempt a task analysis. This involves identifying all the relevant specific neuropsychological requirements of the task. Then they must devise tasks that measure components. The idea is that if any deficits appear there is a strong likelihood that the person cannot perform the task. The advantage of this method is that it may use paper-and-pencil measures and small, portable tasks to simulate the cognitive components. These tests can also be standardized using large populations. If the patient performs specific aspects of the test poorly, that pinpoints the deficits, which can be targeted for rehabilitation. The disadvantage is that this analytic approach may not totally capture the requirements of the whole task. The second method is to actually do the task or closely simulate it. Many rehabilitation hospitals use driving simulators to test driving skills. They may also build kitchens or apartments to directly test the functional skills of meal preparation or laundry, for example. If tasks can be recreated in a controlled environment, then the huge advantage is that they come closest to mimicking real life. Then performance on the task as an integrated whole can be assessed. Of course, the primary disadvantage is the initial expense of installing an entire working kitchen or a driving simulator. In addition, unless the key cognitive components of the task can be teased apart, doing poorly on a meal preparation task, for example, may not yield much information on how to intervene in training. Finally, because each kitchen is different, and the components of meal preparation may differ on any given day, success does not automatically translate into success at home.

Treatment Methods for Neuropsychological Rehabilitation

Neuropsychologists use two primary approaches to brain injury rehabilitation that hearken back to our earlier discussion of restitution versus substitution of functioning: (1) approaches that stress retraining of an impaired skill, such as attention or memory; and (2) those that focus on searching for adaptations to the person's environment in the context in which the person will use them (Diller, 1994).

The first approach is cognitive remediation, or cognitive retraining. In this case, for example, computers may be used to provide practice exercises to attempt to strengthen memory or attention. In many instances, the underlying hope is that the brain may be able to rebuild axonal connections through retraining; that is, restitution. Approaches to cognitive remediation, however, do not necessitate proving structural changes to achieve functional success. For those functions that appear lost, cognitive remediation may focus on finding adaptive means, or "work-arounds," for lost memory or lost expressive speech, for example. In other words, the idea is to find compensatory strategies for the lost process. Cognitive remediation approaches are usually practiced in a laboratory setting. They vary a great deal in the degree to which they seek to simulate real-life situations and in which situations they might generalize.

Cognitive retraining rests on theories of learning and pedagogy. Learning or relearning a skill or behavior is a building process that depends on an adequate base for establishing higher order skills. If the aim is restitution, some neuronal functioning must be left. Whyte (1986) provides a useful hierarchical conceptualization for training. Basic mental activities such as focused attention or auditory processing represent the first level of cognitive operations. Cognitive processes, the next step, are combinations of cognitive operations. Flexible problem solving and word fluency are two examples. A skill such as performing mental arithmetic or writing requires coordination of cognitive processes. Even more complex are metaskills that require the ability to sequence skills together, or to apply old skills

to new situations. Finally, global functions such as working, driving, or managing a household are the most complex and integrative activities that depend on the integrity of the lower functions. The idea is to train in sequence from lower to higher order operations.

Context-driven approaches (Diller, 1994) emphasize treatments that either involve actually training the person in his or her home or work environment or are specifically tailored to the person's future needs outside the hospital, even though he or she may practice them in the rehabilitation hospital. This is a relatively newer area of rehabilitation than is cognitive retraining. After it became evident that many people with brain injury fail to generalize or translate what they have learned in the laboratory environment to their own home or work environment, neuropsychologists recognized the need to train specific skills relevant to an individual's environment. Some of the approaches that train "in place" include the use of job coaches and supported employment, driver training, family training to aid in the home, or computers to assist scheduling or memory. Patients can also practice additional relevant skills for daily life in group therapy situations, in which groups of individuals with similar impairments may concentrate on social, orientation, or organizational skills (to name a few). Although, in some cases, the planners of training in the context where the skills will be used may hope to restore function, usually the aim is compensatory.

Review of various treatment approaches makes apparent that practical, "ecologically valid," or contextual approaches to rehabilitation are increasingly the focus of many treatment programs. However, currently, there remains little outcome research to demonstrate their effectiveness. The largest number of studies has focused on such cognitive mediation efforts as documenting improvements in deficits such as attention or memory (Diller, 1994). Also, most approaches to rehabilitation combine deficit retraining and contextual methods in a more eclectic model. However, unless the neuropsychologist takes a conceptual approach toward the rehabilitation program, a combination of methods may be criticized for its resemblance to a shotgun approach to treatment (throw everything at the problem and see if something hits).

PSYCHOTHERAPY IN REHABILITATION

Neuropsychological rehabilitation is concerned not only with rehabilitating cognition but also with personality, emotion, and awareness. Of course, the brain is also the mediator of these functions. Altered self-awareness and personality after brain injury may, in fact, represent some of the most complicated and higher order brain processes

Neuropsychology in Action 13.4

It Is More Than a Black Box

Cecil R. Reynolds Ph.D., Department of Educational Psychology, Texas A&M University, College Station, TX

A popular means of treating disorders of learning and behavior in children is behavioral therapy and derivative approaches that capitalize on changing behavior by implementing specific reinforcement programs. Clinically, this approach derived from work by the Russian physiologist Ivan Pavlov on classical conditioning (known sometimes as Pavlovian conditioning) and the American psychologist B. F. Skinner, who developed theories of operant conditioning (Skinnerian conditioning). Pavlov is best known for teaching, quite by accident, a dog to salivate on hearing the sound of a bell. Skinner taught rats to press levers for food and pigeons to peck keys to be fed. Early clinicians such as Joseph Wolpe were able to take these phenomena and translate them into methods to cause humans to alter their behavior by altering the so-called reinforcement systems they believe control a specific person's behavior.

As behavioral approaches to treating disorders of learning and behavior grew in schools and clinics around the world, peaking in the late 1970s, understanding brain functioning faded into the background. Skinner and other radical proponents of behavior therapies argued that what went on in the brain was irrelevant. Only input and output were important, and people need not understand the brain's function further; it was treated as a black box, a euphemism for a space in which some transformation may occur through processes not understood but also that are irrelevant to the understanding of behavior and learning. As late as 1977, I had a professor in graduate school, teaching a course in learning, make the pronouncement in class that "the brain has nothing to do with learning; learning is all accomplished through change or continuance of reinforcement paradigms." Such views were not uncommon.

Behavioral approaches to the management and alteration of behavior in children with developmental disorders are often, but far from always, effective. And as it turns out, brain systems are crucial in mediating reinforcement schedules and learning. Let me provide an example. At age 11, Deanna attended a program for gifted and talented children at her local public school, with a measured IQ in excess of 130. She played piano and had won a trophy as star player of her soccer team a year earlier. In spring of that year, Deanna was riding in the passenger seat of her dad's car when a drunk driver ran a stop sign, striking the car at Deanna's door. She suffered many injuries, including a broken pelvic bone and numerous cuts and bruises. Most devastating, however, was her head injury. Deanna had suffered a massive right frontal lobe injury, producing a large subdural hematoma that was evacuated in neurosurgery. Her cerebral bleeding extended through the right superior parietal areas, and much microscopic shearing and tearing of neurons occurred throughout her brain. She spent 11 days in a deep coma, and her parents were warned that she might not even recognize them if she came out of

---

that a neuropsychologist and rehabilitation team attempts to treat (for a case discussion, see Neuropsychology in Action 13.4). Psychotherapy can aid by discussing frustrations in progress and providing motivational strategies. But more importantly, and more profoundly, individuals with brain damage who have suffered more than mild impairment often report they no longer feel "normal" and have to go through a readjustment process to adapt to their new level of functioning. Those who have suffered brain injuries report that their social life has declined (Elsass & Kinsella, 1987) and rank loneliness as their most frequent complaint (Thomsen, 1974). Relatives and significant others often describe a "personality change" (Jennett & Teasdale, 1981). Poor social interaction is evident in ratings of close others and direct behavioral observations (Newton & Johnson, 1985). These losses are perhaps the most tragic and far-reaching aspects of brain injury.

Frontal lobe damage, as we discussed earlier in this book, is a common result of moderate to severe head injury due to bony skull projections and shearing. Frontal lobe damage is typically suspect when certain qualities of psychosocial functioning are observed after injury. Among the difficulties co-occurring with frontal lobe injury are impulsivity, disinhibition, lack of initiation, rigidity, loss of abstract attitude, poor social judgment, and loss of personal and social awareness (Lezak, Howieson, & Loring, 2004). Prigatano (1992; also see Prigatano, 1999) argues that self-awareness requires the highest integration of "thought" and "feeling" areas of the brain, combining inputs from sensorimotor, limbic, and paralimbic areas. The common perception that people with CHIs have an "egocentric" or "unempathic" attitude is usually attributed to various manifestations of these and frontal lobe difficulties. The specific inability to see a situation from another's viewpoint may be one of the cognitive dysfunctions underlying apparent egocentric or unempathic behavior. This skill, labeled cognitive perspective taking, varies among moderately to severely injured people (Spiers, Pouk, & Santoro, 1994; Santoro & Spiers, 1994). The

the coma at all. Deanna did revive and had a miraculous recovery.

After 6 months in a rehabilitation hospital, Deanna returned to school. Over the next 2 years, additional cognitive recovery was evident. Her IQ, measured in the 60s (mentally deficient) 6 months after injury, gradually increased to nearly 100 (average), and her academic skills in reading, writing, and arithmetic came to grade level. A far cry from their prior, or premorbid, status, but all in all, a positive outcome. However, this once popular, socially adept young girl was now ostracized by her peers due to her now obnoxious behavioral patterns.

She had few social skills and just did not appear to know how to interact positively with others. She was extremely impulsive, as she acted most often without thought, was constantly reaching out to touch whomever she talked to, and had no clear sense of personal space. Her social judgment was severely impaired, and she often blurted inappropriate and embarrassing comments to others. Deanna came to my attention after a consult request from the University Clinic, where a doctoral student had been working with the family for more than a year to develop a behavioral treatment plan to change these many socially inappropriate behaviors. Such problems are common among patients

of all ages with frontal lobe damage, especially prefrontal and orbitomedial damage, all of which were present in this case. The early images of her brain injury, taken via magnetic resonance imaging (MRI) in the first few weeks and months after her injury, documented these lesions well. However, Deanna appeared resistant to behavioral intervention.

After a careful review of her case, another MRI scan was requested and obtained, now more than 30 months after injury. The new images showed an injury that had not appeared before. Deanna had a lesion and scar tissue on the posterior portion of her hippocampus just above the fourth ventricle of the brain. The importance of such a lesion may not be immediately obvious; however, the hippocampus is a component of the limbic system and is crucial to memory functions. These brain systems, the frontolimbic system and particularly the hippocampus, are significantly involved in learning reinforcement systems. Individuals with posterior hippocampal damage are especially resistant to reinforcement schedules that are anything less than a one-to-one ratio reinforcement schedule.

The mediation systems that allow reinforcement to be recalled and to mediate learning had been irreparably damaged in Deanna. Despite the protestations of the

devotees of Skinnerian conditioning, the brain does matter! Behavior therapies can be effective in treating TBI and developmentally disordered children with behavior problems, even with frontal lobe systems that are impaired. However, once limbic system and specifically hippocampal functions are also damaged, such interventions fail.

With this knowledge and evidence, Deanna's insurance carrier was persuaded to fund a different, more intensive intervention. An in vivo therapeutic approach was devised in which a therapist went with Deanna to local shopping malls for several hours several times a week. Deanna's behavior was constantly monitored and redirected in this setting by a therapist, who also devised a set of verbal cues and self-talk strategies. In doing so, we took advantage of her stronger verbal skills, given that most of her injuries were in the right hemisphere, as Deanna learned social skills in real-life settings, in vivo, or "on the job," so to speak. Being a teenager is a tough job; being a teenager with frontal lobe injury who does not respond to changes in the reward-and-punishment systems of life is nearly impossible. Deanna did graduate from high school, a year late, and is now employed in a clerical assistant position at a university library. She still hopes to attend college.

general ability to recognize and appreciate one's own functional and cognitive changes also varies over individuals and time since injury. However, those who have greater awareness of their dysfunction typically show higher levels of emotional distress (Nockleby & Deaton, 1987).

Psychotherapy in the rehabilitation setting often targets these neuropsychology-based issues of self-awareness, egocentricity, and empathy. Psychotherapy can be useful not only to aid coping and adjustment but also for practical rea-

sons. Difficulty in psychosocial functioning and poor self-awareness is one of the prime reasons for poor vocational outcomes. If therapy targeting affective issues is provided, another 20% to 30% of patients may become productive workers (Prigatano, 1992). Beh-Yishay and Prigatano (1990) found that three factors largely predicted vocational outcome: involvement with others, ability to regulate affect, and acceptance of cognitive limitations. All three of these factors are mainly influenced by psychotherapy.

Summary

Neuropsychologists play an important role in evaluating the cognitive profile of patients who have suffered from a TBI and are actively involved in the rehabilitation for these conditions. Neuropsychologists are most interested in how such conditions result in specific neuropsychological deficits and disabilities in adaptive behaviors. Research in this area not only improves the patient's care but also provides new knowledge on the normal functioning brain. Rehabilitation is clearly becoming one of the major areas of practice for neuropsychology. The rehabilitation process is complex and depends on many mechanisms, including biological, personal, and environmental factors. The assessment and evaluative methods used necessarily focus on functional or "real-life" tasks of daily living. Treatment requires that patients and families be active in rehabilitation and work as "trainees" of the team. In rehabilitation, assessment is an ongoing process, monitoring the progress of treatment and aiding decision making regarding the effectiveness of interventions and the prognosis for long-term outcome.

The methods of treatment currently being developed by neuropsychologists provide exciting and creative ways to help ameliorate dysfunction of individuals with brain impairments. With specialized knowledge of the brain and behavior, as well as technical advances, neuropsychologists are uniquely positioned to guide individuals and their families to their highest potential for recovery and functioning. Chapters 14, 15, and 16 focus on the relation between diffuse neuropsychological deficits and dementing conditions such as encountered in Alzheimer's disease and disorders of consciousness.

Critical Thinking Questions

- Can a head injury change a person's life?
- What is the potential for the human brain to adapt and recover after brain injury?
- What are the challenges for rehabilitation in the twenty-first century?

Key Terms

Tensile strength	Countercoup injury	Subdural hematoma	Diaschisis
Retrograde degeneration	Glasgow Coma Scale	Extradural hematoma	Restitution
Anterograde degeneration	(GCS)	Epidural hematoma	Plasticity
Penetrating head injury	Coma	Post-traumatic amnesia	Physical therapist
Closed head injury	Edema	(PTA)	Occupational therapy
Acceleration	Intracranial pressure (ICP)	Retrograde amnesia	Speech therapist
Deceleration	Brain herniation	Anterograde amnesia	Dysarthria
Impact injury	Transtentorial herniation	Substitution	Therapeutic recreation

Web Connections

http://www.tbilaw.com
Brain Injury Information Page—provides information about brain injury, concussion, and head injury.

http://www.neuropsychologycentral.com
Neuropsychology Central—a great site that keeps you up to date on the latest in neuropsychological links and resources. Internal search engine allows you to determine what topic you would like to focus on and provides you with detailed summaries of each link that has been found. Provides links to neuropsychological assessment, forensics, treatment, and other related areas.

http://www.tbims.org
Traumatic Brain Injury (TBI) Model Systems—learn about TBI's National Database, the diagnosis of TBI, the Center for Outcome Measures, and more.

http://www.healthpsych.com
Health Psychology and Rehabilitation Web Site—comprehensive site that provides information on health and rehabilitation psychology.

http://www.neuro.pmr.vcu.edu
National Resource Center for Traumatic Brain Injury (TBI)—guide for TBI survivors; tips on rehabilitation and on living and working productively with TBI.

Chapter 14

NORMAL AGING AND DEMENTIA: ALZHEIMER'S DISEASE

In one's youth every person and every event appear to be unique. With age one becomes much more aware that similar events recur. Later on one is less often delighted or surprised, but also less disappointed than in earlier years.

—*Albert Einstein*

Normal Aging

Mild Cognitive Impairment

Defining Dementia

Alzheimer's Disease

Treatment

Neuropsychology in Action

14.1 The Discovery of Alzheimer's Disease

14.2 Differentiating between Symptoms of Alzheimer's Disease and Normal Aging

Keep in Mind

■ Is dementia inevitable? How does healthy "normal" aging differ from dementia?

■ Are dementia and Alzheimer's disease synonymous?

■ Does Alzheimer's disease selectively affect "memory" structures of the brain?

■ Why is Alzheimer's disease so difficult to diagnose?

Overview

Elderly adults are the fastest growing segment of the U.S. population. In 1900, 4% of the population was older than 65. As of the 2000 census, this number has mushroomed to 12.4%, or 34.9 million people. In the year 2030, estimates suggest 20% of the population will be older than 65, constituting approximately 70 million people (Administration on Aging, 2000). The 85-and-older group is expected to double its current size. This trend toward an aging population is found throughout Western industrialized countries. These numbers reflect increased life expectancy and medical advances. However, diseases of aging become a great concern.

Tremendous research effort is focused on understanding the neurologic conditions that target older people. Among these conditions are a group of disorders, collectively known as the **dementias,** that cause global declines in cognitive and behavioral functioning. They have no one cause, and most causative factors are still not fully understood. Moreover, many dementias have no known cure. Dementia is often progressive, eventually affecting numerous higher mental facilities. It is often considered a "thief of the mind," first robbing one aspect of cognition such as memory, communication ability, or visuospatial skills, but then returning to steal other aspects of mental functioning.

With a top-heavy population of aging baby boomers, the problem of identifying dementia and providing medical and psychological services to patients and families is becoming increasingly important. About 10% of Americans older than 65 live in specialized settings (such as residential care facilities or assisted living), and more than 1 million live in nursing homes. Older people account for more than 40% of hospitalization days in acute-care hospitals. They buy 25% of all prescription drugs and use 30% of the total health budget. Clinical neuropsychologists contribute valuable assessment skills to distinguish normal aging from dementia. They also play an important role in health care decision making, helping match level of care to an older patient's actual needs.

This chapter examines the differences among normal aging, mild cognitive impairment (MCI), and dementia, and addresses questions regarding the aging brain and neuropsychological functioning. For example, is there an inevitable cognitive decline with age? This question can be addressed by considering the neuropsychological profiles of both healthy older adults and those with dementia. We examine dementias in both this and the next chapter. This chapter presents an in-depth evaluation of the most common dementia syndrome: Alzheimer's disease (AD). This cortical dementia is examined from a neuropathologic, neuropsychological, and behavioral perspective. Chapter 15 presents the subcortical dementias of Parkinson's disease, Huntington's disease, and Creutzfeldt–Jakob disease.

Normal Aging

Defining "normal aging" is a challenge. Stereotypes and concerns abound as people face getting older. Socially, we may fear becoming isolated with adjustment to retirement and death of friends or a spouse. Physically, age brings the threat of increased ailments and chronic illness. Cognitively, the possibility of memory problems, mental slowing, and dementia looms. These concerns are often amplified by myths of aging, painting people older

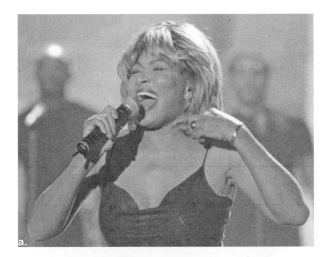

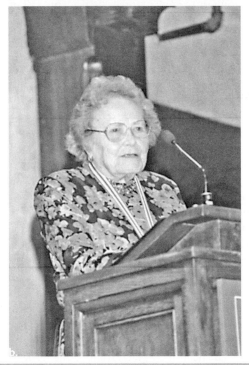

Figure 14.1 (a) Tina Turner, one of the world's success-ful female rock artist, performs at age 65. (b) Dr. Ruth Patrick, one of the world's leading biologists, is still active at age 94. ([a] © Heinz Award photo/Lynn Keith; [b] REUTERS/Alexandra Beier.)

than 65 as unattractive, dull, sickly, and unproductive (Dychtwald & Flower, 1989). Stereotypes of aging, how-ever, can be shattered by examples of highly functioning people. From rock performers such as Tina Turner to renowned scientists like Ruth Patrick (Figure 14.1), we witness the great range of physical, social, and mental ability of people older than 65 and ask, What can we learn from those who age well?

One of the challenges for brain scientists is that the range of cognitive variation for people older than 65 is wide compared with people in their 20s, 30s, 40s, and 50s. Some of this increased variation is due to the inci-dence of brain diseases of aging, such as the dementias or strokes, and some of this may be due to "age-related" de-clines in cognition that affect people differentially as they age. A large part of what clinical neuropsychologists are asked to do is to aid in determining the difference between normal cognitive declines due to the aging brain and brain diseases. Inherent in this is whether problems such as forgetting of names can be considered "normal age-related" or as the harbinger of AD. Scientists have won-dered whether age-related declines in cognition will inevitably lead to dementia (that is, is normal aging and de-mentia on a continuum?) or whether there is a qualitative difference between a disease state and the aging brain. This issue is explored within this chapter and in Chapter 15.

This section reviews both cognitive and brain changes associated with normal aging in humans. By considering both cross-sectional and longitudinal studies, as well as studies that compare normal aging with dementia, a pic-ture of normal aging, cognition, and the brain emerges.

COGNITIVE CHANGES ASSOCIATED WITH AGING

Why is there such a range of functioning in people older than 65? Does everyone lose some cognitive functions even if they do not have degenerative brain disease? Is cog-nitive decline uniform, or are certain areas more likely to decline than others? What is the trajectory of cognitive decline? Finally, are there protective factors against cogni-tive decline and disease?

Numerous examples exist of people who stay active and working in their fields well past the age of retirement. Whether a scientist, a musician, or a mechanic, these peo-ple have developed an expertise and an accumulated body of knowledge related to their work. In fact, all people are likely to develop areas of expertise over their lifetimes re-lated to work, hobbies, or talents. This **crystallized intel-ligence** consists of stored knowledge and habitual ways of acting or solving problems built up over a lifetime. By re-hearsal, practice, and use, certain domains of knowledge become strengthened and are more easily accessible and perhaps less subject to decay. Verbal scales of intelligence tests typically measure general crystallized intelligence not related to a specific work domain. They measure factual knowledge, such as vocabulary definitions, or general information learned in school. Crystallized intelligence represents an accumulation of acquired skills and general information and is more related to formal education or diverse social experiences. Research using the Wechsler Adult Intelligence Scales (WAIS-R) suggests that levels of crystallized intelligence show only slight changes as we age (Kaufman, Reynolds, & McLean, 1989). It has also been theorized that higher levels of crystallized intelligence or general knowledge may provide a protective factor, or "functional reserve" (in this case, a "cognitive reserve"), against dementia that allows the brain to compensate in the presence of declines presented by aging or disease.

Two series of studies lend credence to the idea that a protective cognitive reserve may start early in life. The first of these is provided by the longitudinal study of aging and AD called the *Nun Study*. David Snowdon of the University of Kentucky has followed 678 Roman Catholic sisters who agreed to regular cognitive and medical assessments and brain donation at death. Snowdon and his colleagues seek to shed light on the factors that lead to increased longevity, as well as on the determinants of AD and other brain disorders such as stroke. What is unique about this research is the availability of records from young adulthood and throughout the time each nun resided in the convent. In one study, Snowdon and colleagues (1999) examined the linguistic complexity of autobiographies written as the nuns entered the convent between ages 18 and 32. Women who scored lower on "idea density" (that is, the number of different ideas discussed) early in life also showed lower cognitive functioning after age 75. Also, autopsies of a small sample of nuns indicated that the women who had brain markers of AD showed lower "idea complexity" as young women than those who did not have brain pathology.

Snowdon's studies used "idea density" as a proxy for intelligence, but researchers from Scotland (Whalley, Starr, Athawes, Hunter, Pattie, & Deary, 2000) were able to actually assess the relation between a standardized general intelligence test, administered at age 11, and signs of dementia more than 50 years later. Children who had higher mental ability were less likely to have dementia when they were located again at age 72. Interestingly, there was no relation between mental ability and decline for those who had been diagnosed with an early-onset (before age 65) dementia. Early-onset dementias, as discussed later, may be caused by disease processes that are different than late-life cognitive decline.

Both the Nun studies and the Scottish studies show a correlational link between early intelligence and the health of the aging brain. One possible explanation is that a "cognitive reserve" serves as a reservoir to resist the effects of aging. If this is so, it is not yet known whether cognitive reserve is, for example, a reflection of having more neurons and glial cells in crucial areas or the result of wider or more efficient semantic networks. In addition, the positive correlation between intelligence and the aging brain may be related to other factors associated with longevity. Those with higher intelligence may be more likely to seek and follow health information, have higher paying jobs, adhere to a better diet, and have better access to health care.

Even people who show little signs of cognitive decline, however, are likely to notice changes in **fluid intelligence.** Areas of fluid intelligence involve novel reasoning and the efficiency of solving new problems or responding to abstract ideas. Fluid intelligence has also been conceptualized as a measure of adaptability. Fluid intelligence is most directly related to the influences of changing biological factors and is relatively unaffected by higher levels of experience or education. The most reliable declines in cognition show up in three areas of intellectual activity, all of which are considered fluid markers of intelligence: (1) processing speed, (2) abstract and complex new problem solving, and (3) memory and new learning.

Tests of fluid intelligence (for example, Wechsler's Digit Symbol and Block Design) generally require both novel processing and the ability to complete a task quickly. Studies of aging suggest that performance on tests of this type declines across the life span (Salthouse, 1991). Behavioral slowing also occurs and may partly contribute to poorer performance on a number of tests of fluid intelligence where speed is a factor, but age-related decline is still observed on novel problem-solving tasks even in the absence of speed demands.

Studies of aging suggest that older people are more likely to have more difficulties in many aspects of memory. Early research in aging and memory suggested that the main problem for older people was information retrieval. Poorer performance occurs with free recall, compared with recognition, with less contextualized information, and when more effort is involved. However, new learning may also be difficult because of problems in encoding, particularly with intentional encoding. In fact, some of the retrieval issues relating to poorly remembered contextual information may be due, in part, to poor encoding of context at the outset. Once information is encoded, however, healthy older adults seem to show similar semantic storage in long-term memory as younger adults. Semantic storage can be conceptualized as drawing more heavily on crystallized intelligence and knowledge structures (Bäckman, Small, Wahlin, & Larsson, 2000). There also appears to be little effect of aging on procedural and implicit memory tasks, although these may be performed more slowly.

It has been predicted that older adults would perform more poorly on prospective memory tasks because of a high degree of self-initiation required in remembering to do something in the future (for example, McDaniel &

Einstein, 2000). However, because prospective memory requires both remembering "what" is to be done and "when," it appears that older people have more trouble with the "what" or content that may have more to do with basic encoding, storage, and retrieval mechanisms in retrospective memory (for review, see Henry, MacLeod, Phillips, & Crawford, 2004). Although older people may perform more poorly on laboratory prospective memory tasks, they do much better on real-life tasks, such as keeping appointments or remembering to post mail or return phone calls; tasks for which motivation may be different or external reminder aids may come into play (for review, see Henry et al., 2004).

A number of researchers suggest that working memory (WM) capacity declines with age. Interestingly, short-term memory, or the ability to recall strings of digits, does not appear to decline with age. However, this is a more passive task than WM, where information must not only be held but also manipulated and processed in a more complex manner.

How stable is cognitive functioning among those 75, 85, or older? Does the pattern look the same as one continues to get older? Do initial losses of function stabilize, is there a gradual decline, or is there an acceleration of loss in some areas of functioning? In a review of studies of longitudinal aging, it appears that the pattern of preserved crystallized intelligence over fluid intelligence does not hold in those adults older than 75 (Bäckman et al., 2000), and all intellectual abilities show a decline in group studies.

However, a series of interesting studies conducted in Sweden document the neuropsychological performance of the oldest segment of the population. In one study, researchers gave neuropsychological tests twice, 2 years apart, to more than 300 people between the ages of 84 and 90 (Johansson, 1991). This study of the oldest old (84–90 years old) found surprising stability in neuropsychological functioning between the first and second test sessions. Researchers expected that functioning of people at this advanced age would decline over 2 years. However, two thirds of the sample (66%) remained at the same cognitive level, whereas 31% declined (Johansson, Zarit, & Berg, 1992). Almost half (42%) remained in the normal range of functioning during the 2-year time period. This finding was surprising not only in that a large portion of the sample showed stability of cognitive function over time but also that a significant portion of quite elderly adults still had "normal" cognitive function.

Johansson and his colleagues (Johansson, 1991) suggest that cognitive changes were more related to terminal decline, or proximity to death, than to chronologic age. Among other neuropsychological tests, these examiners administered the digit span task, at regular intervals, to normally aging Swedes older than 70. This requires repeating increasingly longer series of digits either in sequential or reverse order, respectively, until the testee misses them. For the 70- to 88-year-olds studied over time, Johansson examined two groups: those who died before age 85 and those still living. Those alive at age 85 showed a consistent performance as they aged; those who died before age 85 started showing a drop in backward digit span by age 75 and marked declines in both forward and backward span lengths by age 79.

What then is the secret of people who are active and productive well into their later years? In recent years, much focus has been on what can be termed the "use it or lose it" hypothesis. This idea suggests that by keeping mentally active, or by increasing mental exercise, older people may be able to stave off mental decline and diseases of aging. The question is, does mental exercise, such as doing crossword puzzles, starting a new hobby, or memory training help to slow or reverse the affects of aging? This hypothesis has also been called the *differential-preservation* hypothesis (Salthouse, Babcock, Skovronek, Mitchell, & Palmon, 1990) because it is assumed that the large age differences in cognitive functioning seen in the oldest adults are due to differences in their current levels of mental activity and mental exercise. This is in contrast with the *preserved-differentiation* hypothesis (Salthouse et al., 1990) that is more in line with the idea of "cognitive reserve" discussed earlier in this section. In other words, it may be that the range of cognitive differences found among older people are because those who showed higher cognitive ability to begin with continue to show this pattern as they age. In a recent review and commentary on this issue, Salthouse (2006) suggests that the research on "mental exercise" or training as a strategy has not yet demonstrated convincing results. For example, research focused on training people on various cognitive tasks, although showing some immediate benefits in targeted task performance, has not shown to be generalizable to other tasks, often in the same cognitive domain. Also, the effects of training are not convincingly sustained over time compared with those who were not trained. Therefore, although there is much optimism in the popular press about our potential ability to stave off the general effects of aging through mental exercise, this idea does not yet appear to be supported.

Although the mechanisms are not yet known, people who continue to be active well into their 70s, 80s, and 90s may be the best at resisting both declines in fluid and crystallized intelligence. They may have started out with a higher level of crystallized intelligence, and thus are provided with a certain degree of cognitive reserve. They may have learned a great deal in their life, which also provides them with strong crystallized semantic networks. Although aspects of fluid intelligence such as speed and flexibility of thought may decline, many older people do maintain an active and independent lifestyle well into their later years.

BRAIN CHANGES ASSOCIATED WITH AGING

Variation in functional abilities with aging is a clue that the brain may not decline in a uniform manner. But how does it age, and when is change noticeable? By reviewing both global (structural and neuronal) and regional brain changes affected by aging, as well as considering the trajectory of decline and factors that impact brain aging, a picture emerges of how the brain changes as people grow older.

The aging brain undergoes visually apparent gross structural changes such as diminution in size and weight, flattening of the cortical surface, and expansion of the cerebral ventricles. The loss of weight and volume occurs in a general linear trajectory (for review, see Raz, 2000). One of the first recognizable global indexes of brain health or shrinkage is widening of the ventricles. If the brain loses volume in any area, the ventricles reflect this. However, this gross marker does not necessarily imply that the brain loses volume equally across all areas.

Concomitant changes occur at the neuroanatomic and biochemical levels. Neurons undergo significant structural changes with aging. Aging cells may shrink and die, lose some of their dendritic processes, and develop a yellowish brown pigment that accumulates in cells of the cortex and cerebellum and may have to do with "wear and tear" (Bourne, 1973; Kemper, 1994). Observations of cortical thinning may have led to one of the myths of human neurobiology, namely, that throughout adulthood people lose a great number of neurons from their brains each day. Better measurement methods indicate that this is exaggerated, and that much cortical thinning may be due to neuronal shrinkage rather than loss (for review, see Haug, 1985). Although some markers of neuronal abnormalities such as **neurofibrillary tangles** and **senile plaques** (see Figures 14.6 and 14.7) are hallmarks of AD and other dementias, they also occur in older people without frank evidence of cognitive dysfunction.

Images of aging brains often show white matter abnormalities indicating attenuation of myelin around the axons of neurons. This observation has led a number of researchers to question whether white matter (that is, myelinated axons) or gray matter (that is, cell bodies) may succumb more quickly to the aging process. Cerebrovascular disease and hypertension, both more common in older

adults, are associated with white matter abnormalities (for example, Strassburger et al., 1997), but these comorbid problems of aging do not appear to fully explain white matter aging. In an analysis of studies across the life span, gray matter suffers a linear decline from infancy through old age, whereas white matter shows an inverted U-shaped function with increasing white matter into young to middle adulthood, followed by a plateau and then a decline into old age (for review, see Raz, 2005).

The brain shows differential changes with aging. Although some brain areas appear more vulnerable to the effects of aging, there are islands of relative preservation. The hippocampus, the frontal lobes, and specific association areas of the temporal and parietal lobes are more vulnerable, whereas the occipital and somatosensory cortices are relatively preserved. The frontal cortex is one of the cortical areas most affected by aging. The most likely set of age-related neuronal changes specifically affects the prefrontal cortex (Esiri, 1994). Neuronal loss in this area may account for some of the fluid intelligence changes in cognitive functions occurring in older people.

Because cognitive functioning varies widely among older people, it is also reasonable to assume that there is a range of individual variability in physical brain changes. When assessing the degree of cortical **atrophy** caused by advancing age, gross inspection of the brain demonstrates wide variation (Figure 14.2). In the Swedish study (Johansson, 1991), 85% of elderly adults' brains appeared to have little to no evidence of cerebral atrophy. However, all did show some neuropathologic markers usually associated with dementia, including signs of ischemia (that is, insufficient blood supply), neurofibrillary tangles, and senile plaque formations. In individuals older than 85, gray matter atrophy is often apparent on computed transaxial tomography (CT) in both demented and nondemented people. White matter attenuation (thinning of the white matter) relates to cognitive changes associated with fluid intelligence, such as slowed speed of behavior, poorer spatial ability, poorer arithmetic, and memory recognition skills (Johansson, 1991).

Genetic and environmental factors also play a role in an individual's vulnerability to brain aging. A variety of genetic factors have been implicated in the dementias discussed in this and the next chapter. Some of these genetic factors may also prove to accelerate the aging process in people who do not develop a full-blown dementia. For example, a specific allele of apolipoprotein E (that is, ApoE4) has been implicated in some forms of AD. However, ApoE4 may also be implicated in general problems of white matter maintenance through its action on the cholesterol system of the fatty oligodendrocytes that make up the myelin sheath and through a disruption in the

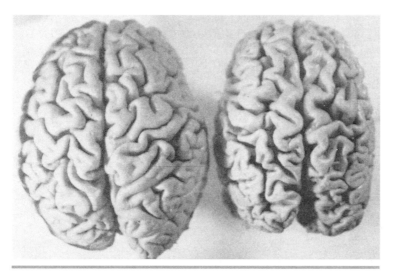

Figure 14.2 Normal brain (left) and brain showing widespread cortical atrophy (right). Note the thinner gyri, wider sulci, and widening of the interhemispheric fissure on the right. Cortical atrophy indicates loss of neuronal connections but not necessarily clinical dementia. (Reproduced from Bigler, E. D. [1987]. The clinical significance of cerebral atrophy in dementia. *Archives of Clinical Neuropsychology, 2,* 178, by permission. Copyright © 2000 Elsevier Science.)

maintenance of intracellular calcium balance (Masliah, Mallory, Veinbergs, Miller, & Samuel, 1996; Raz, 2000).

It is generally accepted that prolonged stress has negative effects on health. However, studies of stress and aging suggest that stress may age both immune and brain cells. Immune cells contain chromosomes with end caps termed *telomeres.* Telomeres shorten as cells reproduce and are a measure of the life of the cell. In a study of women who were continually under high stress levels because of caring for chronically ill children, it was found that their telomeres had undergone the equivalent of 10 more years of aging as compared with women who were living less stressful lives (Epel et al., 2004). Stress also appears to affect certain brain areas. For example, people who have high basal cortisol levels (a biochemical marker of stress) show reduced hippocampal volumes over time (Lupien et al., 1998).

Whereas stress may negatively impact the brain and cognition, aerobic activity appears to enhance it. Older people who engage in regular aerobic activity perform better than sedentary people on a wide range of cognitive tasks (for review, see Colcombe & Kramer, 2003). In direct measures of brain density, it has also been reported that exercising older adults showed reduced loss of gray matter in frontal, temporal, and parietal areas, as well as less reduction in white matter tracts in both anterior and posterior brain areas (Colcombe et al., 2003).

 ## Mild Cognitive Impairment

People who show more than age-related cognitive decline, but do not meet the criteria for dementia, have been the focus of active research interest in recent years. The term ***mild cognitive impairment*** **(MCI),** although somewhat controversial and nonspecific, has come to imply an intermediary, and perhaps transitional, stage between normal aging and dementia. The use of this term has been somewhat controversial because it may be used in an overgeneralized fashion to refer to any number of cognitive changes, but it can be useful if it is well defined. Research also suggests that the presence of MCI is a risk factor for dementia.

Theoretically, MCI can affect many areas of cognition, but most research has focused on memory, or the *MCI-amnestic* type. This criterion identifies memory impairment (for example, Petersen et al., 1999) as the primary cognitive abnormality. In comparison with age-matched control participants, those with MCI-amnesia show deficits in both encoding and retrieval (Bennett et al., 2002; Wang & Zhou, 2002). In comparison with individuals with AD, those with MCI show similar memory deficits but do not show the same level of decline in other areas of cognition (Petersen et al., 1999). Following the initial focus on the MCI-amnestic group, other non-amnestic MCI subtypes have been identified based on other variations in cognitive decline (Petersen, 2004, 2005). Imaging studies also suggest that this MCI group shows hippocampal and brain atrophy that is worse than would be expected in normal aging but is not as marked as that seen in AD (Jack et al., 2000, 2004, 2005).

A major reason for targeting those with MCI is to determine their risk for progressing to AD or another dementia. Indeed, longitudinal research has suggested that the MCI-amnestic group is at a greater risk for development of a dementia at an accelerated rate (Bennett et al., 2002; Daly et al., 2000; Flicker, Ferris, & Reisberg, 1991; Ganguli, Dodge, Shen, & DeKosky, 2004; Lopez et al., 2003). Through the identification of this group, at a high risk for dementia, therapeutic interventions can potentially be started earlier and biomarkers for various types of dementias can be studied.

SUMMARY

The findings from various researchers in aging and cognition suggest that both crystallized and fluid intelligence are important for successful functioning in advanced age. Ability, level of education, and knowledge gained early in life appear to provide some buffer against later brain disorders. Not everyone ages cognitively at the same rate, and many people retain high abilities into advanced age. Some individuals may suffer devastating effects, both physical and cognitive, whereas others suffer relatively few effects. Therefore, among groups of older people, age is not the only, or best, predictor of cognitive decline or mortality. The process of aging increases the probability of cognitive problems. Aging also results in brain and neuronal changes, but physical changes do not by themselves always differentiate between normal aging and dementia because of a wide range of individual differences and differences in functional cognitive reserve. Different measures of functional capacity may well be the key to identifying those at greatest risk for cognitive impairment. Advanced imaging methods correlated with neuropsychological functioning hold promise for more precisely relating structure to function. This will also aid in identifying people at greatest risk for development of dementia, such as those with MCI, and in ultimately answering the following question: What is the difference between normal aging and dementia?

Defining Dementia

With public and scientific attention focused on dementia, one might expect general agreement when referring to dementia and subtypes of dementia such as AD. Given the cornucopia of terms used to refer to dementia

Table 14.1 *Representative Causes of Dementia*

Progressive Dementias	Potentially Reversible Dementias
Cortical dementias	*Systemic illness*
Alzheimer's disease	Severe anemia
Motor neuron disease	Uremia
Pick's disease	
Progressive aphasia	*Deficiency states*
Wilson's disease	B_{12} deficiency
Subcortical dementias	*Endocrine disorders*
Huntington's disease	Addison's disease
Parkinson's disease	Thyroid disorders
Progressive supranuclear palsy	
AIDS dementia	*Drug toxicity*
Creutzfeldt–Jakob disease	Anticholinergics
	Antipsychotics
Mixed dementias	
Lewy body dementia	
Vascular dementias	
Binswanger's disease	
Potentially Static Dementias	
Toxic conditions	
Alcoholic dementia	
Heavy metal poisoning (such as lead and mercury)	
Infectious conditions	
Herpes encephalitis	
Miscellaneous conditions	
Tumor	
Normal pressure hydrocephalus	
Trauma	

and subtypes of dementia, however (Table 14.1), there can be confusion. Professionals and laypeople alike may confuse dementia—the behavioral syndrome—with one particular condition, such as AD. Patients and families often label dementing conditions as "hardening of the arteries," "senility," or "old-timers' disease," which often reflects a perception that the problem is inevitable in aging. In the most generic sense, dementia refers to a behavioral syndrome, and not one disease or cause. It denotes conditions that may have a variety of causes. Some dementias may be treatable, and others may not be treatable. Some stem from disease processes that inevitably become worse, and some from toxic exposure or injury, resulting in a behavioral decline that plateaus.

The dementia syndrome is a cluster of behavioral symptoms that may or may not point to a disease, but dementia is not a disease entity in and of itself. The various subcategories of dementia usually relate to the suspected disease, cause, or primary site of damage (for example, cortical versus subcortical). Researchers have found well over 50 causes of dementia (see Table 14.1). Among the most well known are the degenerative dementias caused by a progressive and unrelenting disease process such as AD or Parkinson's disease. Neurologists traditionally have categorized these disease processes as cortical, subcortical, or mixed, depending on the degree to which they affect gray or white matter areas of the brain. Vascular, infectious, and toxic conditions, as well as a variety of other brain conditions, may also result in dementia.

Some of these conditions are progressive, whereas others, such as the dementia resulting from herpes encephalitis, may be static, rarely worsening over time. Although most dementing conditions encountered by neuropsychologists represent persistent or progressive states, or both, researchers have also documented "reversible" or temporary dementias. Reduced metabolic efficiency accompanies aging, making older adults especially susceptible to conditions and substances that they might have tolerated when younger. For example, symptoms of dementia can stem from adverse reactions to medications (such as sedative-hypnotics and anticholinergic drugs), nutritional disorders (such as thiamine deficiency and pernicious anemia), metabolic disorders (hypoglycemia, hypercalcemia, kidney failure), psychiatric disorders (severe mood disorders, psychosis), and other conditions such as anesthesia or surgery. However, when these conditions are treated, the dementia is usually reversible and the patient returns to baseline.

DIAGNOSTIC CRITERIA FOR DEMENTIA

No one set of criteria represents definitive agreement regarding the diagnosis of dementia. Somewhat varying diagnostic standards are described in the *Diagnostic and Statistical Manual* (4th ed., revised; DSM-IV-R) and by the National Institute of Neurological and Communicative Disorders and Stroke-Alzheimer's Disease and Related Disorders Association (NINCDS-ADRDA) (McKhann et al., 1984) (Table 14.2). However, experts agree about some of the major features of dementia. The first is that dementia results in a *loss of cognitive or intellectual function*. This feature implies a decline that is acquired and unusual. It is acquired because people born with impaired intellectual function, having developmental disorders such as mental retardation, do not have dementia simply by virtue of poor intellect, although they too can experience development of dementia. The loss of cognitive or intellectual functioning must also be unusual or outside of the realm of what would be expected with normal aging. As we have discussed, aging may bring about some cognitive decline, particularly in memory and areas of fluid intelligence. But the decline associated with dementia represents a marked change from previous levels of intellectual and memory ability. Although the most well known subtypes of dementia

Table 14.2 *Diagnostic Criteria for Dementia*

Criteria	DSM-IV-R	NINCDS-ADRDA
Memory impairment	R	R
Impairment of additional area of cognition (such as language, construction, praxis, or executive functioning)	R	D
Confirmed on mental status tests	NS	R
Impaired/decline in social or occupational function	R	NS
State of consciousness unclouded	R	R
Evidence of specific organic factor etiologically related to the disorder or absence of conditions other than organic mental syndrome	R	NS

Note: DSM-IV-R = *Diagnostic and Statistical Manual of Mental Disorders,* Fourth Edition, Revised; NINCDS-ADRDA = National Institute of Neurological and Communicative Disorders and Stroke-Alzheimer's Disease and Related Disorders Association; R = required; D = desirable but not required; NS = not specified.

Source: Adapted from Rebok, G. W., & Folstein, M. F. (1993). Dementia. *Journal of Neuropsychiatry and Clinical Neurosciences, 5,* 265–276; and Katzman, R., Lasker, B., & Bernstein, N. (1988). Advances in the diagnosis of dementia: Accuracy of diagnosis and consequences of misdiagnosis of disorders causing dementia. In R. D. Terry (Ed.), *Aging and the brain* (Vol. 32, pp. 17–61). New York: Raven Press.

have a predilection for the elderly and result in progressive deterioration, this broad definition of dementia could hypothetically refer to the sudden loss of intellectual function from head injury in a 17-year-old.

Although patterns of impairment may differ, the second area of diagnostic agreement in dementia involves *multiple areas of cognitive impairment*. The abilities impaired in dementia may represent all cognitive functions or may present different patterns of neuropsychological disability. Both sets of criteria for dementia identify memory impairment as a prominent and necessary feature. However, it is the multiple and often diffuse cognitive decline that characterizes dementia. It is not uncommon to see impairment in abstract thinking and problem solving, impaired judgment, and other problems of higher cortical functioning.

In summary, the term *dementia* in its broadest sense refers to a group of conditions and diseases that share some similar neuropsychological and behavioral symptoms, although the underlying causes may vary widely. The prime identifying feature is a decline in multiple areas of cognitive functioning, including memory. Beyond this initial definition of dementia, however, lies what is probably most important in working with patients with dementia—an understanding of the different neuropsychological presentations of dementia subtypes.

SUBTYPES AND CLASSIFICATIONS OF DEMENTIA

Cortical versus Subcortical

Traditionally, the primary demarcation among subtypes of dementia has followed the attempt to distinguish between cortical and subcortical dementias. **Cortical dementias** primarily affect, or start out by affecting the cerebral cortex, or gray matter. AD is typically included within this category. With **subcortical dementias,** the disease state predominantly affects the white matter, or neuronal connections between cortical areas, and gray matter structures below the cortex. The term *subcortical* was first used to describe the neuropathology and accompanying pattern of cognitive deficits associated with progressive supranuclear palsy (Albert, Feldman, & Willis, 1974). Since that time, it has expanded to include Huntington's and Parkinson's diseases and may also refer to diseases such as acquired immune deficiency syndrome (AIDS)–related dementia and some depressions. The difficulty with this differentiation, both neuroanatomically and behaviorally, is that these disorders do not conform to strict cortical–subcortical boundaries in the brain. For example, AD typically causes significant cortical neuronal loss and atrophy, but also specifically attacks the hippocampus, a subcortical limbic system structure. In contrast, diagnosticians usually identify Parkinson's disease by the subcortical structure that it targets, the substantia nigra, although evidence suggests that it also affects some higher cortical functions such as executive functioning. Even when evidence indicates that a disease targets only subcortical structures, "cortical" effects may appear because of the disconnection of neural pathways in the white matter that connect the gray matter areas. Although we use the terms *cortical* and *subcortical* dementia as general categories, you must loosely interpret them to imply a major or primary area of damage rather than an exclusive area of damage.

Static versus Progressive

All dementias that result from a disease process are progressive. Diseases such as AD, Pick's, Huntington's, or Creutzfeldt–Jakob inevitably follow a continuous cognitive and behavioral decline. Other conditions, however, may cause a static or steady-state cognitive disorder. A neurotoxic substance (such as lead or alcohol) or infection (such as herpes encephalitis) continues to cause brain damage as long as it is present. But when the condition is arrested, the resultant dementia usually plateaus.

Both static and progressive dementias can begin with a sudden change of functioning, over days or weeks, or a more insidious or gradual onset, over the course of months or years. Lead poisoning may impact the brain for a period of years before obvious impairment appears. Herpes encephalitis, in contrast, is an acute infectious condition with sudden and dramatic effects on the brain. Progressive dementias can also vary in their course. The progression, as in the case of AD, is gradual. However, there may be long periods during which the decline plateaus. Vascular dementias often produce a stepwise progression, as **multiple infarcts (multi-infarct dementia)** or strokes occur at different times. Only repeated neuropsychological testing and keen observation by the neuropsychologist, patient, or family can demonstrate the progression of the dementia.

Reversible versus Irreversible

Researchers have focused primarily on irreversible and progressive dementias. However, clinicians are likely to see a variety of patients with dementia-like symptoms that may remit with time. Part of the diagnostic problem with the so-called reversible dementias is that these people may actually have **delirium** rather than dementia. Delirium does not signal dementia, but rather is a transient cognitive problem associated with an acute confusional state. Typically, individuals with delirium have poor attention, disorganized thinking, perceptual disruption, disorientation, memory impairment, and an altered state of consciousness. Because delirium and dementia share memory impairment and disorientation, they can be easily confused. However, with delirium, the symptoms develop over a period of days or hours and are caused by specific organic problems such as overmedication or an acute or worsening medical condition. Many medical problems listed in Table 14.1 as potentially reversible dementias cause delirium. Moreover, it is not uncommon for patients with dementia to experience development of delirium. For example, a person might be admitted to the hospital to have surgery or to be treated for an acute medical condition. Perhaps an already reduced cognitive capacity causes vulnerability to the cognitive effects of general metabolic dysfunction. People who become delirious for short periods and then recover should not be diagnosed with dementia, even a reversible one. One difference in presentation is that people with dementia, other than in the late stages, are alert and can respond to what is going on around them. People with delirium are grossly confused and disoriented to their surroundings. A true "reversible dementia" should meet the behavioral criteria for dementia discussed earlier; that is, the individual must show dementia in the absence of a delusional state.

Research continues on the question of reversibility. Several possibilities exist. For example, anticholinergic drugs impair memory functioning. Perhaps, reduced cognitive functioning caused by large doses of a medication can, indeed, permanently reverse when the person stops taking the medication. Or perhaps, dementia symptoms stemming from overmedication indicate the early stages of dementia in an already compromised brain, so that discontinuing the drug only temporarily increases cognitive functioning.

The remainder of this chapter focuses on AD. This represents the most scrutinized and researched dementia. We focus on the epidemiology of AD, diagnostic issues, clinical presentation, and neuropsychological profile and treatment.

Alzheimer's Disease

Alzheimer's disease (AD), named after its discoverer, Alois Alzheimer (Neuropsychology in Action 14.1), is a progressive cortical dementia that is irreversible and thus results in an inevitable decline. It is the most devastating and prevalent of the dementias, representing the eighth leading cause of death overall for people older than 65 (Hoyert & Rosenberg, 1997) and more than 50% of diagnosed dementia cases (Kay, 1995). The number of new cases of AD increases with age from 1% of the population aged 65 to 75 years to 6% to 8% of adults older than 85. The rate of survival varies widely between 2 and 20 years with a median survival rate of between 3 and 4 years after diagnosis (Helmer et al., 2001; Wolfson et al., 2001). The prevalence, or number of people living with AD at any one time, increases with age and survival rate. It is estimated that between 10% and 30% of people around the world older than 85 have AD (for example, Bowirrat, Treves, Friedland, & Korczyn, 2001; Gurland et al., 1999; Stevens et al., 2002; Wang et al., 2000). Based on the 2000 census, it is estimated that between 3 and 4 million people older than 65 have AD (Mayeux, 2003).

There appears to be no single cause for AD, and in most cases, the causative factor remains unknown. AD is linked to increased age, which has led some to speculate that it is a disease of "accelerated aging"—implying that if we all lived long enough, AD would be inevitable. Over a lifetime, women are about twice as likely to experience development of dementia or AD as men (Seshadri et al., 1997), but this may be partly accounted for by that women have a longer life expectancy (Mayeux, 2003). People with more education appear less likely to experi-

ence development of AD, but again, this is probably a marker of larger cognitive reserves acting as a buffer between neuropathology and disease manifestation.

AD does not have a clearly identified genetic component in most cases. A variation exists that is autosomal dominant, meaning the family pedigree shows about 50% of the family members as having AD, but this type probably affects less than 150 families worldwide. The most likely chromosomal culprits in genetically established AD appear to be chromosomes, 1, 14, and 21. Interestingly, people born with Down's syndrome, or trisomy 21 (named because the disorder results from an abnormality on chromosome 21), inevitably develop a dementia, usually by age 40. The associated brain changes corresponding to AD (neurofibrillary tangles and senile plaques) appear years before clinical diagnosis. In summary, although the biomedical research searching for causes and markers of the disease appears promising, scientists still know little about the actual causes of AD.

DIAGNOSTIC PROBLEM OF ALZHEIMER'S DISEASE

A definitive diagnosis of AD requires the behavioral presence of dementia and the identification of neuropathologic markers of AD. No single medical test, imaging procedure, or behavioral test can positively identify AD (for example, Mayeux, 2003), short of a brain biopsy showing the characteristic neurofibrillary tangles and neuritic plaques, which are most predominant in the hippocampus and cortical association areas. Because biopsy is not a procedure to which most people would submit, a definitive diagnosis cannot be made until autopsy. AD is difficult to diagnosis because there are other dementias that have may have similar symptoms, especially in the later stages of the disease. In diagnostic accuracy studies, where physicians have to choose the correct diagnosis among several types of dementias, AD disease tends to be overdiagnosed, meaning that other progressive dementias may be misdiagnosed as AD (Lopez et al., 1999). A recent Chinese study that analyzed both the clinical features and brain markers of various dementias at autopsy found that the agreement rate between clinical diagnosis of dementia and pathologic findings was 64.5% of cases (Wang, Zhu, Gui & Li, 2003). Concordance between clinical and biological findings was strongest for vascular dementias (66.7%) and less strong for degenerative dementias (40%).

The clinical diagnosis of AD depends largely on evidence related to behavioral and neuropsychological profiles

Neuropsychology in Action 14.1

The Discovery of Alzheimer's Disease

by Mary V. Spiers

A piece of neuropsychology history puts to rest doubts about Auguste D., the first case of Alzheimer's disease (AD) ever described. After having gone missing for nearly 90 years, Alois Alzheimer's blue cardboard file was found by psychiatrists in the archives of the University of Frankfurt, Germany, in 1996. Among the 32 sheets were Alzheimer's handwritten interview notes, samples of Auguste D.'s "amnestic writing disorder," and a report of the course of the disease. Alzheimer's first notes are as follows:

Nov. 26, 1901

She sits on the bed with a helpless expression. What is your name? *Auguste.* Last name? *Auguste.* What is your husband's name? *Auguste, I think.* Your husband? *Ah, my husband.* She looks as if she didn't understand the question. . . .

What is this? I show her a pencil. *A pen.* A purse and a key, diary, cigar are identified correctly. At lunch she eats cauliflower and pork. Asked what she is eating, she answers *spinach.* . . .

When objects are shown to her, she does not remember after a short time which objects have been shown. In between she always speaks about twins. When she is asked to write, she holds the book in such a way that one has the impression that she has a loss in the right visual field. Asked to write *Auguste D,* she tries to write *Mrs.* and forgets the rest. It is necessary to repeat every word. (Maurer, Volk, & Gerbaldo, 1997, p. 1547)

Dementia had been described before, with terms such as *paralytic dementia, atherosclerotic dementia,* and *senile dementia.* What made Auguste so unusual was that she was so young, only 51. After 4 1/2 years,

Auguste died. When Alzheimer published his description of this case (1907, 1987), he had examined her brain and could describe the unique histologic findings of neurofibrillary tangles: "The nucleus and the cell have fallen apart and only a tangled bundle of fibrils points to the place in which there was once a ganglion cell" (Alzheimer, 1907, 1987). He had even drawn pictures of Auguste D.'s neurofibrillary tangles (Figure 14.3). To Alzheimer, this represented a new entity of "presenile dementia." In 1910, Kraepelin included the new syndrome of *Alzheimerische Krankheit* (Alzheimer's disease) in his famous textbook of psychiatry.

A controversy erupted after their discovery of Alzheimer's file because the original autopsy findings also indicated that Auguste D.

had arteriosclerosis in smaller blood vessels, a fact that today is a criterion excluding pure AD. Other scientists argued that she may have had a metabolic disorder. Finding Auguste D.'s brain would be the only way to resolve whether she had what we now recognize as AD. After a 2-year search, yet another group of German researchers found more than 250 slides of Auguste's brain in the basement of the University of Munich. German researchers have been able to confirm the two classic signs of AD in the brain of Auguste D.: neurofibrillary tangles and amyloid, or senile, plaques. This puts to rest the notion that Auguste D. might have had a disease process other than AD. However, whether she had a coexisting vascular problem is likely to fuel debates for some time.

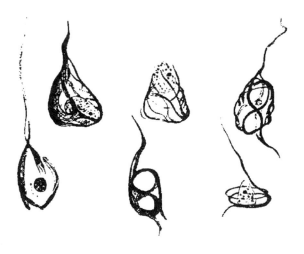

Figure 14.3 Alzheimer's drawings of neurofibrillary tangles from the brain of Auguste D. (From K. Maurer, S. Volk, & H. Gerbaldo, "August D. and Alzheimer's Disease," *The Lancet,* 1997, 349, Figure 5, p. 1549. Reprinted by permission of Elsevier.)

and on ruling out all other identifiable causes of dementia, such as those listed in Table 14.1. The clinical diagnoses of "probable" and "possible" AD reflect, in large measure, the certainty with which other causes of

dementia can be excluded. This chapter also refers to probable AD as "senile dementia of the Alzheimer's type" (SDAT), to reflect the probable nature of the diagnosis.

NEUROPATHOLOGY OF ALZHEIMER'S DISEASE

Major Brain Structures Affected by Alzheimer's Disease

Two interesting facts exist regarding the neuropathology and pathophysiology of AD. First, the disease targets specific regions of the brain. Second, disease-targeted structures sustain neuronal loss and atrophy. Although AD is a "cortical dementia," because major areas of the cerebral cortex show brain shrinkage, this disease does not respect cortical boundaries. It greatly affects major subcortical limbic system structures such as the hippocampus and amygdala. Most pathologic changes occur in the cortical temporoparietal association areas and the *subcortical limbic cortexes*. Specifically, the disease destroys the major pathways to and from the hippocampus, cutting off direct connections to association cortices.

Gross postmortem inspection of the brain often finds cortical atrophy. In Figure 14.4, the most marked atrophy is in the frontal, temporal, and parietal areas. The gyri are thinned, and the sulci are noticeably widened. Researchers estimate that in AD about half of the large neurons deteriorate (Terry, Peck, deTeresa, Schecter, & Horoupian, 1981), resulting in a loss of volume. Specifically, these neurons lose dendritic arborization, or branching. The ventricles also enlarge, because of cortical thinning (Figure 14.5). Although dementia severity increases with increased cell death, longitudinal comparisons of global cerebral atrophy with dementia severity do not reliably indicate dementia (Bigler, 1987; Johansson, 1991).

A closer look at specific structures reveals that they sustain massive cell loss. In fact, SDAT appears to follow structural borders. Chief among these are the parietal and temporal cortices, the hippocampus and the structures leading to it (entorhinal cortex and the perforant neural path), the amygdala, and specific nuclei of the thalamus (Van Hoesn & Damasio, 1987). In addition, certain subcortical

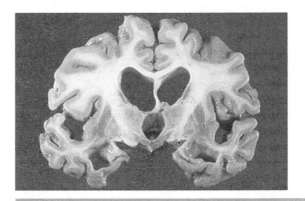

Figure 14.5 Coronal view of an Alzheimer's disease brain, showing widened ventricles. In particular, note also the thinning of the temporal lobes (bottom). (Reproduced from WebPath. Courtesy Edward C. Klatt, M.D., Department of Pathology, University of Utah, Salt Lake City, UT.)

frontal areas are implicated, such as the nucleus basalis of Meynert and the olfactory areas. Noticeably spared are the primary motor and sensory areas (tactile, auditory, visual) and the basal ganglia. The affected structures correspond to areas of higher cognitive functioning and memory, leaving relatively untouched more basic sensory and motor abilities.

HISTOLOGIC MARKERS

The two neuropathologic findings that Alzheimer (1907, 1987) identified, still considered the primary markers of the disease, are neurofibrillary tangles and neuritic, or senile, plaques. These are evident by microscopic inspection of brain tissue obtained at autopsy. Neurofibrillary tangles resemble entwined and twisted pairs of rope within the cytoplasm of swollen cell bodies (see Figures 14.3 and 14.6). Tangles consist of proteins, termed tau proteins, that are believed to accumulate as a result of abnormal phosphorylation. The excessive collection creates tangles that are dispersed throughout the brain but disproportionately in the areas just listed, including the temporoparietal areas and the hippocampal complex. The specificity of structural deterioration in AD extends to the cellular layers of the cortex. For example, within the six-layered isocortex of the cortical association areas, tangles and plaques devastate layers 3 and 5, whereas other layers are relatively spared (Van Hoesn & Damasio, 1987).

Alzheimer described neuritic plaques as "clump-like deposits in the neuropil." They are round aggregates of "cellular trash" that have a particular affinity for the regions where the majority of synapses lie (the neuropil).

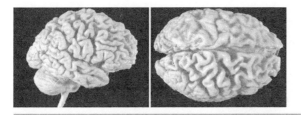

Figure 14.4 Lateral and superior views of cortical atrophy in the postmortem brain of a patient with Alzheimer's disease. (Reproduced from WebPath. Courtesy Edward C. Klatt, M.D., Department of Pathology, University of Utah, Salt Lake City, UT.)

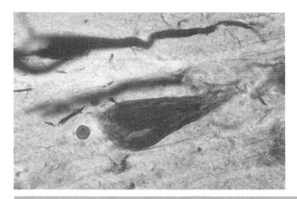

Figure 14.6 Twisted neurofibrillary tangles are a major histologic marker of Alzheimer's disease. (Reproduced from WebPath. Courtesy Edward C. Klatt, M.D., Department of Pathology, University of Utah, Salt Lake City, UT.)

The synapses eventually disintegrate, leaving holes and neurites (that is, pieces of axons and dendrites) where there were once active connections (Figure 14.7). Plaques are likely to concentrate in the frontal and temporal regions (Zubenko, Moossy, Martinez, Rao, Kopp, & Hanin, 1989) and are numerous around the hippocampal formation. As we discussed earlier, tangles and plaques are not specific to AD. They also appear in normally aging individuals without evidence of dementia, as well as in other degenerative diseases. It is the pattern and quantity of these markers that defines AD.

An exciting recent discovery is that the substance of neuritic plaques and tangles may lead to hypotheses regarding possible causes of and treatments for AD. The neuritic plaques found in AD contain an amino acid peptide protein core termed **beta-amyloid (β-amyloid).** As

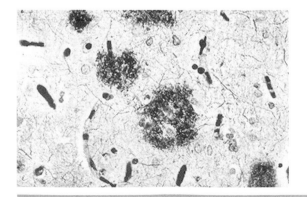

Figure 14.7 The round clumps of "cellular trash" form the neuritic plaques of Alzheimer's disease. (Reproduced from WebPath. Courtesy Edward C. Klatt, M.D., Department of Pathology, University of Utah, Salt Lake City, UT.)

a result, these neuritic plaques are also called *amyloid plaques.* Bradshaw and Mattingly (1995) review several possibilities for how β-amyloid may operate. First, it is coded on chromosome 21, the same chromosome responsible for Down's syndrome. The behavioral significance of this is that if they live past 30 years, people with Down's syndrome often show AD-like dementia symptoms. Therefore, chromosome 21 may be responsible for both problems. Second, there is debate on the function of β-amyloid. Is it a cause of the disease, a by-product of the disease, a "protective reactant," or an autoimmune response?

As we discussed earlier in this chapter, genetic research has focused on the protein ApoE4, which may be associated with both WM aging and AD. This additional protein in plaques and tangles has been studied for its importance in AD. ApoE4 is one of four possible variants, or alleles, of the protein ApoE. Seventy-five percent of people in the population have the ApoE3 variant (Corder et al., 1993), but risk for development of AD increases to 90% if a person inherits the ApoE4 variant from both parents. In addition, a double set of ApoE4 alleles also reduces the mean age of onset. ApoE4 is responsible for ferrying cholesterol into the brain; however, researchers are currently investigating how this protein may operate in AD. It appears on yet another chromosome, chromosome 19, which binds with β-amyloid in cerebrospinal fluid. The exact mechanism for this binding process is not yet known; however, researchers hypothesize that ApoE4 may not be the direct or sole cause of the disease (see Bradshaw & Mattingly, 1995); rather, the protective factors that ApoE2 or ApoE3 provide may be lost. However, there is not yet consensus whether it can serve as a specific or sensitive marker of the disease (Mayeux et al., 1998), and there are no genetic markers of AD that have yet been established for diagnostic purposes (Knopman et al., 2001). Researchers have also examined the CSF of patients with potential AD to examine potential β-amyloid deficiencies or the presence of tau proteins in cerebrospinal fluid. Although a combination of some of these biomarkers holds promise in aiding diagnosis, that some biomarkers are sensitive to more than one condition precludes their routine use in determining the diagnosis of AD (Knopman et al., 2001).

Neurotransmitter Systems Altered by Alzheimer's Disease

AD may impact multiple neurotransmitter systems. However, the most consistent evidence of a neurotransmitter with a direct effect on memory processes in AD is **acetylcholine (ACh).**

In the brain, ACh is synthesized in a group of neurons called the *basal forebrain cholinergic complex (BFCC)*. The cell bodies of these neurons lie in the basal forebrain structures of the nucleus basalis of Meynert, the diagonal band of Broca's area, and the globus pallidus. These axons project to the hippocampus and the cerebral cortex, primarily the frontal and temporal cortexes. The BFCC is a subcortical component of the limbic system and the major source of choline for the hippocampus and cortex (Coyle, 1985). Researchers have long known that ACh plays a role in memory. Drachman (1977) demonstrated that blockage of receptors causes memory loss even in young adults. In AD, the devastation of the BFCC neurons profoundly depresses brain levels of ACh, perhaps as much as 60% to 90% (Terry & Davies, 1980; Bowen, Benton, Spillane, Smith, & Allen, 1982).

Some of the other neurotransmitters implicated in AD are the catecholamines, the amino acid glutamate, and the neuropeptides somatostatin and corticotrophin. However, at this juncture, none of these neurotransmitters appears to play a clear role in AD. Researchers have reported that all are reduced in AD, but their reduction may be secondary to the disease process. For example, general stress also reduces somatostatin. As you might imagine, research in this area is progressing quickly because of the push to find appropriate pharmacologic treatments.

Neuroimaging in Alzheimer's Disease

Gross neuroimaging of the brain in patients with AD may indicate cerebral atrophy on CT or magnetic resonance imaging (MRI). The electroencephalograms of patients with AD are likely to show generalized slowing (LaRue, 1992). Degree of atrophy or slowing taken in isolation is not reliably associated with degree of neuropsychological impairment (for example, see Bigler, 1987), but the degree of ventricular enlargement seen over time as the cortex atrophies accompanies increasing cognitive impairment (Burns, Jacoby, & Levy, 1991) but is only a gross index of general brain health. Special imaging procedures demonstrate the enlarged hippocampal fissure that results from neuronal loss, tangles, and plaques that begin early in the disease process. Also characteristic of AD is a pattern of metabolic or vascular insufficiency, or both, seen in the temporoparietal area, which shows up on positron emission tomography (PET) and single-photon emission computed tomography (SPECT) scans. This hypometabolism can be either unilateral or bilateral and depends on factors such as severity of illness, sex, and age at onset (for review, see Forstl & Hentschel, 1994).

CTs and MRIs are primarily useful, not to confirm a diagnosis of AD, but to rule out other conditions such as tumor or vascular causes of dementia seen as multiple small strokes or ischemic attacks. However, promising new methods of analyzing volume and ratio of specific structures through structural imaging may help confirm diagnosis of AD. PET and SPECT scans appear most sensitive for detecting the characteristic patterns of SDAT. These imaging measures are then correlated with neuropsychological measures to provide a dynamic picture of the disease process.

CLINICAL PRESENTATION AND NEUROPSYCHOLOGICAL PROFILE OF ALZHEIMER'S DISEASE

The clinical presentation of patients with AD can vary, but many share characteristic patterns (Neuropsychology in Action 14.2). The most consistent deficits across patients with autopsy-documented AD are memory and fluent anomic aphasia (for example, see Price et al., 1993). Visuospatial difficulties are also characteristic. These deficits correspond with neuroimaging studies showing patterns of hypometabolism in limbic and association areas in early stages of the disease. In this classic presentation, some frontal areas of the brain appear relatively spared. This also corresponds with neuropsychological testing and clinical observation indicating that, despite severe memory impairment, many patients with AD retain an appropriate "social facade," do not have a Broca-type (nonfluent) aphasia, and retain normal strength and simple motor speed until the end stages of the disease. However, the impairments progress over time, gradually affecting all higher mental functions of the brain. What follows is a description of the neuropsychological and behavioral performance, according to functional area, typical of those with the SDAT variant. Because memory dysfunction is the hallmark of AD, we devote more discussion to this problem than to the other functional areas.

Memory

AD globally and profoundly impairs memory. New declarative learning problems at all levels (encoding, storage, and retrieval) and retention over time are usually noticed first. In addition, structures of the brain that hold previously well-learned semantic knowledge information in organized associational frameworks begin to deteriorate. Finally, short-term memory span, names of family members, and familiar stories fragment. The only type of learning that appears to persist lies outside the corticolimbic system, with certain types of nondeclarative learning.

Neuropsychology in Action 14.2

Differentiating between Symptoms of Alzheimer's Disease and Normal Aging

by Mary V. Spiers

Although memory impairment is the hallmark of Alzheimer's disease (AD), those older than 65 (the time of life when AD is most likely to manifest) often decline in memory ability. The key is to differentiate between general complaints of forgetfulness and lowered cognitive functioning that accompany normal aging and cognitive indicators of incipient dementia. Consider the following two scenarios, which are compilations of cases seen by the authors.

Case 1: Mrs. C

Mrs. C is a 90-year-old woman from a small midwestern town who has lived by herself for the past 10 years since her husband died. She is active in her church and volunteers at a local thrift shop. At home she spends most of her time reading, keeping up with correspondence to family and friends, and talking with neighbors on the phone. She drove her car until a year ago, when after increasing restrictions on night driving due to failing eyesight, she agreed with her physician that she should give it up. She tells her family that her memory is quite poor. She can read through a whole book, but says if she picked it up again it would be "just like reading a new book." She watches the news daily and is interested in following the elections and candidates for office. Mrs. C has a definite opinion regarding who she likes, although she does not remember many of the details of current events and says the news "goes in one ear and out the other." However, she does remember major life events, if asked about them by her children. She can recount episodes from her teens and 20s quite well and tells old family stories from her childhood with incredible detail and animation. For the first time in her life she has had to start taking several prescription medicines for heart problems. At first she needed nearly constant prompting to remember to take her three daily doses at the right times. However, over the course of 2 to 3 months,

she learned her medication routine. She always remembered to take her pills when she got up and before bed, but frequently forgot the 11 A.M. pill.

Case 2: Mrs. R

Mrs. R is a 75-year-old woman who is married and lives with her husband. Mr. and Mrs. R have always had an active social life, getting together with friends quite often to go dancing or play bridge in their retirement community. Within the past several years, Mr. R has noticed that his wife does not seem to be paying attention when they play bridge anymore. She has made wrong bids and makes mistakes keeping score. She usually makes a joke about these things, saying to her friend, "Lucy, you're just trying to distract me so you'll win." Everyone has a big laugh, which seems to just egg her on. Mrs. R particularly likes to tell stories of when she was young, and she has a lot of them to entertain everyone. When the conversation turns to the day's news, Mrs. R seems to have little comment on current events, although she and her husband have always watched the news together every night. She seems to get news stories mixed up. Mrs. R says she just does not have too much use for the news and that "it goes in one ear and out the other." A new couple has joined their dancing club, and much to Mr. R's embarrassment, Mrs. R keeps reintroducing herself to them even after 4 months. After a while it became comical, and Mrs. R says she does it on purpose for a joke. Mrs. R has taken medication for the past 15 years and has always managed well. But now her husband feels like he must remind her to take her pills because he noticed she often does not put it out by her plate as she used to do. She resents being reminded and says accusingly, "I put it out. Are you sure you didn't just take it and put it away when you cleared the table?" This behavior is upsetting to Mr. R, but the thing that bothers him most is that his wife, who had been a good cook, is now very

disorganized in the kitchen. After he noticed that a cake tasted salty, he watched her as she prepared other things. She often added ingredients twice or totally left out essentials of her recipes.

Both Mrs. C and Mrs. R have trouble remembering in areas in which they were previously more able, and they appear to have declined from their own former levels of ability. In some respects, both show a similar pattern of memory loss in that remote memory, or information learned many years ago, such as stories from childhood or facts related to work or home persist remarkably well in comparison with new learning. Difficulty remembering what the news commentator said or learning a new medication routine or a new name presents more of a problem in both cases. These similarities between normal aging and dementia can prompt dread in people who see themselves as less able to rely on their powers of memory. However, these two cases have several notable differences. First, Mrs. C appears to have some insight into her memory difficulties, whereas Mrs. R rationalizes, jokes, and blames others for her poor memory. Second, Mrs. C learns and retains some new things, even though the learning may take longer.

Mrs. R, in contrast, not only is showing difficulty learning new things but appears to be losing her ability to perform previously well-learned tasks, such as cueing herself to take her own medication or to cook. Finally, there is a suggestion that Mrs. R's problems seem more pervasive, in that she may also have problems in concentration, attention, calculation skills, and name finding. Mrs. R's memory difficulties are characteristic of dementia, possibly AD, and may appear paradoxic to patients' families, who can see that their family member is socially appropriate and retains remote and overlearned information quite well. It is easy to discount the importance of cognitive problems.

Long-Term Declarative Memory—As in other conditions that produce "amnesia," SDAT results in profound difficulties in learning new declarative information. As discussed in Chapter 9, declarative memory can be loosely divided into episodic and semantic memory; people with SDAT have deficits in both. One of the first and most prominent symptoms of AD is a deficit in new declarative learning (sometimes termed *anterograde amnesia* to differentiate it from retrograde amnesia [deficit in remote recall]). On neuropsychological testing, patients with SDAT in the mild to moderate stages of the disease typically show marked impairment on both verbal and visual learning tasks, although the progression may begin with one area being of greater deficit. Performance on list learning over trials usually does not progress much beyond an immediate memory span length. That is, if a person has a memory span of four or five items, five attempts to learn a nine-word list often reveals a flat learning curve beginning with recall of four to five items and ending with recall of four to five items. Verbal recall of stories and word lists shows a large number of perseveration and intrusion errors (among others, see Butters et al., 1988). For example, the person may repeat words from the same list as if recalling them for the first time or may recall one aspect of a design that is presented, such as a dot in a box as five or six dots in a box. The person may recall specific events or stimuli across situations, intruding elements from one story into another story or remembering elements of one design as part of another. Although all people with classical amnesia show profound difficulties in new learning, this repeating and confusion of memory differs from most other amnestic dysfunctions that the corticolimbic circuit causes. Intrusions and perseverations are most common in two conditions, AD and Korsakoff's amnesia, which also involve similar patterns of frontal lobe involvement. Butters (for example, see Butters et al., 1988) hypothesizes that the similar pattern of intrusion and perseveration errors in SDAT and alcoholic Korsakoff's amnesia may be caused by a significant loss of cholinergic neurons in the basal forebrain area.

Although many healthy elderly people may forget, they can often remember lost thoughts with the help of retrieval cues. This facilitation of memory by retrieval cues also characterizes Huntington's disease, but the memory problem in AD is more global and profound. People with AD show impairment in encoding, consolidation, and retrieval. The constellation of memory deficits in AD greatly hinders retrieval because it depends on proper encoding, organization, and consolidation of material to be remembered. Thus, retrieval cues will not aid AD patients' recall of information, suggesting that encoding and

consolidation have not occurred. Besides that patients with SDAT show flat learning curves (demonstrating little to no ability to profit from practice), any information that the patient may have remembered immediately after presentation quickly disappears. As the disease progresses, information is lost faster and faster. Although many people benefit from practice over days and weeks, patients with SDAT do not appear to show this consolidation of declarative learning.

Breakdown of Semantic Knowledge—People afflicted with AD have another fundamental problem of memory, which pervades the entire organization of knowledge. As discussed earlier in this book, the brain stores information at the site where it was first processed. That is, most visuospatial information is stored in the posterior areas of the cortex, primarily the parietal and posterior temporal lobes. Auditory information is stored in the temporal lobes, and so on. The dominant theory of memory consolidation, simply put, is that the hippocampus, which has afferent and efferent projections to most areas of the cortex receives to-be-remembered information, codes it for storage, and sends it back to the original processing site (Squire, 1987). Researchers believe memory for information and facts is not stored as separate and complete units (for example, all information about robins stored in one node). Rather, they hypothesize that the brain contains associations of meaning, "semantic networks," whose individual nodes may contain pieces of information or attributes, such as "bird," "wings," "small," and "red breast," which when activated as a pattern lead to the recognition of "robin."

Most amnestic patients, although they cannot encode new information, have an intact semantic organizational network for information. In AD, the memory disorder is much more pervasive, involving a progressive disintegration of this associational network, eventually even for old learned information. The evidence for this loss of knowledge through semantic degradation rests on several findings. First, neuropsychologists noticed that patients with AD do not organize new information semantically as they are attempting to learn it. Thus, if presented with word lists that have inherent semantic categories, such as fruits, vegetables, and items of clothing, most people learn and recall information within semantic categories, clustering the information together. This "semantic clustering" is deficient or nonexistent among patients with AD, who instead show a serial ordering or primacy/recency effect. Second, patients with AD appear to lose conceptual knowledge. Fluency tasks often reveal an interesting pattern. Asked to name as many animals as possible in

60 seconds, people with AD often can retrieve superordinate and high-frequency category exemplars such as cat or bird, but show difficulty retrieving subordinate category exemplars such as leopard or robin. This degradation appears to be more than just a problem in retrieving semantic information from long-term memory. This degradation has been shown to be consistent across tasks, so that the patient may also have difficulty in defining "robin" or naming a picture of a robin (Hodges, Salmon, & Butters, 1991). These difficulties represent neuropathologic changes of higher order intermodal association cortices strongly involved in semantic networking (for example, posterotemporal, inferior parietal), rather than classical language problems associated with the frontal operculum (Broca's area), superior temporal gyrus, or supramarginal gyrus. As the disease progresses, these connected memories or knowledge structures appear to break down to such a degree that even the identity and association of family members eventually become confused in the patient's mind.

In this discussion of memory in AD, we have focused primarily on the encoding, storage, and retrieval processes of declarative long-term memory. These are undoubtedly the areas of the most recognizable and profound memory difficulty. Two areas of memory that appear less affected by AD are short-term memory span and nondeclarative long-term memory.

Relatively Spared Memory Systems—On short-term memory tasks such as length of digit span forward, patients with AD perform relatively well in the early stages of the disease. In later stages, short-term memory retention declines. However, if the examiner looks closely at short-term memory capacity, or WM, it is typically compromised.

Patients with AD perform relatively well on some nondeclarative memory tasks. Separate nondeclarative memory systems exist outside of the subcortical limbic system. The workings of these systems for the most part appear implicit, or outside consciousness. Learning skills with a large motor and practice component, such as riding a bike or typing, or learning psychomotor tests, such as pursuit rotor or mirror tracing, appear to be part of a motor skills learning system. It is not yet clear whether other systems controlling classically conditioned responses and priming represent yet other nondeclarative memory networks, or if they are subcomponents of a single nondeclarative network.

People with AD show normal performance on some nondeclarative tasks and impairment on others. Soliveri (Soliveri, Brown, Jahanshahi, & Marsden, 1992) describes the pattern of nondeclarative memory performance in various neurologically impaired groups. Most people with AD perform well on motor learning tasks that researchers think represent an unimpaired striatal system. However, the picture is different with priming tasks. The methodology of priming, discussed in Chapter 9 with the discussion of memory, assumes that previous exposure to an item will facilitate its future processing. Word stem completion priming tasks typically first present a list of words, such as *there, church,* and *leaf.* Later, they present three-letter stems such as *the___, chu___* and *lea__.* Typically amnestics—even though they have not been able to demonstrate learning of the words through declarative means, namely, spontaneous recall—are likely to produce the targeted words on word stem completion tasks. People with AD usually cannot perform these tasks well. Interestingly, on perceptual priming tasks that present complete and incomplete figures, patients with AD appear to perform better in some instances. Because of this pattern, researchers suggest that patients with AD confront a specific difficulty in implicit verbal priming whereas maintaining nondeclarative learning abilities in perceptual priming and in attaining motor skills. Why would this be so? Verbal implicit priming tasks are probably another pointer to the AD breakdown of the semantic network. Motor skill learning is intact because it is controlled by the striatum, which is relatively unaffected in AD. Perceptual priming appears to point to a relatively more intact visual object recognition system, which may not be affected until late in the disease process.

Language/Speech

Patients with AD do show language problems, but these cannot be neatly characterized with other classic aphasias. In fact, the aphasia progressively worsens both in degree and type. Early in the disease process, AD patients show an anomic aphasia, characterized chiefly by word-finding and naming difficulties (Cummings, Benson, Hill, & Read, 1985). A confrontation naming test (such as the Boston Naming Test), in which the person must retrieve the exact name of an item from line drawings, often results in semantic and circumlocution (talking around) errors. A patient with AD is more likely to say "tool" for "hammer" or "some type of musical instrument" for "harmonica," indicating that he or she recognizes the semantic category but can retrieve only the general category or the wrong exemplar from the same category (for example, see Hodges, Salmon, & Butters, 1991). This type of anomia, together with the difficulty in semantic fluency tasks discussed earlier, suggests a semantic anomic aphasia. As the dementia progresses, language problems become more profound. Comprehension problems begin to appear, followed by problems in repeating information, and last, declines in fluent conversational output may appear that resemble a global aphasia (Zec, 1993; Cummings et al., 1985).

Visuospatial Functioning

Visuospatial problems crop up by the middle stages of AD, if not before. Mr. T, a 70-year-old retired salesman and a patient of ours, came in for neuropsychological evaluation at the request of his wife and neurologist. When they moved to a new retirement community in Florida, Mr. T's wife noticed a change. He started getting lost while driving in the neighborhood, sometimes ending up at the other end of town; embarrassed and angry, he would have to call his wife. Even though they had been there for nearly a month, he kept losing his way and blamed it on that "all those tract houses built in the 60s look alike." Accompanied by his wife, Mr. T could follow the correct route; however, Mrs. T was a bit nervous about riding with her husband. She reported he had a tendency to drift to the left, and on several occasions she had to shout at him to avoid hitting another car. What was most disconcerting to Mrs. T, however, was that Mr. T seemed disoriented in his own home, often heading out to the kitchen to use the bathroom.

The problems Mr. T is showing demonstrate two things. First, he has marked visuospatial impairments in his daily life. Most obviously, he cannot orient himself in his environment, either in the neighborhood or at home. He does not have good spatial sense when he is driving. He veers to the left and appears to have lost his "inner compass." Second, moving to a new residence may unmask a condition that was not evident in a more familiar environment. Mr. T did not have a stroke or some other neurologic event that occurred suddenly. His wife discovered his spatial problems when they moved. Although Mr. T would still have been able to function in his old home, as his dementia progressed, it would have been only a matter of time before he was getting lost in his old, familiar neighborhood and becoming disoriented in his home of 15 years.

On neuropsychological examination, patients with AD usually show poor performance on a number of visuospatial measures. As in the other functional domains, the degree of impairment corresponds to the stage of dementia. Tests of line orientation (for example, the Benton Judgment of Line Orientation Test), spatial construction tasks (such as the WAIS-R Block Design), copying (such as the Rey–Osterreith Complex Figure Test, Bender Gestalt), drawing (such as the Clock Drawing Test), and visual integration (such as the Hooper Visual Organization Test)

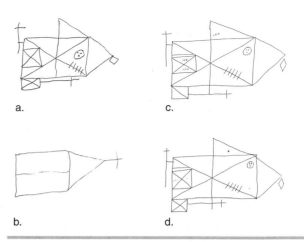

Figure 14.8 Drawing and memory performance on a modified Rey–Osterreith figure drawn by a patient with Alzheimer's disease (AD) and a normal elderly adult: (a) AD copy, (b) AD immediate recall, (c) normal control copy, and (d) normal control immediate recall. (Courtesy David Libon, Ph.D.)

are the most likely to be affected (for review, see Zec, 1993). Complex tasks such as the Rey–Osterreith appear more sensitive to impairment in the early stages of the disease than are simple drawing tasks. Figure 14.8 shows drawing performance in a patient with autopsy-confirmed AD. The patient made these drawings in the early stages of the disease. The more complex Rey figure is somewhat impaired even on the copy. As the dementia progresses, copying designs also becomes distorted.

General Intellectual Functioning

Experts often say that AD, like other dementias, results in a "decline in general cognitive functioning." However, as noted earlier, all functions do not decline at the same rate; thus, it is more useful to consider the subcomponents of measures of global intellectual functioning. We focus here on verbally mediated tasks of abstract reasoning, judgment, crystallized intelligence, and speed of cognitive processing.

The ability to abstract a higher order construct is often impaired in even mild SDAT (Zec, 1993). Verbally, the patient may be unable to say how two objects or concepts are alike, such as a phone and a radio (for example, on the WAIS-R Similarities Test). Visually, the person may be unable to state a common principle that relates multiple figures (for example, on the Category Test or the Ravens Progressive Matrices). This deficit is a problem in conceptualization and abstract reasoning. Thus, people with AD do poorly on a number of tasks that require reasoning and problem solving.

Crystallized intelligence (see earlier discussion) refers to accumulated knowledge over the life span. Often, neuropsychologists measure this via tests of vocabulary knowledge (for example, WAIS-R Vocabulary) or overlearned information. For example, someone who has lived in the United States for several years should know in what month Memorial Day falls. However, few formal tests measure specific areas of expertise that may accumulate from a person's line of employment. This knowledge store is one of the few areas that remain preserved until the later stages of the disease.

Although patients with SDAT are slower on speeded complex tasks (for review, see Zec, 1993), they do not exhibit the **bradyphrenia,** or extremely slow information processing speed characteristic of patients with subcortical dementias.

Executive Functioning

Although deficits are subtle early on, difficulties in executive control are evident to caregivers. For example, in an attempt to compensate for memory loss, a person may keep notes. But without an adequate executive strategy, increased disorganization may show up in notes found in various places around the house and in tasks started but left unfinished. Family members often notice perseveration of thought because the person tells stories over and over or asks questions repeatedly. The person may be less flexible than before. Many apparent "personality" changes may actually stem from frontal impairment. Repeated behaviors, such as checking and rechecking, may emerge from the combined effect of a poor memory and increased perseveration.

An interesting aspect of dysfunctional executive ability is that many patients with AD appear to lose **metacognitive awareness,** or the inability to self-monitor their own behavior and performance. Many clinicians describe patients with AD as having little insight into their own deficits. Often, they appear generally unaware or unconcerned about the magnitude or consequences of their deficits. Is this psychological response understandable as a defense mechanism against the devastating effects of the disease? Not in the typical sense. Many patients with AD appear truly unaware of their difficulties, and consistently overestimate their abilities to accomplish things.

Problems in the ability to organize, plan, and use appropriate strategies for problem solving in patients with AD often appear on tests designed for evaluating strategic processing (such as Tower of London or Tower of Hanoi) and qualitatively on tests designed for other purposes such as visuospatial problem solving (such as the Block Design Test of WAIS-R). Intrusions and perseverations often show up on memory tests. Perseveration is evident as an inability to shift sets on tests that require flexible problem solving (for example, Wisconsin Card Sorting Test or Trails Making Test B).

Orientation, Attention, and Level of Consciousness

AD is not an altered state of consciousness, such as delirium. General orientation and selective attention persist until late in the course of the disease. However, more complex forms of attention such as divided and alternating attention decline from the early stages. Orientation for person, time, and place is generally intact until the moderate to severe stages of AD.

Motor and Sensory Function

In relation to other areas of functioning, motor and sensory abilities are relatively preserved throughout the course of AD. Simple motor speed and strength persist until late in the course of the dementia. However, more complex motor behavior, which may involve coordination or skilled movement, declines earlier.

The disease process appears to spare sensory functioning—that is, visual, auditory, and tactile acuity. Olfaction is the only primary sensory area affected; sense of smell is compromised even in the mild stages of the disease (Jones & Richardson, 1990). Many patients with AD report visual disturbances such as difficulty in reading, interpreting pictures, and recognizing familiar people. Although ophthalmologists often find good acuity and full visual fields, neuropsychological testing often reveals visual-perceptual and visuospatial deficits, which may cause the self-reported visual disturbances.

Mood, Emotion, Personality, and Insight

As with Alzheimer's (1907, 1987) famous patient, clinicians may first refer people for psychiatric symptoms. In some cases, these symptoms stem from the cognitive difficulties that accompany AD, but in other cases, the symptoms, such as depression, may represent an additional disorder. Suspiciousness of others and frank paranoid delusions can manifest memory dysfunction. One 70-year-old woman tearfully related that her husband had begun accusing her of stealing his glasses and other personal items. After 50 years of marriage, he also accused her of having an affair. On questioning, it became apparent that he was accusing her of taking things he was misplacing. Because of his impaired time estimation, not uncommon in AD, 5 minutes could seem like an hour, or an hour like 5 minutes. So when she went to the grocery store on a quick errand, it seemed like an eternity to him.

He had little insight into his memory difficulties, and in trying to make sense of a frustrating situation, he externalized the problem and blamed his wife.

Symptoms that herald a significant about-face in personality usually raise a red flag for family members. Such patients are most likely to be seen by mental health professionals. However, psychiatric symptoms that are exacerbations of premorbid personality styles make recognizing change extremely difficult. A woman always considered impulsive and distractible, flighty or disorganized, may at first appear simply eccentric when she begins to lose track of daily memories. When attempting to deal with memory loss, the person is likely to carry on with coping styles and defense mechanisms characteristic of earlier times. As memory becomes less reliable, a person concerned with order, timeliness, or organization may obsessively check dates, doctor's appointments, medications, memos, and lists.

Depression and Dementia—A common problem in making a differential diagnosis of behavioral disturbances among the elderly is to distinguish psychological depression from global loss of intellectual function. The most effective way to make these diagnostic determinations is to obtain formal psychometric testing from a neuropsychologist, who can describe the patient's cognitive functioning in detail, recognize normal and abnormal patterns of performance, and establish a baseline of performance against which to measure any changes over time. In addition, more subjective guidelines may include the depressed patient's tendency to exaggerate memory problems when compared with the demented patient's tendency to deny or minimize them. It is important to query for information regarding any situational/environmental life crisis that might have precipitated a depressive reaction, but that would not be expected to trigger a dementia process. Because some elderly patients are heavily medicated, it is also important to review all prescriptions to determine whether any, alone or in combination, interfere with optimal cognitive functioning. Of course, depression may also coexist with a cognitive disorder. Approximately 40% of people with AD may also suffer from depression or symptoms of depression, although major depressive episodes are relatively rare (Cummings, 1994).

A common differential diagnostic issue with which consulting neuropsychologists deal is the referral to distinguish between depression and dementia in elderly patients. Following is a possible scenario:

When asked about her husband's behavior during an initial interview, Mrs. S related that her husband no longer appears interested in his daily activities and hobbies.

He used to tinker with their cars and had a hobby of building wooden clocks. He has gradually given both of these up over the past year and a half and says he is no longer interested in them. He spends much more of his day sleeping than he used to, although he is up a lot at night. He has also lost weight and doesn't seem to have a strong interest in eating. In fact, says his wife, Mr. S doesn't seem to have a strong interest in anything. "If it wasn't for me," she says, "he'd probably spend his whole day sitting in his chair. I try to give him things to do, like crossword puzzles or little things to fix, but when I come back, he hasn't gotten anywhere. We don't see our friends anymore because he just doesn't seem to have much to say." Mr. S agreed that he had given up most of his former hobbies, saying he just wasn't interested in them anymore, although he wasn't sure why. He didn't admit to feeling particularly sad or discouraged about these or any other events. Largely, he appeared to be apathetic, not particularly moved in any direction either to be excited and motivated to accomplish things, or to be despondent about his situation. Although he didn't seem to display internal motivation, Mrs. S did say that her husband would accompany her on outings when she planned them. Recently, they had gone to New England on a four-day chartered bus trip with members of their church. Mr. S went along on all the activities and did not spend time sleeping during the day.

At first glance, Mr. S appears to suffer from symptoms suggestive of depression: He has lost interest in previously enjoyable hobbies and activities, and his eating and sleeping habits have changed. Curiously, however, he does not admit to depressed mood or show other subjective or affective signs of depression. He also will become involved in some activities. At this point, three possibilities need to be considered: (1) Mr. S may have primary depression, (2) a dementing process may explain Mr. S's depressive symptoms, or (3) Mr. S may have both progressive dementia and depression. Further discussion of depressive symptoms and testing for depression may show motivational and affective difficulties, perhaps a reaction to a more sedentary lifestyle after retirement, or problems related to his current life situation over the past several years. Chronic medical problems, if they exist, are likely to result in decreased energy, a loss of vitality, and depressed mood. However, it is also possible that these symptoms may be largely explained by dementia. Mr. S may have given up former hobbies such as clock building because he no longer has adequate visuospatial functioning or the organizational and planning abilities to successfully approach novel or complex problems. He also may suffer from "cognitive inertia." If this is the case, what appears to be poor motivation may be an inability to structure and organize in such a manner as to accomplish tasks. Although at first only complex projects may be affected, later in the disease, even straightforward tasks such as washing dishes or taking out the garbage may be difficult to begin, because the affected person does not know where to start. Other possibilities to consider, consistent with AD, are that he may have little insight into his difficulties and thus may appear vague and somewhat detached when speaking about himself. Certainly, further interviewing and testing concerning memory and other cognitive problems are warranted. The primary objective here is not to differentiate between dementia and depression based on a brief description of Mr. S's difficulties. Rather, the point is to consider that, especially when psychiatric symptoms present themselves for the first time in older patients, these may signal underlying cognitive problems. Although changes in personality and mood occur with some frequency in AD, they are not necessary or particular to this disease.

Treatment

No currently available treatments can reverse, halt, or slow the progression of AD. We simply do not yet know enough about the neurophysiology and causes of the disease to develop medical treatments tailored to attack the underlying mechanisms. What, then, does treatment focus on? First, there is a big push for psychopharmacologic investigators to develop drugs that will enhance cognitive functioning. Many drugs are in the experimental stages, and a few have made it to market. Most target the cholinergic system, and therefore memory. Second, both pharmacologic and behavioral interventions are aimed at ameliorating psychiatric symptoms and excess disability (that is, additional cognitive and psychiatric impairment not directly attributable to the disease). With each of these treatments, the goal is to improve quality of life for both the AD sufferers and their caregivers. This section provides an overview of psychopharmacologic and behavioral approaches to intervention.

TREATMENTS FOR COGNITIVE ENHANCEMENT

As discussed earlier, ACh is the neurotransmitter system that holds the most promising physiological link to AD. Many drugs that target the cholinergic system seek to increase its production or action and, therefore, to compensate for the impaired cholinergic production in the basal forebrain, including the nucleus basalis. Researchers have tried varied approaches to augment levels of brain ACh. One approach is to increase the availability of ACh precursors such as choline. Because large quantities of choline are found in lecithin, a substance contained in foods such as egg whites and chocolate, researchers once thought that by increasing dietary choline, they might also elevate brain levels of ACh. However, no clear improvements in memory have materialized from this or other approaches. Other pharmacologic approaches have attempted to target the synaptic transmission itself. One method increases ACh by blocking its breakdown by inhibiting acetylcholinesterase. Other methods strive to directly increase the output of ACh or stimulate the postsynaptic cholinergic (muscarinic) receptors to increase firing. Physostigmine (Synapton) was one of the first cholinergic augmenting drugs that clinical trials tested with AD patients in the mid-1980s. Although some studies suggested improvement, this gain appeared minimal in light of overall declining functioning. But there is some indication that longer term use may result in more gain (for review, see Ashford & Zec, 1993). In the mid-1990s, tacrine (Cognex), which is a long-acting acetylcholinesterase inhibitor, received a flurry of attention. It appeared to show some positive effects, but also resulted in a side effect of liver toxicity. To date, no fewer than 10 drugs have been designed specifically to enhance cholinergic activity in the brain. At this point, however, the search is still on to find the right combination of noticeable memory enhancement coupled with tolerable side effects.

Alternative experimental approaches aimed at understanding the pathophysiology of AD hold the promise of future therapeutic benefit. Nerve growth factor (NGF) is a method being researched to increase cholinergic neuronal functioning. NGF is part of a family of **neurotrophins,** or neuron-feeding nutrients, that researchers have long known sustain neural viability in the autonomic nervous system. The cholinergic system neurons in the basal forebrain also have specific receptors for NGF. In animals, antibodies to NGF result in neuronal shriveling and death. Also in animals, introducing NGF appears to increase ACh functioning and learning and memory behavior in those with lesioned brains. NGF may prove therapeutic in AD if it can sustain life and promote growth of surviving cholinergic neurons. Methods suggested include intraventricular infusion of NGF through a pump (Olson, 1990), attachment of NGF to a gene that can specifically target the ACh system through a retrovirus, and direct neural implants of tissue with active NGF (Dunnet, 1991).

A pharmacologic treatment to halt or reverse the memory and cognitive loss suffered in AD is likely to emerge as our understanding of the underlying pathophysiology develops. Probably this will involve a multifaceted approach to treatment, because large areas of the brain are affected. The treatments reviewed here primarily target the most common and prominent symptom of new learning. A truly effective solution will have to conquer the pervasive cognitive decline.

COGNITIVE, BEHAVIORAL, AND PSYCHIATRIC SYMPTOM CONTROL

The other avenue of treatment for AD aims at symptom control. Behavioral, psychiatric, and cognitive difficulties can emerge either associated with the progression of the disease itself or attributable to processes above and beyond those symptoms that can be explained by the disease itself—a condition termed *excess disability*. Attempts to manage these symptoms use either pharmacologic or behavioral tools.

Common behavioral and affective symptoms associated with dementia include depression, insomnia, persecutory ideation, hallucinations, apathy, agitation, irritability, and purposeless or inappropriate activity patterns. Minor tranquilizers or antidepressants may aid depression and insomnia, but pharmacologic treatment of psychotic symptoms such as delusions or hallucinations may cause serious unwanted side effects. Neuroleptics may further impair cognition, increase agitation, and cause other unwanted motor symptoms.

Patients with AD are also susceptible to illness and conditions associated with aging such as respiratory or urinary tract infections and hearing and vision problems. The associated behavioral problems associated with this "excess disability" can include decreased or increased activity levels, delirium, or hallucinations. In the case of illness, when the condition resolves the behavioral problem likewise should subside. Visual or hearing problems may also amplify hallucinations or sensory illusions.

Because of the severe memory deficit, behavioral management strategies based on learning and responding to reinforcement paradigms can easily prove futile. Instead, most management strategies seek to restructure the environment to ensure safety, provide appropriate stimulation, and redirect inappropriate behavior. As the disease progresses, the person needs more constant supervision. Many nursing homes have specially designated Alzheimer's units because of the difficulties of behavioral management. If a patient is living at home, the burden on caregivers can be enormous. Respite care in the form of dementia "day care" programs serves the purpose of providing appropriate activity and behavioral management, as well as a needed break for caregivers.

Summary

Psychological studies of the elderly have established that aging itself does not necessarily cause dementia. Instead, aging produces predictable changes in patterns of abilities in crystallized and fluid intelligence. Healthy and active individuals in their 60s, 70s, and 80s do not necessarily differ substantially from their past level of functioning in the level of their crystallized cognitive skills or abilities. Relatively stable skills include well-learned verbal abilities such as reading, writing, and speaking; simple arithmetic ability; and immediate and long-term memory. In contrast, fluid intelligence, including short-term memory, abstract and novel problem solving, and behavioral slowing are examples of types of functioning that normal aging may compromise. Health care costs, the aging of the U.S. population, and a renewed concern for well-being of older people have hastened inquiries and interest in this area. Although elderly people are at high risk for diseases that impair cognitive functioning (such as AD), cognitive impairment is potentially reversible in 5% to 20% of dementia cases (for example, in nutritional deficiencies). An understanding of precise neuropsychological deficits can improve the medical management even of patients with irreversible dementia. Neuropsychologists play an important role in comprehensive medical, functional, psychosocial, and neuropsychological assessment. Assessment of mental status and cognitive abilities yields valuable information about prognosis, and it is important in monitoring a patient's health or illness and helping the patient make further life plans (Zillmer & Passuth, 1989; Zillmer, Fowler, Gutnick, & Becker, 1990).

Critical Thinking Questions

◼ Will exercising one's mind help ward off dementia? Must one "use it or lose it"?

◼ How is Alzheimer's disease best identified in life?

◼ How can a neuropsychological profile aid dementia sufferers and their families?

◼ How does the concept of self of the patient with Alzheimer's disease change with the progression of the disease?

Key Terms

Dementia	Atrophy	Multiple infarcts (multi-infarct	Acetylcholine (ACh)
Crystallized intelligence	Mild cognitive impairment	dementia)	Bradyphrenia
Fluid intelligence	(MCI)	Delirium	Metacognitive
Neurofibrillary tangles	Cortical dementia	Alzheimer's disease (AD)	awareness
Senile plaques	Subcortical dementia	Beta-amyloid (β-amyloid)	Neurotrophins

Web Connections

http://www.mc.uky.edu/nunnet
Official site of the "Nun Study," a longitudinal study of aging and AD funded by the National Institute on Aging.

http://www.agelessdesign.com
Ageless Design: Smarter, Safer Living for Seniors—Site of the first organization to dedicate its resources, imagination, and heart to creating smarter, safer living for seniors. By recommending logical, cost-effective home modifications, unique ideas, and products, homes can accommodate those dealing with age-related conditions and embrace the special needs of people as they age.

http://www.un.org/esa/socdev/ageing
The United Nations Program on aging around the world.

http://www.alzforum.org
Alzheimer's Forum—a nonprofit foundation that has established this site to serve the scientific and clinical research community.

http://www.informatik.fh-luebeck.de/icd/icdchVF-D-Index.html
ICD-10 Codes for Dementing Disorders—provides a classification system (the ICD-10) of mental and physical disorders used by the World Health Organization. This site includes a brief description and diagnostic criteria for most major brain diseases.

http://pni.med.jhu.edu
Johns Hopkins University Division of Psychiatric Neuro-Imaging—these pages describe quantitative brain analyses of neuropsychiatric disorders such as AD, using MRI, functional MRI, and SPECT imaging.

http://dementia.ion.ucl.ac.uk
Dementia Web—site is based at the National Hospital for Neurology and is supported by The Institute of Neurology and the Division Imperial College School of Medicine. This site provides updates on dementia research, a virtual chat room, a dementia support group, and other links.

http://www.neurologychannel.com/dementia
Neurology Channel—has information about dementia and other neurologic disorders.

http://www.mentalhealth.com/dis/p20-or05.html
Internet Mental Health: Dementia—provides diagnosis, treatment, and research reports for caregivers and specialists.

http://tv.cbc.ca/national/pgminfo/memory/index.html
The National Online: In Search of Memory—provides information on three forms of memory: semantic, procedural, and episodic memory. It relates these memory forms to different dementia disorders.

Chapter 15

SUBCORTICAL DEMENTIAS

Age is not determined by years, but by trouble and infirmities of mind and body.

—*Mark Twain*

Parkinson's Disease
Huntington's Disease
Creutzfeldt–Jakob Disease

Neuropsychology in Action

Keep in Mind

■ How do the cortical and subcortical dementias differ from each other?

■ How do behavioral motor presentations differ among subcortical disorders?

■ What are the symptoms and progression of Huntington's and Parkinson's diseases?

■ How is Creutzfeldt–Jakob disease acquired?

Overview

Subcortical dementias are so named because, although these conditions often affect cortical areas and functioning, the structures that are prominently damaged are subcortical. Parkinson's disease (PD) and Huntington's disease (HD) attack the basal ganglia; PD targets the substantia nigra, and HD targets the caudate nucleus. Creutzfeldt–Jakob disease (CJD) affects yet another noncortical structure, the cerebellum. The common behavioral feature characterizing these and most subcortical dementias is slowed cognitive and motor dysfunction (Neuropsychology in Action 15.1: Understanding Subcortical Dementia). What is interesting is the manner in which each disease affects the motor system in a different way. You can truly appreciate the complexities of the motor system by examining these diseases. Motor problems present great physical limitations and hardship. These dementias, however, do not represent only motor system dysfunction. The dementias we present in this chapter are progressive and involve multiple functional systems. We present PD in greater detail than the other disorders because it is more common, and these patients are more likely to be seen by clinical neuropsychologists.

Parkinson's Disease

Parkinson's disease (PD) is a slowly progressive disease of the dopaminergic system that, like Alzheimer's disease (AD), largely affects older adults. Later stages of the disease are associated with dementia. PD, or idiopathic parkinsonism as it is also known, is the most common manifestation of parkinsonism. **Parkinsonism,** like *dementia,* does not refer to a particular disease, but rather to a behavioral syndrome marked by the motor symptoms of tremor, **rigidity,** and slowness of movement. This cluster of motor symptoms may be caused by PD but also by drugs, encephalitis, toxins such as carbon monoxide and manganese, and injury. Mohammed Ali, the famous boxer, experienced parkinsonian symptoms (called *dementia pugilistica*) after repeated blows to the head (Figure 15.1). Parkinsonism occurring in the absence of PD can be a static condition. Although the cause of PD is unknown, and the disease is therefore called idiopathic, it is known to selectively affect the substantia nigra and the dopaminergic systems of the brain.

PD affects an estimated 1% of the population of the United States that is older than 50 years, with the incidence of new cases increasing with age (Bennett et al., 1999;

Checkoway & Nelson, 1999). PD rarely occurs before age 40, and the public case of actor Michael J. Fox, who developed PD at age 29, is highly unusual. PD appears more common in men than women, although no differences in risk factors have been identified. Dementia in PD, however, does appear to be age related. Between 24% and 31% of those with PD meet the criteria for dementia (for review, see Aarsland, Zaccai, & Brayne, 2005). However, only about 12% of patients with PD who are in their 50s have dementia, compared with about 70% of those older than 80 (Mayeux et al., 1992). Younger patients with PD are likely to function well, but dementia is more likely with increased age and disease severity. People most likely to have dementia appear to be those who have either had the disease for a longer period or are older at the time of diagnosis (Kay, 1995).

NEUROPATHOLOGY OF PARKINSON'S DISEASE

PD is marked by a degeneration of dopaminergic cells and pigmentation in the substantia nigra (black substance) (Figure 15.2). It is also characterized by **Lewy bodies,** which are small, tightly packed granular structures with

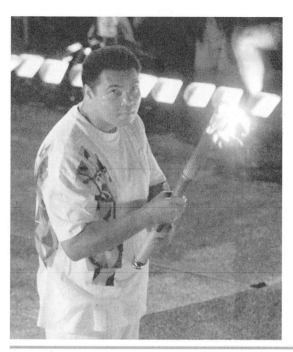

Figure 15.1 Mohammed Ali, who experienced development of Parkinsonian symptoms from injuries that occurred during his boxing career, lit the flame in the 1996 Summer Olympics. (© AP/Wide World Photos.)

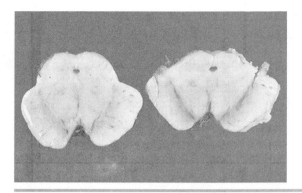

Figure 15.2 The substantia nigra of a patient with Parkinson's disease shows loss of dark pigmentation (left) in contrast with a normal midbrain section (right). (Reproduced from WebPath. Courtesy Edward C. Klatt, M.D., Department of Pathology, University of Utah, Salt Lake City, UT.)

ringlike filaments found within dying cells. Although neurodegeneration and Lewy bodies are pathognomonic markers in cells of the substantia nigra, patients with PD may also have concentrations of them in other pigmented subcortical areas such as the locus ceruleus or unpigmented areas such as the nucleus basalis of Meynert, hypothalamus, cerebral cortex, cranial nerve motor nuclei, and components of the autonomic nervous system (for review, see Olanow & Tatton, 1999). Although the pattern of concentration of Lewy bodies in the substantia nigra indicates PD, the presence of Lewy bodies in the brain is not specific to PD. They may also appear in normally aging people, individuals with AD, and those with other progressive neurodegenerative conditions. This leads to speculation that Lewy bodies are either (1) indicators of a general disease process or (2) markers of cell death.

The darkly pigmented, or melanized, substantia nigra is a midbrain structure that is part of a group of subcortical structures that collectively make up the basal ganglia. The basal ganglia, which reciprocally connect to the premotor cortex and the supplementary motor areas via the thalamus, largely function to control the fluidity of overlearned and "semiautomatic" motor programs (Bradshaw & Mattingly, 1995). The loss of dopamine from the substantia nigra is directly related to the problems of movement initiation and motor rigidity in PD (Bradshaw & Mattingly, 1995). Aging itself takes a toll on the dopamine system, and some cell loss is expected. But the dopaminergic degeneration in PD is several times that of normal aging. Perhaps the reason that noticeable parkinsonian symptoms do not appear in older adults is because there is a "dopamine threshold," estimated to be breached at between 50% and 80% cell loss (Bradshaw & Mattingly, 1995), before symptoms appear.

CLINICAL PRESENTATION AND NEUROPSYCHOLOGICAL PROFILE OF PARKINSON'S DISEASE

When a physician refers patients with PD to a consulting neuropsychologist, the diagnosis has usually been well established from the characteristic **resting tremor** and allied motor symptoms. In this case, the referral is usually to help determine the presence or extent of cognitive decline. However, physicians may refer patients to either a psychotherapist or a neuropsychologist to aid in diagnosis before the "classic" symptoms appear. Unlike stroke, which presents with sudden motor weakness, PD is insidious, slowly sneaking up on its victim. The patient may first sense vague aches and pains and wonder whether arthritis is developing. A general feeling of tiredness or malaise may come first, which could easily be attributed to overwork or "burnout." Other patients with PD may first report feeling irritable or depressed. These symptoms may be met with assurances, a suggestion to undertake medical tests, or a referral to a psychologist to investigate possible psychosomatic problems or depression. As the disease continues to progress, subtle motor

Neuropsychology in Action 15.1

Understanding Subcortical Dementia

by Jeffrey L. Cummings   M.D., Professor of Neurology and Psychiatry, UCLA School of Medicine, Los Angeles, CA

Subcortical dementia is a clinical syndrome characterized by slowness of cognitive processing, executive dysfunction, difficulty retrieving learned information, and abnormalities of mood and motivation. The syndrome is produced by disorders affecting frontal-subcortical circuits, including lesions of the striatum, globus pallidus, and thalamus.

Kinnier Wilson (1912), in his original description of Wilson's disease, recognized the clinical features of subcortical dementia, which von Stockert (1932) described again in the context of discussing postencephalitic Parkinson's disease (PD). Martin Albert and colleagues (Albert, Feldman, & Willis, 1974) reintroduced the syndrome into clinical neurology in descriptions of the subcortical dementia of progressive supranuclear palsy at Boston University in 1975. Substantial controversy centered on this syndrome when researchers first introduced it. Critics of the concept suggested that most dementia syndromes include both cortical and subcortical abnormalities, and that the clinical phenomenology was not distinctive enough to guide differential diagnosis. Subsequent experiences have helped to remold the concept and to account for these criticisms. For example, the subcortical changes in AD in the nucleus basalis of Meynert lead to a cholinergic deficiency that manifests at the cortical level. Thus, although the pathology is subcortical in location, the dysfunction primarily affects the cerebral cortex. Likewise, although there are cortical changes in Huntington's disease, they are minor compared with the marked subcortical abnormalities, and the mental status changes correlate with the subcortical rather than the cortical abnormalities. Thus, even within these mixed syndromes, it is possible to identify cortical and subcortical patterns of dysfunction.

Researchers have increasingly documented the clinical features of subcortical dementia (Cummings, 1986). Slowing of cognition stems from the increased central processing time imposed by subcortical disorders. Patients have prolonged response latencies and slowed complex reaction times. They show executive dysfunction, including difficulty with set shifting, as measured by tests such as the Wisconsin Card Sorting Test or Trails B of the Trail Making Test; reduced verbal fluency on tests of word list generation, such as the number of animals that can be named in 1 minute; impoverished motor programming, as measured by tests such as execution of serial hand sequences; and poor abstracting abilities when asked to interpret proverbs or to distinguish among similar concepts. Memory abnormalities are primarily of a retrieval deficit type. Patients store information at nearly normal rates but have difficulty retrieving the information in a timely way. Thus, on tests of recall they perform poorly, but on tests of recognition memory they may perform in the normal range. This recall deficit includes both recent and remote information. Patients with subcortical dementia show neuropsychiatric and neuropsychological abnormalities. Apathy and depression are particularly prominent. Less common are irritability, disinhibition, mania, and psychosis. Motor abnormalities also accompany most subcortical dementias when the disease involves striatal structures, the substantia nigra, or globus pallidus. Parkinsonism and chorea are the predominant motor manifestations in patients with subcortical dementia.

Recent advances in neuroanatomy contribute to neuropsychological understanding of subcortical dementia syndromes. Five frontal subcortical circuits link regions of the premotor cortex to areas of the striatum, globus pallidus, and thalamus. The dorsolateral prefrontal subcortical circuit mediates executive function and projects from dorsolateral prefrontal regions to the head of the caudate nucleus, globus pallidus, dorsomedial thalamus, and back to the prefrontal cortex. The anterior cingulate region in the medial prefrontal region mediates motivated behavior via a frontal subcortical circuit including the nucleus accumbens, globus pallidus, dorsomedial thalamus, and anterior cingulate. An orbitofrontal subcortical circuit mediates the social governance of behavior and includes orbitofrontal cortex, inferior caudate nucleus, globus pallidus, and dorsomedial thalamus. Dysfunction in the lateral prefrontal-subcortical circuit produces executive dysfunction; abnormalities of the anterior cingulate-subcortical circuit result in apathy; and abnormalities of the orbitofrontal-subcortical circuit produce disinhibited, tactless behavior (Cummings, 1993).

Treatment of patients with subcortical dementia depends on the specific cause of their syndrome. Parkinsonian disorders and PD are treated with levodopa and other dopaminergic agents. The depression syndrome in many patients with subcortical dementia typically responds to antidepressant agents such as selective serotonin reuptake inhibitors. The apathetic syndrome may respond to dopaminergic agonists or psychostimulants such as methylphenidate. Cognitive dysfunction in patients who have a cholinergic disturbance, such as those with PD, may respond to cholinergic therapies such as cholinesterase inhibitors.

symptoms begin to appear. Perhaps the person notices weakness in an arm or leg, including problems in writing, holding a pen, or typing. Voice quality becomes softer and more monotone, and facial expression appears flat to others. If the symptoms are limited to one side of the body, it may appear that the person has suffered a mild stroke. It is nearly impossible to diagnose PD at this stage because the classic motor symptoms have not yet emerged. It would also be rare to even suspect PD, because these initial symptoms could herald a multitude of different problems.

The cognitive profile of those diagnosed with PD is somewhat heterogeneous depending on the presence of dementia and the stage of the disease. Raskin and colleagues (Raskin, Borod, & Tweedy, 1990) suggest two possibilities for the occurrence of dementia in patients with PD. First, demented PD patients may represent a qualitatively different subgroup, experiencing a later onset of symptoms and showing more subcortical and frontal atrophy. The second explanation is that this group may differ only in degree, with a more pronounced progression of cognitive decline. Dementia in patients with PD has been contrasted and compared with both AD and Lewy body dementia (LBD). In LBD, Lewy bodies are prominent throughout the cortex and present a pattern similar to that seen in AD. A magnetic resonance imaging (MRI) study comparing patients with PD with and without dementia with patients with LBD showed that patients with PD with dementia and patients with LBD had widespread cortical atrophy, but patients with PD without frank dementia had atrophy primarily in the frontal lobes (Burton et al., 2004).

This section examines the cognitive profile of nondemented patients with PD. Some authors suggest that the cognitive profile is heterogeneous; that is, there may be several subgroups of PD, possibly pointing to subgroups of neuropathology (Dubois, Boller, Pillon, & Agid, 1991). Others have also raised questions about lateralization of cognitive deficits. Do cognitive deficits in any way parallel the type and degree of motor symptomatology?

Just as memory dysfunction is the hallmark of AD, motor dysfunction is characteristic of PD. Our review of functional systems begins with the clinical presentation and neuropsychological dysfunction of the motor system.

Motor Symptoms

The motor symptoms of PD generally fall into groups of positive and negative symptoms (Table 15.1). Positive symptoms indicate an excess of motor behavior, or abnormal motor reactivity, whereas negative symptoms indicate a diminution or loss of motor functioning. Some experts believe that negative symptoms may manifest before the positive symptoms, although they may be frequently missed. You can think of **bradykinesia** as a poverty of movement that is not only slowed but reduced in magni-

Table 15.1 *Motor Symptoms of Parkinson's Disease*
Positive Symptoms
Resting tremor
Rigidity (cogwheel)
Stooped posture
Impaired righting reflex/poor balance
Negative Symptoms
Bradykinesia: slowness of movement
Hypokinesia: reduced motor initiation
Gait disturbance
Slow
Festinating (rapid small steps)
Freezing
Masked facies: reduced facial expression
Slowed speech
Decreased voice amplitude
Ocular disturbances
Decreased blink rate
Decreased light accommodation
Slowed saccades

tude. Semiautomatic movements such as walking, arm swinging, blinking, swallowing, and facial expressiveness may appear almost frozen, as if the person is robot-like and must consciously think to move. The description of a patient with PD as having **"masked facies"**—denoting a masklike face—captures the essence of an emotionless face. The person's demeanor may seem depressed; a vacant stare may be produced by the combination of reduced facial emotion, slow speech, and decreased eye blinking. In addition to slowness, many movements decline in magnitude. Patients with PD do not take long steps and swing their arms high in the air, but rather exhibit a rapid, small, shuffling, **festinating gait.** Handwriting also gets slower and smaller **(micrographia),** and the voice becomes softer as the ability to project the sound of one's voice becomes increasingly difficult. Patients with PD also describe difficulty in initiating movement, or **hypokinesia,** and may have to consciously think to begin walking, to turn around, or to lift a fork. During the movement, the person may also freeze and may need to "will" the action to continue. Ironically, it may also be difficult to stop an action such as walking or writing, which has led to the suggestion that PD results in a fundamental deficit in initiating and terminating semiautomatic motor programs (for example, see Bradshaw & Mattingly, 1995).

Despite the debilitating effect of the negative symptoms of PD, the positive symptoms of PD are perhaps more noticeable, and most people recognize them as the hallmarks of the disease. Chief among these are a resting tremor and rigidity. Resting tremor, as opposed to a cerebellar intention tremor, is often characterized as "pill rolling." This rhythmic shaking, often first occurring in one hand or the other, looks as if the person might be rubbing or rolling a coin or pill between thumb and forefinger. The tremor stops or lessens with voluntary movements such as reaching, swinging the arm, grasping, or manipulating objects. When the person is sleeping, the tremor usually disappears.

However, with heightened states of alertness, concentration, or nervousness, the tremor is likely to increase. The degree of tremor at any one time is partly due to the voluntary–involuntary nature of the movement, the level of alertness, and the level of stress. It is not always predictable, coming in bursts, but it does increase in speed and may become more violent as the disease progresses. In the early stages of PD, it is not uncommon for the tremor to influence only one side of the body, affecting the hand and foot first and maybe one side of the face. Eventually, it moves to the contralateral side and affects all extremities.

Rigidity, the other major positive symptom, occurs as a tightening of muscles and joints. When a neurologist tries to move the person's wrist, elbow, or knee, there is persistent resistance to this passive movement. Sometimes this resistance appears as a ratcheting movement, as if the person's joint were a cogwheel (cogwheel rigidity). Muscles may appear tense and feel contracted to touch, even when the person is relaxing. This increasing rigidity may result in the characteristic stooped or hunched posture of PD. In addition to a more rigid posture, poor balance and the inability to adjust posture may be evident. The inability to catch oneself quickly, or impaired righting reflex, may appear if the person is pushed or missteps.

On neuropsychological testing of the motor system, patients with PD are extremely slow, with poor reaction times. This is certainly evident on basic tasks that may require simple speeded movement, such as finger tapping. Poor motor performance is also evident on many other tasks that have a speeded motor component such as copying geometric designs with blocks within a specified time limit (such as WAIS-R, Wechsler Adult Intelligence Scale, Revised [WAIS-R] Block Design).

Because PD usually begins as a lateralized motor disorder, some investigators have speculated that the cognitive profile may also show lateralized impairment. Indeed, this may be the case. People with hemiparkinsonism often do show a neuropsychological profile consistent with what would be expected from lateralized cortical damage (Raskin et al., 1990). Exclusively left-sided motor symptoms link to more right hemisphere deficits. Raskin also suggests that this profile may reflect unilateral damage to basal-cortical pathways, resulting in disconnection, rather than unilateral lesions of the basal ganglia.

Motor symptoms may result in lateralized neuropsychological profiles—but is there a relation between the degree of motor impairment and the severity of cognitive dysfunction? Patients with PD followed for up to 10 years did not show evidence of such correspondence (Portin & Rinne, 1986). Although drugs that targeted the motor symptoms, such as levodopa (L-dopa), had great impact on motor performance, they had little effect on cognitive performance.

Visuospatial Deficits

Of nonmotor, higher cognitive functions, visuospatial deficits in nondemented PD are among the most commonly reported in the literature and among the most controversial. Many studies have found that patients with PD perform poorly on spatial tasks that have a motor component. This is not surprising because evidence exists for impairment on visuospatial tasks regardless of whether there is a motor component (for review, see Raskin et al., 1990). However, enough studies show mixed results, or no impairment on visuospatial tasks, to throw the issue of spatial impairment into doubt (for review, see Dubois et al., 1991). To what can we attribute this discrepancy? It may be caused, in part, by the heterogeneity of presentation in patients with PD. Different patients may have somewhat different pathology, and thus different clinical presentations. As discussed earlier, those with more left-sided motor impairment may show more right hemisphere damage (visuospatial deficits). Some studies include patients in more advanced stages of the disease. Some patients with PD may have a comorbid dementia. In any case, factors having to do with possible subgroups of patients with PD continue to cloud the picture of visuospatial functioning.

In nondemented PD sufferers who have visuospatial dysfunction, does such dysfunction point to parietal impairment or some other mechanism? First, patients with PD may report having difficulty orienting themselves in space. For example, when having to walk around the house in the dark without the aid of visible landmarks or outside in a fog, one person relates, "I used to walk alone in the wood, fog or no fog, but when the symptoms of PD appeared, I noticed that I could not orient myself any more, and in case of fog, I got lost" (Dubois et al., 1991, p. 203). Spatial abilities require the person to visualize the relative position of objects in three-dimensional space, and to make a motor response to orient himself or herself or other objects in that space. Therefore, the visual-spatial-motor aspects link in an overall spatial framework. Disease could theoretically disrupt this network in the parietal lobes or anywhere along the visuomotor system. Some investigators have suggested that the basal ganglia play a role in the visuomotor aspects of visuospatial problems in patients with PD (Danta & Hilton, 1975; Dubois et al., 1991). But what about patients who have visual-perceptive difficulty, but no visuomotor problems? For example, a popular test used by neuropsychologists, Benton's Judgment of Line Orientation Test (Benton et al., 1983), requires matching drawings of lines in various orientations to a template (Figure 15.3). It does not require drawing or movement of the body. Yet, many nondemented PD patients have difficulty with this task (Goldenberg, Wimmer, Auff, & Schnaberth, 1986). One explanation is that any disruption in the visual-spatial-motor circuit may impair performance. Another suggestion is that even in tasks in which a person does not use a motor response, he

or she still has an internal representation of a perceptual-motor response (Villardita, Smirni, LaPira, Zappala, & Nicoletti, 1982).

In summary, although it is not clear whether all patients with PD experience visuospatial dysfunction, a sizable proportion does. Certain subgroups of patients, or those in more advanced stages of the disease, for example, may show the most difficulty. The parietal lobes per se do not appear chiefly responsible for the problem. Rather, the basal ganglia are implicated in a larger visuospatial network.

Executive Functioning

Many patients with PD have executive functioning difficulties. Difficulties with specific executive functions can be evident, although most do not have difficulty with abstract thinking (Raskin et al., 1990). These deficits show up early in the disease process, and thus appear to result directly from the disease (for review, see Dubois et al., 1991).

Among executive dysfunctions reported in the literature are difficulties with changing mental sets, maintaining mental sets, and temporal structuring. The inability to switch mental set in response to environmental demands, or perseveration, shows most clearly on neuropsychological testing through measures that require strategy shifts to solve problems (such as the Wisconsin Card Sorting Test) or an alternating response between two different types of stimuli (such as the Trail Making Test B or the Stroop Test). Someone who has set-shifting problems repeatedly tries to use the same strategy, even if it is not working. Investigators have found that patients with PD do not make more total errors on these types of tasks, but the errors they do make are perseverative (Raskin et al., 1990; Dubois et al., 1991). The perseverative problem in maintaining set occurs after the patient tries a new or different strategy. It is a tendency to revert back to a previous strategy after switching "mental set." Some authors have also explained the verbal fluency difficulties of this group as a problem of set maintenance (Dubois et al., 1991). Verbal fluency tasks typically require the person to list as many words as possible that begin with a specified letter or belong to a specified category. The problem appears most evident when the person uses several different letters. First, the task is to name as many words, within a 1-minute time period, that start with the letter *F,* then to name all the possibilities that begin with *A,* then with *S.* In such tasks, during the middle of the *S* sequence, patients with PD may revert to words that begin with *F* or *A* (Lees & Smith, 1983).

A difficulty in "time tagging" events is a problem in temporal structuring. Researchers have reported patients with

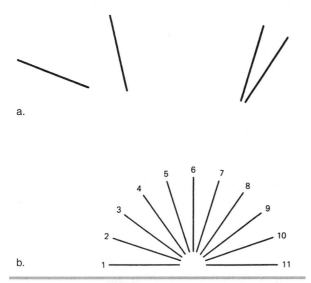

Figure 15.3 The Judgment of Line Orientation Test. Two examples of double-line stimuli (a) to be matched to the template below (b). (Reproduced from Benton, A. L., Hamsher, K. D, Varney, N. R., & Spreen, O. [1983]. *Contributions to Neuropsychological Assessment.* New York: Oxford University Press, by permission.)

PD may have memory for news events without associated memory for the event order (Sagar, Sullivan, Gabrieli, Corkin, & Growdon, 1988). In daily life this can translate into problems remembering "when" medications have been taken or learning the sequence of new tasks. Temporal ordering is an executive problem that interacts with memory.

Not all of the frontal lobe is involved in the dysexecutive problems of PD; rather, the premotor area and the basal ganglia with its associated projections to the frontal lobes are implicated.

Language/Speech

PD typically does not produce classical aphasia. Also, few, if any, linguistic impairments appear involving grammar and sentence structure (Dubois et al., 1991). Thus, general language processing and comprehension are intact. Some researchers indicate that more subtle problems in understanding grammatic complexity may be evident on more sophisticated neuropsychological tests (Levin, Tomer, & Rey, 1992). However, close to 70% of patients with PD have difficulties with articulation and the neuromechanical aspects of speech production (Levin et al., 1992). We have mentioned that patients with PD lose voice amplitude and vocal emotional expression **(dysphonia),** which results in monotonous voice. Other speech irregularities may include segmented accelerated bursts of speech **(tachyphemia)** and compulsive word or phrase repetition **(palilalia).**

Tests that measure aspects of expressive or receptive aphasia show little impairment in patients with PD. However, patients may perform poorly on semantic fluency and word-finding tasks (such as the Boston Naming Test). However, as discussed earlier, these tasks are better conceptualized as belonging in another domain (executive functioning). Behavioral assessment of speech is the method that will demonstrate the characteristic disarticulation problems.

Memory

Compared with AD, memory functioning is relatively spared in PD, even in patients with PD with dementia (Sagar et al., 1988). Digit repetition and block-tapping repetition are usually preserved (for review, see Dubois et al., 1991). On tests involving episodic memory, paired associate learning, auditory verbal learning, and visual reproduction of geometric designs, patients with PD do show a recall deficit but demonstrate encoding and registration of declarative material through recognition tasks (for reviews, see Dubois et al., 1991; Levin et al., 1992). The implication of this pattern is that strategic memory

processes for organization and retrieval of declarative information are defective.

Nondeclarative learning presents a mixed bag in PD. Verbal priming and perceptual-motor adaptation are largely unimpaired in patients with PD without dementia (Crosson, 1992; Heindel, Salmon, Shults, Wallcke, & Butters, 1989). However, nondeclarative learning, which relies on intact motor or executive functioning, is often deficient. The ability to learn new motor skills declines as the disease progresses (Crosson, 1992). This is not surprising, considering the general dysregulation of the motor system. Procedural learning, measured by rule-learning tasks, such as the Tower of London, may be deficient, but results are mixed. At times, patients with PD perform poorly because of a problem in maintaining mental set for the rule, again pointing more to a problem in executive functioning than to a memory registration problem.

Most of the apparent memory difficulties experienced by patients with PD stem from interactions among the executive, the memory registration, and the motor systems. Patients with PD may show difficulty in motor skill acquisition. Patients with PD without dementia can passively register declarative information in short- and long-term memory. However, many have trouble using this information effectively. This includes effectively organizing information to be recalled, maintaining a consistent mental set when trying to learn or retrieve information, and time tagging or knowing not only that something has occurred but "knowing when" it happened.

Mood, Emotion, Personality, and Insight

A large proportion of patients with PD suffer from depression. Debate continues whether the mood disorder is a primary dysfunction of the disease or a secondary result of the medications used to treat the disease. To those suffering from depression, the debate may seem academic. Some researchers also suggest that depression may be a natural reaction to realizing that the patient has PD. Although this probably occurs to some degree, it does not seem to adequately explain the occurrence of depression. Patients with PD appear to be more depressed than patients with many other chronic diseases (Raskin et al., 1990).

Although few standardized neuropsychological tests measure expression of emotion, researchers have studied this in patients with PD. The findings are somewhat equivocal, but some suggest that patients with PD have a dysfunction in emotional expression associated with a right-frontal focus (for example, see Ross, 1985). These patients may have difficulty in showing an angry face or a surprised face but may be able to recognize emotional expression. Does this finding suggest a cortical deficit in emotional expression? Or rather, a problem in the more mechanical aspects of emotional expression? Because of the "masked facies," it is difficult to determine whether emotional expression is lost or just diminished in frequency and intensity. Future research may help answer this question.

TREATMENTS FOR PARKINSON'S DISEASE

Without treatment, patients with PD are souls trapped in the cages of their bodies, unable to command or coax their mutinous muscles into action. Out of the tragedy of this disease, however, has emerged a palette of treatments that are worth examining, not only for addressing PD but because they represent creative and forward-thinking approaches to the treatment of aging-related brain disorders in general. Interestingly, the treatment for PD appears to be traveling full circle from surgery to drugs to surgery. In addition, gene therapies, tissue implants, and various approaches to prevention are on the horizon.

The first surgical approaches to PD in the late 1950s were based on the idea of alleviating symptoms by interfering with what was thought to be "malfunctioning circuitry" in the basal ganglia through heat-induced surgical lesioning of the global pallidus. By 1960, a group of Swedish researchers could demonstrate motor improvement in a significant number of their patients. However, this treatment preceded the advent of computed transaxial tomography (CT) scans, MRIs, and the precision stereotaxic and electrode recording tools needed to locate specific neurons. The imprecision of this surgery made negative side effects likely.

The discovery of L-dopa as a possible treatment for PD in 1961 (Birkmayer & Hornykiewicz, 1961) was revolutionary and heralded a new approach to the treatment of neurodegenerative diseases. With the advent of a seeming miracle drug, surgical approaches fell by the wayside by the late 1960s. Today, there exists a menu of drugs that act not only on the dopaminergic system but also on related neurotransmitter systems.

In Paris in the 1860s, **anticholinergics** extracted from plant sources (such as scopolamine from jimsonweed, black henbane, or deadly nightshade) were the first treatments used for PD. Although the mechanism of action was not known initially, these solanaceous alkaloids acted by blocking the action of acetylcholine, offering some symptomatic control of motor systems for tremor and rigidity. However, the side effects of "anticholinergic intoxication" limit their usefulness. Possible systemic effects, including dry mouth, blurred vision, constipation, weak bladder, and cognitive effects such as memory problems, confusion, slurred speech, and visual hallucinations, can create more than a small nuisance for patients. Physicians now prescribe synthetic anticholinergics of different types, if at all, during the early stages of the disease, and usually in combination with levodopa.

L-Dopa is the left (levo) form of the dopa molecule, a simple amino acid. Prepared as a drug, it is called *levodopa*. Plants and animals manufacture it, and it appears naturally in fava beans and other legumes. Levodopa, being a dopamine precursor, directly metabolizes into dopamine. Cousins of levodopa include dopamine agonists and analogs that mimic the action of dopamine by stimulating its release, whereas reuptake blockers work by preventing reuptake at the synapse to retard metabolic removal. Drugs acting on the dopaminergic neurotransmitter system are still the best family of drugs found to alleviate tremor, bradykinesia, and rigidity. The difficulty with these orally ingested drugs, however, is that they convert to dopamine in the body and do not easily penetrate the blood–brain barrier. Probably less than 1% actually crosses over to be useful to the striatum, causing systemic buildup of dopamine in organs such as the liver and kidneys. Therefore, medications usually combine L-dopa with a decarboxylase inhibitor (such as carbidopa) to prevent the conversion to dopamine until it crosses the blood–brain barrier. Because carbidopa cannot cross the blood–brain barrier, it acts as a protector against conversion in the body until it releases the levodopa into the brain. This arrangement delivers about five times the dopamine to the targeted area, greatly enhancing the effectiveness of the drug.

Physicians may also use other drugs to treat PD, either as adjuncts or to counteract side effects of long-term dopaminergic drug usage. Doctors may add monoamine oxidase B (MAO-B) inhibitors, antidepressants, and agents to counteract the effect of **dyskinesia** to the complex menu, which must be taken at intervals as frequently as every 4 hours. These drugs are extending the survival of patients with PD, but not without a price. The side effects of dopaminergic drugs, including vivid nightmares, disturbed sleep, perceptual illusions, and hypomania can be very disturbing. Also, after a long course of treatment, usually 10 years or so, the drugs lose effectiveness, dopaminergic neurons become hypersensitive, and the therapeutic window becomes shorter in duration, resulting in a severe on/off syndrome. During the "on" phase, the drug exerts its action but may overshoot, resulting in

Neuropsychology in Action 15.2

Pallidotomy Surgery: A Case Report

by Barbara L. Malamut   Ph.D.

The following case report profiles one "typical" patient who underwent right pallidotomy in an attempt to alleviate some of his adverse motor fluctuations. M.J. is a 56-year-old, right-handed man with a 16-year history of Parkinson's disease (PD). His symptoms first began on the left side of his body with abnormal spontaneous movements of his foot, including a rhythmic tapping and an involuntary curling up of his toes. After about 10 years, his motor deficits worsened and he suffered from significant bilateral symptoms including bradykinesia, rigidity, and motor fluctuations. He had dyskinesias when his medication was "on" and freezing when "off." Other than PD, M.J. had no other major medical or psychiatric problems. He was forced to go on medical disability 3 years ago. He has few hobbies, spending his days maintaining the house, walking the dog, doing yard work, and some cooking. M.J. acknowledges a feeling of depression, which increases when he does not feel well.

When he arrived for his presurgical neuropsychological assessment, M.J. presented as an alert, oriented, pleasant, and cooperative man with a stiff, slow gait. Dystonic posturing of his head and upper torso was evident when sitting. Although his facial expression was fixed, he displayed a range of affect. A moderate tremor, which was greater on the left, was also evident. His spontaneous speech was soft in volume, with a choppy cadence, but his language was intact.

No disturbance in thinking was noted during the interview. Results of neuropsychological testing indicated a few areas of mild impairment that were consistent with PD. These included problems with speed of mental processing, working memory for both auditory-verbal and visuospatial information, visual scanning, graphomotor control, and retrieval of verbal and visuospatial material. Recognition memory was intact. Consistent with his self-reported history, M.J. was depressed, socially isolated, and withdrawn.

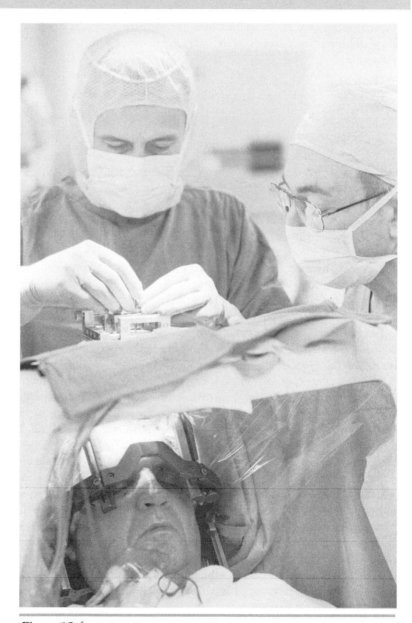

Figure 15.4   In the pallidotomy surgery for Parkinson's disease, the surgeon is using the triangulation of three coordinates of the frame to pinpoint the patient's globus pallidus. (Reproduced from Ueckert, S. [1996, January 22]. In R. SoRelle, "New procedure slows effects of Parkinsons: Surgery can restore balance to system." *Houston Chronicle,* 4a, by permission.)

(continued)

M.J. was a good candidate for pallidotomy because he was generally in good physical and mental health, his neuropsychological profile did not indicate cognitive decline or dementia, and his medications had lost much of their effectiveness. The day of M.J.'s surgery, he was injected with a local anesthetic and fitted with a stereotactic frame necessary to locate the area to be lesioned (Figure 15.4). With the frame in place, a computed transaxial tomography scan was done and compared with his previous magnetic resonance image, to identify the precise placement of critical brain structures. After drilling a tiny hole through M.J.'s skull, the surgeon inserted a small canula, or tube, through the dura mater and snaked a microelectric probe through his brain toward his right pallidum. As the probe approached the area of neuronal hyperactivity, sound bursts became more frequent. The surgeon first stimulated the area to observe motor response. (M.J. was conscious so his responses to stimulation could be tested and any adverse affects on vision or speech could be noted before actual lesions were made.) Being careful not to affect the nearby optic tract, the surgeon then made a small heat-induced lesion to permanently destroy the overactive neurons of the pallidum. After this surgery, M.J. needed a few stitches and was released within 24 hours. M.J. experienced no surgical complications.

Six months later, M.J. returned for a neuropsychological re-evaluation to monitor his cognitive status. He reported that since surgery, his left-sided rigidity had disappeared and he no longer had pain or involuntary movements when walking. On observation, he no longer had dystonic posturing but did continue to walk with a slow, shuffling gait. In addition, his speech was now normal in volume, but he had developed a mild stammer. Overall, M.J. was pleased with the results of his surgery, although he realized this was not a cure. Improvement relative to his preoperative neuropsychological evaluation was noted in speed of mental processing, working memory for both auditory-verbal and visuospatial information, and graphomotor control. M.J.'s problems with depression remained, and he began taking antidepressant medication and agreed to begin psychotherapy.

This case raises several critical and common issues regarding pallidotomy surgery. Although pallidotomy effectively alleviates many motor symptoms and pain associated with later stages of PD, it does not cure the disease or return the patient to preinjury functioning. The long-term benefits and risks of pallidotomy are unknown. Studies currently under way are examining the cognitive sequelae of the pallidotomy procedure in comparison with the natural progression of the disease. The newest procedure, approved by the U.S. Food and Drug Administration in July 1997, is deep thalamic stimulation, which works as a type of electronic pacemaker interfering with the ventral intermediate thalamic nucleus. The surgery, performed like pallidotomy, primarily reduces tremor but may have little effect on the other PD symptoms. This surgery, unlike pallidotomy, does not result in permanent lesions. Other treatment modalities currently being explored, such as gene therapy and fetal implant surgery, may be promising avenues for the future. These procedures may actually arrest or reverse PD, rather than just ameliorate some of its motor symptoms.

---

an effect akin to an overdose. In this phase, severe dyskinesia resembling choreic movements and dystonia involving muscular posturing may result. This may cycle quickly to "off" symptoms, which include the disease symptoms, particularly freezing, severe tremor, and panic.

L-Dopa could not live up to the hopes that pharmacologic substitution of missing dopamine would be sufficient treatment. The debilitating "on/off" drug phenomena led to the return of surgical techniques. These operations currently are intended for those for whom the drug treatments are no longer effective. Now, however, high-tech precision imaging of the brain results in a greater chance of locating the offending neurons. Currently, two types of operations are being conducted. The first operations focus on surgical lesioning of offending neurons. The second wave of surgeries, deep brain stimulation operations, involves nondestructive electrical interference.

Pallidotomy, the PD surgery of the late 1950s, was revived in the early 1990s. Surgeons use it in an attempt to alleviate the abnormal uncontrolled movement of dyskinesia and the frequent on/off symptoms. In pallidotomy, surgeons lesion the ventral (that is, the internal portion) of the globus pallidus by heat-coagulating the neurons.

Studies have shown that the decreased dopamine in the basal ganglia causes the motor portions of the pallidum to become overactive. This hyperfiring, in turn, inhibits the thalamus and portions of the brainstem (which causes bradykinesia and dyskinesia). Lesioning the posteroventral portion of the pallidum arrests this excessive output to the thalamus and brainstem (Neuropsychology in Action 15.2). Surgeons use a second lesioning procedure on a portion of the thalamus, **thalotomy,** to attack tremor. Interestingly, they also use this procedure for patients with tremor caused by multiple sclerosis, essential tremor of old age, cerebellar tremor, and poststroke tremor. These two operations are typically unilateral and not done in combination. In fact, the lesion sites for the two operations are only millimeters apart. Bilateral lesions done at the same time appear to greatly increase the risk for cognitive deficits. In pallidotomy, the risk may be greatest for memory difficulty and confusion. For thalotomy, speech dysfunction appears to be the greatest risk.

Deep brain stimulation procedures represent the newest variation of these surgeries. The target site is the same as in thalotomy, except that instead of a destructive lesion, surgeons transmit electrical interference to the neurons via a permanently implanted lead. An implanted adjustable neurostimulator operates somewhat like a pacemaker and can be turned on and off by the patient.

Although these surgeries represent new hope for patients for whom drugs are no longer effective, they are palliative, not curative. Patients experience relief of symptoms, and about 80% may improve, but they must still take medication. The progression of the disease continues.

Huntington's Disease

Huntington's disease (HD), although rare, has been well studied in the last quarter of the 20th century. Why the resurgent interest in a disease that physicians described more than a century ago and then seemingly left to languish until the 1960s? From 1872, when George Huntington described this "hereditary chorea," until the 1960s, researchers paid little attention to this neurologic disease, which causes adults in the prime of their lives to seemingly "go insane," develop a tendency toward suicide, and suffer devastating motor impairment in the form of chorea. Families of HD sufferers have spearheaded the search for the gene that controls the disease. For neuropsychology, the specificity of this disease offers a window to learn about the widespread behavioral effects of caudate nucleus deterioration.

George Huntington was not the first to describe the twisting, writhing, grimacing choreic movements, which are reminiscent of a puppet at the hands of a sinister master. In the 16th century, "peculiar" families were described, but the hereditary nature of the disease did not appear to come into the medical consciousness until evolutionary theory emerged in the mid-1800s (Wexler, 1995). Other physicians before Huntington hypothesized about the hereditary nature of the disease, but it was young George Huntington, just 22 years old, who in his 1872 article described the disorder most clearly and most completely. He emphasized the emotional and psychological aspects of the disease, describing "the tendency to insanity, and sometimes that form of insanity that leads to suicide." This became the classic account of the disorder, forever after associated with the name Huntington.

The story of the search for the "Huntington's gene" begins in the late 1960s. After years of relatively little scientific interest in this apparently incurable disorder, two families picked up the torch. Marjorie Guthrie, ex-wife of the singer Woody Guthrie, who had HD, founded an organization of HD families to raise money for research. The Wexlers, whose story is told in the book *Mapping*

Fate (Neuropsychology in Action 15.3) were instrumental in pushing basic scientific research toward the search for the gene. Nancy Wexler, at risk for HD herself, was active in the study of colonies of HD families in Venezuela. Largely through the energy generated by these and other at-risk families, researchers pinpointed the offending gene in 1993. This discovery does not translate into an immediate cure or treatment. However, it does provide the first hopeful step in that direction.

HD is a progressive subcortical dementia. This rare disease, which affects about 5 to 10 in 100,000 people, is linked to the gene *ITI5* on chromosome 4 and is passed on by one parent in an autosomal dominant inheritance pattern. As far as genes go, *ITI5* is a big one, with more than 300,000 base pairs, and it is evident in all tissues of the body. People with normal versions of the gene have between 11 and 34 repeats of the trinucleotide CAG (cytosine, adenine, guanine), which codes the gene. However, those with the HD-positive gene have 37 to as many as 100 or more repeats. More repeats entail earlier onset and greater severity of symptoms. Some overlap exists between normal and abnormal functioning, making 35 to 40 a borderline range. When operating normally, *ITI5* produces the amino acid glutamine. It is not clear how the body uses glutamine, or the exact function of *ITI5*, but researchers do know that expanded gene sequence repeats on other genes characterize inherited diseases such as myotonic dystrophy and spinobulbar muscular dystrophy, which affected President Kennedy.

Autosomal dominance translates into a 50% chance of acquiring the disease. Because this disorder runs in families, HD is not suspect unless there is a family history. In those with a family history, a simple genetic test can determine the presence of the disease, but much to the surprise of many scientists, most people at risk have chosen not to be tested (see Neuropsychology in Action 15.3).

NEUROPATHOLOGY OF HUNTINGTON'S DISEASE

Deterioration of the caudate nucleus bilaterally plays a primary role in the neuropathology of HD, although ultimately, HD affects multiple brain systems. The caudate nucleus is one of the structures that comprise the striatum, together with the globus pallidus and putamen. The striatum is part of the basal ganglia, which is responsible for modulating motor activity. However, the role of the striatum is somewhat different from that of the substantia nigra, which is primarily affected in PD. Although the substantia nigra is responsible for the proper initiation and termination of movements, the

Neuropsychology in Action 15.3

Testing Fate: Would You Want to Know If You Were Going to Get Huntington's Disease?

by Mary V. Spiers

Would you take a test to determine whether you would develop an inherited brain disease in the future? This is the question facing family members of people with Huntington's disease (HD), a subcortical dementia with devastating motor and cognitive consequences. Fortunately, the disease is rare, but if it runs in your family, you have a 50% chance of acquiring this autosomal dominant genetic disease. There is no cure and there is no treatment, and if you do have it, you may pass it on to your children. You are also likely to die while in your 50s. Would knowing this help you to plan? Plan not to have children, perhaps plan not to even marry, or perhaps try to pack a lot of living into a short time? Would knowing lessen your worry? Or would knowing be a traumatic experience? Would you consider suicide? Would you always be on guard watching and waiting for the first symptoms to appear?

These questions face the 125,000 people at risk for the disease in the United States. In 1983, researchers discovered a genetic marker that paved the way for the first testing for HD. Then 10 years later, in 1993, researchers located the gene *IT15* (named "Interesting Transcript") on the short arm of chromosome 4, and the test became much more accurate. Only a simple blood test is required. Scientists predicted a flood at testing centers, but there has been only a trickle of people, about 6% of those at risk. Why is this? The answers come from those at risk. Alice Wexler, author of the book *Mapping Fate,* describes the story of her own family, and of her mother, who died of HD. After her mother's diagnosis in 1968, the Wexler family, led by her father and sister, spearheaded one of the most innovative approaches to scientific investigation, bringing scientists and families together in collaborative efforts to search for the HD

gene. The book chronicles the scientific and personal odyssey of the discovery of the gene. Alice Wexler describes her own ambivalence and the feelings of others who have struggled with the idea of getting tested. Some have taken the test, mentioning control and relief from uncertainty as major reasons. Others are concerned about confidentiality of their medical records and possible denial of insurance coverage. For those who have tested positive, the experience is often traumatic and, surprisingly, may not alleviate the anxiety because there is no certainty as to when the symptoms may develop. Even for those who test negative, the result may come as a shock as they realize they have built their lives around the possibility that they might acquire a fatal disease. Alice Wexler, like so many others, has decided against being tested. If you were at risk, you could test your fate. But would you want to?

striatum controls the proper timing, ordering, and sequencing of movement patterns (Bradshaw & Mattingly, 1995). The caudate nucleus has reciprocal projections (afferent and efferent neurons) to a number of limbic and prefrontal areas. Although HD primarily affects the caudate, it may also affect the putamen, other areas of the striatum, and possibly other limbic system structures such as the hippocampus. By the end stages of the disease, the frontal lobes may also shrink by 20% to 30% (Vonsattel, 1992).

In patients with HD who are showing the symptoms of the disease, structural neuroimaging techniques such as CT or MRI clearly reveal the loss of cell mass in the caudate and a widening of the ventricles. On MRI, the volume of the caudate and other basal ganglia structures is clearly reduced. The apparent structural deterioration of the caudate corresponds to a downward progression of behavioral functioning. Functional neuroimaging via positron emission tomography scan is more sensitive to early changes and can show hypometabolism in the frontal and striatal regions before deterioration is evident

structurally (Hasselbalch et al., 1992) and before a clinical diagnosis (Penny & Young, 1993).

CLINICAL PRESENTATION AND NEUROPSYCHOLOGICAL PROFILE OF HUNTINGTON'S DISEASE

How do the symptomatology and neuropsychological functioning of the HD sufferers differ from profiles of AD or PD? HD results in a unique pattern of impairment in which difficulties associated with frontal lobe functioning and motor functioning are prominent. Although PD also results in frontal executive system and motor impairment, the presentation differs in some ways. The caudate nucleus, rather than the substantia nigra, is the main culprit in HD.

Many of the cognitive difficulties of patients with HD likely stem from a breakdown in premotor frontal lobe functioning and the connectivity of the caudate-frontal system. Early in the disease process, patients with HD show characteristic frontal signs of rigidity, perseveration, and difficulty switching mental set in daily life, as well as on neuropsychological testing. Some dysfunctions stem from the impacts that poor executive organizational abilities and attention/concentration problems have on cognitive functioning. For example, the memory difficulties of patients with HD appear largely attributable to poor executive functioning. Capacity for learning new information declines in HD, but the picture differs from the AD profile. Patients with HD demonstrate low levels of free recall but improve greatly if given a recognition test. Why? Apparently they encode new information, or multiple-choice recognition tests would not aid performance. Patients with HD appear to suffer primarily from a retrieval problem caused by ineffective memory search operations. They may have a poor ability to differentiate what they know from what they do not know (for review, see Brandt & Bylsma, 1993). This problem in strategic memory processing and metamemory (knowledge of one's own memory) appears attributable largely to frontal lobe and executive functioning difficulties rather than to hippocampal involvement, although both may interact to some degree. Executive difficulties probably also interact with other cognitive processes such as verbal and spatial conceptualization and processing.

The final manner by which the striatofrontal lobe complex may exert its effects on cognitive functioning is through multiple connections to other areas of the brain. Patients with HD appear to have difficulty orienting themselves in space, which may be a parietal dysfunction. For example, the old-time child's game of blind man's bluff, in which one child is spun around blindfolded and then required to tag others by sound alone as they call out, would be difficult for patients with HD. Potegal (1971) has explained this egocentric spatial disorder as a problem in readjusting, or the ineffectiveness of the caudate in modulating changes in spatial position. Although research has not yet confirmed this interpretation, it appears reasonable, given the role of the striatum in modulating other motor activity.

The emotional difficulties experienced by many patients with HD likely result from prefrontal and limbic system interactions. Patients with HD exhibit a disproportionately high degree of affective disturbance, in the form of depression and manic depression. The suicide rate of 6% (Farrer, 1986) in HD is greater than in other degenerative disorders. Are these emotional disturbances a response to a desperate situation, or perhaps a symptom of frontal-subcortical impairment? Suicide may be an understandable response, given the severe cognitive devastation that people in the early stages of the disease can anticipate. HD sufferers are no strangers to what will befall them. They have seen a parent, a grandparent, aunts, and uncles succumb to the same horrible disease. However, the rate of emotional disturbance in HD is greater than expected. Depression is the most common affective disturbance (Brandt & Bylsma, 1993), but the literature reports a wide range of affective and psychiatric disturbances in patients with HD. These include anxiety, apathy, irritability, impulsivity, aggression, sexual disturbance, schizophreniform thought disorder, and psychosis involving hallucinations and delusions (for reviews, see Brandt & Bylsma, 1993; Bradshaw & Mattingly, 1995). Interestingly, the emotional disturbances often precede motor symptoms. At this point, the affected individual may not even be aware of his or her diagnosis. These emotional symptoms can be best conceptualized as a symptom of the disease, or a predisposition toward symptoms such as depression. However, this is not to say that reactions to the illness do not contribute to the picture of emotional disturbance. A reaction to the severity of the disease can compound a predisposition to depression.

The motor difficulties of HD are characterized by **chorea:** twisting, writhing, undulating, grimacing movements of the face and body. Interestingly, overmedicated PD patients also show choreic movements. This has led to the hypothesis that the dopamine system lies at the root of both these problems. Obviously, this gross-motor dysfunction seriously hinders everyday activity. Like patients with PD, patients with HD are slow motorically (bradykinesia). Also, as in PD, the chorea tends to disappear with sleep and increase with stress. Unlike PD, patients with HD walk with a wide-based gait. Their speech is dysarthric, becoming increasingly erratic in its rate of production and staccato with intermittent pauses. They become clumsy and uncoordinated, unable to do fine-grained work. In testing patients with HD, these severe motor difficulties disrupt performance on other tests that have a motor component, even if the test is designed to measure other functions such as visual problem solving. In assessing the cognitive performance of patients with HD, motor-free tests provide the clearest picture. Currently, no cure exists for HD, and the treatments that exist focus primarily on the relief of emotional symptoms such as depression and hallucinations.

◼ Creutzfeldt–Jakob Disease

Creutzfeldt–Jakob Disease (CJD), a dementia long hidden in obscurity because of its rarity (one that most neuropsychologists have never seen personally in one of their patients), has suddenly leaped into the limelight because of its connection to "mad cow disease" and because of the fear that its incidence is increasing. CJD is a compelling disease, unlike the other dementias we have considered, because of both its speed of progression and mode of transmission. With a malignantly cascading decline over 3 to 4 months, it is the most quickly progressing dementia. Scientists have long known that humans can transmit this disease via transplants of affected neural tissue, cornea transplants, or contamination via medical procedures, but it is now also becoming clear that CJD and its variants can cross species through the consumption of tainted meat containing neural tissue. Extensive spongelike holes appear in the brains of its victims, giving it the fitting name "spongiform encephalopathy" (SE). The mechanism by which the brain becomes infected has eluded scientists for decades because CJD does not manifest the symptoms of typical acute infections. Virologists, biologists, and chemists are joining clinicians to unravel the mysteries of this disease.

In the early 1900s, Bertha, a 23-year-old German woman, was a patient of Hans Gerhard Creutzfeldt. Creutzfeldt, an assistant of Alois Alzheimer at the Munich Psychiatric Clinic, was, like Alzheimer, trying to clarify the differences and similarities between behaviors understood as "psychiatric" and "neurologic." Creutzfeldt noticed that Bertha showed many behaviors typical of other mental illnesses, such as believing she was possessed by the devil, neglecting her hygiene, and posturing strangely. However, other symptoms suggested frank brain impairment. Bertha also had an unsteady gait, twitchy eyes, a voluntary tremor, and a tendency to giggle inappropriately. These latter symptoms, which we now recognize as indicating subcortical motor and emotional dysfunction, were Creutzfeldt's clues. After Bertha died, Creutzfeldt examined her brain tissue under the microscope. What he saw were the little "stars" of astrogliosis (Figure 15.5) dotting her brain. In 1920, he published his article that describes Bertha. With the synchronicity that often occurs in science, Dr. Jakob reported a similar case in 1921. Creutzfeldt and Jakob thus share the distinction of discovery.

CJD is a quickly progressive subcortical dementia estimated to affect only 1 person in 1 million people per year. This is extremely rare even in comparison with HD, which affects 5 to 10 per 100,000 people. CJD appears around the world with the same prevalence and does not appear to vary across groups or cultures. Although Creutzfeldt's patient was young, most cases have been in their 50s or 60s. For the most part, researchers have hypothesized that CJD spontaneously arises as a random mutation. As long as it is not passed on to others, the disease dies out with its victim. Some variants of CJD may

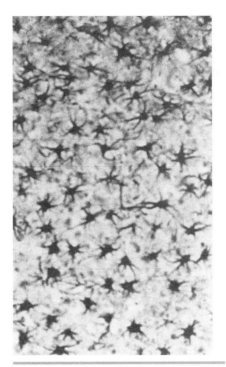

Figure 15.5 The dark stars of astrogliosis. (Courtesy D. Carlton Gajdusek.)

manifest themselves differently in the behavior of those it afflicts. For example, the extremely rare familial CJD variant termed **Gerstmann-Straussler-Scheinker syndrome (GSS),** reported in only a handful of families, results in a "fatal insomnia." This is the only reported incidence of transmission other than through external infection. Researchers believe that in older people CJD incubates for years before manifesting.

One of the most alarming aspects of this disease, and the reason it has been catapulted out of obscurity, is its relation to other SEs. Variations of SE, as mentioned earlier, are aptly named: Portions of the brain actually resemble a sponge, because of the microscopic pattern of holes. Researchers have identified SEs in species from minks to sheep (scrapie) to cows (bovine spongiform encephalopathy [BSE] or "mad cow disease") to humans (CJD and kuru). In his book *Deadly Feasts,* Richard Rhodes chronicles the history of the SEs. He describes the history and current status of research into CJD and kuru. **Kuru** is a SE that the Fore people of Papua New Guinea contract, which presented itself when they began ritually cannibalizing their dead at the beginning of the 1900s. Rhodes (1997) also describes the history of the research, which suggests that SEs can easily leap across species, and that they are probably variations of the same disease process.

In his book *Deadly Feasts* (1997), Richard Rhodes traces the history of spongiform encephalopathies (SEs) in humans and other species. He reflects scientists' views that these diseases are variations of the same infectious process, and that the ingestion or injection of diseased neural tissue can spread many SEs within or across species. He also forecasts an alarming increase in human encephalopathies over the next few years if people do not contain and eliminate the disease in the animal food supply.

How exactly did mad cow disease (bovine spongiform encephalopathy [BSE]) arise and become a threat to humans? Farmers routinely give cattle protein supplements: dairy cows all through their life, and beef cattle for end-stage fattening. As long as farmers fed cattle largely vegetable protein (such as soy) or fish protein together with their diet of grass or hay, and no transmission from randomly affected cattle

occurred, BSE did not arise. However, during the 1980s, a series of events in Great Britain triggered a BSE epidemic. One factor was that, because the pound was devalued, the price of soy and fish meal increased, so the agricultural industry began to rely more heavily on animal sources of protein. Animal protein typically comes from the by-products of slaughterhouses—bones and offal (guts, heads, tails, and blood) are processed into bonemeal pellets or powder and fed to other cattle. As long as the rendering process killed any disease, bonemeal was a good source of protein. During the 1980s in Britain, changes in the rendering process decreased the bonemeal processing temperature and abandoned fat removal, no longer destroying BSE in tissue. By the late 1980s, BSE had spread throughout Great Britain and had infected more than 2000 cattle. Farmers noticed that their cattle were "becoming aggressive, rather nervous, knocking

other cows. . . . and becoming dangerous to handle. . . . If you shooed her, she would stumble, particularly on the back legs, and go down, and then scrabble along" (p. 172). In 1988, the British government ordered milk from affected cows destroyed. However, not until an outbreak in humans occurred in 1996 were massive amounts of beef cattle destroyed. The base rate for CJD is 1 in 1 million people older than 50. CJD cases developing under that age are extremely rare. In the world, there had been only 10 known adolescent cases. Only with kuru-associated cannibalism did researchers notice that young people acquired spongiform encephalopathy with a shortened incubation period. Between 1991 and 1996, 10 cases of a CJD variant of people younger than 40 emerged in Great Britain. According to statistical probability, this is an epidemic. Only time will tell whether awareness has stopped the spread of this disease.

In his book he predicts an alarming increase in the incidence of CJD (Neuropsychology in Action 15.4).

NEUROPATHOLOGY OF CREUTZFELDT-JAKOB DISEASE

The cause of CJD has eluded scientists until recently because it is a transmissible or infectious agent with none of the usual symptoms of acute infection. In fact, scientists first thought that kuru could be genetic, because it occurred primarily among the women and children of the Fore people. However, only the women and children were eating the dead in a mortuary love feast. Men believed contact with women weakened them, and they did not partake in the ritual. Acute infections are easily identified by noticing the body's defensive immune system response. Inflammation, increased numbers of lymph cells in cerebrospinal fluid, and fever are typical, yet none of these symptoms occurs in CJD or any of the SEs.

No one knows from where this infectious agent originally arose. Perhaps it originated from a randomly occur-

ring mutation. This might account for the rarity in the population at large and that CJD occurs with equal frequency throughout the world. However, in the last century, SE has also been transmitted by eating infected neural tissue. This has happened both within species such as cows (BSE or mad cow disease) and across species. SE has developed in mice, hamsters, and even primates injected with kuru. CJD has developed in humans who have eaten infected meat (see Neuropsychology in Action 15.4). Many scientists now believe CJD to be a slow virus that incubates over years, perhaps in the spleen, and is camouflaged in cells so as not to be recognized as an invader. Some have also hypothesized that slow viruses are responsible for AD, PD, and amyotrophic lateral sclerosis (ALS).

What exactly do SEs, specifically CJD, do to the brain? Certain areas of the brain look spongy, taking on a characteristic spongiform pattern. CJD, like kuru, attacks the cerebellum, but it also damages the cerebrum. Microscopically, the "stars" of astrogliosis that Creutzfeldt found were the result of the glial cells, or the "cleanup machines" of the brain, filling in after neuronal tissue had died. Astrogliosis is the aftereffect, not the cause of the disease. Amyloid plaques are also numerous, but as discussed earlier, these are not specific to CJD but are also found in other diseases such as AD.

Patricia Merz, with the aid of her electron microscope, first found small, twisted, sticklike fibers in the cells of tissue samples of sheep with the sheep version of SE, called "scrapie" (Merz, Somerville, Wisneiwski, & Iqbal, 1981). Interestingly, she could then correctly distinguish between healthy control subjects and affected victims with CJD from these scrapie-associated fibrils (SAFs) in spleen and neural tissue samples. Merz hypothesizes that SAFs may be the disease agent, which incubates in the spleen over years before affecting the brain. SAFs have been found in kuru and CJD brains, but not in AD, PD, or ALS brains. This was the first indication of a disease agent specific to SEs such as CJD.

The name that has become popular in referring to SAFs is *prions* (Pruisiner, 1982). Currently, several different variations or strains have been identified. Prion proteins (PrPs), the protein components of prions, which are present in both normal and afflicted individuals, have been the target of research interest in CJD. However, infected PrP resists normal protein digestion via enzymes. Interestingly, both diseased and normal PrP have the same DNA specifications. This helps explain the riddle of why the body's immune system does not attack the infected protein. It does not recognize the protein as foreign! However, one of the unsolved mysteries of this disease is to understand how a normal protein changes to an abnormal protein with the same structural DNA. Several hypotheses exist to explain the mechanism of action. One is that there may be a small virus, termed a *virion,* that has not yet been identified. Proteins are not known to mutate on their own, but perhaps small bits of "naked" nucleic acid infected with the virion, divorced from their cells, attach themselves to proteins and force the mutation. Another explanation involves an interesting nonbiological form of replication. Carleton Gajdusek (1988), who won the Nobel Prize in Medicine, has postulated that something else must be transporting the infectious agent, because even when the nucleic acid is destroyed by radiation, the "infection" persists. He explains this as a crystal nucleation process. Similar to how crystals such as diamonds form in nature, the infection provides the pattern that is the nucleus, or catalyst, for the reaction. Successive proteins then mutate by patterning themselves after the original. If this sounds like science fiction, scientists have already dubbed this the "Ice-9" metaphor after a Kurt Vonnegut novel in which all the water on earth turns to ice, in a crystallization process.

Whether a yet undiscovered virion, nuclear crystallization, or some other process is causing CJD, scientists are pursuing this disease with renewed vigor because of its unfortunate recent resurgence. We now turn to the clinical aspects of CJD.

CLINICAL PRESENTATION AND NEUROPSYCHOLOGICAL PROFILE OF CREUTZFELDT-JAKOB DISEASE

Even though emotional symptoms may be first evident, the hallmark of CJD, as well as other SEs such as kuru, is motor symptomatology. The motor symptoms are those expected of cerebellar and subcortical dysfunction. Movements become uncoordinated, walking resembles a drunken stagger, and speech is slurred and inarticulate. Involuntary tremors and choreiform grimaces emerge, and finally victims cannot swallow and thus may die of starvation. Visual function alters, eventually leading to blindness in some people. These cerebellar and subcortical motor problems may follow initial, emotionally related complaints of mood disorders such as anxiety, depression or hypomania, fatigue, difficulty sleeping, and attention/concentration problems. As with the confusion over Creutzfeldt's patient Bertha, these symptoms may lead one to first believe that a pure mood disorder is present, or in Bertha's case, which was more advanced, a delusional or psychotic disorder. However, the classic motor symptoms quickly reveal themselves.

The dementia of CJD and its variants has a rapid progression, typically less than a year and usually within 3 to 4 months. Kuru has a similar progression. The Fore people of Papua New Guinea categorized the disease (using pidgin) in five stages: (1) *kuru laik i-kamap now* ("kuru like he come up now"), the first stage before motor symptoms are present; (2) *wokabout yet* ("walk-about yet"), motor and gait problems apparent; (3) *sindaun pinis* ("sit down finish"), inability to walk; (4) *slip pinis* ("sleep finish"), stuporous state; and (5) *klostu dai nau* ("close to die now"), final stage during which swallowing is lost (Rhodes, 1997). Some have likened the progression to classical advanced parkinsonism, but it certainly has features of HD as well.

Neuropsychological testing of patients with CJD is rarely done, not only because of the rarity of the disease, but also because of its circumstances. By the time the disorder is identified, patients are untestable. Unfortunately, at this time, there are no treatments and no cure. Perhaps the only fortunate aspect is that the disease dies out if it is not passed along. The level of kuru in the Fore people has decreased dramatically since they have stopped eating infected tissue.

Neuropsychology in Action 15.5

The Neurologic Examination for Dementia

by Allen J. Rubin M.D.

Watching a neurologist at bedside can be perplexing. A process of inference is at work that is not apparent to the onlooker. It begins with history taking, which incorporates as data every symptom the patient describes and the form and pattern of the descriptive process. The physical aspects of examination are selective in some respects and elaborated in others, to serve an incipient process of hypothesis testing at work during the examination. An active set of principles working inwardly guides the conduct of the neurologist. I undertake here to make those inferential processes and those principles explicit, in a general form.

The neurologist examines the central nervous system (CNS) with an attitude that differs from the common attitude toward the body and its symptoms. The neurologist applies an invisible reference "map" derived from neuroanatomy and neurophysiology, and from encounters with past patients and syndromes. She or he seeks to define and localize a symptom as an epiphenomenon of unwitnessed internal mechanisms, respecting the rules of nervous tissue function rather than the culturally validated rules of somatic experience. In the examination of aging and dementia, the neurologist is, in addition, sensitized to a number of pivotal issues in history taking, and pivotal physical signs that narrow the selection of possible causes. A set of diagnostic hypotheses, ranked by priority, is the goal of the examination, then (most often) to be explored by laboratory and neuroimaging investigations, before the neurologist recommends treatments.

The neurologist's attitude is "phenomenologic" in the sense that he or she must "bracket" or hold uninterpreted the symptom the patient presents until a precise neurologic meaning can be attributed to the symptom (we will call these "symptom hypotheses"). Therefore, most of the examination effort focuses on the adept taking of a history, often from observers and family, as well as the patient. The neurologist applies the tools of physical examination to clarify symptoms, achieve more precise localization, and select a favored hypothesis.

The model yielding symptom hypotheses always includes attention to the following seven issues:

1. Clinical Course

Sudden onset (suggesting vascular or pharmacologic causes)
Insidious progression (suggesting metabolic, neoplastic, inflammatory, infectious, or degenerative causes)
Episodic or paroxysmal occurrence (suggesting epileptic or vascular causes)
Exacerbating–remitting course (suggesting inflammatory or demyelinating causes, or disorders deriving from variable systemic illness, or related to neuromuscular junction fatigue)

2. Hierarchical Level of Advancement

Within the nervous system as a whole, symptoms localize to a "level of organization": muscle, neuromuscular junction, peripheral nerve, spinal root, spinal cord, brainstem, or brain. Within the brain "level," symptoms will vary from simple (for example, segmental loss of light perception) to complex (smelling colors, misattributing meaning to objects), from unimodal (for example, primary motor outputs or primary sensory inputs) to heteromodal (for example, converging complex functions, personality, or the flexibility, anticipation, and organizing executive functions of the frontal lobe). The "level" and "complexity" of the symptom lead the inferential process selectively to parts of the nervous system in which these qualities must necessarily be generated.

Within the *CNS, where neuropsychological dysfunction will arise,* elicited history amplifies these issues:

3. "Central Quality" of Symptoms

The presentation of a system may direct the inferential process away from the peripheral nerves to the CNS, the spinal cord and brain. A patient may describe a limb as disobedient or clumsy, rather than weak or limp, and may describe a limb sensory deficit as a regional perversion of normal sensation, rather than numbness. In the visual system, lateralized inattention or distortions (for example, metamorphosis, color alteration, movement or space misperception, or apparitions) are central in origin. Paroxysmal intrusive experiences, seizures, unrealistic experiences, failure of reality testing, or any symptom reporting the disruption of the individual's normal connection to the social or sensory environment raises the specter of brain disease.

4. Lateralization

Co-occurrence of dysfunction in the same-side arm and face may place a suspect lesion contralaterally above the pons, and dysfunction in the same-side leg and arm may place a suspect lesion above the level of synapse within the cervical spinal cord. The presence of "crossed symptoms" (such as right face with left arm) invites exploration of localization within regions of anatomic crossing of specific projections, such as the crossing of paths in the brainstem. Coincidence of multiple lesions may imitate, in some cases, a single lesion in a complex region. Therefore, neuropsychologists must rewrite the logic of inference to entertain all possibilities. Neuroimaging and electrophysiologic tests can corroborate the inference of a focal lateralized hemispheric syndrome, and lateralized neuropsychological findings can substantiate and clarify the diagnosis.

5. Heritable and Risk Factors

Past nervous system insults (such as trauma), vascular disease outside the nervous system (such as coronary disease and cardiac arrhythmia), systemic illnesses (such as immune system compromise, hyperlipidemia, diabetes mellitus, and autoimmune diseases) all narrow the guesswork in selecting a specific pathologic process in brain. Occurrence of CNS diseases in preceding generations (such as dementias, Huntington's disease) renders certain diagnoses more likely.

6. Confluence, Association, Dissociation, Disconnection

Confluence of symptoms (such as ipsilateral motor and sensory findings), *association* (such as right-sided weakness with aphasia, chronic vertigo with loss of facial sensation, right–left confusion with agraphia), or *dissociation* (such as preservation of pain sensation only on the right and preservation of vibratory sensation only on the left; loss of voluntary facial movement but preservation of automatic emotional facial mimicry) all point to a CNS localization. Last, history or examination can identify *disconnection* of cerebral processes, which may be identified by history or examination (for example, alexia without agraphia, conduction aphasia with isolated loss of language repetition) and can place lesions in the interconnecting brain white matter connections.

7. Syndrome Recognition, Including Neurobehavioral Profiles

A neuropsychologist may advance a "diagnostic hypothesis" of a distinct disease syndrome, subject to confirmation with selected laboratory tests (genetic DNA studies, metabolic-hematologic studies, computed transaxial tomography or magnetic resonance neuroimaging, Doppler or contrast angiography, electroencephalography, sensory-evoked responses, cerebral fluid examination, quantitative visual perimetry, and brain biopsy) and neuropsychological consultation.

The following three cases of progressive diseases among the elderly illustrate how the symptoms and findings converge to allow diagnostic hypotheses.

Case 1

At 62, a female patient retired from her work as an effective office manager; at that time she was involved in dancing and was a competitive bridge player as recreation. At 75, she presented with an insidious course of handwriting shrinkage, tremor at rest, stooping, and shuffling in gait. At 79, she had the onset of tiredness and discouragement with lack of motivation and failure of initiative, dysphoric mood, and agoraphobia.

Pertinent examination: Her mental state was normal, with the exception of verbal memory, which benefited by cuing. Orthostatic hypotension was present. She exhibited masked facies and bradykinesia. A resting tremor was observed. Rigidity was present in passive movements. She required the aid of her arms to rise from a chair and walked with diminished arm swing and shortened steps. Coordinated movements were slow but accurate. Reflexes were normal.

Summary: An insidious CNS disorder with predominantly motor impairment respecting a specific degenerative pattern. A disorder of memory retrieval may be emerging.

Principal diagnostic hypothesis: Parkinson's disease with secondary depression and anxiety disorder. Possibly has an early subcortical dementia.

Case 2

At 58, a financial planner found himself taking additional time to perform routine tasks, and found that he could not manage phone transactions. His personality became irritable and obsessive, with reduced frustration tolerance and temperamental flares over trivial matters. He found he could not plan or organize as before, and he had several "near misses" in driving over a short period.

His examination showed slowed velocity of ocular refixation movements (saccades), motor impersistence of tongue protrusion, and poorly sustained grip. His speech was grammatic and expressive, but dysrhythmic. With mental effort, he showed choreic movement in the face and all extremities. His gait was slightly widened in base. His muscle stretch reflexes were hyperactive.

Summary: An insidious progressive brain disorder with frontal executive functional impairment and evolving irritable personality, accompanied by an adult-onset choreic movement disorder. Frontal-subcortical localization is suspected.

Principal diagnostic hypothesis: Huntington's disease. If the family history is negative for this genetic disorder, confirmation of the diagnosis can be sought through DNA testing.

Case 3

A 65-year-old retired judge experiences slowly progressive impairment. He has difficulty in word finding and adopts a "circumlocutory" speech. He misplaces objects and cannot retain the content of his reading. He loses direction when he walks in unfamiliar places, and he finds that he cannot continue his hobby of constructing models. After several years, he loses insight that he is impaired, and accuses his wife of being a malevolent impostor. His memory impairment is not helped by cues or reminders.

The neurologic examination, other than the mental status, is entirely normal, although he has difficulty cooperating with the examiner.

Summary: A progressive disorder manifesting anomic aphasia, visuospatial impairment, and apraxia, all cortical dysfunctions. Memory encoding is impaired and not benefited by recognition. The absence of any motor impairment is striking.

Principal diagnostic hypothesis: A cortical degenerative dementia such as Alzheimer's disease is likely. The medical team will undertake a search for treatable and reversible conditions that imitate this pattern.

Summary

Subcortical dementias primarily target subcortical structures in the brain. The hallmark of these dementias is motor system disorder, but the behavioral impairment also targets many higher cognitive functions. Patients with PD are more likely to experience development of dementia as they age, although dementia is not inevitable. This chapter has examined the neuropsychological profile of patients with PD without dementia. In addition to the characteristic motor symptoms, patients with PD often show lateralized motor dysfunction. Visuospatial and executive dysfunction often are evident. Language difficulties are typically minor, and memory difficulties, in comparison with AD, primarily involve executive aspects of memory. Patients with PD also frequently suffer from a concomitant mood disorder. The pharmacologic and surgical treatments for PD are among the most promising treatments for any of the dementias.

HD is a good example of a contrasting subcortical dementia with motor difficulties different from those of PD. It is also a good example of a progressive hereditary disease. The neuropsychological profile of HD illustrates the executive functioning problems caused by compromise of the striatofrontal lobe complex. Interestingly, patients with HD also show a significant affective disturbance. Finally, CJD, although quite rare, is a good example of a fast-acting dementia that is transmissible via infected neural tissue.

Differential diagnosis among dementia subtypes can be quite complex. This chapter, as well as Chapter 14, discusses only some of the major exemplars of dementia. Practicing neuropsychologists must come to recognize and differentiate many more subtypes. The study and recognition of dementias requires much experience with a number of dementia subtypes, and careful assessment and observation of behavioral differences. In this endeavor, neuropsychologists work in close conjunction with neurologists who specialize in geriatrics. We end this chapter with a look at how neurologists approach evaluation and diagnosis in differentiating dementia subtypes (Neuropsychology in Action 15.5).

Critical Thinking Questions

- It may soon be possible to test for many neurologic diseases. Would you want to be tested for the possibility of future dementia?
- How is the behavioral quality of subcortical motor disorders presented in this chapter similar or different from the cortical motor disorders such as apraxia presented in Chapter 7?
- How do the subcortical and cortical motor systems work together?
- What are the ethical and scientific issues in the treatment of dementias?

Key Terms

Subcortical dementia	Bradykinesia	Tachyphemia	Huntington's disease (HD)
Parkinson's disease (PD)	Masked facies	Palilalia	Chorea
Parkinsonism	Festinating gait	Anticholinergics	Creutzfeldt–Jakob disease (CJD)
Rigidity	Micrographia	Dyskinesia	Gerstmann-Straussler-Scheinker
Lewy bodies	Hypokinesia	Pallidotomy	syndrome (GSS)
Resting tremor	Dysphonia	Thalotomy	Kuru

Web Connections

http://www.parkinson.org/site/pp.asp?c=9dJFJLPwB&b=71117
National Parkinson's Foundation—PD information and research.

http://www.ninds.nih.gov/disorders/huntington/huntington.htm
National Institute of Neurological Disorders and Stroke (NINDS) Huntington's Disease Information Page.

http://www.ninds.nih.gov/disorders/cjd/cjd.htm
NINDS Creutzfeldt–Jakob Disease Information Page.

Chapter 16

ALTERATIONS OF CONSCIOUSNESS

Each mind fabricates itself. We sense its limits, for we have made them.
—*Rainer Maria Rilke*

If we cannot understand such global and major changes in the state of the brain-mind as occur in sleep, what chance will we have with the far more subtle changes in consciousness that trouble our patients?
—Attributed to *Edward Evarts,* by J. Alan Hobson (1995)

Understanding Consciousness
Rhythms of Consciousness
The Brain and Mind in Sleep
Runaway Brain: Seizure Disorders

Neuropsychology in Action

16.1 Self in the Mirror
16.2 The Case of the Last Coronation
16.3 Lucid Dreaming: A Paradox of Consciousness
16.4 Déjà Vu and Epilepsy
16.5 Epilepsy and the Case of the Sweeping Lady

Keep in Mind

▪ Can "brain" states differ from "mind" states?

▪ How can awareness and consciousness be defined?

▪ What brain mechanisms are responsible for the "paradox" of rapid eye movement sleep?

▪ What alterations of consciousness are represented by different seizure types?

▪ Do alterations in conscious alertness result from similar biological mechanisms?

Overview

Consciousness can be conceptualized in a number of ways. Awareness, level of mental alertness, and level of attention are common representations. Consciousness can also imply the mind's subjective experience of brain states and processes that are available to perception. These various definitions point to a number of different functional anatomic areas depending on the aspect of consciousness under consideration. Disorders of these disparate functional systems also result in a variety of disorders of consciousness. For example, we have discussed alterations in conscious "knowing," or agnosias of the visual system. The total unawareness of one side of the body, or neglect, is a dramatic dysfunction of normal conscious awareness. These disorders of lowered, distorted, or piecemeal awareness can occur in any sensory modality. Synesthesia, or the abnormal melding of sensory-perceptual experiences, represents yet another alteration of consciousness covered in this book.

This chapter revisits questions of brain and mind by considering conceptualizations of consciousness particularly for awareness and alertness. We discuss both normal and disordered aspects of consciousness through a discussion of normal sleep, sleep disorders, and seizure disorders. Throughout the day and night, alertness fluctuates according to preset **circadian** (derived from Latin, meaning "about a day") **rhythms.** The study of these daily rhythms, as people move from waking to sleeping and dreaming, offers lessons in the limits of normal brain alterations of consciousness. Disrupted flow of these brain rhythms can result in a variety of sleep disorders. Some, such as the rare circadian rhythm disorder (see Neuropsychology in Action 16.2) can threaten life itself. Others, such as **narcolepsy,** show major disruptions of the REM (rapid eye movement sleep) cycle and result in sleep intrusions into wakefulness. Most sleep disorders disrupt cognition in some way. In sleep apnea, for example, memory and concentration difficulties are prevalent.

Seizures represent another set of disorders of consciousness. Seizure events of various types represent alterations of daytime alertness and awareness. These internally generated brainstorms of activity manifest differently, largely according to the location of the seizure focus in the brain. Typically, neurologists categorize them as either generalized or **partial seizures,** depending on the extent of brain involvement during the seizure episode. We present these in the context of a general seizure classification scheme. Seizures can occur as a result of a variety of causes. Neurologists consider most people with repeat seizures to have an **epileptic syndrome.** This, of course, is potentially more threatening to brain function than is an isolated seizure event. We discuss the neuroanatomy and neurophysiology of **epilepsy,** as well as the neuropsychological consequences and types of treatments available.

Understanding Consciousness

What is consciousness? What makes human consciousness different from that of other animals? What sorts of brains or brain activity are necessary for conscious experience? Is self-awareness a mind process, as William James thought, or a mind state? These questions have tantalized philosophers, theologians, and scientists throughout time. Brain science has taken up the challenge of deciphering consciousness. This was once the domain of psychology, spearheaded by Wilhelm Wundt and the early structuralists at the turn of the century; the strong behavioral movement in U.S. psychology later cast aside the study of consciousness as too subjective for serious study. Observable behavior was now paramount, and the brain was merely a "black box." Psychologists now know that consciousness is fundamentally important to understanding the human condition. Conscious experience, however, is difficult to measure and observe because of its highly private nature. Nobel prize laureate Francis Crick (Crick and James Watson discovered the structure of DNA) admonishes scientists not to worry too much over aspects of the problem that they cannot solve scientifically or, more precisely, cannot solve solely by using existing scientific ideas. Perhaps the only sensible approach is to press the experimental attack until scientists confront dilemmas that call for new ways of thinking (Crick & Koch, 1990).

Here we are concerned with defining the concept of consciousness, the mind–brain relation, and current theories related to how the brain represents consciousness. After considering the "how" of consciousness, we turn to theorist David Chalmer's question related to the "why" of consciousness. Even if we can explain how the brain represents conscious experience, we need to know *why* this is important to human functioning. Why are we not unthinking and unfeeling automatons?

To begin, most people agree that consciousness implies awareness. This is the primary dictionary definition. The term *consciousness* also refers to a certain level of mental alertness and attention. It also connotes what one's inner self knows or feels. Consciousness is above all a subjective and highly personal reckoning of external and internal events. Measuring it has also relied largely on the person's ability to manifest internal experiences through verbal expression. The issue of awareness raises interesting questions for neuropsychology. If the mind is the subjective experience of brain states and processes, then the mind reflects awareness of brain and body functioning. Because of either external or internal stimulation, sometimes the mind may be able to show more awareness, whereas at other times it seems totally oblivious to the workings of the physical brain and body. One of the main questions that brain science must answer (to put it in what is now the common vernacular) is, What distinguishes the conscious mind from the subconscious or unconscious mind?

MIND AND BRAIN

Popular culture often represents the brain in mechanistic terms, like a type of giant computer, reminiscent of Newtonian physics. However, machines can self-regulate behavior but do not have self-awareness or a subjective experience

of consciousness. Another interesting question is to what extent do animals show self-awareness (Neuropsychology in Action 16.1). An interesting theoretical question relates to whether computers will someday imitate the human brain, and presumably become conscious. Will *artificial intelligence (AI)* mimic human consciousness, as in the imagined character HAL, the supercomputer in the science fiction movie *2001: A Space Odyssey?* During a space shuttle to Mars, HAL starts to display "his" own awareness and decision-making capability, finally killing off the shuttle crew.

Conceptualizing the brain as a computer has only limited usefulness. After all, brains have built computers, not the other way around. It appears more useful to conceptualize the brain as attached to the person, as a biological entity. The level of consciousness of biological entities partly responds to biological and cosmic rhythms, as evidenced in the sleep/wake cycle and the rhythm of the sun. Consciousness also changes in response to internal physiology and chemistry, with inputs from food and drugs. The term *mind* is used to reflect subjective experience, and therefore consciousness, of the emanations of the brain and the body together. Can we assume that every state of mind links to a brain state, and that every state of brain reflects a mind state, be it conscious or unconscious?

Scientists have often wondered whether split-brain patients, who have had the two hemispheres of their brain surgically disconnected, are "of two minds." In an older method of treating seizures, surgeons cut the half-billion axons that allow interhemispheric cross-talk in many patients with intractable seizures. Are these two hemispheres still conscious of each other? Do split-brain patients retain one consciousness, or do two separate realities or even two separate personalities exist? Immediately after surgery, some split-brain patients report having two competing hemispheres. When getting dressed, the right hand may reach for a blue shirt whereas the left hand is grabbing a red shirt. These apparently competing programs, however, usually resolve within a matter of weeks. After that, split-brain patients typically report a unified conscious experience. In daily life their actions are not recognizably different from their presurgery state. Only specialized testing that presents information to only one hemisphere at a time continues to show differences. In effect, this testing appears to reveal more differences between right and left hemisphere processing than it shows a fundamental division of consciousness in those who have had a split-brain operation.

The stumbling block is that we usually document awareness via our ability to verbalize, a province largely of the left hemisphere. In individuals with an intact corpus callosum, the right hemisphere—and therefore the

Neuropsychology in Action 16.1

Self in the Mirror

by Steven M. Platek

Have you ever caught your cat (or dog) shaving? Have you ever wondered why your (male) pet might not shave? Well outside of the fact that it is likely difficult to shave with no opposable thumb and challenging to balance yourself on two limbs when you are used to moving about on four, there is another, neurocognitive reason why your pets do not shave. They cannot recognize themselves in the mirror! That's right, your pet (that is unless you own a pet chimpanzee) does not have the cognitive capacity to recognize itself in the mirror; in fact, your pet likely sees its mirror reflection as another member of the same species and reacts as such (for example, hisses, piloerection for cats).

In 1970, a comparative psychologist named Gordon Gallup (Gallup, Nash, Potter, & Donegan, 1970) was investigating the behavior of animals in front of mirrors as a way to measure social behavior systematically when he stumbled on the fact that most organisms react to their mirror reflection as if it were a member of the same species; that is, they responded to their mirror reflection with species-specific social behaviors (threats, attempts to mate, spitting, barking, feces throwing, among other reactions). To scientifically test this notion, Gallup developed the "mark test," which entails marking areas of an animal's body that cannot be seen without the mirror. Animals that can recognize themselves in mirrors ought to use the mirror to examine their newly marked anatomy. It turns out that only our closest

living relatives—the great apes (chimpanzees, orangutans, and gorillas)—posses the ability to use their mirror reflection like humans do (Gallup, 1982).

What is the importance of mirror self-recognition for neuropsychology, and who cares whether chimps can do it? It turns out that the ability to recognize yourself in a mirror is strongly related to your sense of self, or self-awareness, which allows you to engage in a number of adaptive social behaviors, for example, empathy, sympathy, deception, and so on (Gallup, 1982). In addition, great apes' frontal lobes are the most encephalized, second only to humans. Meaning relative to other parts of their brain and their body, great ape frontal lobes are larger than would be expected by chance. Therefore, the investigation of self-recognition in nonhuman primates provides us with insights into the neuropsychological and possible clinical underpinnings of self and consciousness in humans.

If I were to ask you: "Does everyone recognize themselves in a mirror?" You'd likely answer, "Of course!" Not true. In fact, there are several neuropsychological conditions that are marked by deficits in self-processing. The most notable is a condition known as "mirror sign," or mirror self-misidentification syndrome (Breen, Caine, & Coltheart, 2001). Patients with mirror sign are able to use mirrors to recognize objects, and even other people, but when asked about their own reflection, they often

respond as if their mirror reflection was a stranger who was following him or her around. Usually untroubled by their disorder, family members report that patients act "funny" or "strange" at home, often surprising themselves as they walk past mirrors. Some patients do complain that their new counterpart does not talk to them, which does create some frustration. Neuropsychologically, these patients are marked primarily by right hemisphere dysfunction, which suggests that the capability to process information about the self may be localized to regions of the *right* frontal lobe. This notion has recently been confirmed by several functional magnetic resonance imaging investigations of self-face recognition (Platek, Keenan, Gallup, & Mohamed, 2004; Platek et al., 2005).

Several other neuropsychological conditions are marked by subtler deficits in self-processing. For example, patients with schizophrenia make many errors when asked to distinguish their own face from family members' faces and are more likely than control subjects to classify unknown faces as being their own face.

Collectively. these data—from comparative, nonhuman studies to neuropsychiatric patient findings—suggest that the frontal lobes, and perhaps specifically the right frontal lobe, are involved in self-processing and when damaged or compromised might result in impairments in self-awareness and corresponding social intelligence.

consciousness of the right hemisphere—is accessible to left hemisphere verbalizations. Split-brain patients must reformulate a sense of completeness by making their experiences accessible to both halves of their brains through external cross talk. They can largely do this by moving their eyes to capture both visual fields and verbalizing out loud so that each hemisphere hears what is available to the other hemisphere. Within us, many brain and body processes are either automatic or unavailable, and thus

typically remain unconscious to the mind. For split-brain patients, the hemispheres are physically unavailable to each other. The brain is not communicating internally, but the subjective experience is of one mind. The challenge for the split-brain patient is to consciously integrate each half of the cerebral hemispheres that have been made surgically unconscious of each other.

Most people with intact brains agree that large areas of potential experience remain below the level of conscious experience. The common saying "we only use 10% of our brain" might be better thought of as "our conscious mind may be aware of only a percentage of what our brains do and are capable of." Our brains control and monitor the entire nervous system of our bodies and respond to physiological mechanisms in the body, such as those of the endocrine system, to maintain a state of brain–body homeostasis. Many of these processes are automatic and reflexive. They are unconscious. But they can be brought into awareness via techniques such as biofeedback, and can then be modified by the conscious mind. Many have wondered what might be possible if aspects of the unconscious mind became conscious. What hidden potential could people then develop, such as becoming conscious during the "unconscious" state of sleep or developing senses and perception beyond what is now commonly thought possible? This may sound like the stuff of science fiction, but researchers have documented **lucid dreaming** (see later). It is also reasonable to assume that scientists will find ways to study the limits of sensory-perceptual experiences. Boundaries between the concepts of the conscious mind and the unconscious mind are blurring. The challenge now before brain science is to understand the workings of these aspects of mind and to relate them to brain states and processes.

ANATOMIC CORRELATES OF CONSCIOUSNESS

How are states of consciousness represented in brain anatomy and physiology? René Descartes thought the pineal gland was the center of conscious experience, but researchers have found no single location for consciousness. After several hundred more years, this question may still be somewhat premature, because brain science has not yet clearly defined the operations and boundaries of consciousness. Different areas of the brain may play roles in specific aspects of conscious perception and alertness. Brain science is also now providing interesting clues to how the brain "binds" disparate fragments of information from different cortical and subcortical regions into a subjective sense of coherent unity.

The candidates for brain regions or functional areas that have a role in conscious behavior have, depending on the behavior in question, included numerous areas of the brain, both cortical and subcortical. The various definitions of consciousness suggests that different brain correlates are implicated depending on whether the focus is on notions of awareness or perception, notions of alertness or attention, or notions of what is felt or known by one's

inner self. Perceptual awareness, "knowing," and therefore, perceptual consciousness, build up through modality-specific sensory systems of vision, audition, proprioception, olfaction, and taste. The brain correlates of sensory-perceptual consciousness depend on the integrity of each of these systems. Therefore, it is possible for one sensory modality to block access to "knowing," whereas still showing awareness through other sensory modalities. Such is the case with the agnosias, as we have discussed in Chapters 7 and 8, which can occur after damage to any of the sensory systems. When speaking of level of consciousness, or alertness, researchers often identify the **reticular activating system (RAS)** in the midbrain as responsible for arousal, which we discuss in regard to sleep. Finally, if the self-referential, self-evaluative, and metacognitive aspects of consciousness are the focus, then researchers can consider aspects of executive system and frontal lobe functioning.

Brain researchers and theorists have been most intrigued by how the brain creates a unitary experience of consciousness at one particular moment in time. This can be referred to as the *binding problem.* What is the mechanism that binds disparate neural elements together? A unitary experience of consciousness is an operation of the highest order and, therefore, requires a cortex. Thus, the more sophisticated the cortex, theoretically, the greater the ability for subjective experience and self-awareness.

Let us examine the role of the cortex in consciousness more closely. Neuroscientists commonly describe experiences represented in the cortex as stable spatial patterns. For example, vision is a complex constructional process resulting in object recognition by building and binding elements related to color, form, movement, and spatial position. This binding may occur as a simple structural pattern. Experience in seeing your grandmother increasingly hardwires the synaptic conjunctions between the neurons from various cortical areas forming the pattern that defines "grandmother." This way of thinking is an advance over conceptualizations that first postulated the existence of single "grandmother" cells in which the recognition of grandmother, although the culmination of many processes, was ultimately embodied in one neuron or neuron group. Brain scientists soon realized that the model of single cumulative grandmother cells was grossly inefficient, because separate cells would have to be available for every possible combination and permutation of people and objects. Even though the brain consists of billions of neurons, it would soon run out of neurons for every possible permutation of a memory. Having grandmother represented in a large cortical neuronal assembly is a more efficient conceptualization in terms of processing. Individual neurons can participate in different assemblies, one representing grandmother, another father, another a teacher, and so on. The firing pattern within the web of neurons takes precedence over any individual neuron. If the pattern is disrupted at crucial points, the brain loses recognition of the person.

The neocortex unquestionably plays a major role in evaluating external and internal experiences, but subcortical structures, and particularly the thalamus, may play a crucial role in orchestrating the higher cortical symphony. Francis Crick and Christof Koch (1990), in their study of visual consciousness, have postulated that the upper layers of the cortex are largely unconscious, whereas the pyramidal neurons in layer 5 may be "conscious." Their reasoning is that this is the only layer that "projects right out of the cortical system." Layer 5 also shows an unusual propensity to fire in bursts. Others have also noted this important observation that groups of neurons fire together in bursts, which appears to be an important clue to the binding problem. Researchers know that many cell assemblies throughout the brain fire in synchronous oscillations. For example, in the motor system, the inferior olive of the brainstem sends information in packets of bursts at an oscillation of 10 cycles/sec to the cerebellum. Much as with frames of a movie, the movement only appears fluid because we cannot discriminate the fine breaks in continuity.

The thalamus, the sensory relay station of the brain, may also play a crucial role in synchronizing cortical processes. In an alert state, an electroencephalograph (EEG) records in the gamma frequency range (35–80 cycles/sec), averaging 40 cycles/sec from the cortex. This normal frequency decreases with relaxed wakefulness to 8 to 10 cycles/sec and with deep sleep and coma to 0.5 to 4 cycles/sec. Faster frequencies are asynchronous, whereas slower frequencies become increasingly synchronized and rhythmic. Rodolfo Llinas of New York University (cited in Becker & Seldon, 1985) postulates that the EEG frequency represents a binding wave that continuously sweeps the cortex like a huge radar arm. As the wave scans the brain, the brain synchronizes and interprets all information in that sweep as a unified experience. This action, then, could bind packets of information from widely distributed and noncontiguous regions of the cortex by synchronizing them in time. The implication is that more hardwired spatial patterns of neurons do not act as the prime binding mechanism. Researchers have postulated this theory as a general explanation for how consciousness operates, as well as a specific explanation for how aspects of visual consciousness such as visual object recognition work (Bressler, Coppola, & Nakamura, 1993; Crick & Koch, 1990).

If there is a "binding wave," from where does this frequency emanate? It appears as if the intralaminar nucleus of the thalamus generates a cortical binding signal every 12.5 thousandths of a second (that is, every 0.0125 second) (Llinas cited in Becker & Seldon, 1985). As mentioned earlier, nearly all sensory and motor systems route through the thalamus. The thalamus is in constant two-way communication with the cortex through a feedback system of millions of thalamocortical loops. A number of investigators believe this system, which reaches throughout the cortex, is intimately involved with conscious experience. Because nearly all information channels through the thalamus, it can act as the integrator, selecting, packaging, and tagging information that occur together in time from all areas of the brain, and sending it back for the cortex to record as an object or an event. The thalamus and the thalamocortical projection system play an important role in arousal, sleep, and seizure disorders. It may also play a role in remapping phantom sensations. A temporal binding system, whether through the thalamus or other structures, would be highly efficient, because it could register any number of novel neural code combinations together and be experienced instantly without relying on the hardware of contiguous, linear cortical connections. These findings suggest that, indeed, there is no single organ of consciousness; instead, the frequencies of temporal binding may coordinate experience. This would indicate that the whole brain can contribute to awareness depending on which systems activate at any one time to signal the effect of an experience. This view implies a dynamic quality to the brain and conscious experience that is infinitely more flexible than former conceptualizations.

According to theorist David Chalmers (1996), the "how" question of consciousness is not the difficult question. The difficult question is not how conscious processes bind together, but how a subjective experience of mind arises from the functioning brain and its synchronized and bundled oscillations. By looking deeper into people's direct subjective experiences, some of which are explicit and some of which are implicit, researchers will learn more about the relation of brain to mind.

People customarily link consciousness of external events with the tangible. Even our vocabulary reflects this: "I know something to be true because I saw it with my own eyes, I can feel it, I can sense it." Most of what people experience they know by way of senses of smell, taste, sight, sound, and touch—the springtime smells of lilacs and freshly mown grass, the sight of children running across the yard, the sound of laughter, and the squeeze of a hand. But external realities exist that most of us cannot perceive directly through our senses. At the turn of the

20th century, people were just becoming aware that sound could travel through long distances, even through bodies, yet people cannot perceive such sound directly without a little box called a radio. In the animal world, whales, dogs, and bats communicate within their own species on different frequencies than humans can "consciously" perceive. We now know that low- and high-frequency sound exists, because we have instruments that can measure and transmit these "unconscious" ranges of sound. In the same vein, people know that electrical fields and microwave energy exist. In 1933, Enrico Fermi, a physicist, predicted the presence of neutrinos, or energy particles, which permeate the universe and freely flow through bodies without leaving a trace. In 1956, physicists definitively identified neutrinos. What else might exist that people cannot consciously perceive? Modern science may be just beginning to unravel the mysteries that lie beyond limited human sensory abilities.

The Western empirical, materialistic tradition of science takes the stance that if something cannot be observed and measured it does not exist. To study the full range of consciousness, this archaic and human-centered view must give way to the possibility that the range of reality extends beyond ordinary human sensory-perceptual experience. Brain dysfunction can truncate, extend, or otherwise bend sensory-perceptual experience. Many cases we present in this book certainly stretch the bounds of ordinary conscious experience. Supersensory abilities may also be possible. Some Chinese health practitioners diagnose and heal by working with only the energy fields of the body. Fortunately, new technologies may bring into awareness many aspects of sensory experience that are out of range to the "naked senses." Scientists may now experimentally verify awareness of both pathologically altered and exceptional sensory perception, although few studies have considered these issues.

Previously, the limited means of measuring subjective experience have hampered scientists in studying consciousness. Primarily, they have had to rely on direct experience of the senses and on language to reveal consciousness. In other words, people could demonstrate awareness if they could hear, see, taste, smell, or touch something and be able to describe it. Because the left hemisphere is more specialized for spoken words, some have characterized it as the seat of consciousness. But that simplistic notion equates awareness with an ability to describe the phenomenon. Many people can probably recall experiences in which they had a sense of knowing without the ability to verbalize or touch what they felt.

Also, some processes that are now implicit may be made explicit. People can demonstrate implicit knowledge through their actions based on that knowledge. Scientists also know that subliminal sound and scent, under the level of detectable awareness, can affect brains in a predictable manner. Similarly, scientists will also be able to determine whether some individuals can detect electrical energy fields of which most are not conscious. On the internal side of the coin, many of what are considered *automatic processes,* such as breathing and heart rate, churn along without conscious awareness or control. But the means already exist to bring many of these processes into conscious awareness through various biofeedback technologies such as heart-rate monitoring, galvanic skin response measurement, and EEG. Although these technologies present a recent tool for more conscious body and mind control, masters of meditation have long exerted amazing control over many brain and body states. Given the increased ability to gain a window into automatic and subconscious processes through vivid functional brain imaging techniques, whole new areas of research are opening up that may now allow neuropsychologists to learn not only about the workings of the brain but also how to consciously control various brain states. The possibilities available for extending the range of normal conscious experience represent an exciting frontier in brain science.

This chapter visits daily aspects of consciousness, as well as disorders of consciousness. What happens when the fundamental experiences of consciousness run amok because of brain dysfunction? The daily rhythms of alertness and arousal people all move through from waking to sleeping and dreaming provide directions for studying the limits of normal brain alterations of consciousness. Disrupted flow of these brain rhythms can cause a variety of sleep disorders, of which one of the more interesting is narcolepsy. Finally, seizures represent an alteration of consciousness that also affects level of alertness—an internally generated brainstorm of synchronized activity.

Rhythms of Consciousness

Cyclic changes are inherent in the passing of seasons, in weather patterns, in tidal ebbs and flows, and in the rising and setting of the sun. In humans, mood and energy levels respond to seasonal shifts, menstruation cycles follow monthly rhythms, and sleep and wakefulness cycles oscillate daily in a circadian rhythm. Humans also respond to shorter **ultradian** 90-minute cycles of heightened and lowered brain arousal. The autonomic system of the brain controls the rhythms of heart rate and respiration. The brain itself is a web of neuronal circuitry with a frequency measured in cycles per second on an EEG (see

---

Neuropsychology in Action 16.2

The Case of the Last Coronation

He was Italian, 53 years old, and an industrial manager whose health had been fine except for some problems with high blood pressure. Much to his misfortune, he was destined to show researchers how dire things can get when the body's internal clock runs amok.

In 1985, the man experienced development of insomnia. His sleep fell to only 2 or 3 hours a night, he became impotent, and he began to have difficulties with his digestion and developed a high temperature. Within 2 months, he could sleep for only 1 hour a night and was often observed rising from his bed, standing, and giving a military salute. He told his family that he was dreaming of a coronation. By the time the man was admitted to the hospital in Bologna, he had ceased to sleep normally at all. He was alert when spoken to, but when left alone would drift into a stupor in which he would gesture as if communicating in a dream. His doctors tried to treat him with a variety of strong drugs, none of which had a lasting effect. In the eighth month of his illness, the man's stupor was relieved only by episodes in which he screamed and thrashed about. In the ninth month, he died.

Examining his otherwise normal brain, doctors found that certain regions of the thalamus had degenerated. The man's rare disease supported suspicions that sleep, at least nondreaming **NREM** (non–rapid eye movement sleep) sleep, is affected by chemical processes in the thalamus. Just below that structure, near the base of the brain, is a bean-sized region known as the *hypothalamus.* The hypothalamus sends out signals that regulate basic processes such as hunger and sex and affect emotions such as anger. It is also a central control for the biological clock that controls sleep; when the hypothalami of mice are damaged, the mice lose any semblance of orderly or regular sleep.

This man's misfortune also displayed the genetic nature of this sleep disorder. The doctors learned from one of the man's relatives, also a doctor, that in the last 6 generations of the man's family at least 14 relatives, including his sisters, had died of the same bizarre condition.

Source: Adapted from The Case of the Last Coronation. (1988, March–April). *Hippocrates.*

Chapter 2 for a detailed discussion of EEG). It alternates between periods of brain asynchronicity, usually indicative of an alert brain state, and periods of "altered consciousness" synchronicity, in which groups of neurons oscillate rhythmically. Some of these synchronous oscillations, such as those occurring during sleep, represent normal variations. Others, which occur during seizures and coma, may suggest pathology. Many of the normal internal rhythms of the body and brain, such as sleep, are calibrated in response to external environmental changes such as the light/dark cycle. Scientists do not yet understand a great deal about the complex interplay between the many human rhythms and external environmental rhythms that affect human functioning.

In addition to these questions, neuropsychology is interested in how brain states, measurable via dynamic imaging means such as EEG and positron emission tomography, correspond to mind states in both ordinary and pathological functioning. In **absence seizures,** slow-wave synchronous activity abruptly interrupts the normally asynchronous waking state. It would appear, then, that slow synchronous brain activity heralds pathology. But absence seizures in children, which are marked by brief lapses in consciousness, show the same 3 cycles/sec synchronous brain waves characteristic of normal delta-stage sleep. The EEGs of people in coma also show this slow synchronous wave. Masters of meditation, however, can produce delta waves and remain seemingly "conscious." Although the EEG can record similar brain states in two different people, mind states and awareness can range considerably. Therefore, similar brain-wave frequencies can imply pathologic "unconscious" mind states, normal sleeping mind states, or fully conscious mind states. Although the EEG provides clues as to *whether* one is thinking, it does not capture the subjective experience of the mind.

Many interesting questions of consciousness revolve around alertness and level of arousal. We examine sleep in some depth in this chapter because of its rhythmic brain activity and the paradoxical and fascinating nature of the dreaming **REM** (rapid eye movement) stage. Deep within the hypothalamus, a biological clock—in conjunction with the visual system—calibrates the sleep/wake cycle. A case example illustrates how chaotic sleep and health can become without this clock (Neuropsychology in Action 16.2). Sleep disorders such as narcolepsy also illustrate the manner in which sleep/wake rhythms may become confused, resulting in daytime sleep intrusions and fragmented nighttime sleep.

Scientists are just beginning to understand the brain mechanisms underlying neuronal rhythm in sleep and in seizures. At a neuronal level, neurons and neuronal systems maintain a fine balance between excitatory and inhibitory balance. An individual neuron may receive both excitatory and inhibitory messages from the neurons that synapse on it. Whether the neuron fires depends on how these messages add up. Excitatory and inhibitory neurons may also synapse with each other in a loop and oscillate in their intercommunication. The thalamus, a powerful pacemaker, has afferent and efferent neural connections reaching throughout the cortex. At a cell assembly level, the same sort of oscillation, the *thalamocortical loop,* operates between the thalamus and the cortex. Interestingly, the thalamus appears able to initiate thalamocortical synchronous oscillations without external input. Although researchers know that peculiarities in the ion channels of thalamic cell membranes allow these cells to generate and sustain a rhythm, it is unclear what triggers this behavior. In general, scientists can describe how certain local groups of cells begin to oscillate, and how certain widespread cortical brain-controlling mechanisms, such as the thalamus, generate rhythm, but why this occurs is a matter of speculation. Studying rhythmic brain activity in behaviors such as sleep and seizures may help to elucidate these mechanisms.

The Brain and Mind in Sleep

Is sleep unconscious? As a laptop computer goes "to sleep," it shuts down—it is unresponsive, and the hard disk spins down until it is "awakened" again with a touch. But the machine analogy of a steady state does not do justice to the complex ebbs and flows of the sleeping human brain. Sleep is a drifting down into deeper levels of unawareness of the world, which then lighten and deepen in a rhythmic pattern during the night. Seemingly unresponsive to the majority of external sensory stimuli, intense emotions and hallucinations arise created by the spontaneous firings of the brain itself. How conscious are we or can we be during sleep? Delta waves at a frequency of 0.5 to 4 cycles/sec represent the deepest stage of sleep. Yet what of expert mediators who can produce delta waves and remain conscious? They describe their change in awareness of themselves as progressing from the experience of "self" to a "point of still awareness" (Kenyon, 1994). During REM sleep, dreams occur, but people are usually quite oblivious to that they are in a dream state and usually forget the dream. Some people, however, are "lucid" dreamers, knowing they are dreaming during their

dream, and able to influence theme and outcome, thoughts, and emotions (Neuropsychology in Action 16.3). There is much to learn in the emerging area of brain function during sleep. This section explores how consciousness, awareness, and arousal operate through the window of sleep and dreaming. We discuss the known brain mechanisms that govern levels of arousal through the neurology and physiology of normal sleep, and finally, sleep disorders of particular interest to neuropsychology.

SLEEP ARCHITECTURE

The cycle of brain activity during sleep is embedded within the larger circadian rhythm of wakefulness and sleep. The sleep rhythm is a 90-minute cycle of descending and ascending states of cortical arousal. It is punctuated at the end of each cycle by periods of such intense brain activity that the sleeping brain appears active, almost in a waking state. This general pattern is highly stable across people, although much variability exists in the amount of time spent in each phase, depending on such factors as age, physical condition, and other individual variables.

The two general stages of sleep are known as REM and NREM (non–rapid eye movement sleep). Both have characteristic EEG patterns and physiological correlates (Table 16.1). As discussed in Chapter 2, scientists describe EEG waves by their amplitude, which is a measure of microvoltage, and their frequency or speed, measured as the cycles per second of a complete wave. Scientists may also describe the overall characterization, or pattern of waves, as synchronous or asynchronous (arrhythmic), according

Table 16.1 *Electroencephalographic Sleep Stage Characteristics in Adults*

Stage Time	Frequency (cycles/sec)	Amplitude (microvolts)	Waveform	%
NREM (non-rapid eye movement)				
1	4–8	50–100	Alpha, theta	5
2	8–15	50–150	Theta, sleep spindle	45 K complex
3	2–4	100–150	20–50% delta	12
4	0.5–2	100–200	>50% delta	13
REM (rapid eye movement)	Mixed	50–100	"Sawtooth"	25

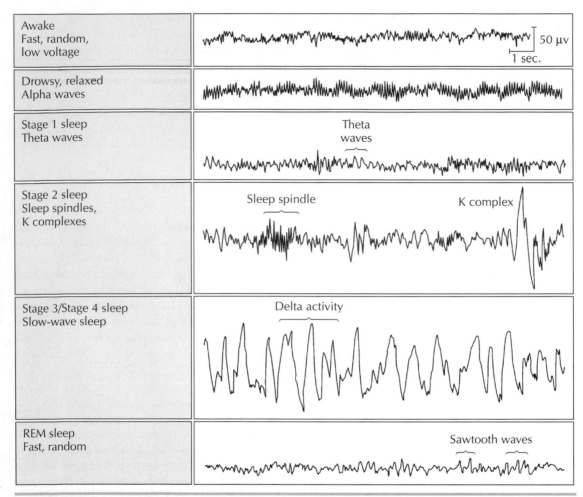

Figure 16.1   Electroencephalographic (EEG) patterns representative of stages of sleep. As a person moves into deeper stages of sleep, the characteristic EEG pattern moves from low-amplitude fast waves to high-amplitude slow waves. REM (rapid eye movement) sleep more closely resembles waking. (Reproduced from Nairne, J. S. [1997]. *The adaptive mind* [p. 216, Figure 6.5]. Pacific Grove, CA: Brooks/Cole, adapted from Hauri, P. [1982]. *Current concepts: The sleep disorders*. Peapack, NJ: Pharmacia & Upjohn.)

to the degree or tendency of neural circuits to fire together in rhythm. The EEG provides a dynamic view of activity in the sleeping brain. Figure 16.1 portrays the characteristic EEG waves and patterns of each stage of sleep. Notice that as EEG slows, wave amplitude correspondingly increases. For each stage of sleep, there are characteristic waveforms, such as alpha, theta, and delta, and for REM, a form that looks like a sawtooth. In addition, certain forms may be superimposed, such as sleep spindles and K complexes in stage 2 sleep. During the waking state, the neural circuits fire in a characteristic 40-cycle/sec, low-voltage, desynchronized pattern. Merely closing the eyes starts a shift toward coordinated rhythmic neural circuit oscillation. Synchronized bursts of alpha waves (8–12 cycles/sec)

appear superimposed on the background of the faster brain rhythm. The person literally descends into sleep as the EEG waves become slower, higher, and more rhythmic with each stage. Finally, in the deepest (stage 4) sleep, EEGs show 50% or more delta waves. This high-amplitude (100–200 microvolts), slow-wave (0.5–2 cycles/sec) rhythm indicates that the cortical circuits are oscillating at the slowest periodicity. It is not surprising that if one is awakened from stage 4 sleep, which is likely to occur about 60 minutes after sleep onset, one takes several minutes to recover from deep-sleep grogginess.

NREM and REM sleep represent different states of consciousness. Progressing through the stages of NREM sleep, the person becomes increasingly difficult to arouse.

ent. The scientific study of lucid dreaming
ay well represent the next wave of research
understanding the brain processes
ed to levels of consciousness.

nly a small proportion of REM
s variation in the developmen-
nswer may lie in the functions
in growth and development.
s, the pituitary gland, under
s, releases somatotrophin
e 4 sleep, and the immune
During rapid growth and
be more necessary. Stage 4
ive sleep because it also

REM and REM

REM
Greater in second half of night
Rapid, conjugate
Dreams
Vivid, emotional
Inhibited
Atonic
Benign paralysis
High
ow
creases
Low
High

s differ
ners
and height-
only visual
kinesthetic as
ng bright light, and
and exhilaration often
ams. What often triggers
ss of inconsistency or
r abruptly shifts into con-
sometimes accompanied
expansion and greater
at is interesting in com-
ry dreams is that lucid
jointed, lacking in judg-
. The dreamer has control
e sense of deciding where to
o, but cannot totally control
come. For example, the
ay decide to travel to a certain
meet various people, but may be
sed by what occurs. The person may
decide to use the dream to face prob-
of living, which has ramifications for the
y of lucid dreams in a healing or thera-
ic manner. A person with a fear of water
rted the following dream:

In reality I have a great fear of water, and
swimming was one of the possible choices for
me to try in a lucid dream. In the dream I'm in
my backyard and am immediately aware that
I'm dreaming. I decide that it would be great fun
to swim. Instantly there is water all around me. I
swim several hundred feet and make many
adjustments to my swimming form.
I start to stand up in what is chest deep
water and start to feel fearful. I remind myself
that in a dream there is no reason to fear. I
immediately feel comfortable and start to

lk back around the house, when I observe
that the water has disappeared. (LaBerge,
1990, p. 260)

The study of lucid dreams has revealed
that dreams occur in real time, not in an
instant or a blink of the eye. As dreamers,
people may take shortcuts and transport
themselves from place to place, but the
story line of dream action occurs at ordinary
speed. This is known because sleep researchers, such as the group at Stanford
Sleep Research Center, have been able to
correlate eye movement during lucid dreams
with dream reports. First, a prearranged
signal is set—for example, a light embedded
in eye shades worn by the sleeper will flash
three times when EEG recordings detect
REM sleep. If the dreamer detects the light
and becomes aware that this is the signal,
he or she returns a signal by moving the
eyes in a pattern that was practiced before
sleep onset. This methodology is quite
ingenious, because during the benign
paralysis of REM sleep, the only way for the
dreamer to signal to the external world is
through the eyes. One lucid dreamer reported that in his dream he was walking
along a beach when suddenly he saw the
sun rise and set, rise and set, rise and set.
He kept walking, and then suddenly thought
how odd that was. In an "aha" experience,
he recognized that this was the prearranged
signal and was able to signal back to the
researchers with his eyes. His report of the
dream and the time period between the
signal and the dreamer's response corresponded to the eye movement tracings.
Are lucid dreams a melding of the
conscious and unconscious mind states?
During lucid dreams, the dreamer has
knowledge of normally available waking
thoughts and memories, as well as an
awareness of the dream illusion. What is
normally unconscious has become conscious. Lucid dreams have been described,
and they may reasonably be thought of as

(continued)

(continued)

a cocreation between the two mind states, sometimes marked by intense pleasure, but with a different twist from the Freudian

idea of a naughty "id" in that the dreamer often experiences these as mind-expanding growth opportunities filled with personal insight and a sense of personal accomplish-

It takes a bit of commotion to wake someone from stage 4 NREM sleep. The brain is less active and becomes less capable of organized activity. Some individuals may vocalize, but this speech usually does not seem logical. Some motor behavior may occur as well, and sleepwalking sometimes accompanies NREM sleep. Although NREM sleep is associated with a sleeping brain, curiously the body is "awake," twitching and turning. Sometimes the twitching is so strong that the person may kick. This is called **nocturnal myoclonus** (restless leg syndrome) and can be so strong that it may wake up the person.

After the first descent into deep sleep, there is a progressive lightening that culminates at 90 minutes after sleep onset in the first REM period (named for the prominence of rapid eye movements). REM sleep shows many contrasts with NREM sleep (Table 16.2). The most striking feature is the relatively high level of alertness during REM sleep, much like stage 1 sleep. In fact, the first time sleep researchers measured REM sleep via EEG they thought the subject had awakened.

The characteristic REM EEG pattern of low-voltage, random, fast "sawtooth" waves is a dynamic representation of the sleeper's internally generated heightened cortical arousal and is associated with intensive processing of the internal mind state of dreaming. The first REM period may be quite short, lasting less than 5 minutes. Thus, in REM sleep, the brain is active and seemingly awake. A person awakened during REM sleep often reports dreams. However, the body is immobile during REM sleep. In fact, all voluntary muscles are temporarily "paralyzed" from the neck down. Both female and male individuals show sexual response (lubrication or erection). As the night progresses, Figure 16.2 illustrates how REM periods lengthen at the end of each 90-minute cycle. Correspondingly, sleep stages 3 and 4 taper off in the early morning hours. In general, normal sleepers spend 75% in NREM and 25% in REM sleep over a night's sleep.

What we have just described is normal adult sleep. Variability in this cycle depends on age and several other factors (Figure 16.3). Infants, in contrast, spend 50% of their sleep time in REM sleep, and a large proportion of their NREM sleep in stage 4 sleep. By late middle age, most people have lost all of this physiologically restorative

stage 4 sleep and retain o
sleep. Why this tremendo
tal qualities of sleep? The a
various types of sleep serve

Among other phasic even
control of the hypothalam
(growth hormone) during sta
system is particularly active.
development, stage 4 sleep may
sleep is often termed restorat

| Table 16.2 | Comparison of N |
| | Sleep Events |

Event	NREM
Occurrence	Greater in first half of night
Eye movement	Slow, rolling
Mentation	Short, ordinary
	Fragmented
Sensory processing	Lowered
Motor response	Relaxed
Autonomic nervous system variability	Low
GSR variability	High
CNS temperature	Decreases
Sexual response	
Neurotransmitter activity	
Aminergic	High
Cholinergic acetylcholine	Low
Hormonal secretion rate	
Growth hormone	High
Parathyroid hormone	High
Luteinizing hormone	Low

NREM = non–rapid eye movement; REM = rapid eye m
response; CNS = central nervous system.

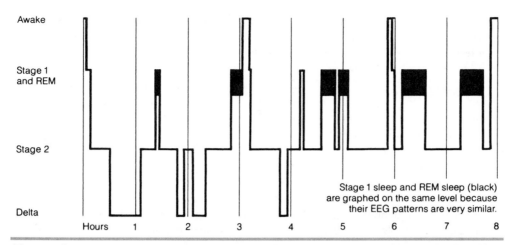

Figure 16.2 Polysomnograph of a typical night of adult sleep. At the beginning of the night, rapid eye movement (REM) periods (in black) are short and delta sleep (stages 3 and 4) is longer. As the night progresses, delta periods become shorter and REM periods become longer. (Reproduced from Hauri, P. [1977]. *Current concepts: The sleep disorders* [p. 8, Figure 2]. Peapack, NJ: Pharmacia & Upjohn.)

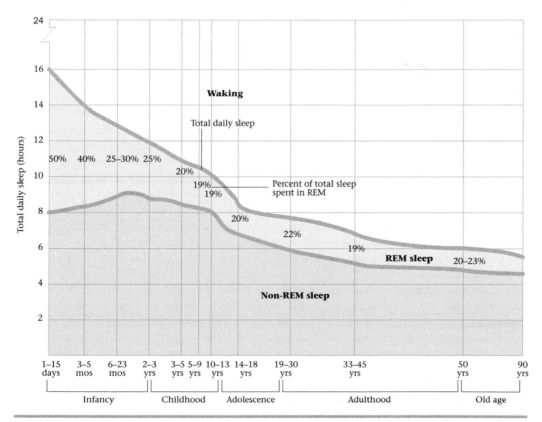

Figure 16.3 Average changes in sleep stage percentages over the life span. Average daily sleep stage percentages are greatest in infancy, decline during childhood, and then are fairly stable throughout middle adulthood. (Reproduced from Weiten, W. [1998]. *Psychology: Themes and variations* [4th ed., Figure 5.8, p. 187]. Pacific Grove, CA: Brooks/Cole, originally adapted from Roffwarg, H. P., Muzio, J. N., & Dement, W. C. [1966]. Ontogenetic development of human sleep–dream cycle. *Science, 152,* 604–619, by permission.)

increases in adults in response to intense physical exertion. At older ages, this growth-and-tissue-repair function of growth hormone becomes less available.

SLEEP ANATOMY AND PHYSIOLOGY

Circadian clocks (derived from Latin, meaning "about a day," as noted earlier), which set the daily pattern of sleep and wakefulness, are intrinsic to most living organisms. This clock might have been patterned in ancient times and embedded in DNA as all life on earth learned to respond to the rhythms of the cycles of days, months, seasons, and years. Even plants have a rudimentary circadian triggering mechanism. The heliotrope folds its leaves at night and opens them in the morning, but it is not directly guided by the light of the sun. Even in a dark room it continues opening and closing, according to daily cycles and according to some internal timing mechanism.

In humans, and all mammals, a more specialized circadian clock nestles in the **suprachiasmic nucleus (SCN)** of the hypothalamus. If the SCN is removed from the brain, the neurons continue to fire according to the programmed daily rhythms. However, if the SCN were totally dependent on genetic programming, what would happen when traveling to the other side of the world? The daily internal clock must have a way to resynchronize according to the light/dark cycle. That, indeed, is the case. In fact, if left without any natural light cues, humans will revert to about 25-hour/day cycles of waking and sleeping. Natural light, or in some cases an alarm clock, apparently resynchronizes the human circadian clock each day for functioning in accord with a 24-hour day. The halves of the SCN lie just above the optic chiasm and receive light via neural input from the two visual fields as they cross hemispheres to the opposite sides of the brain (Figure 16.4). When this internal clock runs amok, sleep patterns can be greatly, even fatally, disrupted (see Neuropsychology in Action 16.1).

Scientists do not yet know how the human circadian clocks signal sleep onset each night and awakening each morning—perhaps through qualitatively different signals, or via a gradual change in the release of neurotransmitter molecules. Clifford Saper, of Harvard University, and his colleagues (Saper, Chou, & Scammell, 2001) have suggested that the ventrolateral preoptic area of the hypothalamus may be the "master switch" to arousal (see Figure 16.3). Researchers have observed this somnolence region to be the only brain center that is more active during sleep than wakefulness. Other researchers have identified a peptide molecule named "factor S" and claim it may

be one of the neurotransmitters most directly responsible for setting off the downward drift into sleepiness. Injected into the hypothalamus, factor S induces sleep and increases body temperature. It also appears to trigger the release of interleukin-1, which raises many interesting questions about the immunoprotective function of sleep. This collective evidence points to a strong role for the hypothalamus as the "biological sandman."

When activated, the hypothalamus sends its molecular message to the thalamus and the RAS of the lower brainstem. Gradually, the brain moves from a state of processing external sensory information to a closing off of inputs from vision, hearing, and touch. During alertness, the thalamus relays inputs from most sensory systems, except for smell. The thalamus constantly communicates with the cortex through a feedback system of millions of thalamocortical loops. With high alertness, neuronal firing is frequent and finely tuned. Any external sensory "noise" against this background is easily picked up because the brain discriminates it from the high-frequency background rhythm by its irregularity or novelty. As alertness drops, at a certain point the thalamocortical loops start oscillating to their own rhythm, in a sort of internal dance between the thalamus and the cortex.

On an EEG, this is also when the sleep spindles (12–14 cycles/sec) emerge, typical of stage 2 sleep. With the slowed frequency of thalamocortical firing, orientation to and processing of external stimuli is less likely. The brain turns inward, attention drifts, and the sleeper becomes oblivious to his or her surroundings. Currently, the thalamocortical loop stands as the primary mechanism in sleep onset and in maintenance of reduced attention to external stimuli. As sleep continues to deepen, responsiveness to the outward environment lessens even further. Yet many parents of newborns apparently maintain vigilance to their baby's stirrings while sleeping. Perhaps future research will reveal whether another mechanism monitors the environment during sleep, or whether sleep remains lighter for those who must remain alert. Animals in the wild, which must retain more alertness to danger, show lighter and more fragmented sleep than zoo and domestic animals. Perhaps this is also the case with humans.

RETICULAR ACTIVATING SYSTEM AND RAPID EYE MOVEMENT SLEEP

Approximately every 90 minutes, and lengthening throughout the night, a sleeper enters REM stage sleep. The cortical activity of high-frequency sawtooth EEG

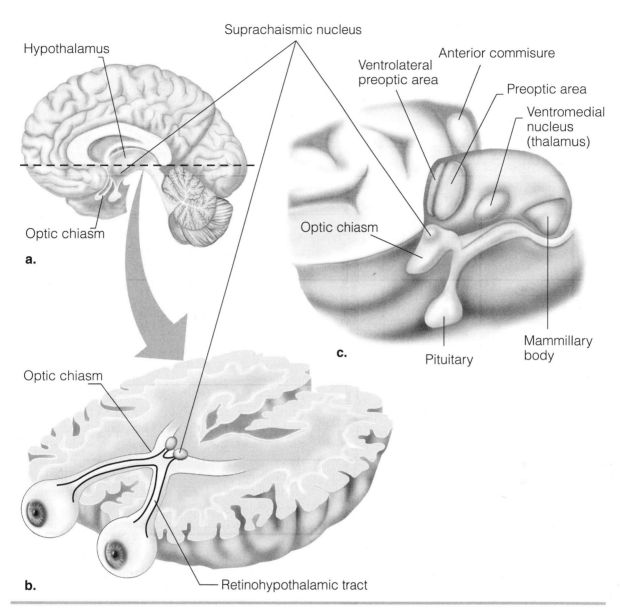

Figure 16.4 The suprachiasmic nucleus (SCN) of the hypothalamus. A (a) sagittal and (b) horizontal section of the human brain showing the SCN in relation to the optic chiasm; (c) exploded view of the hypothalamus showing the SCN in relation to other nuclei. (a: Adapted from Kalat, J. W. [1998]. *Biological psychology* [6th ed., Figure 9.6c]. Pacific Grove, CA: Brooks/Cole, by permission; b, c: modified from Pinel, P. J., & Edwards, M. [1998]. *A colorful introduction to the anatomy of the human brain* [p. 195, Figure 11.6]. Boston: Allyn & Bacon, by permission.)

waves in the theta range nearly resembles a waking brain state, yet the sleeper is turned inward. The view is an internal movie as scenes and images flash by and fall away. Willful movement is impossible, because the motoneurons have temporarily lost communication with the spinal cord. Sensation from the outside world is turned down to its lowest point. For all practical purposes, more than any other stage of sleep, the sleeper is in a cocoon, insulated from the outside world and unable to act on it, yet with a very active mind. What brain mechanisms are responsible for this paradox? Although science does not yet understand the complete workings of REM sleep, it is evident that the RAS is the primary mechanism for turning REM sleep on and off. This section discusses both the mechanical aspects and the chemical transmitters that play a role in REM sleep.

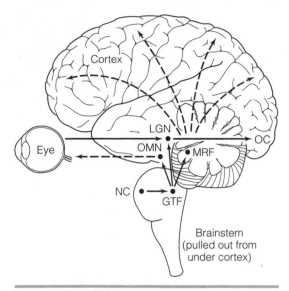

Figure 16.5 Schematic diagram of the rapid eye movement (REM) system. OMN = oculomotor nuclei; MRF = midbrain reticular formation. (From Hauri, P. [1977]. *Current concepts: The sleep disorders* [p. 15, Figure 5]. Peapack, NJ: Pharmacia & Upjohn.)

The RAS maintains cortical arousal. It arises from deep within the brainstem (Figure 16.5). During wakefulness, the high activity in the ascending RAS stimulates the brain via projections into many different neurologic systems in the cortex. The nuclei of the gigantocellular tegmental field (GTF) located in the higher pons appear to generate these brain waves. Left unchecked, they fire spontaneously, producing a high level of activity. During stages 1 and 2, the nucleus ceruleus (NC) becomes active and acts as an inhibitory control on the GTF, dampening the firing. Cortical activation continues to slow through stages 3 and 4. Then, during REM sleep, the NC releases its inhibition of the GTF, leaving it free to activate again, sending spikes through the cortex and activating the cortex into a higher level of arousal. One particular set of discharges is termed PGO spikes because they travel from the pons (P) to the lateral geniculate nucleus (LGN) of the thalamus to the occipital cortex (OC). The lateral geniculate nucleus is part of the visual pathway from the retina to the occipital cortex. The internally generated PGO spikes intercept this pathway midway. Interestingly, the PGO spikes fire in pulsating bursts. This is an additional indication that the thalamus may be synchronizing brain rhythms. Although it also happens during waking hours, PGO bursts are more active in REM sleep. The stimulation that finally reaches the occipital cortex creates dream images and the corresponding rapid REM charac-

teristic of this stage. The occipital lobes are therefore excited without external visual input. Given this scenario, it is curious that eyes move. But they appear somehow calibrated to move in conjunction with scene changes of dreams. Researchers think that bursts from the pons also stimulate nearby oculomotor neurons, resulting in corresponding eye movements (Hobson, 1995).

Areas other than the occipital lobes also activate during REM sleep. In rats, rabbits, and cats, single-neuron recording has demonstrated that the theta rhythm emanates from the hippocampus, specifically in the dentate gyrus and the entorhinal cortex (Winson, 1972). However, the signal to activate the theta rhythm has its trigger in the brainstem within the RAS. This hippocampal activation during REM sleep has ramifications for proposing a role for memory within REM sleep. We discuss this issue further in considering the functions of REM sleep.

Many of the REM sleep occurrences listed in Table 16.2 have brainstem mechanisms. **"Sleep paralysis"** occurs because it is simply too dangerous to act out dreams. Although we may see or sense movement in dreams, through active central motoneuronal activity, the motoneurons responsible for actually carrying out the action are "turned off" at the level of the spinal cord. The active reticular firing in the medulla during REM sleep inhibits the spinal motor pathways. This greatly reduces muscle tone **(atonia),** and for all practical purposes paralyzes the sleeper. When researchers surgically turned off cats' medullar inhibitory mechanism, the cats actually became physically active during REM. They stalked, attacked, hissed, and otherwise acted out the drama of their dreams.

REM sleep dampens external sensory stimulation. The pontine excitement also inhibits peripheral nerve pathways where they synapse with the spinal cord. During all stages of sleep, after an initial increase in the first 2 hours, respiration rate and body temperature gradually diminish. Body movement and systolic blood pressure also increase during the night. These changes continue during REM but tend to fluctuate more than during NREM sleep. As the night progresses and REM periods lengthen, fluctuations become more variable from REM period to REM period.

As with all behavior, REM sleep combines structural and functional processes. The neurophysiological processes provide the fuel for the mechanical processes we have just discussed. Many brain neurotransmitters decline only slightly during REM sleep. The question is, Do certain neurotransmitters operate differently during REM sleep? This is apparently true. Researchers have observed within the locus ceruleus a cluster of neurons, which they labeled "REM off" cells, that completely stop firing during REM sleep (Hobson, 1995). Because these cells otherwise release norepinephrine and serotonin, the consequence is a relative unavailability of these substances to the brain during REM. J. Alan Hobson (1995) hypothesizes that the lowering of these aminergic transmitters plays a role in the "lack of self-reflective awareness, disorientation, and logical fallacy" in verbal reports of dreaming during REM sleep. Hobson also postulates that serotonin and norepinephrine act as long-term neuromodulators on the brain. As NREM sleep commences, "REM off" cells begin to slow their firing rate, with the functional result of slowly releasing their hold on the "rational" cortex. The mind becomes more disinhibited during sleep but is especially free to wander during REM because of a now complete lack of aminergic transmission. At the end of the REM cycle, the cells "turn on," activating at a higher level of serotonin and norepinephrine. This level then tapers off, leading to the next REM period. From this information, it is possible to speculate that lengthening REM periods during the night may result from progressively lower levels of aminergic neurotransmitter release during the night.

Another neurotransmitter of interest in REM sleep is acetylcholine (ACh). Interestingly, ACh increases during REM sleep in animals and can trigger "spectacularly long and intense" REM periods when administered in high doses. As discussed in Chapters 4 and 9, ACh is important in facilitating memory processing. The next section explores the role of REM in memory consolidation.

FUNCTIONS OF RAPID EYE MOVEMENT SLEEP

Scientists know that slow-wave delta sleep is physically restorative, but the debate over the purpose of REM sleep has ranged from postulations that it serves as a type of mental "garbage dump" to Freud's assertion that dreams are the "royal road to the unconscious." Science is now aware of at least two behavioral functions that REM sleep may serve. The first is memory consolidation. The second function is the intrapsychic function of dreaming. With a nod to Freud, neuropsychologists now conceptualize the psychological function of dreaming somewhat differently from Freud. Because scientists have again blessed the study of personal internal conscious processes, the study of dream function is once more opening up. Next, we introduce an area of study that is likely to provide many insights into the functioning of the conscious and subconscious minds.

Memory Consolidation and Rapid Eye Movement Sleep

The physiological means by which long-term memory storage occurs is most likely through long-term potentiation (LTP) of special glutamate neurotransmitter receptors (*N*-methyl-D-aspartate [NMDA] receptors) in the hippocampus. Memory consolidation may also be inhibited by gamma-aminobutyric acid (GABA). The hippocampus actively produces theta waves during REM sleep, as well as during stage 1 and 2 sleep. The important link between sleep and memory is that LTP in the hippocampus occurs during the production of theta rhythms (Larson & Lynch, 1986). Researchers have long thought that memory consolidates during sleep, because people can remember more after sleep. Sleeping pills may interfere with this process. However, it has been difficult to know whether sleep or REM itself accounts for the memory boost, or whether people just remember better when other information does not interfere. Now animal and human experiments have provided more evidence that memory is processed during sleep. Using rats, a team of researchers have recorded from individual neurons of the hippocampus (Pavlides & Winson, 1989). While the rats were awake, and moving about learning their position, only specific spatial coding neurons fired. Later during sleep, and particularly during production of the theta rhythm, these same neurons, and *only* these same neurons, fired at an even higher rate than during waking learning. This finding suggests that rats were reprocessing and strengthening the information during sleep.

In another experiment, a group of Israeli researchers studied memory consolidation and sleep under three different conditions. The task involved having to identify perceptual targets embedded in a visually noisy background. With learning and practice, people can usually improve their speed in picking out targets. In the first condition, researchers let people sleep normally after their initial practice session. In the second condition, researchers awakened people each time they entered REM sleep, effectively depriving them of REM sleep. In the same manner, in the third condition, researchers deprived people of delta sleep within stages 3 and 4. The two groups that were allowed REM sleep showed enhanced task learning on awakening. All those who underwent REM sleep deprivation, in contrast, showed either less improvement or an actual decrement in performance (Karni, Tanne, Rubenstein, Askenasy, & Sagi, 1994). Together, the findings from both animal and human research suggest that stage REM sleep plays a role in memory consolidation. However, whether REM plays a unique role in memory consolidation is still a matter of debate. This is a promising area of research for neuropsychologists and neuroscientists interested in the relations among REM, ACh, and hippocampal consolidation through LTP.

The Dreaming Mind

The aspects of consciousness discussed thus far involve the mind looking out. Dreams reflect the mind looking in. There is almost no physical input or output. Brains and minds are temporarily suspended from bodies. This is an amazing state, seemingly disjointed and illogical. Except for those who are "lucid" dreamers, dreaming minds wander from scene to scene with no conscious guidance. Dreamers are detached from their own self-consciousness and more critical selves. Dreams may be intensely emotional to strangely devoid of emotion. After a history of much debate on the function that dreams may serve, scientists are returning to the premise that dreams have a psychological core.

Aspects of the mind state of dreams may correlate with the physical aspects of a brain temporarily divorced from a body. Noted sleep researcher J. Alan Hobson (1995) has suggested that dreamers may feel they move effortlessly during dream states because they are being moved or guided by internally generated states and active central motoneurons. Perhaps in some measure, dream experiences of floating or flying also result from the brain being allowed to "float free" from the body, or perhaps in combination with, as Hobson suggests, spontaneous stimulation of orientation and position control centers in the brain. Hobson notices that when dreamers try to "will" dream movement while trying to escape from a pursuer, their feet and bodies may become leaden because of the conflicting motor messages of "voluntarily commanded movement (saying go) and the involuntarily clamped muscles (saying stop)." He further suggests that this standoff may suddenly break off the dream, thrusting the person into wakefulness and vivid dream recall. Awakening from a particular terrifying dream is called a "sleep anxiety attack." In fact, a large percentage of reported dreams are "hostile," and the most frequent themes are those of being chased and falling.

Many other correspondences probably exist between brain–body states and mind states in dreaming. This is an interesting area of study in its own right, and work in it will help to explain "how" people dream. Another question fundamental to understanding consciousness is "why" people dream. The brain activity occurring during REM sleep, such as memory consolidation, does not require conscious awareness. Biological functions of the brain could all occur without being brought to waking attention. Many dreams are not recalled. But why do some dreams bubble to the surface? This has been a matter of theoretical interest since Freud's revolutionary *The Interpretation of Dreams,* written in 1899. Since Freud's time, the history of dream theory has gone through a cycle from Freud's ideas that dreams represented unconscious sexual and aggressive urges, to the behaviorist movement totally turning away from the study of subjective states. Francis Crick's utilitarian housekeeping notion that dreams may just be the images that float by as the brain rids itself of the day's mental garbage suggests that dreaming is nothing more than a random firing of neurons. But many dream researchers have come back to a version of psychological interpretations.

Freud laid some of the basic groundwork in thinking about the psychological function of dreams from which other theories could spring. Today, most dream theorists do not attribute the same negative sexual and aggressive motivations to dream images that Freud did, but some of his methods and ideas may still be useful in uncovering the psychological meaning of dreams for the dreamer. With expansion from recent conceptualizations, researchers may be closer to a neuropsychological understanding of dreaming. Freud divided mental processing into conscious and unconscious processes. He saw unconscious processes as primitive, ancient, and disguised. Dreams, he felt, arose from these "unconscious" areas of the brain. This conceptualization is not unlike recent ideas of explicit versus implicit information processing. That which is explicit is available to verbal conscious awareness. However, as in memory processing and in some disorders such as neglect, a level of processing and recognition may exist outside conscious awareness. Is this not unlike the unconscious or the subconscious? Freud did not have the ability to look deep into the brain, but his ideas that unconscious thoughts emerge from more primitive areas of the brain are not inconsistent with theories of implicit processing taking place in the more primitive subcortical and limbic centers of the brain.

Perhaps where modern dream interpretive approaches have advanced most is in moving away from Freud's idea that even remembered dream content is unavailable psychologically to the dreamer unless interpreted by someone, such as an analyst, who can slice through the manifest content, defense mechanisms, and symbols, to uncover the latent meaning. This is not to say that the perspectives of others regarding the meaning of one's dreams are useless. In fact, such perspectives may be quite revealing and helpful. However, some of the greatest understanding available of the meaning in a dream involves self-interpretation in light of personal current life circumstances. After all, the dream was generated by the person dreaming it. Self-interpretation may involve not only the content, but the associated emotion that the dream invokes.

Troubling life circumstances provide the fodder for sleep researcher Rosalind Cartwright (Cartwright, Lloyd, Knight, & Trenholme, 1984; Cartwright, Kavits, Eastman, & Wood, 1991). Her volunteers, all going through separation or divorce, agreed to go through psychological testing that examined coping styles, and they consented to be awakened during REM sleep to report their dreams. Cartwright found that dream content and topics differed among subjects, but the themes were congruent with the waking response to the problem. Indeed, the content and themes of dreams may be useful in helping to solve many personal problems. But sometimes dreams accompany remarkable changes in waking life. We once treated depression in a patient who was also a smoker trying to kick the habit. During one therapy session he reported a dramatic dream he had had. In his dream, his whole body was turned grotesquely inside out, showing his lung, which was full of tumors and pus, to the outside world. After this dream the patient quit smoking.

An interesting exercise in exploring your own "dream consciousness" is to keep a dream journal for collecting and analyzing the content and themes of your dreams. What sensory processes are operating? Do you see, hear, feel, taste, or smell things in your dreams? As we mentioned earlier, sleep researcher J. Alan Hobson reminds us that the absurdity of dreams and the temporary "impairment" of judgment and cognition that occur during dreaming are common phenomena. Temporary disinhibition of the cortex may very well represent a physiological disconnection of aspects of the frontal lobes from other cortical and limbic centers. This may help to explain our often bizarre logic and lack of self-reflection during dreams. But what of those brain-impaired individuals who have structural damage resulting in waking disinhibition? Will we find that their dreams are even more disinhibited? This is a question for future research.

SLEEP DISORDERS

For most people, sleep is a pleasurable event. For some people, however, sleeping can become a medical emergency, as during sleep apnea, or intrude into wakefulness, as in narcolepsy.

Sleep Apnea

Sleep apnea has become the most common disorder the sleep literature describes and the most common presenting problem that sleep disorder centers evaluate (Guilleminault, 1982). **Sleep apnea syndrome (SAS)** is a serious disorder resulting from frequent episodes of apnea (cessation of airflow) during sleep. **Apnea** literally means "lack of breath." It is normal for muscles to relax during REM sleep. In some people, however, excessive muscle relaxation may disrupt breathing. The sleep apnea patient may actually stop breathing while asleep. This, of course, presents an immediate crisis for the body, because of the danger of **hypoxia** and of increased rapid heart rate and blood pressure. The apnea finally stops when, in an effort to breathe, the patient arouses, gasping for air. Each gasp for air is associated with a mini-awakening, as recorded on the EEG. If repeated apnea and awakening occur more than five times an hour, the patient is diagnosed with sleep apnea (Figure 16.6).

Patients with SAS may actually experience hundreds of apnea episodes per night, lasting up to a minute or longer. Serious cases may show more than 500 apneas per night, each one lasting more than 10 to 120 seconds and terminating with at least partial arousal. In addition to markedly disrupted sleep characterized by a significant absence of the normal progression of sleep stages, dangerously low levels of oxygen to the brain may result. Apnea periods usually produce declines in sleep-related blood oxyhemoglobin saturation and increases in carbon dioxide. This condition, known as hypoxia, is associated with below-average levels of oxygenated blood, often below 60% (normal is 95%). These changes have a profound impact on numerous body systems. It is impossible to hold one's breath indefinitely, even when a person is sleeping. Essentially, a reflex controls breathing. But in young children, this reflex has not yet developed, and cessation of breathing

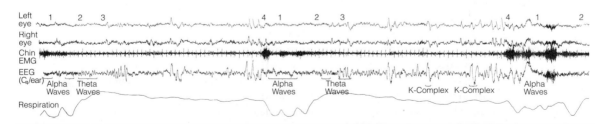

Figure 16.6 An electroencephalogram (EEG)-recorded episode of sleep apnea. The patient is fully awake at point 1 (EEG alpha waves). At point 2, he is starting to fall asleep (EEG theta waves). At point 3, the patient is fully asleep (notice the relaxation of the chin electromyogram and absence of breathing). At point 4, the patient awakens and breathing resumes. The cycle then repeats. (Reproduced from Hauri, P. [1977]. *Current concepts: The sleep disorders.* Peapack, NJ: Pharmacia & Upjohn.)

during sleep may result in death. This is one of the possible causes of **sudden infant death syndrome (SIDS);** SIDS most often occurs between the ages of 2 and 4 months.

Two primary mechanisms are involved in sleep apnea. The first one is the more common **obstructive sleep apnea.** Apneas occur most often during REM sleep when either the upper airway collapses, not allowing air to pass, or the body weight of the patient on the chest compromises respiratory effort. In each case, the consequence is disordered breathing. In the second mechanism of sleep apnea, **central sleep apnea,** disordered breathing is related to the brain failing to send the necessary signals to breathe. This may reflect brainstem abnormalities that manifest only during sleep. In either case, the disorder is serious and often associated with severe O_2 desaturation. The terms *central* and *obstructive* do not represent a strict dichotomy, because obstructive sleep apnea may impair CNS control of muscles, and episodes of obstructive sleep apnea often precede central apnea. Such episodes are called *mixed apnea.* Complications of apnea result in poor physical health and associated neuropsychological deficits of poor concentration and memory (Barth, Findley, Zillmer, Gideon, & Surrat, 1993).

The cause of sleep apnea is not well understood, although age, obesity, and being male are all risks. Generally, researchers consider sleep apnea episodes to be caused by a complex interaction of physiologic and anatomic factors. Clinical features that are characteristic of the syndrome include excessive daytime sleepiness, heart failure, hypertension, headaches, disturbing snoring, irritability, sleep disruption, and personality changes. The hypoxia of sleep apnea markedly affects central neurotransmitter function and cellular metabolism, disrupting the biochemical and hemodynamic (pertaining to blood circulation) state of the CNS. Hypoxia may also lead to disturbed fluid and electrolyte distribution within the sodium-potassium pump, and it alters brain adenosine levels in animals. In addition, in patients with sleep apnea, cerebral blood flow studies demonstrate abnormally decreased blood flow, which may further compromise neuropsychological functioning because of decreased neuronal activity (Guilleminault & Dement, 1978). Sleep apnea can have serious psychosocial effects as well, including significant changes in adaptive functioning (Zillmer, Ware, Rose, & Bond, 1989).

Most treatment efforts focus on relief of apneas through surgical and mechanical means. The most effective treatment is continuous positive airway pressure (CPAP), which is a mask that "forces" air through the nose or mouth while sleeping. CPAP is not considered a "cure," but it abolishes sleep apnea by maintaining upper airway flow during sleep. One of the most successful and least invasive treatments for SAS, CPAP acts as a pneumatic splint to prevent upper airway collapse during the night. CPAP must be used every night by the patient but has few side effects as long as one can actually sleep (one patient described CPAP as analogous to holding your head out of the car window while driving at 50 miles/hour). Losing weight can also help, because obesity is a major risk factor in sleep apnea. More controversial treatments include surgery to increase the dimensions of the pharynx via **uvulopalatopharyngoplasty (UPPP)** and tracheotomy, to completely bypass the upper airway obstruction during sleep (Williams & Karacan, 1978). UPPP involves removing the uvula, the small, fleshy tissue hanging from the center of the soft palate, which may relax and sag, obstructing the upper airway. However, this treatment is not as successful as CPAP and may also alter the subject's voice. Patients who have undergone treatment for SAS often report an improvement in their cognitive functioning.

Narcolepsy

The most notable disorder resulting from impaired CNS control of the sleep/wake cycle is narcolepsy (derived from Greek meaning "a taking hold of numbness"). Narcoleptics are afflicted with irresistible daytime "sleep attacks." They can fall asleep while at work, while driving a car, or during a conversation. Such sleep attacks can last from a few seconds to more than 30 minutes. **Excessive daytime sleepiness** is the primary symptom of narcolepsy, although patients are also subject to narcoleptic sleep attacks, **cataplexy,** sleep paralysis, and **hypnagogic hallucinations.** Narcolepsy is a central nervous system disorder of the region in the brainstem that controls and regulates sleep and wakefulness. Once the disorder is established, it typically persists for one's entire life. Narcolepsy occurs in 1 of 1000 people. Symptoms typically begin to appear between the onset of puberty and age 25.

Excessive Daytime Sleepiness—Pathologic daytime sleepiness is often the first sign to emerge in narcolepsy, typically associated with normal amounts of sleep at night. Many narcoleptics are asleep or sleepy during much of the day. They often report poor concentration and memory. Especially during the afternoon, after a meal, or when watching TV, narcoleptics are at risk for falling asleep. It is as if no amount of sleep could satisfy the patient's frequent and irresistible need for sleep. Excessive daytime sleepiness is the most prominent and troublesome component of narcolepsy. The patient is typically miserable and fatigued, often demonstrating inappropriate sleep.

Cataplexy—Cataplexy is the most debilitating of the narcoleptic symptoms. Cataplexy is a brief (seconds to

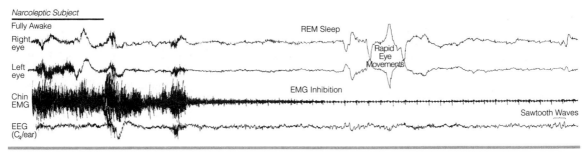

Figure 16.7 The narcoleptic goes quickly into rapid eye movement sleep. (Reproduced from Hauri, P. [1977]. *Current concepts: The sleep disorders*. Peapack, NJ: Pharmacia & Upjohn.)

minutes) episode of muscle weakness, actual paralysis, or both. In a benign form of cataplexy, only the face and the head may droop. In a severe attack, all the muscles may become limp, resulting in the victim falling to the floor. After the attack, the patient quickly regains alertness and muscle tone. Cataplectic attacks occur during periods of sudden excitement and emotional change, including laughter, anger, and athletic activity. The sleep paralysis of cataplexy is always associated with pathologic REM sleep. If a cataplectic attack lasts long enough, it often becomes full-blown REM sleep. Thus, you can think of cataplexy as an inappropriate attack of REM sleep. The pathologic intrusion of REM sleep and associated motor inhibition relates to a variety of nervous system dysfunctions, including massive nonreciprocal excitation of spinal inhibitory interneurons and active inhibition of motoneurons.

Hypnagogic Hallucinations—Hypnagogic hallucinations are also a symptom of narcolepsy and occur in the transition between wakefulness and sleep onset. Most people do not experience imagery during the transition from waking to sleep, because they are moving into NREM sleep, a period of little imagery. Narcoleptics, in contrast, can experience hypnagogic hallucinations during their shorter transition from waking to REM sleep. Thus, narcoleptics may experience vivid, dreamlike intrusions into wakefulness. The hallucinations can be mundane or nightmarish, and they can cause great anxiety.

Sleep Paralysis—Sleep paralysis is the momentary paralysis on awakening or at sleep onset. Although the person may be able to see what is happening in the room, the body is totally unable to move for seconds to minutes. People without narcolepsy have also described this sleep paralysis on awakening from a REM period in the early morning hours. To "break out" of this paralysis, they may start by moving their eyes, then willfully moving a finger. As soon

as the voluntary muscles engage, the person breaks out of the REM-controlled sleep paralysis.

Narcolepsy can be best conceptualized as an imbalance among the wake, REM, and NREM systems. In such patients, wakefulness is weak, and REM sleep, or parts thereof, can intrude into it. This imbalance among the three stages can range from mild to severe. Narcolepsy is not a psychological disorder, although the socioeconomic and psychological toll on the patients can be great. The casual observer often thinks narcoleptic attacks are related to epilepsy, but they are not. The cause is generally unknown, although a minority of patients manifests parts of the syndrome after encephalitis, severe head injury, or brain tumor. Clinicians often make the differential diagnosis in a sleep disorder center using a procedure known as the *multiple sleep latency test (MSLT)*. Interestingly, narcoleptics are asked to arrive at the sleep disorder center, not in the evening, but during the morning. Around 10 A.M. they are put to "rest." The reason for this is that the early morning would be the least likely time for most well-rested people to fall asleep and proceed into REM sleep. The subject must fall asleep in less than 5 minutes (normal sleep latency is 15 minutes at nighttime) and must show at least two sleep-onset REM periods to diagnose narcolepsy (Figure 16.7). Treatment of narcolepsy includes counseling for patient and family, developing good sleep habits including frequent naps, and the administration of medication, typically stimulants (such as amphetamines) for sleepiness and tricyclics (such as imipramine) for cataplexy. Although narcolepsy cannot be cured, its symptoms can be controlled with proper behavioral and medical therapy.

Runaway Brain: Seizure Disorders

Seizures, like sleep, are reversible alterations of consciousness. But seizures occur suddenly during periods of expected wakefulness and are abnormal. For reasons not fully explainable, groups of neurons fire excessively in synchronous oscillation, as opposed to their normal pattern of relatively independent electrical activity. During a seizure, the firing rate of neurons may be as high as 500 times a second, which is more than 6 times faster than the normal rate of 80 firings per second (National Institute of Neurological Disorders and Stroke [NINDS], 2004). Seizures are transient alterations in consciousness and can be provoked by external stimuli such as pulsing lights or sounds, or internal triggers such as psychological and physical stress, sleep deprivation, high fever, and hormonal changes. Although there are many types of seizures that can be categorized by focus, behavior, and the extent of abnormal brain activity, there are two main categories of seizures. If the abnormal firing is confined to a particular brain area, the result will be a partial or focal seizure. If the abnormal discharge involves both hemispheres, the event is termed a **generalized seizure.** Episodes can also begin as a partial seizure and secondarily generalize to involve the whole brain.

The causes of seizures are varied. Seizures that first appear in infants and young children may manifest due to genetic and developmental abnormalities of the brain, infections, fever, or other disorders in metabolism. In people of all ages, seizures may also be caused by traumatic brain injury, brain infections, tumors, vascular abnormalities, alcohol and drug use or withdrawal, or environmental toxins. In about half of the seizures reported, however, there is no clearly identifiable cause.

Epilepsy is not a disease itself, but a syndrome in which brain seizure activity is a primary and chronic symptom. Older diagnostic schemes stated epilepsy could be diagnosed only if the seizures were recurrent (at least two separate seizures) and unpredictable. Newer consensus definitions state that people can be diagnosed with epilepsy after suffering only one seizure if they also have an "enduring" alteration of the brain that makes it highly likely they will suffer future seizures (Fisher et al., 2005). Many people who have had a seizure, in fact, do not show the full epileptic syndrome (Hauser, 1992). Adults may suffer "nonepileptic episodes" from such events as hyperventilation breath holding, migraines, ischemic attacks, drug toxicity, narcolepsy, and extreme emotion such as anger. In summary, a person must have at least two seizures, or the high *potential* for more than one seizure, that cannot be attributed to another medical condition to be diagnosed with epilepsy.

Epilepsy affects approximately 1% of the U.S. population (NINDS, 2004) with an age-related increase in incidence to 3% by age 75. Many more people or approximately 10% of the population may suffer a seizure during their life (Epilepsy Foundation, n.d.).

CLASSIFICATION OF SEIZURE TYPES

Previously, classification of seizures was based on the original French classification scheme and was categorized according to behavioral observations of what happened during a seizure. For example, **grand mal** or "big bad" seizures were named for the most violent motoric abnormalities of stiffening (**tonic**) and jerking (**clonic**) episodes and the accompanying loss of consciousness. The **petit mal** or "little bad" seizures, in contrast, were considered seizures that do not result in violent physical loss of control but do cause an altered state of consciousness. Current seizure classifications depend on what is known of the origin or focus of the seizure within the brain. The current taxonomies are divided into two primary classifications: generalized and partial seizures. Generalized seizures involve both cortical hemispheres at the onset, whereas partial seizures are confined to a specific area. Partial seizures may be further divided into two types: simple partial and complex partial. In simple partial seizures, consciousness is preserved, whereas in **complex partial seizures,** consciousness is impaired. In addition, a partial seizure can spread out, resulting in a secondary generalized seizure, which is a seizure that started being partial—limited to a specific brain area—and later generalized to both hemispheres. As you may imagine, besides the consciousness factor that divides partial seizures into simple or complex, there are many different variations of partial seizures, depending on the site of origin. Generalized seizures can also be classified into different types. The epilepsy classification scheme presented in Table 16.3 shows the seizure types of both groups.

Regardless of the primary seizure type, up to 70% of people report having an **aura** before a seizure. This happens in **prodromal phase,** or precursory phase, of the episode, in which one may experience odd transient symptoms such as nausea, dizziness, or numbness. Sensory

Table 16.3   *Seizure Classification*

Generalized Seizures	Partial or Focal Seizures
1. Absence	1. Simple: focal motor, somatosensory or special-sensory, psychic, and autonomic
2. Myoclonic	2. Complex partial: psychomotor, temporal lobe
3. Clonic	3. Secondarily generalized
4. Tonic	
5. Tonic-clonic	
6. Atonic	

smell may halt the seizure (Efron, 1957). We explore this aspect of seizure control further in our discussion of epilepsy treatment.

After a seizure episode is a **postictal phase** in which the person gradually emerges into full consciousness. Often symptoms of confusion, disorientation, depression, headache, or fatigue follow. Less common, the person may bite his or her tongue or lose bladder control. This phase may be momentary or may last for hours, somewhat depending on seizure type.

The following sections discuss seizure types according to the epilepsy classification scheme of Table 16.3. Clinical descriptions correlate with what is known of their neurologic counterparts. A more generalized discussion of the brain mechanisms responsible for seizure activity follows.

Generalized Seizures

Generalized seizures, formally known as *grand mal seizures,* are bilaterally symmetric episodes characterized by a temporary lack of awareness. The brain origin of these seizures has traditionally been considered unknown or generalized. Behaviorally, they typically have a motor component that onlookers consider frightening. The motor discharge is likely to consist of any combination of a *tonic* or *clonic* form. Some seizures have only the tonic component, others only the clonic component, and a number of seizures involve both aspects. In these *tonic-clonic* seizures, the behavior that alerts others to a seizure onset is the tonic stage. Patients describe passing out, and onlookers are likely to witness a stiffening of the person's whole body, jaw clenching, and a blue appearance to the face. The blueness may look like a respiratory arrest, but during a seizure this actually occurs because peripheral blood vessel constriction allows more blood to flow to the brain. In any case, breathing stops only temporarily. After seconds to minutes, the second clonic stage appears. The body begins a rhythmic jerking of limbs and may involve the whole torso. This is followed by abrupt limpness (or atonia) and a gradual regaining of conscious awareness. Generalized seizures may take several forms, but usually include components of irregular motor discharge in the form of tonic and/or clonic movement.

Other types of generalized seizures resulting in abnormal muscular symptoms are myoclonic and atonic seizures. **Myoclonic seizures** manifest in arrhythmic bursts of jerky motor movements that usually do not last more than a second and tend to occur in clusters over a short period. People who experience them sometimes describe them as "jumps." **Atonic seizures,** in contrast, are characterized by a sudden loss of muscle tone and may result in a fall. They last no longer than 15 seconds while the person remains conscious.

Absence seizures appear in some classification schemes as a partial seizure and in others as a generalized seizure. This may represent differences related to the brain areas responsible and the extent of cortical involvement. As seen in the following case example described by a neurologist, the typical gross-motor involvement of generalized absence seizures is not present and is replaced by ictal **automatisms.**

[A] mother brought her delightful red-headed eight-year-old daughter to see me. Because the girl seemed so attentive, intelligent, and well-behaved, it was hard for me to believe that she was having a difficult time at school. Her teacher reported that she made frequent mistakes on the blackboard and was often unable to answer simple questions. In my office, I asked her to take some rapid shallow breaths. After thirty seconds, she stared vacantly into space with her eyelids fluttering. Ten seconds later, she was back to her usual self. I had witnessed a classic absence seizure. Her EEG showed a pattern of 3 cycles/sec spike and dome activity during overbreathing, typical of absence epilepsy. (Richard & Reiter, 1990, p. 30)

In the above case, the doctor precipitated a seizure by having the girl hyperventilate. This girl's fluttering eyelids are an important behavioral clue to seizure activity. Additional automatisms may include stereotyped hand movements or facial tics. Less typical for this type of seizure is a sudden myoclonic jerk or atonic loss of muscle tone. At the approach of an attack, some individuals may just stop talking midstream, stare blankly into space for the duration of the attack, and then resume without noticing any lapse in consciousness. Absence attacks characteristically affect children from age 4 to 14. Interestingly, many children with absence attacks "outgrow" them, suggesting that a delay or anomaly in brain development plays an important role in their occurrence. It is rare for adults with no seizure or trauma history to develop absence attacks.

Partial Seizures

Partial or focal seizures may take several forms, but they always begin as a local neuronal discharge that may generalize across the corpus callosum, eventually involving the entire brain in a secondarily generalized seizure. This seizure category represents the most common type, affecting about 800,000 people in the United States (Cascino, 1992). These seizures can be more frequently localized than generalized seizures, but still only a third of those afflicted have identifiable causes. Head trauma, stroke, and viral brain diseases such as meningitis and encephalitis are a few of the conditions that may lead to partial seizures.

Partial seizures consist of three main types. First, **simple seizures** are focal events that may involve sensorimotor expression or psychic expression (mood, emotion, or

Neuropsychology in Action 16.4

Déjà Vu and Epilepsy

by Karen B. Friedman

We have all some experience of a feeling, that comes over us occasionally, of what we are saying and doing having been said and done before, in a remote time—of our having been surrounded, dim ages ago, by the same faces, objects, and circumstances—of our knowing perfectly what will be said next, as if we suddenly remember it!

—Charles Dickens, David Copperfield

Have you ever been in a situation where suddenly everything seems familiar, the place, the objects, the layout of the setting . . . even the movements taking place. . . and then, when you are still perplexed by such a bizarre feeling, it goes away? Then you probably are like the two thirds of the population who has experienced at least one déjà vu experience in their lifetime.

The phenomenon of déjà vu caught the attention of philosophers and writers for ages, and more recently has become the subject of scientific study. The most common definition for déjà vu ("already seen" in French) was proposed by V. M. Neppe (1983): "Any subjectively inappropriate impression of familiarity of a present experience with an undefined past." This definition implies that there is a certain insight into the nature of the impossibility of the situation.

Interestingly, a considerable number of patients with temporal lobe epilepsy report déjà vu auras. In the late 1800s, Hughlings Jackson first observed that seizures that arose in the medial temporal lobe could result in a "dreamy state" described as vivid memory-like hallucinations and/or the sense of having previously lived through the exact same situation. Later, other researchers have tried to evoke that "dreamy state" by electrically stimulating different regions of the temporal lobe such as the lateral temporal neocortex, the hippocampal formation, and the amygdala (Mullan & Penfield, 1959; Halgren, Walter, Cherlow, & Crandall, 1978). Gloor (1990) proposes that this dreamy state could be evoked by lateral temporal lobe stimulation, but only if the brain activity spread medially toward the limbic system, thus emphasizing the importance of limbic rather than temporal neocortical structures. After much debate, in 1994, Bancaud and his colleagues studied 16 patients with temporal lobe epilepsy with presurgically implanted electrodes; measured the electrical activity of the temporal lobe, the amygdala, and the hippocampus; and at the same time, attempted to stimulate those areas of the brain. They found that déjà vu could be experimentally evoked by stimulation of any of those three sites, and that there was no one single place that was solely responsible for the experience in every epilepsy patient. However, they did find that the stimulation of the deeper structures (amygdala and hippocampus) was 10 times more likely to evoke those states, concluding that the temporal neocortex probably plays a secondary but still important role in the déjà vu experience.

Another area of interest in the field of déjà vu and epilepsy is that of lateralization, because the presentation of a déjà vu cou eventually help neurologists diagnose the of seizure onset for those who present this type of aura. Mullan and Penfield (1959) suggest that déjà vu occurs in the nondor nant temporal lobe—usually, but not alwa the right temporal lobe for right handed people. In accordance with this idea, Glo (1990) asserts that having an aura of déj would be sufficient to localize the focus o seizure to the right temporal lobe. Howev Weinand and colleagues (1994) later fou that right-handed seizure patients with preictal déjà vu all had seizures arising in their left hemispheres. They concluded th handedness rather than language domi- nance appears to be a more consistent predictor of ictal déjà vu lateralization.

Many people have experienced at lea one déjà vu experience, and this does no imply that they have epilepsy. However, connection to the temporal lobe and lim structures may exist, as well as a brief a mal firing, which gives a false sense of familiarity. Researchers have suggested positive correlation of déjà vu with highe socioeconomic level, more education, m travel, and better dream recall (Brown, 2003). The range of possible explanatio for this fascinating phenomenon is exter but not yet fully understood. Perhaps by better understanding déjà vu we will be to discover more about the oddities of th brain and how our memories and experi- ences are processed and retrieved.

---

alterations or hallucinations in any sensory domain may appear. For example, chemical sense disruptions may manifest as unpleasant metallic tastes or foul odors. Some people recognize their aura as an emotional change such as fear or anxiety. Others experience a temporary aphasia or a sense of forced thinking. Yet others describe auras as an otherworldly or surreal dream state, or a sense of déjà vu (Neuropsychology in Action 16.4). These symptoms are highly idiosyncratic but are likely to be consistent within a person. Most seizure sufferers become adept at re nizing their own auras; however, some auras occur w out awareness, although they may be recognized by ers. Auras may point to the genesis, or the **epileptog focus,** of the seizure within the brain (Cascino, 19 Interestingly, some people are also able to arrest the gression of a seizure during this prodromal phase by le ing to counteract the sensation with its opposite. For ample, if a foul smell is part of an aura, a strong plea

altered consciousness). The behavior experienced reflects the area from which the seizure emanates. For example, discharges from the motor strip can cause sudden or stereotypic movement, such as jerking or twitching. People have reported that their eyes may move to a certain position or that they turn their heads involuntarily. Occipital lobe foci can result in seeing vivid images or flashing lights. Memory and personality alterations can be a result of temporal lobe foci, and intensive mood experiences can occur with limbic system foci. The behavioral results vary widely from person to person but are closely tied to the site of seizure focus. Because there is no further involvement, the person can also experience these events as an aura.

The second type of partial seizure is complex partial seizures, the most common forms being **psychomotor** or **temporal lobe epilepsy.** These are more "complex" than simple partial seizures in that they have an element of altered psyche or awareness in addition to sensory or motor components. About half of those with complex partial seizures experience an aura (Cascino, 1992). Complex partial seizures typically emanate from the temporal lobes but can also occur as the result of a frontal lesion. The alteration of consciousness can take several forms. It may include a sense of déjà vu ("already seen") in new environments or jamais vu ("never seen") in a familiar place. The person may experience a sense of forced thinking, illusions, panic, terror, or even ecstasy. The motor changes during the ictal phase often take the form of odd, catatonic-like posturing and automatisms such as lip smacking or undoing buttons. The shift into the ictal phase is abrupt, usually commencing with a motionless stare. The postictal period of confusion and drowsiness can be quite long with complex partial seizures. The case of the "sweeping lady" is a good example of what may happen with complex partial seizures (Neuropsychology in Action 16.5).

The third type of partial seizure, a **secondarily generalized seizure,** is actually a variation of the first type. If a simple seizure spreads, this spreading can generalize throughout the whole brain as in the case of **Jacksonian seizures.** Jacksonian seizures involve motor areas and have been called "marching seizures," because they begin with jerking or tingling of a single body area and spread to other areas. The symptoms reflect their corresponding brain regions; thus, diagnosticians consult maps of the motor homunculus.

NEUROANATOMY AND NEUROPHYSIOLOGY OF SEIZURES

Partial and secondarily generalized seizures are the most likely to be localized because both the aura and the behavior during a seizure can point to a seizure's epileptogenic focus (the anatomic site of onset). Generalized seizures are difficult to localize, because they quickly disrupt the entire range of behavior involving all cortical neurons and may arise from a central mechanism capable of having a global effect on the brain. If there is an identifiable seizure focus, EEG recording is useful in locating it if a seizure occurs spontaneously or can be induced during EEG monitoring.

Seizures are a symptom, similar to the concept of fever, that something is going on in the brain. A seizure may be localized to a particular anatomic area of the brain, and technicians may be able to image a corresponding structural pathology such as a lesion, a tumor, a vascular disease, or other anomaly. For example, the cause of some childhood seizures may be malformed brain tissue (Figure 16.8).

Because seizures also arise from metabolic disturbances and infections that affect the delicate physiological balance of the brain, neurologists cannot always find a structural location of injury or neuronal destruction in the brain. Although many normal people may experience a seizure, the occurrence may indicate significant brain pathology and medical consultation should always be sought.

Normally, the brain maintains a balance of neuronal firing between excitatory discharges and inhibitory control of excessive firing. Single neurons and neuronal circuits fire according to their own direction and processing in what appear to be random patterns. Because so many different patterns are occurring simultaneously, and because the EEG represents a summation of neuronal firing, the resultant EEG tracing is fast and asynchronous. Seizures occur due to excessive excitatory synchronous neuronal firing. If you have ever been caught up in a "wave" in a packed football stadium, the analogy to the brain is similar. All the people represent individual neurons and are initially involved in their own behaviors. At first, although small groups of people may be involved in a rhythmic "give and take," the summation of "stadium behavior" appears random, with occasional synchronous bursts of cheering from one side or the other. But if a small group of people successfully initiate a wave, before long the entire stadium of 50,000 people synchronizes in a rhythm that sweeps through the crowd.

Absence seizures provide a good example of a generalized seizure that arises from a central mechanism. EEGs of classical absence seizures show characteristic synchronous bilateral spike-and-wave discharge with a 3 cycles/sec frequency. This EEG frequency is within the same range as delta waves, characteristic of deep sleep. A reasonable description of absence seizures is that they force a temporary disconnection within the arousal system of the RAS, thus pushing the whole cortex into a temporary sleeplike state.

Neuropsychology in Action 16.5

Epilepsy and the Case of the Sweeping Lady

by Thomas L. Bennett Ph.D., Professor of Psychology, Colorado State University, Clinical Director, Brain Injury Recovery Program, Fort Collins, CO

Epilepsy is a common neurologic disorder, currently affecting more than 2 million people in the United States (for a detailed discussion of epilepsy, see Bennett, 1992). Diagnosis of epilepsy depends on clinical interview and EEG assessment showing abnormality in the interictal (between seizures) scalp electrode EEG tracings. The interictal spike is a marker for this disorder (McIntosh, 1992).

When psychic alterations occur, the seizures are called complex partial seizures. For neuropsychologists, these are the most interesting epileptic disorders (Bennett, 1987). They may be associated with motor automatisms consisting of stereotyped, repetitive movements such as chewing, blinking, lip smacking, pointing, or picking at one's clothes. Complex partial seizures, because of their frequent temporal lobe and limbic system focus, may have an emotional

component to the psychic alterations. The most common emotion is fear, but the person may also report pleasure, sadness, or vague familiarity. Individuals with complex partial seizures also commonly report sensory hallucinations or misperceptions. These sensations may range throughout the spectrum of visual, gustatory, olfactory, auditory, or somatic perceptions. Olfactory sensations are the most common type of sensory aura reported. These are typically quite displeasing (such as the smell of burning or rotting flesh), but may on occasion be pleasant (such as the smell of roses).

In the course of a complex partial seizure, the person may utter meaningless speech, laugh, or cry. Complex motor responses may also occur, including compulsive, purposeless writing and even running. During a complex partial seizure, a person may be unaware of or unresponsive to her or his

environment, failing to respond to questions by others. The person may be vaguely aware of what is going on but unable to control it. While in a state of altered consciousness during a seizure, he or she may go into another room, wander through a public place, or leave a store and wander down the street. Imagine how upset you would be to find yourself in a different place from where you "just" were and to have lost several minutes or even hours of time, not knowing what you did during the interim. This is illustrated by the case of the sweeping lady.

This individual—let us call her Alice—has been a client of mine for almost 15 years. We meet on occasion as she continues to deal with the impact of her epilepsy on her life. Alice's epilepsy has never been completely controlled by antiepileptic drugs, a far too common experience for those with complex partial seizures. She has had to alter her

Both animal and human studies point to the thalamocortical circuitry as the source for the primary aberrant mechanism involved in absence attacks. As we have discussed, during an alert state, neurons in the thalamocortical loop are involved in continuous tonic firing. This allows signals from the external environment to pass through the thalamus to the cortex. External transmission to the cortex dampens when neurons begin firing according to an internally generated oscillating rhythm. Neurologists think that a group of neurons within the thalamus, the **nucleus reticularis thalami (NRT),** regulates oscillatory behavior of the thalamocortical loop. Direct recordings indicate that this is the source of rhythmic burst firing when the EEG becomes synchronized and also is a source of asynchronous firing during wakefulness. The NRT also project to the contralateral dorsal thalamus, and thus have the ability to influence both hemispheres. The NRT mainly consist of GABAergic neurons that project to each other within the NRT and other areas of the thalamus.

One of their main functions is in controlling cerebral excitability. Researchers report that during early development, one form of GABA receptors—the GABA-b type—increases and later is pruned to adult levels. Researchers also know that GABA agonist drugs make absence seizures worse. Some investigators believe that absence seizures in children may result from an error in development, resulting in a temporary overabundance of GABA receptors and, therefore, a temporary imbalance in the excitatory/inhibitory forces of the brain (Snead, 1995). They think what happens within this system of neurons that affects a shift between asynchronous and synchronous rhythms is a change in the calcium potential of the cellular membrane. This may explain why some antiepileptic drugs such as ethosuximide and trimethadione, which act on the calcium current of the membrane, are effective.

In addition to the GABAergic neurons within the thalamus, numerous neurotransmitter systems may be involved in generalized absence seizures, because the ascending

lifestyle and goals in life significantly; but overall, she has adapted well to her disability. Before the onset of her seizure disorder in her early 20s, she was active in sports and the community, and she planned to return to college to complete a bachelor's degree.

ice has two daughters. She has worked in a
le of settings, but overstimulation and
e can increase seizure frequency, and
rently is not working. Diagnostic
cephalograms (EEGs) have pro-
e normal and some abnormal
nal EEGs are also observed in
mplex partial seizures, showing
G does not rule out
ure pattern is interesting,
ontains many of the
cussed.
nent of her epilepsy,
e less frequent with
l, Alice typically
tions ("butter-
ea during the
nomenon,
led her to
al
res
time
g

e episode.
ed after a
es not expe-
e occasions,
and therefore
ther time the
nvolve com-
to as the in-
his is particu-
mplex seizures
epilepsy/partial
effect of remov-
guage and mem-
Wada (Wada &
olves the injection
m amytal, through
ize one hemisphere
heres are connected
amytal reaches only
on both sides of the
de makes the barbitu-
is to test the function

As the abnormal electrical activity spread and overt signs of the seizure pattern began to develop, Alice experienced olfactory/gustatory sensations, including detecting the odor of putrid, burning flesh, olfactory sensations, and the taste of soap. A blank stare preceded her motor automatisms, and she lost clear awareness of her surroundings at this point. She then began purposeless pacing and hand rubbing for 2 to 3 minutes. She reported that she was vaguely aware of these things happening, but she could not control them. She would typically emit a series of grunting and gasping sounds, which sounded to others as if she were having trouble getting enough air. Grimacing contorted her face. She laughed uncontrollably for several minutes, and then cried and rocked back and forth for several minutes more. The sequence ended when the spread of epileptic activity caused a generalized tonic contraction and she lost consciousness. This case illustrates the wealth of events that can occur during a complex partial seizure episode.

Several times Alice lost all awareness of what she had done for several hours. This happened when she went into a grocery store or large department store during the day when things were busy, noisy, and visually overstimulating. She later discovered that she must have just aimlessly wandered through the store, perhaps repeatedly examining objects, because she had lost up to 2 to 3 hours of time for which she had no recollection. One of the most unusual experiences she had during a complex partial seizure occurred several years ago. I have thought of this as the "great fugue," or the "case of the sweeping lady."

It was the middle of the day in late spring or early summer, and Alice was home alone. She remembers that she was in her kitchen and had decided to sweep the floor. She vaguely remembers starting to sweep the floor, but nothing of the next 45 to 60 minutes. Apparently, she swept across the kitchen, down the hall, through the entryway, and out the front door! Her next memory was that she was lying on a stranger's porch. At first, she did not know who she was or where she was. Over the next few minutes, she became reoriented and realized she was on someone's porch. She stood up, walked down the sidewalk into the street, and recognized a friend's house several houses away. That enabled her to reorient to where she was. It turned out that she had walked several blocks from her home, crossing several intersections, without awareness, while in an extended complex partial seizure fugue!

cholinergic, no-
rgic neurons.
from the nu-
rousal apart
lation and
resent a
vstems.

seizure onset. For example, if a person shows impaired memory for a list of words, this may indicate an abnormality in the left temporal region. Testing can also help determine the extent to which emotional components and stress may stem from seizures and help discriminate between neurologically based epilepsy and pseudoseizures arising from a somatoform disorder. As with any other neurologic disorder, neuropsychological testing can demonstrate a pattern of individual cognitive strengths and weaknesses to make appropriate recommendations for better adjustment to daily life.

One of the most frequent uses of a neuropsychological evaluation in epilepsy is in the context of a presurgical evaluation. When medication or other treatment has proved ineffective to reduce or eliminate the seizures, then the resection of the possible epileptogenic focus is considered. To perform a surgery of this type, the neurosurgeon needs to perform a series of tests to determine with precision the site of the focus and to assess whether the person would not suffer undue loss of function from removal of

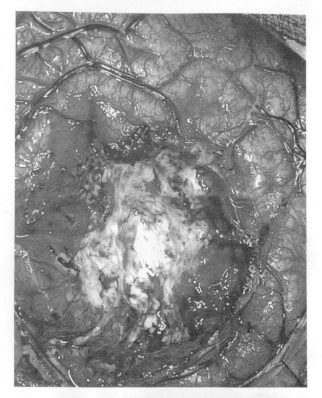

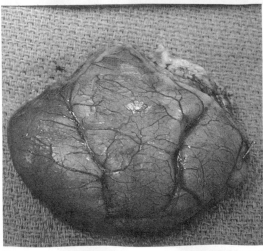

Figure 16.8 Malformed tissue, present and growing from birth, was the cause of seizures. After removal this person has been seizure free and able to attend college. (Courtesy H. McNiece.)

the affected brain area. A neuropsychological evaluation is in order; first, because it provides a baseline of the person's level of performance, and second, because as mentioned earlier, it can help by providing clues as to where the focus of the seizures might be through analysis of the patterns of

dysfunction. To determine and localize brain impairment, the neuropsychologist will analyze the facts obtained by such an evaluation in conjunction with other sources of information such as clinical observation and structural and functional brain imaging. A procedure that is usually performed in a presurgical evaluation is inpatient video EEG monitoring (Figure 16.9). EEG monitoring is either done through noninvasive scalp electrodes (such as those used for sleep EEGs) or through depth electrodes that are surgically implanted. EEG and behavior (via video recording) are then continuously recorded together 24 hours a day. The purpose is to localize the seizure onset and learn as much as possible about the individual behavioral seizure characteristics. Even though the ultimate goal is to eliminate the seizures, this is a point in the treatment course where involved want a seizure to happen! If a seizure does occur spontaneously (as we mentioned earlier, interi periods can take months, even years), actions can be ta within this controlled environment to provoke a sei such as reduce the antiepileptic medication or induce deprivation or hyperventilation.

The presurgical neuropsychological evaluator looking for any fluctuations in consciousness or b that may herald a seizure. If seizures occur during and if the patient is conscious and not in dang jury, an assessment of consciousness and memo made. For example, after the seizure is over, t can be asked to recall what happened or to what was said or shown to them during th Sometimes an evaluation can be continu seizure if the person recovers quickly and do rience many postictal symptoms; but on sor the person may show signs of confusion, the evaluation needs to be continued at an

Neuropsychologists are also typically administration of a specialized presurgery monly called the *Wada test* (it is also refer *tracarotid amobarbital procedure [IAP]*). larly useful before surgeries for partial involving the temporal lobe (temporal lob complex seizures), to determine the likel ing brain tissue on the functions of lar ory. Named after its developer, Juhn Rasmussen, 1960), this procedure inv by a radiologist of a barbiturate, sodiu the patient's carotid artery to anesthe at a time. Even though the two hemis and irrigated by arteries, the sodium one side because of equal pressure brain. The blood pressure on one s rate stay on the other side. The ain

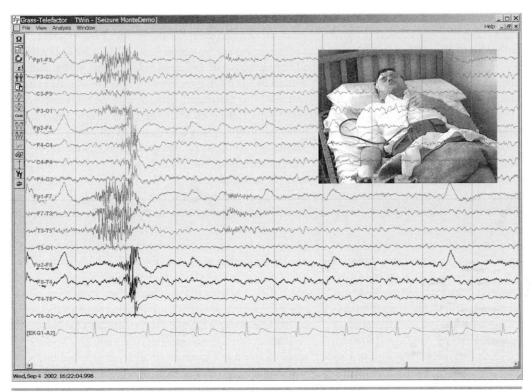

Figure 16.9 Inpatient electroencephalographic and video monitoring of a patient during a seizure. (Courtesy Astro-Med, Inc.)

of each hemisphere individually for its relative dominance for language and its ability to support memory functioning before temporal lobectomy. During the 6 to 8 minutes while one hemisphere remains "paralyzed," the neuropsychologist tests the functioning of the "awake" hemisphere to model functioning without the other hemisphere. This is a gross measure of loss of function, typically focusing on speech and memory. If, for example, the Wada test shows that speech is atypically represented in the right hemisphere, then right temporal lobectomy is contraindicated.

Many variations of the procedures are used during the Wada test, but the core involves brief testing of both expressive and receptive language and short- and long-term memory in both the verbal and visuospatial domains. The premise behind this assessment procedure is that the neuropsychological testing shows the distribution of brain function and can help predict the sparing of memory and language functioning after temporal lobe resection. This aspect is usually quite helpful; however, some controversy exists over whether sodium amytal injections indeed anesthetize memory functions. For one reason, the injection into the anterior carotid artery only perfuses into the anterior portion of the hippocampus, leaving posterior aspects free to function. To handle this problem, some medical

centers also selectively inject the middle or posterior cerebral artery, although this is more risky. The change in a patient undergoing a Wada procedure is usually quite dramatic, in that the brain anesthetizes quickly and speech abruptly halts if the dampened hemisphere is dominant for speech. Because many patients being considered for epilepsy surgery have a long-standing history of epilepsy, often dating back to early developmental years, cerebral representation of speech can show a variety of patterns, presumably because the brain, responding to seizures, may have developed atypically. For example, there could be reversed dominance for speech with both expressive and receptive aspects controlled by the right hemisphere, equal disruption in each hemisphere, or a dissociation of expressive speech in one hemisphere and receptive speech in the other (for review, see Jones-Gotman, 1996).

Neuropsychological presentation of seizures is highly individualistic, depending on seizure locus, type of seizure, and chronicity of disorder. No typical pattern of cognitive dysfunction is associated with epilepsy, and some patients may show few to no discernible problems. However, many seizure sufferers exhibit attention and memory problems. This is particularly evident in tests that require sustained or divided attention. In general, cognitive functioning tends to be more impaired with longer duration (younger age of onset) and increased frequency of seizures (Haynes & Bennett, 1990). Lowered cognitive functioning is also linked with greater EEG abnormality. In general, the type of seizure activity parallels the functional deficits expected. For example, generalized tonic-clonic seizures are more likely to result in widespread functional impairment of both hemispheres. Partial seizures (which have not generalized) are most likely to be associated with lateralized impairment related to the side of abnormal discharge. As mentioned earlier, behavior during auras and the type of motor or sensory behavior evident during a seizure can also provide clues to seizure locus and are likely to correspond to neuropsychological assessment.

People with complex partial seizures that involve the temporal lobe show the most consistent neuropsychological and behavioral pattern. This group most commonly reports problems with learning, memory, and language and is less affected by attentional difficulties. Verbal fluency and verbal retrieval deficits are common manifestations of the interaction between memory and language. However, all aspects of memory encoding, organization, and retrieval may be affected. Emotional and behavioral disturbances, although prevalent among seizure sufferers in general, are most common with those who have complex partial seizures that involve the temporal lobe.

TREATMENT OF EPILEPSY

The treatment of epilepsy is a collaborative effort between the patient and various health care professionals. As in many chronic diseases, patients are often the best experts on the symptoms of their conditions and the situations most likely to provoke a seizure. The various treatments available for epilepsy range from behavioral management, to nutritional therapy, to pharmacologic treatments, to neurosurgery; however, medication remains the most widely used form of treatment, and for most patients, seizures can be controlled with medication.

The decision to take regular medication for seizures requires a neurologist's full evaluation as to its necessity, as well as a commitment from the patient. As we have discussed, seizures may occur in isolation, but epilepsy denotes a pattern of seizure activity. If a neurologist can establish a diagnosis of epilepsy, then a physician often prescribes specific drugs according to seizure type. For example, generalized tonic-clonic seizures often respond to anticonvulsants that prolong the inhibitory action of GABA in the brain. These drugs include phenytoin (Dilantin), carbamazepine (Tegretol), or sodium valproate (Depakote) barbiturates and **benzodiazepines.** As de-

scribed earlier, absence seizures appear to involve a mechanism that is pharmacologically different from GABA. Absence seizures are worsened by GABAergic drugs such as Dilantin, Tegretol, or barbiturates (Snead, 1995) and are treated by GABA-b antagonists ethosuximide (Zarontin), but may also be treated with Depakote. Physicians may treat partial seizures with the preceding drugs or, for seizures involving motor disturbances, often use clonazepam (Klonopin) or acetazolamide (Diamox). In instances when drugs have not effectively controlled seizures, surgery as a treatment method has also been used. The pathologic brain area, if it can be localized, is simply cut out. This is where the neuropsychological evaluation, and specifically the Wada test, can be particularly useful in advising the surgeon as to areas of function, such as speech and memory, that might be affected by the procedure.

In recent years, a dietary treatment called the "ketogenic diet" has been gaining popularity. It was first developed in the 1920s based on anecdotal reports about the effectiveness of strict dietary regimens that date back even to Biblical times. It was not until the early 1990s when interest in this diet was renewed after a 2-year-old boy with intractable seizures was treated successfully at the John Hopkins Hospital. This diet mimics the effects of biochemical changes that occur during fasting (acidosis, dehydration, and ketosis). It is mainly a very "low-carb" diet, based on an intake of proteins, fat, and little carbohydrates. Its mechanism of action is not fully understood yet, but scientists consider that calorie restriction, acidosis, ketosis, or dehydration may be possible mediators of its effect on seizure control. This treatment is generally used when seizures are difficult to control; when the patient responds poorly to medication; or when there is adequate control, but the drug's side effects are not well tolerated. A recent study has shown that 37% of patients have a 90% reduction in seizures and an additional 30% experience a 50% to 90% reduction (Thiele, 2003). It has also been suggested that even though this treatment works for adults, it appears to be more effective in children (Vining, 1999).

Some people with seizures have also learned to control their attacks by noticing their auras and arresting the seizure before the ictal episode fully materializes. One pioneer in seizure research, Wilder Penfield, made the following observation: "When an attack is just beginning, strong stimulation of the part threatened may avert the further development of a seizure" (Penfield, 1975, p. 39). Sensory auras including smell, touch, and taste appear particularly amenable to natural arrest. For example, if the aura involves the sensation of a putrid smell, countering this with a pleasant smell may interrupt the progression of a seizure. In an early case study, Robert Efron (1957) reports that one of his patients, a concert singer, had seizures preceded by the aura of a bad smell. He gave her a vial of essential oil of jasmine to sniff at the onset of her aura. The jasmine served as a natural counteractant to the hallucinated bad smell and apparently stopped the seizure. Through behavioral conditioning, Efron also taught the patient to arrest her seizures by imagining the odor of jasmine. In a similar vein, some patients find that they can halt gustatory auras such as metallic tastes by eating something pleasant tasting. Tactile auras have been stopped by such methods as tickling and squeezing. It is reasonable to assume that because the type of aura experienced by any one person is highly individual, patients would need to experiment to find what works for them. Efron's patient was able to control her seizures well enough that her medications could be reduced. In another interesting example (Pritchard, Holmstrom, & Giacinto, 1985), a patient with complex partial seizures developed his own technique of blinking or shutting his eyes and visualized himself fishing. What was most striking was that EEG monitoring corroborated that he could arrest his seizure through this specific visualization, but not through other mental tasks suggested to him such as mental arithmetic or reading.

In addition to these self-control methods, other behavioral techniques have been explored to control seizures. These involve stress reduction measures, as well as biofeedback. Because seizures have often been associated with increased levels of stress, progressive relaxation techniques have offered some effectiveness (Rousseau, Hermann, & Whitman, 1985). This technique involves tightening and relaxing isolated muscle groups and also learning how to apply this procedure when facing situations and feelings that are associated with a high risk for seizure activity (Dahl, Melin, & Lund, 1987). Besides the notion that stress can, on some occasions, precipitate seizures, it has also been suggested that sudden changes in arousal may be associated with seizure upsurge. Therefore, a technique called "countermeasures" has been applied to fight the onset of seizures. With this technique, the goal is to change the arousal level when early signs of a seizure appear. For example, if a person experiences drowsiness at the time of the seizure onset, the objective of the countermeasure technique would be to teach the person to heighten the arousal level at this point to prevent the progression of the seizure (Dahl, Brorson, & Melin, 1992). Biofeedback based on galvanic skin response has also been used to reduce seizure frequency. This practice is based on the notion that an increase in sympathetic arousal (galvanic skin response) is associated with reduced abnormal cortical activity present in epilepsy (Nagai, Goldstein, Fenwick, & Trimble, 2004).

EEG biofeedback is another method that has been used to attempt seizure reduction, particularly for those who do not respond to conventional drug treatments. The idea of neurofeedback is for the person to learn to identify the EEG patterns that may lead to seizures. The EEG signals occurring in real time are "fed back" to the person in a form that is easily understood. While being monitored, a person could, for example, receive feedback via a tone that would sound lower on the musical scale if the direction of the neuronal pattern was to de-emphasize seizure activity and sound higher if seizure activity was more likely. By training people to recognize their brain and mind states, the idea is that they can also learn to control them. The purpose of this technique is to apply "operant conditioning" principles to brain activity. In addition to tones, this is often done by presenting to the patient his or her own brain activity in a creative way and providing rewards whenever the brain signals move in the desired direction. For example, some protocols of neurofeedback for children use spaceship races in which each spaceship represents a type of brain wave captured by the EEG and the goal is to make the desired spaceship "win the race," which, in fact, means that the targeted brain activity measured by the EEG is moving in the desired direction. Overall, EEG biofeedback or "neurofeedback" for the treatment of epilepsy has shown positive results along the years; however, no consensus has been reached as to which particular protocol works the best, because few studies are available, and the ones that exist are quite variable in subject selection and also lack rigorously controlled designs. Nevertheless, recent improvements in quantitative EEG (qEEG) may facilitate this endeavor. qEEG uses digital technology to capture brain-wave activity, which is recorded and converted into a color map of brain functions. The advantages of qEEG as compared with a regular EEG are that data can be more easily interpreted and a patient's performance can be compared statistically with its own or with that of a large population database. With this technology a new window of opportunity is opened for the development of neurofeedback, because it becomes easier to target and quantify particular sites of abnormal brain activity for each individual and also detect incoherences in neuronal firing between different brain locations that may contribute to seizure activity. A preliminary study by Walker and Kozlowski (2005) has reported several cases for whom qEEG biofeedback was applied where seizures decreased considerably and many of the subjects even become medication free. Controlling seizures by learning how to recognize and manipulate brain activation is an exciting field that deserves further exploration.

Summary

Consciousness is a frontier of brain science that presents some of the most intriguing puzzles of the human mind. Although issues of changing alertness, such as sleep and sleep disorders, may be easier to map out and understand within the workings of the brain, issues of awareness, particularly understanding of the brain mechanisms of self-awareness and unity of experience, still present many mysteries. Throughout this book, we have considered many brain disorders that result in altered states of awareness. In this chapter, we went further into defining normal consciousness and considered two types of disorders of consciousness: sleep disorders and seizure disorders.

With normal alertness, circadian peaks and valleys occur on about a 24-hour cycle in accordance with the sleep/wake cycle. In general, EEG indicates level of alertness, as seen in normal sleep and wakefulness patterns. However, EEG, which is the outward measure of brain rhythm, is not necessarily an accurate indicator of mind state. Two people may show similar EEG patterns but have very different levels of conscious alertness. For example, although sleep is often called "unconscious," some people show "lucidity" during REM sleep. Slow delta waves accompany deep sleep and coma, but accomplished meditators can also produce this "deep" brain state whereas maintaining a more alert "mind" state. The mind state of dreaming during the brain state of REM has fascinated philosophers and scientists alike as they endeavor to understand potential connections to problem solving, memory, and psychological adjustment.

The hypothalamus, the thalamus, and the RAS are particularly important in the sleep/wake cycle. When this clocklike rhythm is disrupted, sleep disorders such as life-threatening insomnia or narcolepsy can occur. Excessive daytime sleepiness occurs with most sleep disorders, often associated with patient reports of poor memory and concentration.

Seizures suddenly alter consciousness during wakefulness and often result in abnormal movement and mentation. Seizures are the outward behavioral manifestation of excessive excitatory synchronous neuronal firing. The behavioral symptoms of seizures relate to the scope and the location of the brain focus, and the classifications of generalized and partial seizures are well documented. Neuropsychologists assess seizure patients for treatment planning and surgical evaluations. Although treatment of seizures primarily relies on medications, behavioral interventions may also be possible in the future as scientists and individuals learn more about controlling aspects of their own consciousness.

Critical Thinking Questions

- What is the biological or psychological function of "rhythms" of consciousness?
- How fluid are the boundaries between conscious and subconscious awareness?
- How do REM sleep and dreaming change in people who have various neurologic disorders?
- In what ways might neuropsychology be able to contribute to treatments for people with sleep disorders or epilepsy?

Key Terms

Consciousness	Ultradian	Sleep apnea syndrome	Excessive daytime
Circadian rhythm	Absence seizures	(SAS)	sleepiness
Narcolepsy	REM (rapid eye movement)	Apnea	Cataplexy
Seizures	sleep	Hypoxia	Hypnagogic hallucinations
Partial seizures	NREM (non–rapid eye	Sudden infant death syndrome	Generalized seizure
Epileptic syndrome	movement) sleep	(SIDS)	Grand mal seizure
Epilepsy	Nocturnal myoclonus	Obstructive sleep apnea	Tonic
Lucid dreaming	Suprachiasmic nucleus (SCN)	Central sleep apnea	Clonic
Reticular activating system	Sleep paralysis	Uvulopalatopharyngoplasty	Petit mal seizure
(RAS)	Atonia	(UPPP)	Complex partial seizure

Aura	Myoclonic seizures	Psychomotor or temporal lobe	Jacksonian seizure
Prodromal phase	Atonic seizures	epilepsy	Nucleus reticularis thalami
Epileptogenic focus	Automatisms	Secondarily generalized	(NRT)
Postictal phase	Simple seizure	seizure	Benzodiazepines

Web Connections

http://www.stanford.edu/~dement/sleepinfo.html
Stanford University Sleep Center—a complete guide to various sleep disorders including all the disorders discussed In the text. In addition, discussions of the relation of sleep disorders to specific psychiatric and medical diagnosis may provide an interesting link between previously discussed disorders and sleep disturbances.

http://www.sleepnet.com/disorder.htm
SleepNet—provides an overview of sleep, including sleep disorders, research, sleep labs, and more.

http://www.efa.org
Epilepsy Foundation—presents research as well as advocacy information.

http://neuro.med.cornell.edu/NYH-CMC/ne-general.html
Cornell University Epilepsy Center—this overview of epilepsy covers the basics, such as the definition of a selzure, to more advanced discussions of treatment options and surgical procedures available for patients with epilepsy.

http://neurosurgery.mgh.harvard.edu/epilepsy.htm
Harvard Epilepsy Site—not only is this site an excellent source for discussions of surgical options in epilepsy, it also provides general resources and other links on this topic, as well as the more general topic of epilepsy as a whole.

REFERENCES

Aarsland, D., Zaccai, J., & Brayne, C. (2005). A systematic review of prevalence studies of dementia in Parkinson's disease. *Movement Disorders, 20*(10), 1255–1263.

Adams, R. D., & Victor, M. (1993). *Principles of neurology* (4th ed.). New York: McGraw-Hill.

Administration on Aging. (2000). *A profile of older Americans.* Washington, DC: Author.

Adolphs, R., Tranel, D., & Damasio, A. R. (1998). The human amygdala in social judgment. *Nature, 393,* 470–474.

Agnew, J., Bolla-Wilson, K., Kawas, C., & Bleeker, M. L. (1988). Purdue Pegboard age and sex norms for ages forty and older. *Developmental Neuropsychology, 4,* 29–35.

Alarcón, M., Pennington, B. F., Filipek, P. A., & DeFries, J. C. (2000). Etiology of neuroanatomical correlates of reading disability. *Developmental Neuropsychology, 17,* 339–360.

Albert, M. L., Feldman, R. G., & Willis, A. L. (1974). The "subcortical dementia" of progressive supranuclear palsy. *Journal of Neurology, Neurosurgery, and Psychiatry, 37,* 121–130.

Alexander, M. P., & Stuss, D. T. (2000). Disorders of frontal lobe functioning. *Seminars in Neurology, 20,* 427–437.

Alsobrook, J. P., & Pauls, D. L. (1999). Molecular genetics of childhood psychiatric disorders. In D. S. Charney, E. J. Nestler, & B. S. Bunney (Eds.), *Neurobiology of mental illness* (pp. 749–760). New York: Oxford University Press.

Alvarez-Buylla, A., & Garcia-Verdugo, J. M. (2002). Neurogenesis in adult subventricular zone. *Journal of Neuroscience 22*(3), 629–634.

Alvarez-Buylla, A., & Lois, C. (1995). Neuronal stem cells in the brain of adult vertebrates. *Stem Cells, 13*(3), 263–272.

Alzheimer, A. (1907). Über eine eigenartige Erkrankung der Hirnrinde. *Allgemeine Zeitschrift für Psychiatrie, 64,* 146–148.

Alzheimer, A. (1987). About a peculiar disease of the cerebral cortex. *Alzheimer's Disease and Associated Disorders, 1,* 7–8.

Amedi, A., Raz, N., Pianka, P., Malach, R., & Zahory, E. (2003). Early visual cortex activation correlates with superior verbal memory performance in the blind. *Nature Neuroscience, 6,* 758–766.

American Psychiatric Association. (1980). *Diagnostic and statistical manual of mental disorders* (3rd ed.). Washington, DC: Author.

American Psychiatric Association. (1987). *Diagnostic and statistical manual of mental disorders* (3rd Rev. ed.). Washington, DC: Author.

American Psychiatric Association. (1994). *Diagnostic and statistical manual of mental disorders* (4th ed.). Washington, DC: Author.

Amin, Z., Constable, R. T., & Canli, T. (2005). Gender differences in the implicit processing of emotional faces: A region of variance approach. *Journal of Cognitive Neuroscience, B141*(Suppl.), 65–66.

Andersen, R. A., Snyder, L. H., Li, C. S., & Stricanne, B. (1993). Coordinate transformations in the representation of spatial information. *Current Opinions in Neurobiology, 3,* 171–176.

Anderson, G. M. (2002). Genetics of childhood disorders: XLV. Autism, part 4: Serotonin in autism. *Journal of the American Child and Adolescent Psychiatry, 41,* 1513–1516.

Anderson, S. W., & Tranel, D. (2002). Neuropsychological consequences of dysfunction in human dorsolateral prefrontal cortex. In F. Boller, J. Grafman (Series Eds.), & J. Grafman (Vol. Ed.), *Handbook of neuropsychology: The frontal lobes* (Vol. 7, 2nd ed., pp. 145–156). New York: Elsevier.

Anderson, V., Jacobs, R., & Harvey, A. S. (2005). Prefrontal lesions and attentional skills in childhood. *Journal of the International Neuropsychological Society, 11,* 817–831.

Anderson, V., Levin, H. S., & Jacobs, R. (2002). Executive functions after frontal lobe injury: A developmental perspective. In D. T. Stuss & R. T. Knight (Eds.), *Principles of frontal lobe function* (pp. 504–527). New York: Oxford University Press.

Anderson, V., Northam, E., Hendy, J., & Wrennall, J. (2001). *Developmental neuropsychology: A clinical approach.* Philadelphia: Taylor & Francis.

Anderson, V. A., Anderson, P., Northam, E., Jacobs, R., & Catroppa, C. (2001). Development of executive functions through late childhood and adolescence in an Australian sample. *Developmental Neuropsychology, 20,* 385–406.

Anderson, V. A., Anderson, P., Northam, E., Jacobs, R., & Mikiewicz, O. (2002). Relationships between cognitive and behavioral measures of executive function in children with brain disease. *Child Neuropsychology, 8,* 231–240.

Andreasen, N. C. (1988). Brain imaging: Applications in psychiatry. *Science, 239,* 215–226.

Annett, M. (1985). *Left, right, hand and brain: The right shift theory.* London: Lawrence Erlbaum Associate.

Annett, M. (2002). *Handedness and brain asymmetry: The right shift theory.* East Sussex, United Kingdom: Psychology Press.

Archibald, S. J., & Kerns, K. A. (1999). Identification and description of new tests of executive functioning in children. *Child Neuropsychology, 5,* 115–129.

Archibald, S. J., Mateer, C. A., Kerns, K. A. (2001). Utilization behavior: Clinical manifestations and neurological mechanisms. *Neuropsychology Review, 11,* 117–130.

Armony, J. L., & LeDoux, J. E. (2000). How danger is encoded: Toward a systems, cellular, and computational understanding of cognitive-emotional interactions in fear. In M. S. Gazzaniga (Ed.), *The new cognitive neurosciences* (2nd ed., pp. 1067–1079). Cambridge, MA: MIT Press.

Armstrong, C., Corn, B., Ruffer, J., Pruitt, A., Mollman, J., & Phillips, P. (2000). Radiotherapeutic effects on brain function: Double dissociation of memory systems. *Neuropsychiatry, Neuropsychology, & Behavioral Neurology, 13*(2), 101–111.

Armstrong, R. J., Watts, C., Svendsen, C. N., Dunnett, S. B., & Rosser, A. E. (2000). Survival, neuronal differentiation, and fiber outgrowth of propagated human neural precursor grafts in an animal model of Huntington's disease. *Cell Transplantation, 9,* 55–64.

Armstrong-Hickey, D. (1991). A validation of lucid dreaming in school age children. *Lucidity, 10,* 250–254.

Ashford, J. W., & Zec, R. F. (1993). Pharmacological treatment in Alzheimer's disease. In R. W. Parks, R. F. Zec, & R. S. Wilson (Eds.), *Neuropsychology of Alzheimer's disease and other dementias.* New York: Oxford University Press.

Asperger, H. (1991). "Autistic psychopathy" in childhood (U. Frith, Trans.). In U. Frith (Ed.), *Autism and Asperger's syndrome* (pp. 32–97). New York: Cambridge University Press.

Atkinson, J., Braddick, O., Anker, S., Curran, W., Andrew, R., Wattam-Bell, J., et al. (2003). Neurobiological models of visuospatial cognition in children with Williams syndrome: Measures of dorsal-stream and frontal function. *Developmental Neuropsychology, 23,* 139–172.

Atkinson, J., King, J., Braddick, O., Nokes, L., Anker, S., & Braddick, F. (1997). A specific deficit of dorsal visual stream function in Williams syndrome. *NeuroReport, 8,* 1919–1922.

Aylward, E. H., Reiss, A. L., Reader, M. J., Singer, H. S., Brown, J. E., & Denckla, M. B. (1996). Basal ganglia volumes in children with attention-deficit hyperactivity disorder. *Journal of Child Neurology, 11,* 112–115.

Babinski, J., & Joltran, E. (1924). Un nouveau cas d'anosognosie. *Revue Neurologique, 31,* 638–640.

Bachevalier, J. (1994). Medical temporal lobe structure and autism: A review of clinical and experimental findings. *Neuropsychologica, 32,* 627–648.

Backman, L., Small, B. J., Wahlin, A., & Larsson, M. (2000). Cognitive functioning in very old age. In F. I. M. Craik & T. A. Salthouse (Eds.), *Handbook of aging and cognition* (2nd ed., pp. 499–558). Mahwah, NJ: Erlbaum.

Baddeley, A. (1986). *Working memory.* New York: Oxford University Press.

Baddeley, A. D. (2000). The episodic buffer: A new component of working memory? *Trends in Cognitive Sciences, 4,* 417–423.

Baddeley, A. D. (2001). Alan D. Baddeley award for distinguished scientific contributions. *American Psychologist, 56,* 849–864.

Baddeley, A. D. (2002). Fractionating the central executive. In D. T. Stuss & R. T. Knight (Eds.), *Principles of frontal lobe function* (pp. 246–260). New York: Oxford University Press.

Baddeley, A. D., & Hitch, G. J. (1994). Developments in the concept of working memory. *Neuropsychology, 8,* 485–493.

Bailey, A., Phillips, W., & Rutter, W. (1996). Autism: Towards an integration of clinical, genetic, neuropsychological, and neurobiological perspectives. *Journal of Child Psychology and Psychiatry, 37,* 89–126.

Balasubramanian, V., & Ranamurthi, B. (1970). Stereotaxic amygdalotomy in behavior disorders. *Confinia Neurology, 32,* 367.

Ball, G. F., & Hulse, S. H. (1998). Birdsong. *American Psychologist, 53,* 37–58.

Bancaud, J., Brunet-Bourgin, F., Chauvel, P., & Halgren, E. (1994). Anatomical origin of deja vu and vivid 'memories' in human temporal lobe epilepsy. *Brain, 117*(Pt 1), 71–90.

Banich, M. T. (1997). *Neuropsychology: The neural basis of mental function.* New York: Houghton Mifflin.

Bannister, R. (1992). Disorders of the cerebral circulation. In R. Bannister (Ed.), *Brain and Bannister's clinical neurology* (7th ed.). New York: Oxford University Press.

Barakat, L. P., & Kazak, A. E. (1999). Family issues. In R. T. Brown (Ed.), *Cognitive aspects of chronic illness in children* (pp. 333–354). New York: Guilford Press.

Barakat, L. P., Kazak, A. E., Meadows, A. T., Casey, R., Meeske, K., & Stuber, M. L. (1997). Families surviving childhood cancer: A comparison of posttraumatic stress symptoms with families of healthy children. *Journal of Pediatric Psychology, 22*(6), 843–589.

Barch, D. M., Braver, T. S., Sabb, F. W., & Noll, D. C. (2000). Anterior cingulated and the monitoring of response conflict: Evidence from an fMRI study of overt verb generation. *Journal of Cognitive Neuroscience, 12,* 298–309.

Barkley, R. A. (1990). *Attention deficit hyperactivity disorder.* New York: Guilford Press.

Barkley, R. A. (1997a). *ADHD and the nature of self-control.* New York: Guilford Press.

Barkley, R. A. (1997b). Behavioral inhibition, sustained attention, and executive functions: Constructing a unifying theory of ADHD. *Psychological Bulletin, 121,* 65–94.

Barkley, R. A. (1997c). Update on a theory of ADHD and its clinical implications. *The ADHD Report, 5,* 10–16.

Barkley, R. A. (1998). *Attention deficit hyperactivity disorder* (2nd ed.). New York: Guilford Press.

Barnett, H. J., Mohr, J. P., Stein, B. M., & Yatsu, F. M. (1986). *Stroke: Pathophysiology, diagnosis, and management* (Vols. 1 & 2). New York: Churchill Livingstone.

Baron-Cohen, S., O'Riordan, M., Stone, V., Jones, R., & Plaisted, K. (1999). Recognition of faux pas by normally developing children and children with Asperger syndrome or high-functioning autism. *Journal of Autism and Developmental Disorders, 29,* 407–418.

Baron-Cohen, S., Ring, H. A., Bullmore, E. T., Wheelwright, S., Ashwin, C., & Williams, S. C. (2000). The amygdala theory of autism. *Neuroscience and Biobehavioral Reviews, 24,* 355–364.

Baron-Cohen, S., Ring, H. A., Wheelwright, S., Bullmore, E., Brammer, M., Simmons, A., et al. (1999). Social intelligence in the normal and autistic brain: An fMRI study. *European Journal of Neuroscience, 11,* 1891–1898.

Barr, C. L. (2001). Genetics of childhood disorders: XXII. ADHD, part 6: The dopamine D4 receptor gene. *Journal of the American Child and Adolescent Psychiatry, 40,* 118–121.

Barrash, J., Tranel, D., & Anderson, S. W. (2000). Acquired personality disturbances associated with bilateral damage to the ventromedial prefrontal region. *Developmental Neuropsychology, 18,* 355–381.

Barth, J. T., Alves, W. M., Ryan, T. V., Macciocchi, S. N., Rimel, R. E., Jane, J. A., et al. (1989). Mild head injury in sports: Neuropsychological sequelae and recovery of function. In H. S. Levin, H. M. Eisenberg, & A. L. Benton (Eds.), *Mild head injury.* New York: Oxford University Press.

Barth, J. T., Findley, L. J., Zillmer, E. A., Gideon, D. A., & Surrat, P. M. (1993). Obstructive sleep apnea, hypoxemia, and personality functioning: Implications for medical psychotherapy assessment. *Advances in Medical Psychotherapy, 6,* 29–36.

Barth, J. T., Macciocchi, S. N., Boll, T. J., Giordani, B., Jane, J. A., & Rimel, R. W. (1983). Neuropsychological sequelae of minor head injury. *Neurosurgery, 13,* 529–533.

Basso, A., Spinnler, H., Vallar, G., & Zanobio, M. E. (1982). Left hemisphere damage and selective impairment of auditory verbal short-term memory: A case study. *Neuropsychologia, 20,* 263–274.

Bates, E. (1999). Plasticity, location and language development. In S. Broman, & J. Fletcher (Eds.), *The changing nervous system* (pp. 214–253). New York: Oxford University Press.

Bates, E., & Roe, K. (2001). Language development in children with unilateral brain injury. In C. A. Nelson & M. Luciana (Eds.), *Handbook of developmental cognitive neuroscience* (pp. 281–308). Cambridge, MA: MIT Press.

Bear, M. F., Connors, B. W., & Paradiso, M. A. (1996). *Neuroscience: Exploring the brain.* Baltimore: Williams & Wilkins.

Beatty, J. (1995). *Principles of behavioral neuroscience.* Chicago: Brown & Benchmark.

Bechara, A., Tranel, D., & Damasio, A. R. (2002). The somatic marker hypothesis and decision-making. In F. Boller, J. Grafman (Series Eds.), & J. Grafman (Vol. Ed.), *Handbook of neuropsychology: The frontal lobes* (Vol. 7, 2nd ed., pp. 117–144). New York: Elsevier.

Bechara, A., Tranel, D., & Damasio, H. (2000). Characterization of the decision-making deficit of patients with ventromedial prefrontal cortex lesions. *Brain, 123,* 2189–2202.

Bechara, A., Tranel, D., Damasio, H., & Damasio, A. R. (1996). Failure to respond autonomically to anticipated future outcomes following damage to prefrontal cortex. *Cerebral Cortex, 6,* 215–225.

Becker, R. O., & Seldon, G. (1985). *The body electric: Electromagnetism and the foundation of life.* New York: William Morrow.

Beeman, J. J., & Chiarello, C. (1998). Complementary right- and left-hemisphere language comprehension. *Current Directions in Psychological Science, 7,* 1–8.

Beh-Yishay, Y., & Prigatano, G. P. (1990). Cognitive remediation. In E. Griffith & M. Rosenthal (Eds.), *Rehabilitation of the adult and child with traumatic brain injury* (2nd ed.). Philadelphia: F. A. Davis.

Bell, M. A., & Fox, N. A. (1994). Brain development over the first year of life: Relations between electroencephalographic frequency and coherence and cognitive and affective behaviors. In G. Dawson & K. W. Fischer (Eds.), *Human brain and the developing brain* (pp. 314–345). New York: Guilford Press.

Bender, B. G., Linden, M. G., & Robinson, A. (1994). Neurocognitive and psychosocial phenotypes associated with Turner syndrome. In S. H. Broman & J. Grafman (Eds.), *Atypical cognitive deficits in developmental disorders* (pp. 197–216). New York: Oxford University Press.

Bender, L. (1938). *A visual motor gestalt test and its clinical use.* New York: American Orthopsychiatric Association.

Benes, F. M. (1997). Corticolimbic circuitry and the development of psychopathology during childhood and adolescence. In N. A. Krasnegor, G. R. Lyon, & P. S. Goldman-Rakic (Eds.), *Development of the prefrontal cortex: Evolution, neurobiology, and behavior* (pp. 211–240). Baltimore: Paul H. Brookes.

Bennett, D. A., Beckett, L. A., Murray, A. M., Shannon, K. M., Goetz, C. G., Pilgrim, D. M., & Evans, D. A. (1996). Prevalence of parkinsonian signs and associated mortality in a community population of older people. *New England Journal of Medicine, 334,* 71–76.

Bennett, D. A., Wilson, R. S., Schneider, J. A., Evans, D. A., Beckett, L. A., Aggarwal, N. T., et al. (2002). Natural history of mild cognitive impairment in older persons. *Neurology, 59*(2), 198–205.

Bennett, T. L. (1987). Neuropsychological aspects of complex partial seizures: Diagnostic and treatment issues. *International Journal of Clinical Neuropsychology, 9,* 37–45.

Bennett, T. L. (1992). *The neuropsychology of epilepsy.* New York: Plenum Press.

Bensen, D. F. (1991). The role of frontal dysfunction in attention-deficit hyperactivity disorder. *Journal of Child Neurology, 6,* S9–S12.

Benton, A. L. (1972). The "minor" hemisphere. *Journal of History of Medicine and Allied Sciences, 27,* 5–14.

Benton, A. L. (1994). Four neuropsychologists. *Neuropsychology Review, 4,* 31–44.

Benton, A. L., & Hamsher, K. D. (1989). *Multilingual aphasia examination.* Iowa City, IA: AJA Associates.

Benton, A. L., Hamsher, K. D., Varney, N. R., & Spreen, O. (1983). *Contributions to neuropsychological assessment.* New York: Oxford University Press.

Berch, D. B., & Bender, B. G. (2000). Turner syndrome. In K. O. Yeates, M. D. Ris, & H. G. Taylor (Eds.), *Pediatric neuropsychology: Research, theory and practice* (pp. 252–274). New York: Guilford Press.

Berg, E. A. (1948). A simple objective treatment for measuring flexibility in thinking. *Journal of General Psychology, 39,* 15–22.

Berlin, L., Bohlin, G., Nyberg, L., & Janols, L. O. (2004). How well do measures of inhibition and other executive functions discriminate between children with ADHD and controls? *Child Neuropsychology, 10,* 1–13.

Bernstein, J. H., & Waber, D. P. (1997). Pediatric neuropsychological assessment. In T. E. Feinberg & M. J. Farah (Eds.), *Behavioral neurology and neuropsychology* (pp. 721–728.). New York: McGraw-Hill.

Beuren, A. J., Schulze, C., Eberle, P., Harmjanz, D., & Apitz, J. (1964). The syndrome of supravalular aortic stenosis, peripheral pulmonary artery stenosis, mental retardation and similar facial appearance. *American Journal of Cardiology, 13,* 471–483.

Bigler, E. D. (1987). The clinical significance of cerebral atrophy in dementia. *Archives of Clinical Neuropsychology, 2,* 177–190.

Bigler, E. D. (1996). *Neuroimaging* (Vols. 1 & 2). New York: Plenum.

Bigler, E. D., & Snyder, J. L. (1995). Neuropsychological outcome and quantitative neuroimaging in mild head injury. *Archives of Clinical Neuropsychology, 10*(2), 159–174.

Birch, S., & Chase, C. (2004). Visual and language processing deficits in compensated and uncompensated college students with dyslexia. *Journal of Learning Disabilities, 37,* 389–410.

Birkmayer, W., & Hornykiewicz, O. (1961). Der L-dioxyphenalalanin L-DOPA Effekt bei der Parkinson Akinese. *Wiener Klinische Wochenzeitschrift, 73,* 787–793.

Bisiach, E., & Rusconi, M. L. (1990). Break-down of perceptual awareness in unilateral neglect. *Cortex, 26*(4), 643–649.

Blair, R. J., Morris, J. S., Frith, C. D., Perrett, D. I., & Dolan, J. R. (1999). Dissociable neural responses facial expressions of sadness and anger. *Brain, 122,* 883–893.

Blakemore, C. (1977). *Mechanics of the mind.* Cambridge, United Kingdom: Cambridge University Press.

Blumer, D., & Benson, D. F. (1975). Personality changes with frontal and temporal lobe lesions. In D. F. Benson & D. Blumer (Eds.), *Psychiatric aspects of neurological disease* (pp. 151–170). New York: Grune & Stratton.

Boles, D. B. (2005). A large-sample study of sex differences in functional cerebral lateralization. *Journal of Clinical and Experimental Neuropsychology, 27,* 759–768.

Boller, F., & Vignolo, L. A. (1966). Latent sensory aphasia in hemisphere-damaged patients: An experimental study with the Token Test. *Brain, 89,* 815–831.

Bornstein, R. A., King, G., & Carroll, A. (1983). Neuropsychological abnormalities in Gilles de la Tourette's syndrome. *Journal of Nervous and Mental Disease, 171,* 497–502.

Borod, J. C. (1993). Cerebral mechanisms underlying facial, prosodic and lexical emotional expression: A review of neuropsychological studies and methodological issues. *Neuropsychology,* 445–463.

Borod, J. C., Haywood, C. S., & Koff, E. (1997). Neuropsychological aspects of facial asymmetry during emotional expression: A review of the normal adult literature. *Neuropsychology Review, 7,* 41–60.

Bourne, G. H. (1973). Lipofuscin. In D. H. Ford (Ed.), *Neurobiological aspects of maturation and aging* (pp. 189–201). Amsterdam: Elsevier.

Bowen, D. M., Benton, J. S., Spillane, J. A., Smith, C. C., & Allen, S. J. (1982). Choline acetyltransferase activity and histopathology of frontal neocortex from biopsies of demented patients. *Journal of Neurological Science, 57,* 191–202.

Bowirrat, A., Treves, T. A., Friedland, R. P., & Korczyn, A. D. (2001). Prevalence of Alzheimer's type dementia in an elderly Arab population. *European Journal of Neurology, 8*(2), 119–123.

Bradshaw, J. L. (2001). *Developmental disorders of the frontostriatal system: Neuropsychological, neuropsychiatric and evolutionary perspectives.* Philadelphia: Taylor & Francis.

Bradshaw, J. L., & Mattingly, J. B. (1995). *Clinical neuropsychology: behavioral and brain science.* San Diego, CA: Academic Press.

Brandt, J. A., & Bylsma, F. W. (1993). The dementia of Huntington's disease. In R. W. Parks, R. F. Zec, & R. S. Wilson (Eds.), *Neuropsychology of Alzheimer's disease and other dementias* (pp. 265–282). New York: Oxford University Press.

Brazier, M. A. (1959). The historical development of neurophysiology. In J. Field, H. W. Magoun, & V. E. Hall (Eds.), *Handbook of physiology* (Vol. 1). Washington, DC: American Physiological Society.

Breen, N., Caine, D., & Coltheart, M. (2001). Mirrored-self misidentification: Two cases of focal onset dementia. *Neurocase, 7*(3), 239–254.

Bressler, S. L., Coppola, R., & Nakamura, R. (1993). Episodic multiregional cortical coherence at multiple frequencies during visual task performance. *Nature, 366,* 153–156.

Brewer, V. R., Fletcher, J. M., Hiscock, M., & Davidson, K. C. (2001). Attention processes in children with shunted hydrocephalus versus attention deficit-hyperactivity disorder. *Neuropsychology, 15,* 185–198.

Brickenkamp, R., & Zillmer, E. A. (1998). *d2 Test of Attention.* Göttingen, Germany: Hogrefe & Huber.

Broca, P. (1861). Perte de la parole. *Bulletin de la Société Anthropologique, 2,* 235–238.

Brodal, A. (1981). *Neuroanatomy in relation to clinical medicine* (3rd ed.). New York: Oxford University Press.

Brodmann, K. (1909). *Vergleichende Lokalisationslehre der Grosshirnrinde in ihren Prinzipien dargestellt auf Grund des Zellenbaues.* Leipzig: Barth.

Brookshire, B. L., Fletcher, J. M., Bohan, T. P., Landry, S. H., Davidson, K. C., & Francis, D. J. (1995). Verbal and nonverbal skill discrepancies in children with hydrocephalus: A five-year longitudinal follow-up. *Journal of Pediatric Psychology, 20,* 785–800.

Brown, A. S. (2003). A review of the deja vu experience. *Psychological Bulletin, 129*(3), 394–413.

Brown, G., Baird, A. D., & Shatz, M. W. (1986). The effects of cerebrovascular disease and its treatment on higher cortical functioning. In I. Grant & K. M. Adams (Eds.), *Neuropsychological assessment of neuropsychiatric disorders.* New York: Oxford University Press.

Brown, G. L., & Linnoila, M. I. (1990). CSF serotonin metabolite 5-HIAA studies in depression, impulsivity, and violence. *Journal of Clinical Psychiatry, 54,* 31–41.

Brown, R. T., & Ivers, C. E. (1999). Gilles de la Tourette syndrome. In S. Goldstein & C. R. Reynolds (Eds.), *Handbook of neurodevelopmental and genetic disorders in children* (pp. 185–215). New York: Guilford Press.

Brown, W. E., Kesler, S. R., Eliez, S., Warsofsky, I. S., Haberecht, M., Patwardhan, A., et al. (2002). Brain development in Turner syndrome: A magnetic resonance imaging study. *Psychiatry Research: Neuroimaging, 116,* 187–196.

Bruce, D. (1985). On the origin of the term "neuropsychology." *Neuropsychologia, 28,* 813–814.

Buchanan, L., Pavlovic, J., & Rovet, J. (1998). A reexamination of the visuospatial deficit in Turner syndrome: Contributions of working memory. *Developmental Neuropsychology, 14,* 341–368.

Bundick, W. T., Zillmer, E. A., Ives, D., & Beadle-Lindsay, M. (1995). Neurobehavioral sequelae and neurological complications of acute Lyme disease: Case studies of two adults. *Advances in Medical Psychotherapy and Psychodiagnosis, 8,* 145–160.

Burns, A., Jacoby, R., & Levy, R. (1991). Computed tomography in Alzheimer's disease: A longitudinal study. *Biological Psychiatry, 29,* 383–390.

Burt, A. M. (1993). *Textbook of neuroanatomy.* Philadelphia: W. B. Saunders.

Burton, E. J., McKeith, I. G., Burn, D. J., Williams, E. D., & O'Brien, J. T. (2004). Cerebral atrophy in Parkinson's disease with and without dementia: A comparison with Alzheimer's disease, dementia with Lewy bodies and controls. *Brain, 127*(Pt 4), 791–800.

Burton, L. A., Henninger, D., & Hafetz, J. (2005). Gender differences in relations of mental rotation, verbal fluency, and SAT scores to finger length ratios and hormonal indexes. *Developmental Neuropsychology, 28,* 493–506.

Butters, N., Salmon, D. P., Munro Culum, C., Cairns, P., Troster, A. I., Jacobs, D., et al. (1988). Differentiation of amnestic and demented patients with the Wechsler Memory Scale-Revised. *The Clinical Neuropsychologist, 2,* 133–148.

Cabeza, R., & Nyberg, L. (2000). Imaging cognition II: An empirical review of 275 PET and fMRI studies. *Journal of Cognitive Neuroscience, 12,* 1–47.

Cahill, L., Haier, R. J., White, N. S., Fallon, J., Kilpatrick, L., Lawrence, C., et al. (2001). Sex-related difference in amygdala activity during emotionally influenced memory storage. *Neurobiology of Learning and Memory, 75,* 1–9.

Cahill, L., & McGaugh, J. L. (1998). Mechanisms of emotional arousal and lasting declarative memory. *Trends in Neuroscience, 21,* 294–299.

Cajal, R. (1937). *Recollections of my life. Memoirs of the American Philosophical Society* (Vol. 8). (Original work published 1901–1917.). Boston: MIT Press.

Cameron, J. L. (2001). Effects of sex hormones on brain development. In C. A. Nelson & M. Luciana (Eds.), *Handbook of developmental cognitive neuroscience* (pp. 59–78). Cambridge, MA: MIT Press.

Canfield, R. L., Gendle, M. H., & Cory-Slechta, D. A. (2004). Impaired neuropsychological functioning in lead-exposed children. *Developmental Neuropsychology, 26,* 513–540.

Canfield, R. L., Henderson, C. R., Cory-Slechta, D. A., Cox, C., Jusko, T. A., & Lanphear, B. P. (2003). Intellectual impairment in children with blood lead concentrations below 10 µg per deciliter. *New England Journal of Medicine, 348,* 1517–1526.

Cannon, W. B. (1927). The James-Lange theory of emotion: A critical examination and an alternative theory. *American Journal of Psychology, 39,* 106–124.

Cantu, R. C., & Mueller, F. O. (2003). Brain injury-related fatalities in American football, 1945–1999. *Neurosurgery, 52*(4), 846–853.

Cantwell, D. P. (1996). Attention deficit disorder: A review of the past 10 years. *Journal of Child and Adolescent Psychiatry, 35,* 978–987.

Cardon, L. R., DeFries, J. C., Fulker, D. W., Kimberling, W. J., Pennington, B. F., & Smith, S. D. (1994). Quantitative trait locus for reading disability on chromosome 6. *Science, 265,* 276–279.

Carey, M. E., Barakat, L. P., Foley, B., Gyato, K., & Phillips, P. C. (2001). Neuropsychological functioning and social functioning of survivors of pediatric brain tumors: Evidence of nonverbal learning disability. *Child Neuropsychology, 7*(4), 265–272.

Carlson, N., & Buskist, W. (1994). *The science of behavior* (5th ed.). Boston: Allyn & Bacon.

Carlson-Green, B., Morris, R. D., & Krawiecki, N. (1995). Family and illness predictors of outcome in pediatric brain tumors. *Journal of Pediatric Psychology, 206,* 769–784.

Carmichael Olson, H., Streissguth, A. P., Sampson, P. D., Barr, H. M., Bookstein, F. L., & Thiede, K. (1997). Association of prenatal alcohol exposure with behavioral and learning problems in early adolescence. *Journal of the American Academy of Child and Adolescent Psychiatry, 36,* 1187–1194.

Carpenter, M. K., Mattson, M., & Rao, M. S. (2003). Sources of cells for CNS therapy. In T. Zigova, E. Snyder, & R. Sanberg (Eds.), *Neural stem cells for brain and spinal cord repair* (pp. 1–44). Totowa, NJ: Humana Press.

Cartwright, R. D., Kravits, D. O., Eastman, C. I., & Wood, E. (1991). REM latency and the recovery from depression: Getting over divorce. *American Journal of Psychiatry, 148,* 1530–1535.

Cartwright, R. D., Lloyd, S., Knight, S., & Trenholme, I. (1984). Broken dreams: A study of the effects of divorce and depression on dream content. *Psychiatry, 47,* 251–259.

Cascino, G. D. (1992). Complex partial seizures: Clinical features and differential diagnosis. *Psychiatric Clinics of North America, 152,* 373–382.

Casey, B. J., Castellanos, F. X., Giedd, J. N., Marsh, W. L., Hamburger, S. D., Schubert, A. B., et al. (1997). Implication of right frontostriatal circuitry in response inhibition and attention-deficit hyperactivity disorder. *Journal of Child Psychology and Psychiatry, 36,* 374–383.

Casey, B. J., Giedd, J. N., & Thomas, K. M. (2000). Structural and functional brain development and its relation to cognitive development. *Biological Psychology, 54,* 241–257.

Casey, B. J., Tottenham, N., & Fossella, J. (2002). Clinical, imaging, lesion, and genetic approaches toward a model of cognitive control. *Developmental Psychobiology, 40,* 237–254.

Castellanos, F. X. (1997). Toward a pathophysiology of attention-deficit hyperactivity disorder. *Clinical Pediatrics, 36,* 381–393.

Castellanos, F. X., Giedd, J. N., Berquin, P. C., Walter, J. M., Sharp, W. Tran, T., et al. (2001). Quantitative brain magnetic resonance imaging in girls with attention-deficit/hyperactivity disorder. *Archives of General Psychiatry, 58,* 289–295.

Castellanos, F. X., Giedds, J. N., Eckburg, P., Marsh, W. L., Vaituzis, C. V., Kaysen, D., et al. (1994). Quantitative morphology of the caudate nucleus in attention deficit hyperactivity disorder. *American Journal of Psychiatry, 151,* 279–281.

Castellanos, F. X., Giedds, J. N., Marsh, W. L., Hamburger, S. D., Vaituzis, A. C., Dickstein, D. P., et al. (1996). Quantitative brain magnetic resonance imaging in attention-deficit hyperactivity disorder. *Archives of General Psychiatry, 53,* 607–616.

Catts, H. W., Gillispie, M., Leonard, L. B., Kail, R. V., & Miller, C. A. (2002). The role of speed of processing, rapid naming, and phonological awareness in reading achievement. *Journal of Learning Disabilities, 35,* 510–525.

Cenci, M. A., Kalen, P., Mandel, R. J., & Bjoerklund, A. (1992). Regional differences in the regulation of dopamine and noradrenaline release in the medial frontal cortex, nucleus accumbens and caudate-putamen: A microdialysis study in the rat. *Brain Research, 581,* 217–228.

Centers for Disease Control and Prevention. (1997). Sport-related recurrent brain injuries—United States. *JAMA: The Journal of the American Medical Association, 277,* 1190–1192.

Chalmers, D. J. (1996). *The conscious mind: In search of a fundamental theory.* New York: Oxford University Press.

Changeux, J. P., & Chavaillon, J. (1995). *Origins of the human brain.* Oxford, United Kingdom: Clarendon Press.

Channon, S., Pratt, P., & Robertson, M. M. (2003). Executive function, memory, and learning in Tourette's syndrome. *Neuropsychology, 17,* 247–254.

Chapman, L. F., & Wolff, H. (1959). The cerebral hemispheres and the highest integrative functions of man. *Archives of Neurology, 1,* 357.

Charman, T. (1997). The relationship between joint attention and pretend play in autism. *Development and Psychopathology, 9,* 1–16.

Checkoway, H., & Nelson, L. M. (1999). Epidemiologic approaches to the study of Parkinson's disease etiology. *Epidemiology, 10*(3), 327–336.

Chen, W. J., Maier, S., Parnell, S. E., & West, J. R. (2004). *Alcohol and the developing brain: Neuroanatomical studies.* Retrieved September 2005, from the National Institute of Alcohol Abuse and Alcoholism of the National Institute of Health Web site: http://pubs.niaaa.nih.gov/publications/arh27-2/174-180.htm

Chow, T. W., & Cummings, J. L. (1999). Frontal-subcortical circuits. In B. L. Miller & J. L. Cummings (Eds.), *The human frontal lobes: Functions and disorders* (pp. 3–26). New York: Guilford Press.

Christensen, A. L. (1979). *Luria's neuropsychological investigation* (2nd ed.). Copenhagen: Munksgaard.

Chugani, H., Muller, R., & Chugani, D. (1996). Functional brain organization in children. *Brain & Development, 18,* 347–356.

Churchland, P. S. (1993). *Neurophilosophy: Toward a unified science of the mind/brain.* Cambridge, MA: MIT Press.

Chusid, J. G. (1982). *Correlative neuroanatomy and functional neurology.* Los Altos, CA: Lange Medical.

Ciesielski, K. T., & Harris, R. J. (1997). Factors related to performance failure on executive tasks in autism. *Child Neuropsychology, 3,* 1–12.

Cirino, P., Chapieski, L., & Massman, P. (2000). Card sorting performance and ADHD symptomatology in children and adolescents with Tourette syndrome. *Journal of Clinical and Experimental Neuropsychology, 22,* 245–257.

Civin, C. I. (2002). Commitment to biomedical research: Clearing unnecessary impediments to progress. *Stem Cells, 20*(6), 482–484.

Cohen, D. J., & Leckman, J. F. (1994). Developmental psychopathology and neurobiology of Tourette's syndrome. *Journal of the Academy of Child and Adolescent Psychiatry, 33,* 2–15.

Cohen, J. D., Aston-Jones, G., & Gilzenrat, M. S. (2004). A system-level perspective on attention and cognitive control: Guided activation, adaptive gating, conflict monitoring, and exploitation versus exploration. In M. I. Posner (Ed.), *Cognitive neuroscience of attention* (pp. 74–76). New York: Guilford Press.

Cohen, J. D., Noll, D. C., & Schneider, W. (1993). Functional magnetic resonance imaging: Overview and methods for psychological research. *Behavior Research Methods, Instruments, & Computers, 25,* 101–113.

Cohen, L. G., Celnik, P., Pascual-Leone, A., Corwell, B., Falz, L., Dambrosia, J., et al. (1997). Functional relevance of cross-modal plasticity in blind humans. *Nature, 389,* 180–183.

Cohen, N. J. (1984). Preserved learning capacity in amnesia: Evidence for multiple memory systems. In L. R. Squire & N. Butters (Eds.), *Neuropsychology of memory.* New York: Guilford Press.

Cohen, R. A. (1993). *The neuropsychology of attention.* New York: Plenum Press.

Colcombe, S., & Kramer, A. F. (2003). Fitness effects on the cognitive function of older adults: A meta-analytic study. *Psychological Science, 14*(2), 125–130.

Colcombe, S. J., Erickson, K. I., Raz, N., Webb, A. G., Cohen, N. J., McAuley, E., et al. (2003). Aerobic fitness reduces brain tissue loss in aging humans. *Journals of Gerontology. Series A, Biological Sciences and Medical Sciences, 58*(2), 176–180.

Committee on the Biological and Biomedical Applications of Stem Cell Research. (2002). *Stem cells and the future of regenerative medicine.* Retrieved October 17, 2006, from http://www.nap.edu/openbook/0309076307/html/7.html.

Connor, P. D., Sampson, P. D., Bookstein, F. L., Barr, H. M., & Streissguth, A. P. (2000). Direct and indirect effects of prenatal alcohol damage on executive function. *Developmental Neuropsychology, 18,* 331–354.

Corder, E. H., Saunders, A. M., Strittmatter, W. J., Schmechel, D. E., Gaskell, P. C., Small, G. W., et al. (1993). Gene dose of apolipoprotein E type 4 allele and the risk of Alzheimer's disease. *Science, 261,* 921–923.

[...] Tactually guided maze learning in man. Effects of unilateral cortical excisions and bilateral hippocampal lesions. *Neuropsychologia, 3,* 339.

Corn, B. W., Yousem, D. M., Scott, C. B., Rotman, M., Asbell, S. O., Nelson, D. F., et al. (1994). White matter changes are correlated significantly with radiation dose. *Cancer, 74,* 2828–2835.

Corwin, J., & Bylsma, F. W. (1993). Translations of excerpts from André Rey's Psychological examination of traumatic encephalopathy and P. A. Osterrieth's Complex Figure Copy Test. *The Clinical Neuropsychologist, 7,* 3–15.

Costello, E. J., Angold, A., Burns, B. J., Stangl, D. K., Tweed, D. L., Erkanli, A., et al. (1996). The Great Smokey Mountains study of youth, goals, design, methods, and the prevalence of DSM-III-R disorders. *Archives of General Psychiatry, 53,* 1129–1136.

Courchesne, E., Carper, R., & Akshoomoff, N. (2003). Evidence of brain overgrowth in the first year of life in autism. *Journal of the American Medical Association, 290,* 337–344.

Courchesne, E., Townsend, J. P., & Saitoh, O. (1994). The brain in infantile autism: Posterior fossa structures are abnormal. *Neurology, 44,* 214–223.

Covassin, T., Swanik, C. B., & Sachs, M. L. (2003). Epidemiological considerations of concussions among intercollegiate athletes. *Applied Neuropsychology, 10*(1), 12–22.

Cowan, W. C. (1979). The developing brain. In W. C. Cowan (Ed.), *The brain* (pp. 56–69). San Francisco: W. H. Freeman.

Cowan, W. M. (1990). The development of the brain. In R. R. Llinas (Ed.), *The workings of the brain: Development, memory, and perception.* New York: W. H. Freeman.

Cowart, B. J., Young, I. M., Feldman, R. S., & Lowry, L. D. (1997). Clinical disorders of smell and taste. In G. K. Beauchamp & L. Bartoshuk (Eds.), *Tasting and smelling.* San Diego: Academic Press.

Coyle, J. T. (1985). The cholinergic systems in psychiatry. In R. E. Hales & A. J. Frances (Eds.), *Psychiatry update: American Psychiatric Association annual review* (Vol. 4). Washington, DC: American Psychiatric Press.

Crick, F., & Koch, C. (1990). Towards a neurobiological theory of consciousness. *Seminars in the Neurosciences, 2,* 263–275.

Crosson, B. (1992). *Subcortical functions in language and memory.* New York: Guilford Press.

Culbertson, J. L., & Edmonds, J. E. (1996). Learning disabilities. In R. L. Adams, O. A. Parsons, J. L. Culbertson, & S. J. Nixon (Eds.), *Neuropsychology for clinical practice: Etiology, assessment, and treatment of common neurological disorders* (pp. 331–408). Washington, DC: American Psychological Association.

Culbertson, W., & Zillmer, E. A. (2005). *TOL-DX Tower of London-Drexel University* (2nd ed.). Toronto, Ontario: Multi-Health Systems.

Culbertson, W. C., & Zillmer, E. A. (1998a). The construct validity of the Tower of London-Drexel University as a measure of the executive functioning of ADHD children. *Assessment, 5,* 215–226.

Culbertson, W. C., & Zillmer, E. A. (1998b). The Tower of London^{DX}: A standardized approach to assessing executive functioning in children. *Archives of Clinical Neuropsychology, 13,* 285–301.

Cullum, C. M., Harris, J. G., Waldo, M., Smernoff, E., Madison, A., Nagamoto, H., et al. (1993). Neurophysiological and neuropsychological evidence for attentional dysfunction in schizophrenia. *Schizophrenia Research, 10,* 131–141.

Cummings, J. L. (1986). Subcortical dementia: Neuropsychology, neuropsychiatry, and pathophysiology. *British Journal of Psychiatry, 149,* 682–697.

Cummings, J. L. (1993). Frontal-subcortical circuits and human behavior. *Archives of Neurology, 50,* 873–880.

Cummings, J. L. (1994). Depression in neurologic diseases. *Psychiatric Annals, 24,* 525–531.

Cummings, J. L., Benson, D. F., Hill, M., & Read, S. (1985). Aphasia in dementia of the Alzheimer type. *Neurology, 35,* 394–397.

Cytowic, R. E. (1993). *The man who tasted shapes: A bizarre medical mystery offers revolutionary insights into reasoning, emotion, and consciousness.* New York: Putnam.

Dahl, J., Brorson, L. O., & Melin, L. (1992). Effects of a broad-spectrum behavioral medicine treatment program on children with refractory epileptic seizures: An 8-year follow-up. *Epilepsia, 33*(1), 98–102.

Dahl, J., Melin, L., & Lund, L. (1987). Effects of a contingent relaxation treatment program on adults with refractory epileptic seizures. *Epilepsia, 28*(2), 125–132.

Daly, E., Zaitchik, D., Copeland, M., Schmahmann, J., Gunther, J., & Albert, M. (2000). Predicting conversion to Alzheimer disease using standardized clinical information. *Archives of Neurology, 57*(5), 675–680.

Daly, G., Hawi, Z., Fitzgerald, M., & Gill, M. (1999). Mapping susceptibility loci in attention deficit hyperactivity disorder: Preferential transmission of parental alleles at DAT1, DBH, and DRD5 to affected children. *Molecular Psychiatry, 4,* 192–196.

Damasio, A. R. (1994). *Descartes' error.* New York: Putnam.

Damasio, A. R. (1998). The somatic marker hypothesis and the possible functions of the prefrontal cortex. In A. C. Roberts, T. W. Robbins, & L. Weiskrantz (Eds.), *The prefrontal cortex: Executive and cognitive functions* (pp. 36–50). New York: Oxford University Press.

Damasio, A. R., Tranel, D., & Damasio, H. (1990). Individuals with sociopathic behavior caused by frontal damage fail to respond autonomically to social stimuli. *Behavioural Brain Research, 41,* 81–94.

Damasio, H., Grabowski, T., Frank, R., Galaburda, A. M., & Damasio, A. M. (1994). The return of Phineas Gage: Clues about the brain from the skull of a famous patient. *Science, 264,* 1102–1105.

D'Andrea, E. A., & Spiers, M. V. (2005a). The effect of familial sinistrality and academic experience on cognition in right-handed women. *Neuropsychology, 19,* 657–663.

D'Andrea, E. A., & Spiers, M. V. (2005b, October 27). *Hormones, cognitive performance, and individual differences.* Paper presented at the Graylyn Conference on Women's Cognitive Health, Winston-Salem, NC.

Danta, G., & Hilton, R. (1975). Judgement of the visual vertical and horizontal in patients with Parkinsons. *Neurology, 25,* 43–47.

Darwin, C. (1968). *On the origin of species.* (Originally published in 1859.) New York: Penguin Books.

Davidson, R. J. (1994). Temperament, affective style, and frontal lobe asymmetry. In G. Dawson & K. W. Fischer (Eds.), *Human brain and the developing brain* (pp. 518–537). New York: Guilford Press.

Dawson, M. E., & Nuechterlein, K. H. (1984). Psycho-physiological dysfunctions in the developmental course of schizophrenic disorders. *Schizophrenia Bulletin, 102,* 204–232.

Dean, R. S., & Reynolds, C. R. (1997). Cognitive processing and self-reported lateral preference. *Neuropsychology Review, 7,* 127–142.

DeAngelis, L., Delattre, J. Y., & Posner, J. (1989). Radiation-induced dementia in patients cured of brain metastases. *Neurology, 39,* 789–796.

Del Bigio, M. R. (2004). Cellular damage and prevention in childhood hydrocephalus. *Brain Pathology, 14,* 317–324.

Demb, J. B., Boynton, G. M., Best, M., & Heeger, D. J. (1998). Psychophysical evidence for a magnocellular pathway deficit in dyslexia. *Vision Research, 38,* 1555–1560.

Denckla, M. B. (1996). A theory and model of executive function: A neuropsychological perspective. In G. R. Lyon & N. A. Krasnegor (Eds.), *Attention, memory, and executive function* (pp. 263–278). Baltimore: Paul H. Brookes.

Denckla, M. B., & Reiss, A. L. (1997). Prefrontal-subcortical circuits in developmental disorders. In N. A. Krasnegor, G. R. Lyon, & P. S. Goldman-Rakic (Eds.), *Development of the prefrontal cortex: Evolution, neurobiology, and behavior* (pp. 283–294). Baltimore: Paul H. Brookes.

Dennis, M., & Barnes, M. (1994). Developmental aspects of neuropsychology: Childhood. In D. W. Zaidel (Ed.), *Neuropsychology* (2nd ed., pp. 219–246). New York: Academic Press.

Department of Health and Human Services. (2001). Stem cells: Scientific progress and future research directions. Retrieved October 17, 2006, from http://stemcells.nih.gov/info/scireport/2001report.htm

Deruelle, C., Mancini, J., Livet, M. O., Casse-Perrot, C., & de Schonen, S. (1999). Configural and local processing of faces in children with Williams syndrome. *Brain and Cognition, 41,* 276–298.

Devinsky, O. (1983). Neuroanatomy of Gilles de la Tourette's syndrome. *Archives of Neurology, 5,* 447–453.

Devinsky, O., Morrell, M. J., & Vogt, B. A. (1995). Contributions of anterior cingulate cortex to behaviour. *Brain, 118,* 279–306.

Diamond, A. (1981). Retrieval of an object from an open box: The development of visual-tactile control of reaching in the first year of life. *Society for Research in Child Development Abstracts, 3,* 78.

Diamond, A. (1991). Neuropsychological insights into the meaning of object concept development. In S. Carey & R. Gelman (Eds.), *The epigenesis of mind: Essays on biology and cognition* (pp. 67–110). Hillsdale, NJ: Erlbaum.

Diamond, A. (2000). Close interrelation of motor development and cognitive development of the cerebellum and prefrontal cortex. *Child Development, 71,* 44–56.

Diamond, A., & Gilbert, J. (1989). Development as progressive inhibitory control of action: Retrieval of a contiguous object. *Cognitive Development, 12,* 223–249.

Dickens, C. (1849). *David Copperfield.* Oxford: Oxford World Classics.

Diller, L. (1994). Finding the right treatment combinations: Changes in rehabilitation over the past five years. In A. Christensen & B. P. Uzzell (Eds.), *Brain injury and neuropsychological rehabilitation: International perspectives.* Hillsdale, NJ: Erlbaum.

Dool, C. B., Stelmack, R. M., & Rourke, B. P. (1993). Event-related potentials in children with learning disabilities. *Journal of Clinical Child Psychology, 22,* 387–398.

Doty, R. L. (1990). Olfaction. In F. Boller & J. Grafman (Eds.), *Handbook of neuropsychology* (Vol. 4). Amsterdam: Elsevier.

Doty, R. L., Shaman, P., & Dann, M. (1984). Development of the University of Pennsylvania Smell Identification Test: A standard microencapsulated test of olfactory function. *Physiology of Behavior, 32,* 489–502.

Douglas, R. J., & Pribram, K. H. (1966). Learning aids and limbic lesions. *Neuropsychologia, 4,* 197.

Dr. Robert Ley's brain. (1946). *Medical Record, 159,* 188.

Drachmann, D. A. (1977). Memory function in man: Does the cholinergic system have a specific role? *Neurology, 27,* 783–790.

Drake, E. B., Henderson, V. W., Stanczyk, F. Z., McCleary, C. A., Brown, W. S., Smith, C. A., et al. (2000). Associations between circulating sex steroid hormones and cognition in normal elderly women. *Neurology, 54,* 599.

Dubb, A., Gur, R., Avants, B., & Gee, J. (2003). Characterization of sexual dimorphism in the human corpus callosum. *NeuroImage, 20,* 512–519.

Dubois, B., Boller, F., Pillon, B., & Agid, Y. (1991). Cognitive deficits in Parkinson's disease. In S. Corkin, J. Grafman, & F. Boller (Eds.), *Handbook of neuropsychology* (Vol. 5, pp. 195–240). Amsterdam: Elsevier.

Duffy, F. H. (1989). Clinical value of topographic mapping and quantified neurophysiology. *Archives of Neurology, 46,* 1133–1135.

Duffy, J. D., & Campbell, J. J. (2001). Regional prefrontal syndromes: A theoretical and clinical overview. In S. P. Salloway, P. F. Malloy, & J. D. Duffy (Eds.), *The frontal lobes and neuropsychiatric illness* (pp. 113–123). Washington, DC: American Psychiatric Publishing.

Dunnet, S. B. (1991). Neural transplants as a treatment for Alzheimer's disease? *Psychological Medicine, 21,* 825–830.

Dychtwald, K., & Flower, J. (1989). Age wave: The challenges and opportunities of an aging America. Los Angeles: Tarcher.

Dykens, E. M. (2003). Anxiety, fears, and phobias in persons with Williams syndrome. *Developmental Neuropsychology, 23,* 291–316.

Eals, M., & Silverman, I. (1994). The hunter-gatherer theory of spatial sex differences: Proximate factors mediating the female advantage in recall of object arrays. *Ethology and Sociobiology, 15,* 95–105.

Ebers, G. C., & Sadovnick, A. D. (1993). The geographic distribution of multiple sclerosis. *Neuroepidemiology, 12,* 1–5.

Echemendia, R. J., & Cantu, R. C. (2003). Return to play following sports-related mild traumatic brain injury: The role for neuropsychology. *Applied Neuropsychology, 10*(1), 48–55.

Eden, G. F., Stein, J. F., Wood, M. H., & Wood, F. B. (1995). Verbal and visual problems in reading disability. *Journal of Learning Disabilities, 28,* 272–290.

Efron, R. (1957). The conditioned inhibition of uncinate fits. *Brain, 80,* 251–262.

Ehlers, S., Nyden, A., Gillberg, C., Sandberg, A. D., Dahlgren, S. O., Hjlemquist, E., et al. (1997). Asperger's syndrome, autism and attention disorders: A comparative study of the cognitive profiles of 120 children. *Journal of the American Academy of Child and Adolescent Psychiatry, 38,* 207–217.

Eiraldi, R. B., Power, T. J., & Nezu, C. M. (1997). Patterns of comorbidity associated with subtypes of attention-deficit/hyperactivity disorder among 6- to 12-year-old children. *Journal of the American Academy of Child and Adolescent Psychiatry, 36,* 503–514.

Eisenmajer, R., Prior, M., Leekam, S., Wing, L., Gould, J., Gelham, M., et al. (1996). Comparison of clinical symptoms in autism and Asperger's disorder. *Journal of the American Academy of Child and Adolescent Psychiatry, 35,* 1523–1531.

El-Hai, J. (2005). *The lobotomist: A maverick medical genius and his tragic quest to rid the world of mental illness.* Hoboken, NJ: John Wiley & Sons.

Elliott, F. A. (1992). Violence-the neurologic contribution: An overview. *Archives of Neurology, 49,* 595–603.

Elliott, T. K., Watkins, J. M., Messa, C., Lippe, B., & Chugani, H. (1996). Positron emission tomography and neuropsychological correlations in children with Turner's syndrome. *Developmental Neuropsychology, 12,* 365–386.

Elsass, L., & Kinsella, G. (1987). Social interaction following severe closed head injury. *Psychological Medicine, 17,* 67–78.

England, M. A., & Wakely, J. (1991). *Brain and spinal cord: An introduction to normal neuro-anatomy.* Aylesbury, United Kingdom: Mosby-Wolfe.

Epel, E. S., Blackburn, E. H., Lin, J., Dhabhar, F. S., Adler, N. E., Morrow, J. D., et al. (2004). Accelerated telomere shortening in response to life stress. *Proceedings of the National Academy of Sciences of the United States of America, 101*(49), 17312–17315.

Epilepsy Foundation. (n.d.). *Epilepsy and seizure statistics, 2005,* from www.epilepsyfoundation.org/answerplace/statistics. cfm.

Erickson, K., Baron, I. S., & Fantie, B. D. (2001). Neuropsychological function in early hydrocephalus: Review from a developmental perspective. *Child Neuropsychology, 7,* 199–229.

Erickson, K., Colcombe, S., Elavsky, S., McAuley, E., Korol, D., Scalf, P., et al. (2005). Interactive effects of fitness and duration of hormone treatment on prefrontal cortex volume and executive function. *Journal of Cognitive Neuroscience, D101*(Suppl.), 123.

Erlanger, D. M., Kutner, K. C., & Jacobs, A. R. (1999). Hormones and cognition: Current concepts and issues in neuropsychology. *Neuropsychology Review, 9,* 175–207.

Ernst, M., Cohen, R. M., Liebenauer, M. A., Jons, P. H., & Zametkin, A. J. (1997). Cerebral glucose metabolism in adolescent girls with attention-deficit/hyperactivity disorder. *Journal of the American Academy of Child and Adolescent Psychiatry, 36,* 1399–1406.

Ernst, M., Liebenauer, L. L., Jons, P. H., & Zametkin, A. J. (1994). Cerebral glucose metabolism in adolescent girls with attention-deficit/hyperctivity disorder. *Journal of the American Academy of Child and Adolescent Psychiatry, 36,* 1399–1406.

Ernst, M., Liebenauer, L. L., King, A. C., Fitzgerald, G. A., Cohen, R. M., & Zametkin, A. J. (1994). Reduced brain metabolism in hyperactive girls. *Journal of the American Academy of Child and Adolescent Psychiatry, 33,* 858–868.

Esiri, M. (1994). Dementia and normal aging: Neuropathology. In F. A. Huppert, C. Brayne, & D. W. O'Connor (Eds.), *Dementia and normal aging* (pp. 385–436). Cambridge, United Kingdom: Cambridge University Press.

Eslinger, P. J. (1996). Conceptualizing, describing, and measuring components of executive function: A summary. In G. R. Lyon & N. A. Krasnegor (Eds.), *Attention, memory, and executive function* (pp. 367–396). Baltimore: Paul H. Brookes.

Eslinger, P. J. (1998). Neurological and neuropsychological bases of empathy. *European Neurology, 39,* 193–199.

Eslinger, P. J., Biddle, K. R., & Grattan, L. M. (1997). Cognitive and social development in children with pre-frontal cortex lesions. In N. A. Krasnegor, G. R. Lyon, & P. S. Goldman-Rakic (Eds.), *Development of the prefrontal cortex: Evolution, neurobiology, and behavior* (pp. 295–336). Baltimore: Paul H. Brookes.

Eslinger, P. J., Flaherty-Craig, C. V., & Benton, A. L. (2004). Developmental outcomes after early prefrontal cortex damage. *Brain and Cognition, 55,* 84–103.

Espeland, M. A., Rapp, S. R., Shumaker, S. A., Brunner, R., Manson, J. E., Sherwin, B. B., et al. (2004). Conjugated equine estrogens and global cognitive function in post-menopausal women. *Journal of the American Medical Association, 291,* 2959–2968.

Espy, K. A., Kaufmann, P. M., Glisky, M. L., & McDiarmid, M. D. (2001). New procedures to assess the executive functions in preschool children. *The Clinical Neuropsychologist, 15,* 46–58.

Ewing-Cobbs, L., Barnes, M. A., & Fletcher, J. M. (2003). Early brain injury in children: Development and reorganization of cognitive function. *Developmental Neuropsychology, 24,* 669–704.

Fan, J., McCandliss, B. D., Sommer, T., Raz, A., & Posner, M. I. (2002). Testing the efficiency and independence of attentional networks. *Journal of Cognitive Neuroscience, 14,* 340–347.

Farah, M. J. (1990). *Visual agnosia: Disorders of object vision and what they tell us about normal vision.* Cambridge, MA: MIT Press/Bradford.

Faraone, S. V., & Biederman, J. (2004). Neurobiology of attention deficit hyperactivity disorder. In D. S. Charney &

E. J. Nestler (Eds.), *Neurobiology of mental illness* (2nd ed., pp. 979–999). New York: Oxford University Press.

Farran, E. K., & Jarrold, C. (2003). Visuospatial cognition in Williams syndrome: Reviewing and accounting for the strengths and weaknesses in performance. *Developmental Neuropsychology, 23,* 173–200.

Farrer, L. A. (1986). Suicide and attempted suicide in Huntington's disease: Implications of preclinical testing for persons at risk. *American Journal of Medical Genetics, 24,* 305–311.

Feifel, D. (1999). Neurotransmitters and neuromodulators in frontal-subcortical circuits. In B. L. Miller & J. L. Cummings (Eds.), *The human frontal lobes: Functions and disorders* (pp. 174–186). New York: Guilford Press.

Fein, D., Joy, S., Green, L. A., & Waterhouse, L. (1996). Autism and pervasive developmental disorders. In B. S. Fogel, R. R. Schiffer, & S. M. Rao (Eds.), *Neuropsychiatry* (pp. 571–614). Philadelphia: Williams & Wilkins.

Feldman, R. S., Meyer, J. S., & Quenzer, L. F. (1997). *Principles of neuropsychopharmacology.* Sunderland, MA: Sinauer Associates.

Fernandez-Duque, D., & Posner, M. I. (2001). Brain imaging of attentional networks in normal and pathological states. *Journal of Clinical and Experimental Neuropsychology, 23,* 74–93.

Fields, R. D., & Stevens-Graham, B. (2002). New insights into neuron-glia communication. *Science, 298,* 556–562.

Filipek, P. A. (1995). Quantitative magnetic resonance imaging in autism: The cerebellar vermis. *Current Opinion in Neurology, 8,* 134–138.

Filipek, P. A. (1996). Structural variations in measures of developmental disorders. In R. W. Thatcher, G. R. Lyon, J. Rumsey, & N. Krasnegor (Eds.), *Developmental neuroimaging: Mapping the development of brain and behavior* (pp. 169–186). San Diego, CA: Academic Press.

Filipek, P. A., Semrud-Clikeman, M., Steingard, R. J., Renshaw, P. F., Kennedy, D. N., & Biederman, J. (1997). Volumetric MRI analysis comparing subjects having attention-deficit hyperactivity disorder with normal controls. *Neurology, 48,* 589–601.

Fisher, N. J., DeLuca, J. W., & Rourke, B. P. (1997). Wisconsin Card Sorting Test and Halstead Category Test performances of children and adolescents who exhibit the syndrome of nonverbal learning disabilities. *Child Neuropsychology, 3,* 61–70.

Fisher, R. S., van Emde Boas, W., Blume, W., Elger, C., Genton, P., Lee, P., & Engel, J. (2005). Epileptic seizures and epilepsy: definitions proposed by the International League Against Epilepsy (ILAE) and the International Bureau for Epilepsy (IBE). *Epilepsia, 46*(4), 470–472.

Fletcher, J. M., Brookshire, B. L., Landry, S. H., Bohan, T. P., Davidson, K. C., Francis, D. J., et al. (1996). Attention skills and executive functions in children with early hydrocephalus. *Developmental Neuropsychology, 12,* 53–76.

Fletcher, J. M., Dennis, M., & Northrup, H. (2000). Hydrocephalus. In K. O. Yeater, M. D. Ris, & H. G. Taylor

(Eds.), *Pediatric neuropsychology: Research, theory, and practice* (pp. 25–46). New York: Guilford Press.

Flicker, C., Ferris, S. H., & Reisberg, B. (1991). Mild cognitive impairment in the elderly: Predictors of dementia. *Neurology, 41*(7), 1006–1009.

Flowers, D. L., Wood, F. B., & Naylor, C. E. (1991). Regional cerebral blood flow correlates of language processes in reading disability. *Archives of Neurology, 48,* 637–643.

Foley, B., Barakat, L. P., Herman-Liu, A., Radcliffe, J., & Molloy, P. (2000). The impact of childhood hypothalamic/chiasmatic brain tumors on child adjustment and family functioning. *Children's Health Care, 29,* 209–223.

Fombonne, E. (2001). Ask the editor: What is the prevalence of Asperger disorder? *Journal of Autism and Developmental Disorders, 31,* 363–364.

Fombonne, E. (2003a). Epidemiological surveys of autism and other pervasive developmental disorders: An update. *Journal of Autism and Developmental Disorders, 33,* 365–382.

Fombonne, E. (2003b). The prevalence of autism. *Journal of the American Medical Association, 289,* 87–89.

Fombonne, E., Bolton, P., Prior, J., Jordon, H., & Rutter, M. (1997). A family study of autism: Cognitive patterns and levels in parents and siblings. *Journal of Child Psychology and Psychiatry, 38,* 667–684.

Ford, C. E., Jones, K. W., Polani, P. E., de Almeida, J. C., & Briggs, J. H. (1959). A sex-chromosome anomaly in a case of gonadal dysgenesis Turner syndrome. *Lancet, 2,* 711–713.

Forrest, B. J. (2004). The utility of math difficulties, internalized psychopathology, and visual-spatial deficits to identify children with nonverbal learning disability syndrome: Evidence for a visual-spatial disability. *Child Neuropsychology, 10,* 129–146.

Forstl, H., & Hentschel, F. (1994). Contribution to the differential diagnosis of dementias: Neuroimaging. *Reviews in Clinical Gerontology, 4,* 317–341.

Fox, P. T., Ingham, R. J., Ingham, J. C., Hirsch, T. B., Downs, J. H., Martin, C., et al. (1996). A PET study of the neural systems of stuttering. *Nature, 382,* 158–161.

Frackowiak, R. S. (1996). Plasticity and the human brain: Insights from functional imaging. In E. L. Bjork & R. A. Bjork (Eds.), *Memory.* New York: Academic Press.

Freedman, A. M., Kaplan, H. I., & Sadock, B. J. (1978). *Modern synopsis of comprehensive textbook of psychiatry II.* Baltimore: Williams & Wilkins.

Freeman, W., & Watts, J. W. (1950). *Psychosurgery in the treatment of mental disorders and intractable pain.* Springfield, IL: Charles C. Thomas.

Freud, S. (1891). *Zur Auffassung der Aphasien.* Vienna: Deuticke.

Freud, S. (1959). On narcissism: An introduction. In S. Freud (Ed.), *Collected papers* (pp. 30–59). New York: Basic Books.

Frith, U. (1989). *Autism: Explaining the enigma.* Cambridge, MA: Blackwell.

Frith, U. (1991). Asperger and his syndrome. In U. Frith (Ed.), *Autism and Asperger syndrome* (pp. 1–36). New York: Cambridge University Press.

Frost, J. A., Binder, J. R., Springer, J. A., Hammeke, T. A., Bellgowan, P. S., Rao, S. M., Cox, R. W. (1999). Language processing is strongly left lateralized in both sexes: Evidence from functional MRI. *Brain, 122,* 199–208.

Fuster, J. M. (1997). *The prefrontal cortex: Anatomy, physiology, and neuropsychology of the frontal lobe* (3rd ed.). New York: Lippincott-Raven.

Fuster, J. M. (2002). Physiology of executive functions: The perception-action cycle. In D. T. Stuss & R. T. Knight (Eds.), *Principles of frontal lobe function* (pp. 96–108). New York: Oxford University Press.

Fuster, J. M., Van Hoesen, G. W., Morecraft, R. J., & Semendeferi, K. (2000). Executive systems. In B. S. Fogel, R. B. Schiffer, & S. M. Rao (Eds.), *Synopsis of neuropsychiatry* (pp. 229–244). Philadelphia: Lippincott Williams & Wilkins.

Gabrieli, J. D., Keane, M. M., & Corkin, S. (1987). Acquisition of problem-solving skills in global amnesia. *Society for Neuroscience Abstract, 13,* 1455.

Gaddes, W. H., & Edgell, D. (1993). *Learning disabilities and brain function* (3rd ed.). New York: Springer.

Gage, F. H. (2000). Mammalian neural stem cells. *Science, 287,* 1433–1438.

Gainetdinov, R. R., & Caron, M. G. (2001). Genetics of childhood disorders: XXIV. ADHD, Part 8: Hyperdopaminergic mice as an animal model of ADHD. *Journal of the American Child and Adolescent Psychiatry, 40,* 380–382.

Gajdusek, D. C. (1988). Transmissible and non-transmissible amyloidoses: Autocatalytic post-translational conversion of host precursor proteins to beta-pleated configuration. *Journal of Neuroimmunology, 20,* 95–110.

Galaburda, A., & Bellugi, U. (2000). Multi-level analysis of cortical neuroanatomy in Williams syndrome. *Journal of Cognitive Neuroscience, 12,* 74–88.

Galaburda, A., & Livingstone, M. (1993). Evidence for a magnocellular defect in developmental dyslexia. *Annals of the New York Academy of Sciences, 682,* 70–82.

Gallup, G. G., Jr. (1982). Self-awareness and the emergence of mind in primates. *American Journal of Primatology, 2,* 237–248.

Gallup, G. G., Jr., Nash, R. F., Potter, R. J., & Donegan, N. H. (1970). Effect of varying conditions of fear on immobility reactions in domestic chickens (Gallus gallus). *Journal of Comparative & Physiological Psychology, 73*(3), 442–445.

Ganguli, M., Dodge, H. H., Shen, C., & DeKosky, S. T. (2004). Mild cognitive impairment, amnestic type: an epidemiologic study. *Neurology, 63*(1), 115–121.

Gazzaniga, M. S. (1966). Interhemispheric communication of visual learning. *Neuropsychologia, 4,* 183.

Gazzaniga, M. S. (2000). Cerebral specialization and interhemispheric communication: Does the corpus callosum enable the human condition? *Brain, 123,* 1293–1326.

Gennarelli, T. A. (1983). Head injury in man and experimental animals: Clinical aspects. *Acta Neurochirugica, 32*(Suppl.), 1–13.

Georgopoulos, A. P., Whang, K., Georgopoulos, M. A., Tagaris, G. A., Amirikian, B., Richter, K., et al. (2001). Functional magnetic resonance imaging of visual object construction and shape discrimination: Relations among task, hemispheric lateralization, and gender. *Journal of Cognitive Neuroscience, 13,* 72–89.

Geschwind, N. (1965). Disconnexion syndromes in animals and man. *Brain, 88,* 237–294.

Geschwind, N., & Levitsky, W. (1968). Human brain: Left-right asymmetries in temporal speech region. *Science, 161,* 186–187.

Giedd, J. N. (2004). Structural magnetic resonance imaging of the adolescent brain. *Annals of the New York Academy of Sciences, 1021,* 77–85.

Giedd, J. N., Blumenthal, J., Mollowy, E., & Castellanos, F. X. (2001). Brain imaging of attention deficit/hyperactivity disorder. *Annals New York Academy of Sciences, 931,* 33–49.

Giedd, J. N., Castellanos, F. X., Casey, B. J., Kozuch, P., King, A. C., Hamburger, S. D., et al. (1994). Quantitative morphology of the corpus callosum in attention deficit hyperactivity disorder. *American Journal of Psychiatry, 151,* 665–669.

Giedd, J. N., Castellanos, F. X., Rajapakse, J. C., Vaituzis, A. C., & Rapoport, J. L. (1997). Sexual dimorphism of the developing human brain. *Progress in Neuropsychopharmacology and Biological Psychiatry, 21,* 1185–1201.

Gilman, S., & Newman, S. W. (1996). *Essentials of clinical neuroanatomy and neurophysiology* (9th ed.). Philadelphia: F. A. Davis.

Gilman, S., & Newman, S. W. (1996). The cerebrospinal fluid. In *Manter & Katz's Clinical neuroanatomy and neuropsychology* (9th ed.) (pp. 259–263). Philadelphia: F. A. Davis.

Giraud, A. I., & Price, C. J. (2001). The constraints functional neuroimaging places on classical models of auditory word processing. *Journal of Cognitive Neuroscience, 13,* 754–765.

Gitelman, D. R., Nobre, A. C., Parrish, T. B., LaBar, K. S., Kim, Y. H., Meyer, J. R., et al. (1999). A large-scale distributed network for covert spatial attention: Further anatomical delineation based on stringent behavioural and cognitive controls. *Brain, 122,* 1093–1106.

Glaser, G. H., & Pincus, J. H. (1969). Limbic encephalitis. *Journal of Nervous Mental Disorder, 149,* 59.

Glidden, R. A., Zillmer, E. A., & Barth, J. T. (1990). The long-term neurobehavioral effects of prefrontal lobotomy. *The Clinical Neuropsychologist, 4,* 301.

Gloor, P. (1990). Experiential phenomena of temporal lobe epilepsy: Facts and hypotheses. *Brain, 113*(Pt 6), 1673–1694.

Gogtay, N., Giedd, J. N., Lusk, L., Hayashi, K. M., Greenstein, D., Vaituzis, A. C., et al. (2004). Dynamic mapping of human cortical development during childhood through early adulthood. *Proceedings of the National Academy of Sciences, 101,* 8174–8179.

Goldberg, E. (2001). *The executive brain: Frontal lobes and the civilized mind.* New York: Oxford.

Goldberg, E., & Costa, L. (1981). Hemispheric differences in the acquisition and use of descriptive systems. *Brain and Language, 14,* 14–22.

Golden, C. J. (1978). *The Stroop Color and Word Test.* Chicago: Stoelting.

Golden, C. J., Zillmer, E. A., & Spiers, M. V. (1992). *Neuropsychological assessment and intervention.* Springfield, IL: Charles C. Thomas.

Goldenberg, G., Wimmer, A., Auff, E., & Schnaberth, G. (1986). Impairment of motor planning in patients with Parkinson's disease: Evidence for ideomotor apraxia. *Journal of Neurology, Neurosurgery, and Psychiatry, 49,* 1266–1272.

Goldman, S., & Nottebohm, F. (1983). Neuronal production, migration, and differentiation in a vocal control nucleus of the adult female canary brain. *Proceedings of the National Academy of Sciences of the United States of America, 80,* 2390–2394.

Goldman-Rakic, P. S. (1987a). Circuitry of primate prefrontal cortex and representation of behavior by representational memory. In F. Plum (Ed.), *Handbook of physiology: The nervous system* (Vol. V). Bethesda: American Physiological Society.

Goldman-Rakic, P. S. (1987b). Development of cortical circuitry and cognitive function. *Child Development, 58,* 601–622.

Goldman-Rakic, P. S. (1988). Topography of cognition: Parallel distributed networks in primary association cortex. *Annual Review of Neuroscience, 11,* 137–156.

Goldman-Rakic, P. S. (1993). Working memory and the mind. In *Mind and brain: Readings from Scientific American.* New York: W. H. Freeman.

Goldman-Rakic, P. S., & Friedman, H. R. (1991). The circuitry to working memory revealed by anatomy and metabolic imaging. In S. Levin, H. M. Eisenberg, & A. L. Benton (Eds.), *Frontal lobe functioning and dysfunction.* New York: Oxford University Press.

Goldstein, E. B. (1994). *Psychology.* Pacific Grove, CA: Brooks/Cole.

Good, C. D., Johnsrude, I., Ashburner, J., Henson, R. N. A., Friston, K. J., & Frackowiak, R. S. J. (2001). Cerebral asymmetry and the effects of sex and handedness on brain structure: A voxel-based morphometric analysis of 465 normal adult human brains. *NeuroImage, 14,* 685–700.

Gordon, A., & Zillmer, E. A. (1997). Integrating the MMPI and neuropsychology: A survey of NAN membership. *Archives of Clinical Neuropsychology, 4,* 325–326.

Gould, E., & Gross, C. G. (2002). Neurogenesis in adult mammals: Some progress and problems. *Journal of Neuroscience 22*(3), 619–623.

Gould, S. J. (1981). *The mismeasure of man.* New York: Norton.

Grabowski, T. J., Damasio, H., Eichhorn, G. R., & Tranel, D. (2003). Effects of gender on blood flow correlates of naming concrete entities. *NeuroImage, 20,* 940–954.

Graf, P., & Schacter, D. L. (1985). Implicit and explicit memory for new associations in normal and amnesic subjects. *Journal of Experimental Psychology: Learning Memory & Cognition, 2,* 501–518.

Grant, D. A., & Berg, E. A. (1948). A behavioral analysis of degree of reinforcement and ease of shifting two new responses in a Weigl-type card sorting problem. *Journal of Experimental Psychology: Learning Memory & Cognition, 38,* 404–411.

Greenberg, D. A., Aminoff, M. J., & Simon, R. P. (2002). *Clinical neurology* (5th ed). New York: McGraw-Hill/Appleton & Lange.

Grigorenko, E. L., Wood, F. B., Meyer, M. S., Hart, L. A., Speed, W. C., Shuster, A., et al. (1997). Susceptibility loci for distinct components of developmental dyslexia on chromosome 6 and 15. *American Journal of Human Genetics, 60,* 27–39.

Grill-Spector, K., & Malach, R. (2004). The human visual cortex. *Annual Review of Neuroscience, 27,* 649–677.

Grön, G., Wunderlich, A. P., Spitzer, M., Tomczak, R., & Riepe, M. W. (2000). Brain activation during human navigation: Gender-different neural networks as substrate of performance. *Nature Neuroscience, 3,* 404–408.

Gronwall, D. M. A. (1977). Paced Auditory Serial-Addition Task: A measure of recovery from concussion. *Perceptual and Motor Skills, 44,* 367–373.

Guilleminault, C. (1982). *Sleeping and waking disorders: Indications and techniques.* Menlo Park, CA: Addison-Wesley.

Guilleminault, C., & Dement, W. C. (1978). Sleep apnea syndromes and related sleep disorders. In R. L. Williams & I. Karacan (Eds.), *Sleep disorders: Diagnosis and treatment.* New York: Wiley.

Gur, R. C., Gur, R. E., Obrist, W. D., Hungerbuhler, J. P., Younkin, D., Rosen, A. D., et al. (1982). Sex and handedness differences in cerebral blood flow during rest and cognitive activity. *Science, 217,* 659–660.

Gur, R. C., Turetsky, B. I., Matsui, M., Yan, M., Bilker, W., Hughett, P., et al. (1999). Sex differences in brain gray and white matter in healthy young adults: Correlations with cognitive performance. *Journal of Neuroscience, 19,* 4065–4072.

Gur, R. E., Levy, J., & Gur, R. C. (1977). Clinical studies of brain organization and behavior. In A. Frazer & A. Winokur (Eds.), *Biological bases of psychiatric disorders.* New York: Spectrum.

Gurland, B. J., Wilder, D. E., Lantigua, R., Stern, Y., Chen, J., Killeffer, E. H., et al. (1999). Rates of dementia in three ethnoracial groups. *International Journal of Geriatric Psychiatry, 14*(6), 481–493.

Guthrie, P. B., Kanappenberger, J., Segal, M., Bennett, M. V. L., Charles, A. C., & Kater, S. B. (1999). ATP release from astrocytes mediates glial calcium waves. *Journal of Neuroscience, 19*(2), 520–528.

Guy, S. C. (1996). Social and emotional responsivity of children with nonverbal learning disabilities. *Dissertation Abstracts International: Section B: The Science and Engineering, 57,* 6573.

Haberecht, M. F., Menon, V., Warosfsky, I. S., White, C. D., Dyer-Friedman, J., & Glover, G. H. (2001). Functional neuroanatomy of visual-spatial working memory in Turner syndrome. *Human Brain Mapping, 14,* 96–107.

Haeger, K. (1988). *The illustrated history of surgery.* New York: Bell.

Hagerman, R. J. (1999). *Neurodevelopmental disorders: Diagnosis and treatment.* New York: Oxford University Press.

Haines, D. E. (1997). *Fundamental neuroscience.* New York: Churchill Livingstone.

Halgren, E., Walter, R. D., Cherlow, D. G., & Crandall, P. H. (1978). Mental phenomena evoked by electrical stimulation of the human hippocampal formation and amygdala. *Brain, 101*(1), 83–117.

Hallgren, B. (1950). Specific dyslexia (congenital word blindness): A clinical and genetic study. *Acta Psychiatrica et Neurologica, 65*(Suppl.), 1–28.

Halpern, D. F. (1992). *Sex differences in cognitive abilities* (2nd ed.). Hillsdale, NJ: Erlbaum.

Halpern, J. M., & Schulz, K. P. (2006). Revisiting the role of the prefrontal cortex in the pathophysiology of attention-deficit/hyperactivity disorder. *Psychological Bulletin, 132,* 560–581.

Halstead, W. C. (1947). *Brain and intelligence: A quantitative study of the frontal lobes.* Chicago: University of Chicago Press.

Hampson, E., Rovet, J. F., & Altmann, D. (1998). Spatial reasoning in children with congenital adrenal hyperplasia due to 21-hydroxylase deficiency. *Developmental Neuropsychology, 14,* 299–320.

Hanson, J. W., Jones, K. L., & Smith, D. W. (1976). Fetal alcohol syndrome: Experience with 41 patients. *Journal of the American Medical Association, 235,* 1459.

Harasty, J., Double, K. L., Halliday, G. M., Kril, J. J., & McRitchie, D. A. (1997). Language-associated cortical regions are proportionally larger in the female brain. *Archives of Neurology, 54,* 171–176.

Hari, R. (1994). Human cortical functions revealed by magnetoencephalography. *Progress in Brain Research, 100,* 163–168.

Harlow, H. F. (1952). Functional organization of the brain in relation to mentation and behavior. In M. M. Fund (Ed.), *The biology of mental health and disease.* New York: Hoeber.

Harlow, J. M. (1868). Recovery from the passage of an iron bar through the head. *Publications of the Massachusetts Medical Society, 2,* 327–347.

Harnadek, M. C. S., & Rourke, B. P. (1994). Principal identifying features of the syndrome of nonverbal learning disabilities in children. *Journal of Learning Disabilities, 27,* 144–154.

Harris, J. C. (1995). *Developmental neuropsychiatry.* New York: Oxford University Press.

Harrower, M. (1991). Inkblots and poems. In C. D. Walker (Ed.), *Clinical psychology in autobiography* (pp. 125–170). Pacific Grove, CA: Brooks/Cole.

Hartlage, L. C., & Gage, R. (1997). Unimanual performance as a measure of laterality. *Neuropsychology Review, 7,* 143–156.

Hartman, D. E. (1995). *Neuropsychological toxicology: Identification and assessment of human neurotoxic syndromes* (2nd ed.). New York: Plenum.

Hasselbalch, S. G., Oberg, G., Sorensen, S., Andersen, A. R., Waldemar, G., Schmidt, J. F., et al. (1992). Reduced regional cerebral blood flow in Huntington's disease studied by SPECT. *Journal of Neurology, Neurosurgery, and Psychiatry, 55,* 1018–1023.

Haug, H. (1985). Are neurons of the human cerebral cortex really lost during aging? A morphometric examination. In J. Tarber & W. H. Gispen (Eds.), *Senile dementia of Alzheimer type* (pp. 150–163). New York: Springer-Verlag.

Hauri, P. (1977). *The sleep disorders.* Kalamazoo, MI: Upjohn Company.

Hauser, P., Zametkin, A. J., Martinez, P., Vitiello, B., Matochik, J. A., Mixon, A. J., et al. (1993). Attention deficit-hyperactivity disorder in people with generalized resistance to thryroid hormone. *New England Journal of Medicine, 328,* 997–1001.

Hauser, W. A. (1992). Seizure disorders: The changes with age. *Epilepsia, 33*(Suppl. 4), S6–S14.

Haynes, S. D., & Bennett, T. L. (1990). Cognitive impairments in adults with complex partial seizures. *International Journal of Clinical Neuropsychology, 12,* 74–81.

Heaton, R. K. (1981). *Wisconsin Card Sort manual.* Odessa, FL: Psychological Assessment Resources.

Heaton, R. K., Chelune, G. J., Talley, J. L., Kay, G. G., & Curtis, G. (1993). *Wisconsin Card Sorting Test manual: Revised and expanded.* Odessa, FL: Psychological Assessment Resources.

Heaton, R. K., Grant, I., & Matthews, C. G. (1991). *Comprehensive norms for an extended Halstead-Reitan battery: Demographic corrections, research findings, and clinical applications.* Odessa, FL: Psychological Assessment Resources.

Hebb, D. O. (1949). *The organization of behavior: A neuropsychological theory.* New York: Wiley.

Hebb, D. O. (1959). Intelligence, brain function and the theory of mind. *Brain, 82,* 260.

Hebb, D. O. (1983). Neuropsychology: Retrospect and prospect. *Canadian Journal of Psychology, 37,* 4–7.

Hécaen, H., & Albert, M. L. (1978). *Human neuropsychology.* New York: Wiley.

Heilman, K. M. (2002). *Matter of mind: A neurologist's view of brain-behavior relationships.* New York: Oxford University Press.

Heilman, K. M., Watson, R. T., & Valenstein, E. (1993). Neglect and related disorders. In K. M. Heilman & E. Valenstein (Eds.), *Clinical neuropsychology* (3rd ed.). New York: Oxford University Press.

Heindel, W. C., Salmon, D. P., Shults, C. W., Wallcke, P. A., & Butters, N. (1989). Neuropsychological evidence for multiple implicit memory systems: A comparison of Alzheimer's and Parkinson's disease patients. *Journal of Neuroscience, 9,* 582–587.

Helland, T., & Asbjørnsen, A. (2000). Executive functions in dyslexia. *Child Neuropsychology, 6,* 37–48.

Heller, K. W. (1996). *Understanding physical, sensory, and health impairments.* Pacific Grove, CA: Brooks/Cole.

Helmer, C., Joly, P., Letenneur, L., Commenges, D., & Dartigues, J. F. (2001). Mortality with dementia: Results from a French prospective community-based cohort. *American Journal of Epidemiology, 154*(7), 642–648.

Henry, J. D., MacLeod, M., Phillips, L., & Crawford, J. R. (2004). A meta-analytic review of prospective memory and aging. *Psychology and Aging, 19,* 27–39.

Hill, D. E., Yeo, R. A., Campbell, R. A., Blaine, H., Vigil, J., & Brooks, W. (2003). Magnetic resonance imaging correlates of attention-deficit/hyperactivity disorder. *Neuropsychology, 17,* 496–506.

Hirsch, H. V. B., & Jacobson, M. (1974). The perfect brain. In M. S. Gazzaniga & C. B. Blakemore (Eds.), *Fundamentals of psychobiology.* New York: Academic Press.

Hobson, J. A. (1995). *Sleep.* New York: Scientific American Library.

Hodges, J. R., Salmon, D. P., & Butters, N. (1991). The nature of the naming deficit in Alzheimer's and Huntington's disease. *Brain, 114,* 1547–1558.

Hoekstra, P. J., Kallenber, C. G. M., Korf, J., & Minderaa, R. B. (2002). Is Tourette's syndrome an autoimmune disease? *Molecular Psychiatry, 7,* 437–445.

Holiger, D. P., McMenamin, D., Sherman, G. F., & Galaburda, A. (2001). *Williams syndrome: Cell packing density and neuronal size in primary auditory cortex* [Abstract]. Society for Neuroscience Annual Meeting, San Diego, CA, 986.4.

Holmes, J., Payton, A., Barrett, J. H., Hever, T., Fitzpatrick, H., Trumper, A. L., et al. (2000). A family-based and a case-control association study of the dopamine D4 receptor gene and dopamine transporter gene in attention deficit hyperactivity disorder. *Molecular Psychiatry, 5,* 523–530.

Honda, H., Shimizu, Y., & Rutter, M. (2005). No effect of MMR withdrawal on the incidence of autism: A total population study. *Journal of Child Psychology and Psychiatry, 46,* 572–579.

Hooper, H. E. (1983). *Hooper Visual Organization Test VOT.* Los Angeles: Western Psychological Services.

Hooper, S. R., Willis, W. G., & Stone, B. H. (1996). Issues and approaches in the neuropsychological treatment of children with learning disabilities. In E. S. Batchelor & R. S. Dean (Eds.), *Pediatric neuropsychology: Interfacing assessment and treatment in rehabilitation* (pp. 211–248). Boston: Allyn & Bacon.

Hopyan, T., Dennis, M., Weksberg, R., & Cytrynbaum, C. (2001). Music skills and the expressive interpretation of music in children with Williams-Beuren syndrome: Pitch, rhythm, melodic imagery, phrasing, and musical affect. *Child Neuropsychology, 7,* 42–53.

Hornak, J. (1992). Ocular exploration in the dark by patients with visual neglect. *Neuropsychologia, 30,* 353–384.

Hornak, J., Rolls, E. T., & Wade, D. (1996). Face and voice expression identification in patients with emotional and behavioral changes following ventral frontal lobe damage. *Neuropsychologia, 34,* 247–261.

Hornsey, H., Banerjee, S., Zeitlin, H., & Robertson, M. (2001). The prevalence of Tourette syndrome in 13–14-year-olds in mainstream schools. *Journal of Child Psychology and Psychiatry and Allied Disciplines, 42,* 1035–1039.

Horwitz, B., Rumsey, J. M., & Donohue, B. C. (1998). Functional connectivity of the angular gyrus in normal reading and developmental dyslexia. *Proceedings of the National Academy of Sciences, 95,* 8939–8944.

Howes, N. L., Bigler, E. D., Burlingame, G. M., & Lawson, J. S. (2003). Memory performance of children with dyslexia: A comparative analysis of theoretical perspectives. *Journal of Learning Disabilities, 36,* 230–246.

Howlin, P. (2003). Outcome in high-functioning adults with autism with and without early language delays: Implications for the differentiation between autism and Asperger syndrome. *Journal of Autism and Developmental Disorders, 33,* 3–13.

Hoyert, D. L., & Rosenberg, H. M. (1997). Alzheimer's disease as a cause of death in the United States. *Public Health Reports, 112*(6), 497–505.

Hubel, D. H. (1988). *Eye, brain, vision.* New York: Scientific American Library.

Hughes, C., Russell, J., & Robbins, T. W. (1994). Evidence for executive dysfunction in autism. *Neuropsychologia, 32,* 477–492.

Hutt, M. L. (1985). *The Hutt adaptation of the Bender-Gestalt Test: Rapid screening and intensive diagnosis* (4th ed.). Orlando, FL: Grune & Stratton.

Huttenlocher, P. R. (1990). Morphometric study of human cerebral cortex development. *Neuropsychologia, 28,* 517–527.

Huttenlocher, P. R. (1999). Dendritic and synaptic development in human cerebral cortex: Time course and critical periods. *Developmental Neuropsychology, 16,* 347–368.

Huttenlocher, P. R., & Dabholkar, A. S. (1997). Developmental anatomy of prefrontal cortex. In N. A. Krasnegor, G. R. Lyon, & P. S. Goldman-Rakic (Eds.), *Development of the prefrontal cortex: Evolution, neurobiology, and behavior* (pp. 69–84). Baltimore: Paul H. Brookes.

Hyde, J. S. (2005). The gender similarities hypothesis. *American Psychologist, 60,* 581–592.

Hynd, G. W., Hall, J., Novey, E. S., Eliopulos, D., Black, K., Gonzales, J. J., et al. (1995). Dyslexia and corpus callosum morphology. *Archives of Neurology, 52,* 32–38.

Hynd, G. W., Hern, K. L., Novey, E. S., Eliopulos, D., Marshall, R., Gonzalez, J. J., et al. (1993). Attention deficit-hyperactivity disorder and asymmetry of the caudate nucleus. *Journal of Child Neurology, 8,* 339–347.

Hynd, G. W., & Hiemenz, J. R. (1997). Dyslexia and gyral morphology variations. In C. Hulme & M. Snowling (Eds.), *Dyslexia: Biology, cognition and intervention* (pp. 38–58). London: Whurr.

Hynd, G. W., Morgan, A. E., & Vaughn, M. (1997). Neurodevelopmental anomalies and malformations. In C. R. Reynolds & E. Fletcher-Janzen (Eds.), *Handbook of clinical child neuropsychology* (2nd ed., pp. 42–61). New York: Plenum Press.

Hynd, G. W., Semrud-Clikeman, M., Lorys, A. R., Novey, E. S., & Eliopulos, D. (1990). Brain morphology in developmental dyslexia and attention deficit disorder/hyperactivity. *Archives of Neurology, 47,* 919–926.

Hynd, G. W., Semrud-Clikeman, M., Lorys, A. R., Novey, E. S., Eliopulos, D., & Lyytinen, H. (1991). Corpus callosum morphology in attention deficit-hyperactivity disorder: Morphometric analysis of MRI. *Journal of Learning Disabilities, 24,* 141–146.

Hynd, G. W., & Willis, W. G. (1988). *Pediatric neuropsychology.* Boston: Allyn & Bacon.

Imperato-McGinley, J., Pichardo, M., Gautier, T., Voyer, D., & Bryden, M. P. (1991). Cognitive abilities in androgen-insensitive subjects: Comparisons with control males and females from the same kindred. *Clinical Endocrinology, 34,* 341–347.

Jack, C. R., Jr., Petersen, R. C., Xu, Y., O'Brien, P. C., Smith, G. E., Ivnik, R. J., et al. (2000). Rates of hippocampal atrophy correlate with change in clinical status in aging and AD. *Neurology, 55*(4), 484–489.

Jack, C. R., Jr., Shiung, M. M., Gunter, J. L., O'Brien, P. C., Weigand, S. D., Knopman, D. S., et al. (2004). Comparison of different MRI brain atrophy rate measures with clinical disease progression in AD. *Neurology, 62*(4), 591–600.

Jack, C. R., Jr., Shiung, M. M., Weigand, S. D., O'Brien, P. C., Gunter, J. L., Boeve, B. F., et al. (2005). Brain atrophy rates predict subsequent clinical conversion in normal elderly and amnestic MCI. *Neurology, 65*(8), 1227–1231.

Jacobson, S. W., Jacobson, J. L., Sokol, R. J., Martier, S. S., & Ager, J. W. (1993). Prenatal alcohol exposure and infant information processing ability. *Child Development, 64,* 1706–1721.

James, E. M., & Selz, M. (1997). Neuropsychological bases of common learning and behavior problems in children. In C. R. Reynolds & E. Fletcher-Janzen (Eds.), *Handbook of clinical child neuropsychology* (2nd ed., pp. 157–189). New York: Plenum Press.

James, T. W., & Kimura, D. (1997). Sex differences in remembering the locations of objects in an array: Location-shifts versus location-exchanges. *Evolution and Human Behavior, 18,* 155–163.

Jarrold, C., Butler, D. W., Cottington, E. M., & Jimenez, F. (2000). Linking theory of mind and central coherence bias in autism and in the general population. *Developmental Psychology, 36,* 126–138.

Jeffries, K. J., Schooler, C., Schoenbach, C., Herscovitch, P., Chase, T. N., & Braun, A. R. (2002). The functional neuroanatomy of Tourette's syndrome: An FDG PET study III: Functional coupling of regional cerebral metabolic rates. *Neuropsychopharmacology, 27,* 92–104.

Jenkins, M. R., & Culbertson, J. L. (1996). Prenatal exposure to alcohol. In R. L. Adams, O. A. Parsons, J. L. Culbertson, & S. J. Nixon (Eds.), *Neuropsychology for clinical practice: Etiology, assessment, and treatment of common neurological disorders* (pp. 407–452). Washington, DC: American Psychological Association.

Jennett, B., & Teasdale, G. (1981). *Management of head injuries.* Philadelphia: F. A. Davies.

Jensen, P. S., Martin, D., & Cantwell, D. P. (1997). Comorbidity in ADHD: Implications for research, practice, and DSM-V. *Journal of the American Academy of Child and Adolescent Psychiatry, 36,* 1065–1079.

Johansson, B. (1991). Neuropsychological assessment in the oldest-old. *International Psychogeriatrics, 3*(Suppl.), 51–60.

Johansson, B., Zarit, S. H., & Berg, S. (1992). Changes in cognitive functioning of the oldest old. *Journal of Gerontology Psychological Sciences, 47,* 75–80.

Johnson, S. C., Bigler, E. D., Burr, R. B., & Blatter, D. D. (1994). White matter atrophy, ventricular dilation, and intellectual functioning following traumatic brain injury. *Neuropsychology, 8,* 307–315.

Jones, A. W. R., & Richardson, J. S. (1990). Alzheimer's disease: Clinical and pathological characteristics. *International Journal of Neuroscience, 50,* 147–168.

Jones, C. M., Braithwaite, V. A., & Healy, S. D. (2003). The evolution of sex differences in spatial ability. *Behavioral Neuroscience, 117,* 403–411.

Jones, E. (1981). *The life and work of Sigmund Freud: The formative years and the great discoveries* (Vol. 1). New York: Basic Books.

Jones, K. L., Smith, D. W., Ulleland, C. N., & Streissguth, A. P. (1973). Pattern of malformation in offspring of chronic alcoholic mothers. *Lancet, 1,* 1267–1271.

Jones-Gotman, M. (1996). Psychological evaluation for epilepsy surgery. In S. Shorvon, F. Dreifuss, D. Fish, & D. Thomas (Eds.), *The treatment of epilepsy.* Oxford, United Kingdom: Blackwell Science.

Jonides, J., Smith, E. E., Koeppe, R. A., Awh, E., Minoshima, S., & Mintun, M. A. (1993). Spatial working memory in humans as revealed by PET. *Nature, 363,* 623–625.

Jurko, M. F., & Andy, O. J. (1973). Psychological changes correlated with thalamotomy site. *Journal of Neurology, Neurosurgery, and Psychiatry, 36,* 846.

Kaemingk, K., & Paquette, A. (1999). Effects of prenatal alcohol exposure on neuropsychological functioning. *Developmental Neuropsychology, 15,* 111–140.

Kagan, J. (1964). *The Matching Familiar Figures Test.* Cambridge, MA: Harvard University.

Kalat, J. W. (1998). *Biological psychology* (6th ed.). Pacific Grove, CA: Brooks/Cole.

Kalat, J. W. (2004). *Biological psychology* (8th ed.). Belmont, CA: Wadsworth/Thomson Learning.

Kandel, E. R., Schwartz, J. H., & Jessell, T. H. (1991). *Principles of neural science* (5th ed.). New York: Elsevier Science.

Kanner, L. (1943). Autistic disturbances of affective contact. *Nervous Child, 2,* 9–33.

Kansaku, K., Yamaura, A., & Kitazawa, S. (2000). Sex differences in lateralization revealed in the posterior language areas. *Cerebral Cortex, 10,* 866–872.

Karmiloff-Smith, A. (1997). Crucial differences between developmental cognitive neuroscience and adult neuropsychology. *Developmental Neuropsychology, 13,* 513–524.

Karmiloff-Smith, A. (1998). Development itself is the key to understanding developmental disorders. *Trends in Cognitive Sciences, 2,* 389–398.

Karmiloff-Smith, A., Brown, J. H., Grice, S., & Paterson, S. (2003). Dethroning the myth: Cognitive dissociation and innate modularity in Williams syndrome. *Developmental Neuropsychology, 23,* 227–242.

Karni, A., Tanne, D., Rubenstein, B. S., Askenasy, J. J. M., & Sagi, D. (1994). Dependence on REM sleep of overnight improvement of a perceptual skill. *Science, 265,* 679–682.

Katzman, R., Lasker, B., & Bernstein, N. (1988). Advances in the diagnosis of dementia: Accuracy of diagnosis and consequences of misdiagnosis of disorders causing dementia. In R. D. Terry (Ed.), *Aging and the brain* (Vol. 32, pp. 17–61). New York: Raven Press.

Kaufman, A. S. (2001). Do low levels of lead produce IQ loss in children? A careful examination of the literature. *Archives of Clinical Neuropsychology, 16,* 303–341.

Kaufman, A. S., Reynolds, C. R., & McLean, J. E. (1989). Age and WAIS-R intelligence in a sample of adults in the 20–74-year age range: A cross sectional analysis with educational level controlled. *Intelligence, 13,* 235–253.

Kaushall, P. I., Zetin, M., & Squire, L. R. (1981). Single case study: A psychosocial study of chronic, circumscribed amnesia. *Journal of Nervous and Mental Disease, 169,* 383–389.

Kawasaki, H., Adolphs, R., Hiroyuki, O., Kovach, C., Damasio, H., Kaufman, O., et al., (2005). Analysis of single-unit responses to emotional scenes in human ventromedial prefrontal cortex. *Journal of Cognitive Neuroscience, 17,* 1509–1518.

Kay, D. W. K. (1995). The epidemiology of age-related neurological disease and dementia. *Reviews in Clinical Gerontology, 5,* 39–56.

Kemper, T. L. (1994). Neuroanatomical and neuropathological changes in normal aging and in dementia. In M. Albert & J. Knoefel (Eds.), *Clinical neurology of aging* (pp. 3–78). New York and Oxford: Oxford University Press.

Kennedy, C. H. (1999). Assessing competency to consent to sexual activity in the cognitively impaired population. *Journal of Forensic Neuropsychology, 1,* 17–33.

Kennedy, C. H. (2003). Legal and psychological implications in the assessment of sexual consent in the cognitively impaired population. *Assessment, 10*(4), 352–358.

Kennedy, C. H., & Niederbuhl, J. (2001). Establishing criteria for sexual consent capacity. *American Journal of Mental Retardation, 106*(6), 503–510.

Kennedy, C. H., & Zillmer, E. A. (2006). *Military psychology: Clinical and operational applications.* New York: Guilford Press.

Kenyon, T. (1994). *Brain states.* Naples, FL: United States Publishing.

Kerns, K. A., Don, A., Mateer, C. A., & Streissguth, A. P. (1997). Cognitive deficits in nonretarded adults with fetal alcohol syndrome. *Journal of Learning Disabilities, 30,* 685–693.

Kerr, D. A., Lladó, J., Shamblott, M. J., Maragakis, N. J., Irani, D. N., Crawford, T. O., et al. (2003). Human embryonic germ cell derivatives facilitate motor recovery of rats with diffuse motor neuron injury. *Journal of Neuroscience, 23,* 5131–5140.

Kertesz, A., & Gold, B. T. (2003). Recovery of cognition (pp. 617–639). In K. M. Heilman & E. Valenstein (Eds.), *Clinical neuropsychology.* New York: Oxford University Press.

Kety, S. S. (1979). Disorders of the human brain. *Scientific American, 241,* 202–214.

Kibby, M. Y., Marks, W., Morgan, S., & Long, C. J. (2004). Specific impairments in developmental reading disabilities: A working memory approach. *Journal of Learning Disabilities, 37,* 349–363.

Kim, Y. H., Gitelman, D. R., Nobre, A. C., Parrish, T. B., LaBar, K. S., & Mesulam, M. M. (1999). The large-scale network for spatial attention displays multifunctional overlap but differential asymmetry. *NeuroImage, 9,* 269–277.

Kimura, D. (1999). *Sex and cognition.* Cambridge, MA: MIT Press.

Kinsbourne, M. (1993). Orientational bias model of unilateral neglect: Evidence from attentional gradients within hemispace. In H. Robertson & J. C. Marshall (Eds.), *Unilateral neglect: Clinical and experimental studies* (pp. 63–86). Hove, United Kingdom: Erlbaum.

Klein, B. P., & Mervis, C. B. (1999). Contrasting patterns of cognitive abilities of 9- and 10-year-olds with Williams syndrome or Down syndrome. *Developmental Neuropsychology, 16,* 177–196.

Kleist, K. (1933). *Gehirnpathologie.* Leipzig: Barth.

Klin, A. (2000). Attributing social meaning to ambiguous visual stimuli in higher functioning autism and Asperger syndrome: The social attribution task. *Journal of Child Psychology and Psychiatry, 41,* 831–846.

Knaus, T. A., Bollich, A. M., Corey, D. M., Lemen, L. C., & Foundas, A. L. (2004). Sex-linked differences in the anatomy of the perisylvian language cortex: A volumetric MRI study of gray matter volumes. *Neuropsychology, 18,* 738–747.

Knecht, S., Deppe, M., Dräger, B., Bobe, L., Lohmann, H., Ringelstein, E. B., et al. (2000a). Language lateralization in healthy right-handers. *Brain, 123,* 74–81.

Knecht, S., Dräger, B., Deppe, M., Bobe, L., Lohmann, H., Flöel, A., et al. (2000). Handedness and hemispheric language dominance in healthy humans. *Brain, 123,* 2512–2518.

Knight, R. T., & Stuss, D. T. (2002). Prefrontal cortex: The present and the future. In D. T. Stuss & R. T. Knight (Eds.), *Principles of frontal lobe function* (pp. 573–598). New York: Oxford University Press.

Knopman, D. S., DeKosky, S. T., Cummings, J. L., Chui, H., Corey-Bloom, J., Relkin, N., et al. (2001). Practice parameter: Diagnosis of dementia (an evidence-based review). Report of the Quality Standards Subcommittee of the American Academy of Neurology. *Neurology, 56*(9), 1143–1153.

Kolb, B. (1995). *Brain plasticity and behavior.* Mahwah, NJ: Erlbaum.

Kolb, B., & Fantie, B. (1997). Development of the child's brain and behavior. In C. R. Reynolds & E. Fletcher-Janzen (Eds.), *Handbook of clinical child neuropsychology* (2nd ed., pp. 17–41). New York: Plenum Press.

Kolb, B., Gibb, R., & Gorny, G. (2000). Cortical plasticity and the development of behavior after early frontal cortical injury. *Developmental Neuropsychology, 18,* 423–444.

Kolb, B., & Whishaw, I. Q. (1990). *Fundamentals of human neuropsychology* (3rd ed.). New York: W. H. Freeman.

Kolb, B., & Whishaw, I. Q. (1996). *Fundamentals of human neuropsychology* (4th ed.). New York: W. H. Freeman and Company.

Koller, K., Brown, T., Spurgeon, A., & Levy, L. (2004). Recent developments in low-level lead exposure and intellectual impairment in children. *Environmental Health Perspectives: Annual Review, 112,* 987–994.

Korkman, M., Kettunen, S., & Autti-Rämö, I. (2003). Neurocognitive impairment in early adolescence following prenatal alcohol exposure of varying duration. *Child Neuropsychology, 9,* 117–128.

Korkman, M., Kirk, U., & Kemp, S. (1998). *NEPSY: A developmental neuropsychology assessment manual.* San Antonio, TX: Psychological Corporation.

Krakauer, J. (1997). *Into thin air.* New York: Villard.

Krech, D. (1962). Cortical localization of function. In L. Postman (Ed.), *Psychology in the making.* New York: Knopf.

Kunin-Batson, A., Primeau, M., Zelko, F., Glanzman, M., Martini, D. R., & Erwin, R. (2002). Effects of methylphenidate on neuropsychological functioning in children with ADHD. *Journal of the International Neuropsychological Society, 8,* 309–310.

Kupfermann, I. (1991). Hypothalamus and limbic system: Peptidergic, neurons, homeostasis, and emotional behavior. In E. R. Kandel, J. H. Schwartz, & T. M. Jessell (Eds.), *Principles of neural science* (pp. 736–749). New York: Elsevier.

LaBerge, S. (1990). *Exploring the world of lucid dreaming.* New York: Ballantine Books.

Lai, Z. (1998). Emotional expression and perception in Williams syndrome. Paper presented at the Cognitive Neuroscience Society, San Francisco, CA.

Lange, C. G. (1922). *The emotions.* Baltimore: Williams & Wilkins.

Larsen, J. P., Hoien, T., & Odegaard, H. (1992). Magnetic resonance imaging of the corpus callosum in developmental dyslexia. *Cognitive Neuropsychology, 9,* 123–134.

Larson, J., & Lynch, G. (1986). Induction of synaptic potentiation in hippocampus by patterned stimulation involves two events. *Science, 232,* 985–988.

LaRue, A. (1992). *Aging and neuropsychological assessment.* New York: Plenum Press.

Lashley, K. S. (1929). *Brain mechanisms and intelligence.* Chicago: University of Chicago Press.

Laws, G., & Bishop, D. (2004). Pragmatic language impairments and social deficits in Williams syndrome: A comparison with Down's syndrome and specific language impairment. *International Journal of Communication Disorders, 39,* 45–64.

Lawson, J., Baron-Cohen, S., & Wheelwright, S. (2004). Emphathising and systemising in adults with and without Asperger syndrome. *Journal of Autism and Developmental Disorders, 34,* 301–309.

Leckman, J. F., & Cohen, D. J. (1996). Tic disorders. In M. Lewis (Ed.), *Child and adolescent psychiatry: A comprehensive textbook* (2nd ed., pp. 622–629). Baltimore: Williams & Wilkins.

Leckman, J. F., Peterson, B. S., Anderson, G. M., Arsten, A. F., Pauls, D. L., & Cohen, D. J. (1997). Pathogenesis of Tourette's syndrome. *Journal of Child Psychology and Psychiatry and Allied Disciplines, 38,* 119–142.

Leckman, J. F., Peterson, B. S., Schultz, R. T., & Cohen, D. J. (2001). Tics: When habit-forming neural systems form habits of their own. In C. A. Nelson & M. Luciana (Eds.), *Handbook of developmental cognitive neuroscience* (pp. 549–560). Cambridge, MA: MIT Press.

LeDoux, J. E. (1992). Brain mechanisms of emotion and emotional learning. *Current Opinion in Neurobiology, 2,* 191–197.

LeDoux, J. E. (1994). Emotion, memory and the brain. *Scientific American, 270*(6), 50–57.

LeDoux, J. (1996). *The emotional brain: The mysterious underpinnings of emotional life.* New York: Touchstone.

Lee, K. T., Mattson, S. N., & Riley, E. P. (2004). Classifying children with heavy prenatal alcohol exposure using measures of attention. *Journal of the International Neuropsychological Society, 10,* 271–277.

Lees, A. J., & Smith, E. (1983). Cognitive deficits in the early stages of Parkinson's disease. *Brain, 106,* 257–270.

Leiguarda, R. C., Merello, M., Nouzeilles, M. I., Balej, J., Rivero, A., & Nogues, M. (2003). Limb-kinetic apraxia in corticobasal degeneration: Clinical and kinetic features. *Movement Disorders, 18*(1), 49–59.

Lemire, R. J., Loeser, J. D., Leech, R. W., & Alvord, E. C. (1975). *Normal and abnormal development of the human nervous system.* New York: Harper & Row.

Lemke, G. (2001). Glial control of neuronal development. *Annual Review of Neuroscience, 24,* 87–105.

Lemoine, P., Harrowsseau, H., Borteryu, J. P., & Menuet, J. C. (1968). Les enfants de parents alcoholiques: Anomalies observees a propos de 127 cas. *Quest Medicale, 21,* 476–482.

Levin, B. E., Tomer, R., & Rey, G. J. (1992). Cognitive impairment in Parkinson's disease. *Neurologic Clinics, 2,* 471–485.

Levin, H. S., Benton, A. L., & Grossman, R. G. (1982). *Neurobehavioral consequences of closed head injury.* New York: Oxford University Press.

Levin, H. S., Culhane, K. A., Hartmann, J., Evankovitch, K., Mattson, A. J., Harward, H., et al. (1991). Developmental changes in performance on tests of purported frontal lobe function. *Developmental Neuropsychology, 7,* 377–395.

Levin, H. S., Eisenberg, H. M., & Benton, A. L. (1989). *Mild head injury.* New York: Oxford University Press.

Levin, H. S., O'Donnell, V. M., & Grossman, R. G. (1979). The Galveston Orientation and Amnesia Test: A practical scale to assess cognition after head injury. *Journal of Nervous and Mental Disease, 167,* 675–684.

Levine, B., Black, S. E., Cabeza, R., Sinder, M., McIntosh, J. P., Toth, J. P., et al. (1998). Episodic memory and the self in a case of isolated retrograde amnesia. *Brain, 121,* 1951–1973.

Levitin, D. J., Cole, K., Chiles, M., Lai, Z., Lincoln, A., & Bellugi, U. (2004). Characterizing the musical phenotype in individuals with Williams syndrome. *Child Neuropsychology, 10,* 223–247.

Levy, J., & Heller, W. (1992). Gender differences in human neuropsychological function. In A. A. Gerall, H. Moltz, & I. L. Ward (Eds.), *Handbook of behavioral neurobiology: Sexual differentiation.* New York: Plenum.

Lezak, M. D. (1995). *Neuropsychological assessment* (3rd ed.). New York: Oxford University Press.

Lezak, M. D., Howieson, D. B., & Loring, D. W. (2004). *Neuropsychological assessment* (4th ed.). New York: Oxford University Press.

Lichter, D. G., & Cummings, J. L. (2001). Introduction and overview. In D. G. Lichter & J. L. Cummings (Eds.), *Frontal-subcortical circuits in psychiatric and neurological disorders* (pp. 1–43). New York: Guilford Press.

Lifton, R. J. (1986). *The Nazi doctors: Medical killing and the psychology of genocide.* New York: Basic Books.

Lisowksi, F. P. (1967). Prehistoric and early historic trepanation. In D. Brothwell & A. T. Sandison (Eds.), *Diseases in antiquity* (pp. 651–672). Springfield, IL: Charles C. Thomas.

Little, S. S. (1993). Nonverbal learning disabilities and socioemotional functioning: A review of recent literature. *Journal of Learning Disabilities, 26,* 653–665.

Lopez, O. L., Jagust, W. J., DeKosky, S. T., Becker, J. T., Fitzpatrick, A., Dulberg, C., et al. (2003). Prevalence and classification of mild cognitive impairment in the Cardiovascular Health Study Cognition Study: part 1. *Archives of Neurology, 60*(10), 1385–1389.

Lopez, O. L., Litvan, I., Catt, K. E., Stowe, R., Klunk, W., Kaufer, D. I., et al. (1999). Accuracy of four clinical diagnostic criteria for the diagnosis of neurodegenerative dementias. *Neurology, 53*(6), 1292–1299.

Lord, C., Risi, S., Lambrecht, L., Cook, E. H., Jr., Leventhal, B. L., DiLavore, P. C., et al. (2000). Autism Diagnostic Observation Schedule-Generic: A standard measure of social and communication deficits associated with the spectrum of autism. *Journal of Autism & Developmental Disorders, 30,* 205–223.

Lowther, J. L., & Wasserman, J. D. (1994, November). *Use of Mirsky's neurocognitive model of attention in identifying DSM-IV disorders of attention.* Poster presented at the annual meeting of National Academy of Neuropsychology, Orlando, FL.

Lupien, S. J., de Leon, M., de Santi, S., Convit, A., Tarshish, C., Nair, N. P., et al. (1998). Cortisol levels during human aging predict hippocampal atrophy and memory deficits. *Nature Neuroscience, 1*(1), 69–73.

Luria, A. R. (1964). Neuropsychology in the local diagnosis of brain injury. *Cortex, 1,* 3.

Luria, A. R. (1966). *Higher cortical functions in man.* New York: Basic Books.

Luria, A. R. (1968). *The mind of a mnemonist.* New York: Basic Books.

Luria, A. R. (1971). Memory disturbances in local brain lesions. *Neuropsychologia, 9,* 367.

Luria, A. R. (1990). *The neuropsychological analysis of problem-solving.* Orlando, FL: Paul M. Deutsch Press.

MacDonald, A. W., Cohen, J. D., Stenger, V. A., & Carter, C. S. (2000). Dissociating the role of the dorsolateral prefrontal and anterior cingulated cortex in cognitive control. *Science, 288,* 1835–1838.

Macintosh, K. E., & Dissanayake, C. (2004). Annotation: The similarities and differences between autistic disorder and Asperger's disorder: A review of the empirical evidence. *Journal of Child Psychology and Psychiatry, 45,* 421–434.

MacLean, P. D. (1949). Psychosomatic disease and the "visceral brain": Recent developments bearing on the Papez theory of emotion. *Psychosomatic Medicine, 11,* 338–353.

MacLean, P. D. (1952). Some psychiatric implications of physiological studies on frontotemporal portion of limbic system (visceral brain). *Electroencephalography and Clinical Neurophysiology, 4,* 407–418.

Macmillan, M. (1996). Phineas Gage: A case for all reasons. In C. Code, C. Wallesch, Y. Joanette, & A. R. Lecours (Eds.), *Classic cases in neuropsychology* (pp. 243–262). Sussex, United Kingdom: Psychology Press.

Mai, J. K., Assheuer, J., & Paxinos, G. (1997). *Atlas of the human brain.* San Diego, CA: Academic Press.

Majovski, L. V. (1997). Mechanisms and development of cerebral lateralization in children. In C. R. Reynolds & E. Fletcher-Janzen (Eds.), *Handbook of clinical child neuropsychology* (2nd ed., pp. 102–119). New York: Plenum Press.

Marie, P. (1971). Pierre Marie's papers on speech disorders. New York: Hafner.

Marino, B. S., Fine, K. S., & McMillan, J. A. (2004*). Blueprints pediatrics* (3rd ed.). Malden, MA: Blackwell Publishing.

Markman, J. A., McKian, K. P., Stroup, T. S., & Juraska, J. M. (2004). Sexually dimorphic aging of dendritic morphology in CA1 of hippocampus. *Hippocampus, 15,* 97–103.

Marshall, J. C., & Halligan, P. W. (1988). Line bisection in a case of visual neglect. *Nature, 336,* 766–777.

Marshall, L. F., & Ruff, R. M. (1989). Neurosurgeon as a victim. In H. S. Levin, H. M. Eisenberg, & A. L. Benton (Eds.), *Mild head injury.* New York: Oxford University Press.

Martin, J. H. (1996). *Neuroanatomy text and atlas* (2nd ed.). Stamford, CT: Appleton & Lange.

Martin, J. H., & Jessell, T. M. (1991). Development as a guide to the regional anatomy of the brain. In E. R. Kandel, J. H. Schwartz & T. M. Jessell (Eds.), *Principles of neural science* (3rd ed., pp. 296–308). New York: Elsevier Science.

Masliah, E., Mallory, M., Veinbergs, I., Miller, A., & Samuel, W. (1996). Alterations in apolipoprotein E expression during aging and neurodegeneration. *Progress in Neurobiology, 50*(5–6), 493–503.

Mason, C., & Kandel, E. R. (1991). Central visual pathways. In E. R. Kandel, J. H. Schwartz, & T. M. Jessell (Eds.), *Principles of neural science* (3rd ed., pp. 420–439). New York: Elsevier.

Mataró, M., Junqué, C., Poca, M. A., & Sahuquillo, J. (2001). Neuropsychological findings in congenital and acquired childhood hydrocephalus. *Neuropsychology Review, 11,* 169–178.

Mattingly, J. B. (1996). Paterson & Zangwill's (1944) case of unilateral neglect: Insights from 50 years of experimental inquiry. In C. Code, C. Wallesch, Y. Joanette, & A. R. Lecours (Eds.), *Classic cases in neuropsychology* (pp. 243–262). Brighton, United Kingdom: Psychology Press.

Mattson, S. N., Lang, A. R., & Calarco, K. E. (2002). Attentional focus and attentional shift in children with heavy prenatal alcohol exposure. *Journal of the International Neuropsychological Society, 8,* 295.

Mattson, S. N., & Riley, E. P. (2000). Parent ratings of behavior in children with heavy prenatal alcohol exposure to alcohol. *Alcoholism: Clinical and Experimental Research, 24,* 226–231.

Mattson, S. N., Riley, E. P., Delis, D. C., Stern, C., & Jones, K. L. (1996). Verbal learning and memory in children with fetal alcohol syndrome. *Alcoholism: Clinical and Experimental Research, 20,* 810–816.

Mattson, S. N., Riley, E. P., Gramling, L., Delis, D. C., & Jones, K. L. (1998). Neuropsychological comparison of alcohol-exposed children with or without physical features of fetal alcohol syndrome. *Neuropsychology, 12,* 146–153.

Mattson, S. N., Riley, E. P., Sowell, E. R., Jenigan, T. L., Sobel, D. F., & Jones, K. L. (1996). A decrease in the size of the basal ganglia in children with fetal alcohol syndrome. *Alcoholism: Clinical and Experimental Research, 20,* 1088–1093.

Maurer, K., Volk, S., & Gerbaldo, H. (1997). Auguste D. and Alzheimer's disease. *Lancet, 349,* 1546–1549.

Mayes, S. D., & Calhoun, S. L. (2001). Non-significance of early speech delay in children with autism and normal intelligence and implications for DSM-IV Asperger's disorder. *Autism, 5,* 81–94.

Mayeux, R. (2003). Epidemiology of neurodegeneration. *Annual Review of Neuroscience, 26,* 81–104.

Mayeux, R., Denaro, J., Hemenegildo, N., Marder, K., Tang, M. X., Cote, L. J., & Stern, Y. (1992). A population-based investigation of Parkinson's disease with and without dementia. *Archives of Neurology, 49,* 492–497.

Mayeux, R., Saunders, A. M., Shea, S., Mirra, S., Evans, D., Roses, A. D., et al. (1998). Utility of the apolipoprotein E genotype in the diagnosis of Alzheimer's disease. Alzheimer's Disease Centers Consortium on Apolipoprotein E and Alzheimer's Disease. *New England Journal of Medicine, 338*(8), 506–511.

McCarthy, R. A., & Warrington, E. K. (1990). *Cognitive neuropsychology.* San Diego, CA: Academic Press.

McCormick, C. M., & Teillon, S. M. (2001). Menstrual cycle variation in spatial ability: Relation to salivary cortisol levels. *Hormones and Behavior, 39,* 29–38.

McDaniel, M. A., & Einstein, G. O. (2000). Strategic and automatic processes in prospective memory retrieval: A multiprocess framework. *Applied Cognitive Psychology, 14,* S127–S144.

McDonough, L., Stahmer, A., Schreibman, L., & Thompson, S. J. (1997). Deficits, delays, and distractions: An evaluation of symbolic play and memory in children with autism. *Development and Psychopathology, 9,* 17–41.

McDougle, C. J., Scahill, L., McCracken, J. T., Aman, M. G., Tierney, E., Arnold, L. E., et al. (2000). Research units on pediatric psychopharmacology (RUPP) autism network: Background and rationale for an initial controlled study of risperidone. *Child and Adolescent Psychiatric Clinics of North America, 9,* 201–224.

McDowell, S., Whyte, J., & D'Esposito, M. (1998). Differential effects of a dopaminergic agonist on prefrontal function in head injury patients. *Brain, 121,* 1155–1164.

McGaugh, J. L. (2004). The amygdala modulates the consolidation of memories of emotionally arousing experiences. *Annual Review of Neuroscience, 27,* 1–28.

McIntosh, G. C. (1992). Neurological conceptualizations of epilepsy. In T. L. Bennett (Ed.), *The neuropsychology of epilepsy.* New York: Plenum.

McKhann, G., Drachman, D., Folstein, M., Katzman, R., Price, D., & Stadlan, E. M. (1984). Clinical diagnosis of Alzheimer's disease: Report of the NINCDS-ADRDA Work Group. *Neurology, 34,* 939–944.

McLardy, T. (1970). Memory function in hippocampal gyri but not in hippocampi. *International Journal of Neuroscience, 1,* 113.

Meador, K. J., Loring, D. W., Lee, G., Nichols, M., & Heilman, K. M. (1999). Cerebral lateralization: relationship of language and ideomotor praxis. *Neurology, 53,* 2028–2031.

Meehl, P. (1973). *Psychodiagnosis: Selected papers.* New York: Norton Press.

Merabet, L. B., Rizzo, J. R., Amedi, A., Somers, D. C., & Pascual-Leone, A. (2005). What blindness can tell us about seeing again: Merging neuroplasticity and neuroprostheses. *Nature Reviews Neuroscience, 6,* 71–77.

Mervis, C. B., & Bertrand, J. (1997). Developmental relations between cognition and language: Evidence from Williams syndrome. In L. B. Adamson & M. A. Rornski (Eds.), *Research on communication and language acquisition: Discoveries from atypical development* (pp. 75–106). New York: Brookes.

Mervis, C. B., Morris, C. A., Klein-Tasman, B. P., Bertrand, J., Kwitny, S., Appelbaum, L. G., et al. (2003). Attentional characteristics of infants and toddlers with Williams syndrome during triadic interactions. *Developmental Neuropsychology, 23,* 243–268.

Mervis, C. B., & Robinson, B. F. (2000). Expressive vocabulary ability of toddlers with Williams syndrome or Down syndrome: A comparison. *Developmental Neuropsychology, 17,* 111–126.

Merz, P. A., Somerville, R. A., Wisneiwski, H. M., & Iqbal, K. (1981). Abnormal fibrils from scrapie-infected brain. *Acta Neuropathologica, 54,* 63–74.

Mesulam, M. M. (1981). A cortical network for directed attention and unilateral neglect. *Annals of Neurology, 10,* 309–325.

Mesulam, M. M. (1985). *Principles of behavioral neurology.* Philadelphia: F. A. Davis.

Mesulam, M. M. (1990). Large-scale neurocognitive networks and distributed processing for attention, language and memory. *Annals of Neurology, 28,* 597–613.

Mesulam, M. M. (2000). *Principles of behavioral and cognitive neurology* (2nd ed.). New York: Oxford University Press.

Meyer-Lindenberg, A., Hariri, A. R., Munoz, K. E., Mervis, C. B., Mattay, V. S., Morris, K. E., et al. (2005). Normal correlates of genetically abnormal social cognition in Williams syndrome. *Nature Neuroscience, 8,* 991–993.

Meyer-Lindenberg, A., Kohn, P., Mervis, C. B., Kippenhan, J. S., Olsen, R. K., Morris, C. A., et al. (2004). Neural basis of genetically determined visuospatial construction deficits in William syndrome. *Neuron, 43,* 623–631.

Meyers, P. S. (1999). *Right hemisphere damage: Disorders of communication and cognition.* San Diego: Singular Publishing Group.

Middleton, F. A., & Strick, P. L. (2001). Revised neuroanatomy of frontal-subcortical circuits. In D. G. Lichter & J. L. Cummings (Eds.), *Frontal-subcortical circuits in psychiatric and neurological disorders* (pp. 44–58). New York: Guilford Press.

Milberg, W. P., Hebben, N., & Kaplan, E. (1986). The Boston process approach to neuropsychological assessment. In I. Grant & K. M. Adams (Eds.), *Neuropsychological assessment of neuropsychiatric disorders.* New York: Oxford University Press.

Miller, E. K., & Cohen, J. D. (2001). An integrative theory of prefrontal cortex function. *Annual Review of Neuroscience, 24,* 167–202.

Milner, B. (1968). Visual recognition and recall after right temporal lobe excision in man. *Neuropsychologia, 6,* 191.

Milner, B., Corkin, S., & Teuber, S. C. (1968). Further analysis of the hippocampal amnesic syndrome: 14 year follow-up study of H.M. *Neuropsychologia, 6,* 215–234.

Minshew, N. J. (1997). Pervasive developmental disorders: Autism and similar disorders. In T. E. Feinberg & M. J. Farah (Eds.), *Behavioral neurology and neuropsychology* (pp. 817–826). New York: McGraw-Hill.

Mirsky, A. F. (1995). Perils and pitfalls on the path to normal potential: The role of impaired attention. Homage to Herbert G. Birch. *Journal of Clinical and Experimental Neuropsychology, 17,* 481–498.

Mirsky, A. F. (1996). Disorders of attention: A neuropsychological perspective. In G. R. Lyon & N. A. Krasnegor (Eds.), *Attention, memory, and executive function* (pp. 71–96). Baltimore: Paul H. Brookes.

Mishkin, M., Malamut, B., & Bachevalier, J. (1984). Memories and habits: Two neural systems. In G. Lynch, J. L. McGaugh, & N. M. Weinberger (Eds.), *Neurobiology of learning and memory.* New York: Guilford Press.

Mishkin, M., Ungerleider, L., & Macko, K. A. (1983). Object vision and spatial vision: Two cortical pathways. *Trends in Neurosciences, 6,* 414–417.

Moffat, S. D., & Hampson, E. (1996). A curvilinear relationship between testosterone and spatial cognition in humans: Possible influences of hand preference. *Psychoneuroendocrinology, 21,* 323–337.

Mohn, K., Spiers, M. V., & Sakamoto, M. (2005, November). Oral contraceptive use and cognitive functioning in young women presented at the annual meeting of the National Academy of Neuropsychology [Abstract]. *Archives of Clinical Neuropsychology, 20,* 846.

Monk, C. S., Webb, S. J., & Nelson, C. A., (2001). Prenatal neurobiological development: Molecular mechanisms and anatomical change. *Developmental Neuropsychology, 19,* 211–236.

Moore, K. L., & Persaud, T. V. N. (1993). *Before we are born: Essentials of embryology and birth* (4th ed.). Philadelphia: W. B. Saunders.

Morgan, A. E., & Hynd, G. W. (1998). Dyslexia, neurolinguistic ability, and anatomical variation of the planum temporale. *Neuropsychology Review, 8,* 79–93.

Morris, C. A., & Mervis, C. B. (1999). Williams syndrome. In S. Goldstein & C. R. Reynolds (Eds.), *Handbook of neurodevelopmental and genetic disorders of childhood* (pp. 555–590). New York: Guilford Press.

Morris, J. S., Öhman, A., & Dolan, R. J. (1998). Conscious and unconscious emotional learning in the human amygdala. *Nature, 393,* 467–470.

Moscovitch, M., & Winocur, G. (2002). The frontal cortex and working with memory. In D. T. Stuss & R. T. Knight (Eds.), *Principles of frontal lobe function* (pp. 188–209). New York: Oxford University Press.

Moser, R. S., & Schatz, P. (2002). Enduring effects of concussion in youth athletes. *Archives of Clinical Neuropsychology, 17*(1), 91–100.

Mostofsky, S. H., Reiss, A. L., Lockhart, P., & Denckla, M. B. (1998). Evaluation of cerebellar size in attention-deficit hyperactivity disorder. *Journal of Child Neurology, 13,* 434–439.

Mullan, S., & Penfield, W. (1959). Illusions of comparative interpretation and emotion; production by epileptic discharge and by electrical stimulation in the temporal cortex. *AMA Archives of Neurology and Psychiatry, 81*(3), 269–284.

Murphy, D. G., DeCarli, C., Daly, E., Haxby, J. V., Allen, G., White, B. J., et al. (1993). X-chromosome effects on female brain: A magnetic resonance imaging study of Turner's syndrome. *Lancet, 342,* 1197–2000.

Murphy, D. G. M., Mentis, M. J., Pietrini, P., Grady, C., Haxby, J. V., De La Granja, M., et al. (1997). A PET study of Turner's syndrome: Effect of sex steroids and the X chromosome on brain. *Biological Psychiatry, 41,* 285–298.

Nagai, Y., Goldstein, L. H., Fenwick, P. B., & Trimble, M. R. (2004). Clinical efficacy of galvanic skin response biofeedback training in reducing seizures in adult epilepsy: A preliminary randomized controlled study. *Epilepsy and Behavior, 5*(2), 216–223.

Nairne, J. S. (1997). *Psychology: The adaptive mind.* Pacific Grove, CA: Brooks/Cole.

National Directory of Head Injury Services. (1992). Southbridge, MA: National Head Injury Foundation.

National Institute of Neurological Disorders and Stroke (NINDS). (2004). *Seizures and epilepsy: Hope through research.* Retrieved December 28, 2005, from www.ninds.nih.gov/disorders/epilepsy/epilepsy.htm.

National Institutes of Health. (2002). Stem cells information. Retrieved from http://stemcells.nih.gov/info/basics/defaultpage.asp.

Naugle, R. I., Cullum, C. M., & Bigler, E. D. (1998). *Introduction to clinical neuropsychology: A casebook.* Austin, TX: Pro-Ed.

Nauta, W. J. H., & Feirtag, M. (1986). *Fundamental neuroanatomy.* New York: W. H. Freeman.

Nedergaard, M., Ransom, B., & Goldman, S. A. (2003). New roles for astrocytes: Redefining the functional architecture of the brain. *Trends in Neurosciences, 26*(10), 523–530.

Nelson, H. D., Humphrey, L. L., Nygren, P., Teutsch, S. M., & Allan, J. D. (2002). Postmenopausal hormone replacement therapy. *Journal of the American Medical Association, 288,* 872–881.

Neppe, V. M. (1983). The concept of déjà vu. *Parapsycholigcal Journal of South Africa, 4,* 25–35.

Newman, A. C., Barth, J. T., & Zillmer, E. A. (1986). Serial neuropsychological assessment in an adult with Tourette's syndrome. *International Journal of Clinical Neuropsychology, 9,* 135–139.

Newton, A., & Johnson, D. A. (1985). Social adjustment and interaction after severe head injury. *British Journal of Clinical Psychology, 24,* 225–234.

Nicolson, R., Craven-Thuss, B., Smith, J., McKinlay, B. D., & Castellanos, F. X. (2005). A randomized double-blind, placebo-controlled trial of metoclopramide for the treatment of Tourette's disorder. *Journal of the American Academy of Child and Adolescent Psychiatry, 44,* 640–646.

Nigg, J. (2001). Is ADHD a disinhibitory disorder? *Psychological Bulletin, 127,* 571–598.

Nigg, J. T. (2006). *What causes ADHD? Understanding what goes wrong and why.* New York: Guilford Press.

Noback, C. R., & Demarest, R. J. (1975). *The human nervous system.* New York: McGraw-Hill.

Nobre, A. C., Coull, J. T., Maquet, C. D., Frith, C. D., Vandenberghe, R., & Mesulam, M. M. (2004). Orienting attention to locations in perceptual versus mental representations. *Journal of Cognitive Neuroscience, 16,* 363–373.

Nockleby, D. M., & Deaton, A. V. (1987). Denial versus distress: Coping patterns in post head trauma patients. *International Journal of Clinical Neuropsychology, 9,* 145–148.

Nordahl, T. E., & Salo, R. (2004). Selected neuroimaging topics in psychiatric disorders. In S. C. Yudofsky & H. F. Kim (Eds.), *Neuropsychiatric assessment* (pp. 155–190). Washington, DC: American Psychiatric Publishing.

Nottebohm, F. (1981). A brain for all seasons: Cyclical anatomical changes in song-control nuclei for the canary brain. *Science, 214,* 1368–1370.

Nuland, S. B. (1993). *How we die.* New York: Vintage.

Nurmi, E. L., Dowd, M., Tadevosyan-Leyfer, O., Haines, J. L., Folstein, S. E., & Sutcliffe, J. S. (2003). Exploratory subsetting of autism families based on savant skills improves evidence of genetic linkage to 15q11-q13. *Journal of the American Child and Adolescent Psychiatry, 42,* 856–863.

Öberg, C., Larsson, M., & Bäckman, L. (2002). Differential sex effects in olfactory functioning: The role of verbal processing. *Journal of the International Neuropsychological Society, 8,* 691–698.

O'Doherty, J., Kringelbach, M. L., Rolls, E. T., Hornak, J., & Andrews, C. (2001). Abstract reward and punishment representatives in the human orbitofrontal cortex. *Nature Neuroscience, 4,* 95–102.

Ogden, J. A. (1985). Anterior-posterior interhemispheric differences in the loci of lesions producing visual hemineglect. *Brain and Cognition, 4,* 59–75.

Ojemann, G. A. (1980). Brain mechanisms for language: Observation during neurosurgery. In J. S. Lockard & A. A. J. Ward (Eds.), *Epilepsy: A window to brain mechanisms.* New York: Raven Press.

Olanow, C. W., & Tatton, W. G. (1999). Etiology and pathogenesis of Parkinson's disease. *Annual Review of Neuroscience, 22,* 123–144.

Oldfield, R. C. (1971). The assessment and analysis of handedness: The Edinburgh inventory. *Neuropsychologia, 9,* 97–113.

Olson, L. (1990). Grafts and growth factors in CNS. Basic science with clinical promise. *Stereotactic Functional Neurosurgery, 54,* 250–267.

Ommaya, A. K., & Gennarelli, T. A. (1974). Cerebral concussion and traumatic unconsciousness. *Brain, 97,* 633–654.

Osborne, L., & Pober, B. (2001). Genetics of childhood disorders: XXVII. Genes and cognition in Williams syndrome. *Journal of the American Child and Adolescent Psychiatry, 40,* 732–735.

Osterrieth, P. A. (1944). Le test de copie d'une figure complexe. *Archives de Psychologie, 30,* 206–356.

Ozonoff, S. (2001). Advances in the cognitive neuroscience of autism. In C. A. Nelson & M. Luciana (Eds.), *Handbook of developmental cognitive neuroscience* (pp. 537–548). Cambridge, MA: MIT Press.

Ozonoff, S., & Griffith, E. M. (2000). Neuropsychological function and the external validity of Asperger syndrome. In A. Klin, F. R. Volkmar, & S. S. Sparrow (Eds.), *Asperger syndrome* (pp. 72–96). New York: Guilford Press.

Ozonoff, S., & Jensen, J. (1999). Specific executive function profiles in three neurodevelopmental disorders. *Journal of Autism and Developmental Disorders, 29,* 171–177.

Ozonoff, S., & Strayer, D. L. (2001). Further evidence of intact working memory ability in autism. *Journal of Autism and Developmental Disorders, 31,* 257–263.

Papalia, D. E., & Olds, S. W. (1995). *Human development* (6th ed.). New York: McGraw-Hill.

Papez, J. W. (1937). A proposed mechanism of emotion. *Archives of Neurology & Psychiatry, 38,* 725–743.

Pargman, D. (1999). *Psychological bases of sport injuries* (2nd ed.). Morgantown, WV: Fitness Information Technology.

Pascual-Leone, A., & Hamilton, R. (2001). The metamodal organization of the brain. *Progress in Brain Research, 134,* 427–445.

Paterniti, M. (2000). *Driving Mr. Albert: A trip across America with Einstein's brain.* New York: Random House.

Paterson, A., & Zangwill, O. L. (1944). Disorders of visual space perception associated with lesions of the right cerebral hemisphere. *Brain, 67,* 331–358.

Paus, T., Otaky, N., Caramanos, Z., MacDonald, D., Zijdenbos, A., d'Avirro, D., et al. (1996). In vivo morphometry of the intrasulcal gray matter in the human cingulate, paracingulate, and superior-rostral sulci: Hemispheric asymmetries, gender differences and probability maps. *Journal of Comparative Neurology, 376,* 664–673.

Pavlides, C., & Winson, J. (1989). Influences of hippocampal place cell firing in the awake state on the activity of these cells during subsequent sleep episodes. *Journal of Neuroscience, 9,* 2907–2918.

Pearson, D. A., Yaffee, L. S., Loveland, K. A., & Norton, A. M. (1995). Covert visual attention in children with attention deficit hyperactivity disorder: Evidence for developmental immaturity? *Development and Psychopathology, 7,* 351–367.

Pelletier, P. M., Ahmad, S. A., & Rourke, B. P. (2001). Classification rules for basic phonological processing disabilities and nonverbal learning disabilities: Formulation and external validity. *Child Neuropsychology, 7,* 84–98.

Pellman, E. J., Lovell, M. R., Viano, D. C., Casson, I. R., & Tucker, A. M. (2004). Concussion in professional football: Neuropsychological testing. *Neurosurgery, 55,* 1290–1303.

Penfield, W. (1975). *The mystery of the mind.* Princeton, NJ: Princeton University Press.

Penfield, W., & Jasper, H. H. (1954). *Epilepsy and the functional anatomy of the human brain.* Boston: Little, Brown.

Penfield, W., & Milner, B. (1958). Memory deficit produced by bilateral lesions in the hippocampal zone. *Archives of Neurology Psychiatry, 79,* 475.

Pennington, B. F. (1991). *Diagnosing learning disorders: A neurological framework.* New York: Guilford Press.

Pennington, B. F. (1997a). Attention deficit hyperactivity disorder. In T. E. Feinberg & M. J. Farah (Eds.), *Behavioral neurology and neuropsychology* (pp. 803–807). New York: McGraw-Hill.

Pennington, B. F. (1997b). Dimensions of executive functions in normal and abnormal development. In N. A. Krasnegor, G. R. Lyon, & P. S. Goldman-Rakic (Eds.), *Development of the prefrontal cortex: Evolution, neurobiology, and behavior* (pp. 265–282). Baltimore: Paul H. Brookes.

Pennington, B. F. (2002). *The development of psychopathology: Nature and nurture.* New York: Guilford Press.

Pennington, B. F., Heaton, R. K., Karzmark, P., Pendleton, M. G., Lehman, R., & Shucard, D. W. (1985). The neuropsychological phenotype in Turner syndrome. *Cortex, 21,* 391–404.

Pennington, B. F., & Ozonoff, S. (1996). Executive functions and developmental psychopathology. *Journal of Child Psychology and Psychiatry, 37,* 51–87.

Pennington, B. F., & Smith, S. (1983). Genetic influences on learning disabilities and speech and language disorders. *Child Development, 54,* 369–387.

Penny, J. B., & Young, A. B. (1993). Huntington's disease. In J. Jankovic & E. Tolosa (Eds.), *Parkinson's disease and movement disorders* (2nd ed., pp. 205–216). Baltimore: Williams & Wilkins.

Petersen, R. C. (2004). Mild cognitive impairment as a diagnostic entity. *Journal of Internal Medicine, 256*(3), 183–194.

Petersen, R. C. (2005). Mild cognitive impairment: Where are we? *Alzheimer Disease Association Disorders, 19*(3), 166–169.

Petersen, R. C., Smith, G. E., Waring, S. C., Ivnik, R. J., Tangalos, E. G., & Kokmen, E. (1999). Mild cognitive impairment: Clinical characterization and outcome. *Archives of Neurology, 56*(3), 303–308.

Petersen, S. E., Robinson, D. L., & Morris, J. D. (1987). Contributions of the pulvinar to visual spatial attention. *Neuropsychology, 25,* 97–105.

Peterson, B. S., Thomas, P., Kane, M. J., Scahill, L., Zhang, H., Bronen, R., et al. (2003). Basal ganglia volumes in patients with Gilles de la Tourette syndrome. *Archives of General Psychiatry, 60,* 415–424.

Petitto, L. A., Zatorre, R. J., Gauna, K., Nikelski, E. J., Dostie, D., & Evans, A. C. (2000). Speech-like cerebral activity in profoundly deaf people processing signed languages: Implications for the neural basis of human language. *Proceedings of the National Academy of Sciences, 97,* 13961–13966.

Petri, H. L., & Mishkin, M. (1994). Behaviorism, cognitivism and the neuropsychology of memory. *American Scientist, 82,* 30–37.

Petrides, M. (1998). Specialized systems for the processing of mnemonic information within the primate frontal cortex. In A. C. Roberts, T. W. Robbins, & L. Weiskrantz (Eds.), *The prefrontal cortex: Executive and cognitive functions* (pp. 103–116). New York: Oxford University Press.

Pfefferbaum, A., Mathalon, D. H., Sullivan, E. V., Rawles, J. M., Zipursky, R. B., & Lim, K. O. (1994). A quantitative magnetic resonance imaging study of changes in brain morphology from infancy to late adulthood. *Archives of Neurology, 51,* 874–887.

Pfrieger, F. W., & Barres, B. A. (1997). Synaptic efficacy enhanced by glial cells in vitro. *Science, 277*(5332), 1684–1687.

Phelps, E. A., O'Connor, K. J., Gatenby, J. C., Gore, J. C., Grillon, C., & Davis, M. (2001). Activation of the left amygdala to a cognitive representation of fear. *Nature Neuroscience, 4,* 437–441.

Phillips, S. M., & Sherwin, B. B. (1992). Effects of estrogen on memory function in surgically menopausal women. *Psychoneuroendocrinology, 17,* 485–495.

Piacentini, J., & Chang, S. (2001). Behavioral treatments for Tourette syndrome and tic disorders: State of the art. In D. J. Cohen & C. G. Goetz (Eds.), *Tourette syndrome* (pp. 319–331). Philadelphia: Lippincott Williams & Wilkins.

Piggot, J., Kwon, H., Mobbs, D., Blasey, C., Lotspeich, L., Menon, V., et al. (2004). Emotional attribution in high-functioning individuals with autism spectrum disorder: A functional imaging study. *Journal of the American Child and Adolescent Psychiatry, 43,* 473–480.

Pincus, J. H., & Tucker, G. J. (1985). *Behavioral neurology.* New York: Oxford University Press.

Pinel, P. J., & Edwards, M. (1998). *A colorful introduction to the anatomy of the human brain.* Boston: Allyn & Bacon.

Piven, J., Berthier, M. L., Starkstein, S. E., Nehme, E., Pearlson, G., & Folstein, S. (1990). Magnetic resonance imaging evidence for a defect of cerebral cortical development in autism. *American Journal of Psychiatry, 147,* 734–739.

Piven, J., Harper, J., Palmer, P., & Arndt, S. (1996). Course of behavioral change in autism: A retrospective study of high-IQ adolescents and adults. *Journal of the American Academy of Child and Adolescent Psychiatry, 35,* 523–529.

Platek, S. M., Keenan, J. P., Gallup, G. G., Jr., & Mohamed, F. B. (2004). Where am I? The neurological correlates of self and other. *Cognitive Brain Research, 19*(2), 114–122.

Platek, Steven M; Loughead, James W; Gur, Ruben C; Busch, Samantha; Ruparel, Kosha; Phend, Nicholas; Panyavin, Ivan S; Langleben, Daniel D. (2006). Neural Substrates for Functionally Discriminating Self-Face From Personally Familiar Faces. *Human Brain Mapping, 27*(2), 91–98.

Pliszka, S. R. (2003). *Neuroscience for the mental health clinician.* New York: Guilford Press.

Polster, M. R. (1993). Drug-induced amnesia: Implication for cognitive neuropsychological investigations of memory. *Psychological Bulletin, 114,* 477–493.

Poppel, E., & Richards, W. A. (1974). Light sensitivity in cortical scotomata contralateral to small islands of blindness. *Experimental Brain Research, 21,* 125–130.

Poppel, E., & vonSteinbuchel, N. (1992). Neuropsychological rehabilitation from a theoretical point of view. In N. vonSteinbuchel, D. Y. von Cramon, & E. Poppel (Eds.), *Neuropsychological rehabilitation* (pp. 3–19). Berlin: Springer.

Popplestone, J. A., & McPherson, M. W. (1994). *An illustrated history of American psychology.* Madison, WI: Brown & Benchmark.

Portin, R., & Rinne, U. (1986). Predictive factors for cognitive deterioration and dementia in Parkinson's disease. *Advances in Neurology, 45,* 413–416.

Posner, M. I. (1992). Attention as a cognitive and neural system. *Current Directions in Psychological Science, 1,* 11–14.

Posner, M. I., & DiGirolama, G. J. (1998). Executive control: Conflict, target detection, and cognitive control. In R. Parasuraman (Ed.), *The attentive brain* (pp. 401–424). Cambridge, MA: MIT Press.

Posner, M. I., & Fan, J. (2004). Attention as an organ system. In J. Pomerantz (Ed.), *Neurobiology of perception and communication: From synapse to society the IVth De Lange conference.* Cambridge, United Kingdom: Cambridge University Press.

Posner, M. I., & Petersen, S. E. (1990). The attention system of the human brain. *Annual Review of Neuroscience, 13,* 25–42.

Postma, A., Izendoorn, R., & De Haan, E. H. F. (1998). Sex differences and object location memory. *Brain and Cognition, 36,* 334–345.

Potegal, M. (1971). A note on spatial motor deficits in patients with Huntington's disease: A test of a hypothesis. *Neuropsychologia, 9,* 233–235.

Powell, M. P., & Schulte, T. (1999). Turner syndrome. In S. Goldstein & C. R. Reynolds (Eds.), *Handbook of neurodevelopmental and genetic disorders of childhood* (pp. 277–297). New York: Guilford Press.

Powers, W. J. (1990.). Stroke. In A. L. Pearlman & R. C. Collins (Eds.), *Neurobiology of disease.* New York: Oxford University Press.

Preston, J. D., O'Neal, J. H., & Talaga, M. C. (1997). *Handbook of clinical psychopharmacology for therapist* (2nd ed.). Oakland, CA: New Harbinger Publications.

Price, B. H., Gurvit, H., Weintrub, S., Geula, C., Leimkuhler, E., & Mesulam, M. (1993). Neuropsychological patterns and language deficits in 20 consecutive cases of autopsy-confirmed Alzheimer's disease. *Archives of Neurology, 50,* 931–937.

Prigatano, G. P. (1992). Neuropsychological rehabilitation and the problem of altered self-awareness. In N. vonSteinbuchel, D. Y. von Cramon, & E. Poppel (Eds.), *Neuropsychological rehabilitation.* Berlin: Springer.

Prigatano, G. P. (1999). *Principles of neuropsychological rehabilitation.* New York: Oxford University Press.

Pritchard, P. B., Holmstrom, V. L., & Giacinto, J. (1985). Self-abatement of complex partial seizures. *Annals of Neurology, 18,* 265–267.

Pruisiner, S. B. (1982). Novel proteinaceous infectious particles cause scrapie. *Science, 216,* 136–144.

Pugh, K. R., Mencl, W. E., Jenner, A. R., Katz, L., Frost, S. J., Lee, J. R., et al. (2000). Functional neuroimaging studies of reading and reading disability (developmental dyslexia). *Mental Retardation and Developmental Disabilities Research Review, 6,* 207–213.

Purves, D., Augustine, G. J., Fitzpatrick, D., Katz, L. C., LaMantia, A., McNamara, J. O., & Williams, S. M. (Eds.) (2001). *Neuroscience* (2nd ed.) Sunderland, MA: Sinauer Associates.

Purvis, K. L., & Tannock, R. (2000). Phonological processing, not inhibitory control, differentiates ADHD and reading disability. *Journal of the American Academy of Child and Adolescent Psychiatry, 39,* 485–494.

Rabinowicz, T., Dean, J. M.-C., Petetot, J. M. C., & de Courten-Myers, G. M. (1999). Gender differences in the human cerebral cortex: More neurons in males; more processes in females. *Journal of Child Neurology, 14,* 98–107.

Ragland, J. D., Gur, R. C., Raz, J., Schroeder, L., Smith, R. J., Alavi, A., et al. (2000). Hemispheric activation of anterior and inferior prefrontal cortex during verbal encoding and recognition: A PET study of healthy volunteers. *NeuroImage, 11,* 624–633.

Raichle, M. E. (1983). Positron emission tomography. *Annual Review of Neuroscience, 6,* 249–267.

Rakic, P., & Lombroso, P. J. (1998). Development of the cerebral cortex: I. forming the cortical structure. *Journal of the American Academy of Child and Adolescent Psychiatry, 37,* 116–117.

Ramachandran, V. S., Rogers-Ramachandran, D., & Steward, M. (1992). Perceptual correlates of massive cortical reorganization. *Science, 258,* 1159–1160.

Raskin, S. A., Borod, J. C., & Tweedy, J. (1990). Neuropsychological aspects of Parkinson's disease. *Neuropsychology Review, 1,* 185–221.

Raz, N. (2000). Aging of the brain and its impact on cognitive performance: Integration of structural and functional findings. In F. I. M. Craik & T. A. Salthouse (Eds.), *Handbook of aging and cognition* (2nd ed., pp. 1–90). Mahwah, NJ: Erlbaum.

Raz, N. (2005). The aging brain observed in vivo: Differential changes and their modifiers. In R. Cabeza, L. Nyberg, & D. Park (Eds.), *Cognitive neuroscience of aging.* New York: Oxford.

Rebok, G. W., & Folstein, M. F. (1993). Dementia. *Journal of Neuropsychiatry and Clinical Neurosciences, 5,* 265–276.

Rees, J. R. (1948). *The case of Rudolf Hess: A problem in diagnosis and forensic psychiatry.* New York: Norton.

Reiss, A. L., Eliez, S., Schmitt, J. E., Straus, E., Lai, Z., Jones, W., et al. (2000). Neuroanatomy of Williams syndrome: A high-resolution MRI study. *Journal of Cognitive Neuroscience, 12*(Suppl.), 65–73.

Reiss, A. L., Mazzocco, M. M. M., Greenlaw, R., Freund, L. S., & Ross, J. L. (1995). Neurodevelopmental effect on X monosymy: A volumetric imaging study. *American Neurological Association, 38,* 731–738.

Reitan, R. M. (1966). A research program on the psychological effects of brain lesions in human beings. In N. R. Ellis (Ed.), *International review of research in mental retardation* (pp. 153–218). New York: Academic Press.

Reitan, R. M., & Davison, L. A. (1974). *Clinical neuropsychology: Current status and applications.* Washington, DC: V. H. Winston.

Reitan, R. M., & Wolfson, D. (1993). *The Halstead-Reitan Neuropsychological Test Battery: Theory and clinical interpretation* (2nd ed.). Tucson, AZ: Neuropsychology Press.

Rey, A. (1941). Psychological examination of traumatic encephalopathy. *Archives de Psychologie, 28,* 286–340.

Rhodes, R. (1997). *Deadly feasts.* New York: Simon and Schuster.

Richard, A., & Reiter, J. (1990). *Epilepsy: A new approach.* New York: Prentice Hall.

Richters, J. E., Arnold, L. E., Jensen, P. S., Abikoff, H., Conners, C. K., Greenhill, L. L., et al. (1995). NIMH collaborative multisite multimodal treatment study of children with ADHD: Background and rationale. *Journal of the American Academy of Child and Adolescent Psychiatry, 34,* 987–1008.

Rilke, R. M. (1996). *Rilke's book of hours: Love poems to God* (A. Burrows & J. Macy, Trans.). New York: Riverhead Books.

Rimel, R. W., Giordani, B., Barth, J. T., Boll, T. J., & Jane, J. A. (1981). Disability caused by minor head injury. *Neurosurgery, 9*(3), 221–228.

Ris, M. D., Kietrich, K. N., Succop, P. A., Berger, O. G., & Bornschein, R. L. (2004). Early exposure to lead and neuropsychological outcomes in adolescence. *Journal of the International Neuropsychological Society, 10,* 261–270.

Roberts, A. C., Robbins, T. W., & Weiskrantz, L. (1998). Discussions and conclusions. In A. C. Roberts, T. W. Robbins, & L. Weiskrantz (Eds.), *The prefrontal cortex: Executive and cognitive functions* (pp. 221–242). New York: Oxford University Press.

Roberts, J. E., & Bell, M. A. (2003). Two- and three-dimensional mental rotation tasks lead to different parietal laterality for men and women. *International Journal of Psychophysiology, 50,* 235–246.

Robinson, B. F., Mervis, C. B., & Robinson, B. W. (2003). The roles of verbal short-term and working memory in the acquisition of grammar by children with Williams syndrome. *Developmental Neuropsychology, 23,* 13–32.

Roeser, R. J., & Daly, D. D. (1974). Auditory cortex deconnection associated with thalamic tumor. *Neurology, 24,* 555.

Roland, P. E., Larsen, B., Lassen, N. A., & Skinholf, E. (1980). Supplementary motor area and other cortical areas in organization of voluntary movements in man. *Journal of Neurophysiology, 43,* 118–136.

Rolls, E. T. (1986). Neuronal activity related to the control of feeding. In R. Ritter & S. Ritter (Eds.), *Neural and humoral controls of food intake.* New York: Academic Press.

Rolls, E. T. (1998). The orbitofrontal cortex. In A. C. Roberts, T. W. Robbins, & L. Weiskrantz (Eds.), *The prefrontal cortex: Executive and cognitive functions* (pp. 67–86). New York: Oxford University Press.

Rolls, E. T. (2002). The functions of the orbitofrontal cortex. In D. T. Stuss & R. T. Knight (Eds.), *Principles of frontal lobe function* (pp. 354–375). New York: Oxford University Press.

Romans, S. M., Roeltgen, D. P., Kushner, H., & Ross, J. L. (1997). Executive function in girls with Turner's syndrome. *Developmental Neuropsychology, 13,* 23–40.

Romine, C. B., & Reynolds, C. R. (2005). A model of the development of frontal lobe functioning: Findings from a meta-analysis. *Applied Neuropsychology, 12,* 190–201.

Rorschach, H. (1942). *Psychodiagnostics: A diagnostic test based on perception.* Bern, Switzerland: Huber.

Rosenblum, J. A. (1974). Human sexuality and cerebral cortex. *Disorder of the Nervous System, 35,* 268.

Ross, E. (1985). Modulation of affect and nonverbal communication by the right hemisphere. In M. M. Mesulam (Ed.), *Principles of behavioral neurology* (pp. 239–257). Philadelphia: F. A. Davis.

Rosvold, H. E., Mirsky, A. F., Sarason, I., Bransome, E. D., & Beck, L. H. (1956). A continuous performance test of brain damage. *Journal of Consulting Psychology, 20,* 343–350.

Rourke, B. B., & Del Dotto, J. E. (1994). *Learning disabilities: A neuropsychological perspective.* Thousand Oaks, CA: Sage.

Rourke, B. P. (1989). *Non-verbal learning disabilities: The syndrome and the model.* New York: Guilford Press.

Rourke, B. P. (1993). Arithmetic disabilities, specific and otherwise: A neuropsychological perspective. *Journal of Learning Disabilities, 26,* 214–226.

Rourke, B. P. (1995). The NLD syndrome and the white matter model. In B. P. Rourke (Ed.), *Syndrome of nonverbal learning disabilities: Neurodevelopmental manifestations* (pp. 1–26). New York: Guilford Press.

Rourke, B. P., Bakker, D. J., Fisk, L. J., & Strang, J. D. (1983). *Child neuropsychology: An introduction to theory, research, and clinical practice.* New York: Guilford Press.

Rourke, B. P., & Conway, J. A. (1997). Disabilities of arithmetic and mathematical reasoning: Perspectives from neurology and neuropsychology. *Journal of Learning Disabilities, 30,* 34–46.

Rourke, B. P., Fisk, J. L., & Strang, J. D. (1986). *Neuropsychological assessment of children: A treatment-oriented approach.* New York: Guilford Press.

Rourke, B. P., & Fuerst, D. E. (1996). Psychosocial dimensions of learning disability subtypes. *Assessment, 3,* 277–290.

Rousseau, A., Hermann, B., & Whitman, S. (1985). Effects of progressive relaxation on epilepsy: Analysis of a series of cases. *Psychology Reports, 57*(3 Pt 2), 1203–1212.

Rovee-Collier, C. (1993). The capacity for long-term memory in infancy. *Current Directions in Psychological Science, 2,* 130–135.

Rovet, J. F. (1993). The psychoeducational characteristics of children with Turner syndrome. *Journal of Learning Disabilities, 26,* 333–341.

Rowe, A. D., Bullock, P. R., Polkey, C. E., & Morris, R. G. (2001). 'Theory of mind' impairments and their relationship to executive functioning following frontal lobe excisions. *Brain, 124,* 600–616.

Rowland, L. P., Fink, M., & Rubin, L. (1991). Cerebrospinal fluid: Blood-brain barrier, brain edema, and hydrocephalus. In E. R. Kandel, J. H. Schwartz, & T. M. Jessell (Eds.), *Principles of neural science* (3rd ed., pp. 1050–1060). New York: Elsevier Science.

Roy, A., De Jong, J., & Linnoila, M. (1989). Cerebrospinal fluid monoamine metabolites and suicidal behavior in depressed patients. *Archives of General Psychiatry, 46,* 609–612.

Rubens, A. B., & Benson, D. F. (1971). Associative visual agnosia. *Archives of Neurology, 24,* 304–316.

Rubia, K., Overmeyer, S., Talyor, E., Brammer, M., Williams, S. C. R., Simmons, A., et al. (1999). Hypofrontality in attention deficit/hyperactivity disorder during higher-order motor control: A study with functional MRI. *American Journal of Psychiatry, 156,* 891–896.

Ruchinskas, R. A., Francis, J. P., & Barth, J. T. (1997). Mild head injury in sports. *Applied Neuropsychology, 4*(1), 43–49.

Rumsey, J. M. (1996a). Neuroimaging in developmental dyslexia. In G. R. Lyon & J. M. Rumsey (Eds.), *Neuroimaging: A window to the neurological foundations of learning and behavior in children* (pp. 57–78). Baltimore: Paul H. Brookes.

Rumsey, J. M. (1996b). Neuroimaging studies of autism. In G. R. Lyon & J. M. Rumsey (Eds.), *Neuroimaging: A window to the neurological foundations of learning and behavior in children* (pp. 119–146). Baltimore: Paul H. Brookes.

Rumsey, J. M. (1998). Brain imaging of reading disorders. *Journal of the American Academy of Child and Adolescent Psychiatry, 37,* 12.

Rumsey, J. M., Andreason, P., Zametkin, A. J., Aquino, T., King, A. C., Hamberger, S. D., et al. (1992). Failure to activate the left temporoparietal cortex in dyslexia. *Archives of Neurology, 49,* 527–534.

Russell, W. R., & Espir, M. L. E. (1961). *Traumatic aphasia.* London: Oxford University Press.

Rutherford, M. D., & Rogers, S. J. (2003). Cognitive underpinnings of pretend play in autism. *Journal of Autism and Developmental Disorders, 33,* 289–302.

Rutter, M., Le Couteur, A., & Lord, C. (2003). *ADI-R Autism Diagnostic Interview-Revised.* Los Angeles, CA: Western Psychological Services.

Sacks, O. (1987). *The man who mistook his wife for a hat.* New York: Harper & Row.

Sacks, O. (1995). *An anthropologist on Mars.* New York: Knopf.

Sadato, N., Ibañez, V., Deiber, M.P., & Hallett, M. (2000). Gender differences in premotor activity during active tactile discrimination. *NeuroImage, 11,* 532–540.

Sadato, N., Pascual-Leone, A., Grafmani, J., Ibañez, V., Deiber, M-P., Dold, G., & Hallett, M. (1996). Activation of the primary visual cortex by Braille reading in blind subjects. *Nature, 380,* 526–528.

Sagar, H., Sullivan, E., Gabrieli, J., Corkin, S., & Growdon, J. (1988). Temporal ordering and short-term memory deficits in Parkinson's disease. *Brain, 111,* 525–539.

Saint-Cyr, J. A., Bronstein, Y. L., & Cummings, J. L. (2002). Neurobehavioral consequences of neurosurgical treatments and focal lesions of frontal-subcortical circuits. In D. T. Stuss & R. T. Knight (Eds.), *Principles of frontal lobe function* (pp. 408–427). New York: Oxford University Press.

Salthouse, T. A. (1991). *Theoretical perspectives on cognitive aging.* Hillsdale, NJ: Lawrence Erlbaum Associates.

Salthouse, T. A. (2006). Mental exercise and mental aging: Evaluating the validity of the "use it or lose it" hypothesis. *Perspectives on Psychological Science, 1,* 68–87.

Salthouse, T. A., Babcock, R. L., Skovronek, E., Mitchell, D. R. D., & Palmon, R. (1990). Age and experience effects in spatial visualization. *Developmental Psychology, 26,* 128–136.

Santoro, J. M., & Spiers, M. V. (1994). Social cognitive factors in brain injury associated personality change. *Brain Injury, 8,* 265–276.

Saper, C. B., Chou, T. C., Scammell, T. E. (2001). The sleep switch: Hypothalamic control of sleep and wakefulness. *TRENDS in Neurosciences, 24,* 726–731.

Sarter, M., Givens, B., & Bruno, J. P. (2001). The cognitive neuroscience of sustained attention: Where top-down meets bottom-up. *Brain Research Reviews, 35,* 146–160.

Saucier, D. M., & Elias, L. J. (2001). Lateral and sex differences in manual gesture during conversation. *Laterality: Asymmetries of Body, Brain, and Cognition, 6,* 239–245.

Schacter, D. L. (1987). Implicit memory: History and current status. *Journal of Experimental Psychology: Learning, Memory and Cognition, 13,* 501–518.

Schacter, D. L., & Curran, T. (2000). Memory without remembering and remembering without memory: Implicit and false memories. In M. S. Gazzaniga (Ed.), *The new cognitive neurosciences* (2nd ed., pp. 829–840). Cambridge, MA: MIT Press.

Schatschneider, C., Carlson, C. D., Francis, D. J., Foorman, B. R., & Fletcher, J. M. (2002). Relationship of rapid automatized naming and phonological awareness in early reading development: Implication for the double-deficit hypothesis. *Journal of Learning Disabilities, 35,* 245–256.

Schiller, F. (1982). *Paul Broca: Explorer of the brain.* New York: Oxford University Press.

Schlaepfer, T. E., Harris, G. J., Tien, A. Y., Peng, L., Lee, S., & Pearlson, G. D. (1995). Structural differences in the cerebral cortex of healthy female and male subjects: A magnetic resonance imaging study. *Psychiatry Research: Neuroimaging, 61,* 129–135.

Schnass, L., Rothenberg, S. J., Flores, M. F., Martinez, S., Hernandez, C., Osorio, E., et al. (2006). Reduced intellectual development in children with prenatal lead exposure. *Environmental Health Perspectives, 114,* 791–797.

Schultz, K. P., Tang, C. Y., Fan, J., Marks, D. J., Cheung, A. M., Newcorn, J. H., et al. (2005). Differential prefrontal cortex activation during inhibitory control in adolescents with and without childhood attention-deficit/hyperactivity disorder. *Neuropsychology, 19,* 390–402.

Schultz, R. T., Gauthier, I., Klin, A., Fulbright, R. K., Anderson, A. W., Volkmar, F., et al. (2000). Abnormal ventral temporal cortical activity during face discrimination among individuals with autism and Asperger syndrome. *Archives of General Psychiatry, 57,* 331–340.

Schultz, R. T., Grelotti, D. J., Klin, A., Kleinman, J., Van der Gaag, C., Marois, R. (2003). The role of the fusiform face area in social cognition: Implications for the pathology of autism. *Philosophical Transactions of the Royal Society of London, 358,* 415–427.

Schultz, R. T., Grelotti, D. J., & Pober, B. (2001). Genetics of childhood disorders: XXVI. Williams syndrome and brain-behavior relationships. *Journal of the American Academy of Child and Adolescent Psychiatry, 40,* 606–609.

Schultz, R. T., Romanski, L. M., & Tsatsanis, K. D. (2000). Neurofunctional models of autistic disorder and Asperger syndrome: Clues from neuroimaging. In A. Klin, F. R. Volkmar, & S. S. Sparrow (Eds.), *Asperger syndrome* (pp. 172–209). New York: Guilford Press.

Schwartz, J. H., & Kandel, E. R. (1991). Synaptic transmission mediated by second messengers. In E. R. Kandel, J. H. Schwartz, & T. M. Jessell (Eds.), *Principles of neural science* (3rd ed., pp. 173–193). New York: Elsevier.

Scott, A. M., Fletcher, J. M., Brookshire, B. L., Davidson, K. C., Landry, S. H., Bohan, T. C., et al. (1998). Memory functions in children with early hydrocephalus. *Neuropsychology, 12,* 578–589.

Scoville, W. B. (1968). Amnesia after bilateral mesial temporal-lobe excision: Introduction to case H.M. *Neuropsychologia, 6,* 211–213.

Scoville, W. B., & Milner, B. (1957). Loss of recent memory after bilateral hippocampal lesions. *Journal of Neurology, Neurosurgery, and Psychiatry, 20,* 11.

Semrud-Clikeman, M., Filipek, P. A., Biederman, J., Steingard, R., Kennedy, D., Renshaw, P., et al. (1994). Attention-deficit hyperactivity disorder: Magnetic resonance imaging morphometric analysis of the corpus callosum. *Journal of the American Academy of Child and Adolescent Psychiatry, 33,* 875–881.

Semrud-Clikeman, M., Hooper, S. R., Hynd, G. W., Hern, K., Presley, R., & Watson, T. (1996). Prediction of group membership in developmental dyslexia, attention deficit hyperactivity disorder, and normal controls using brain morphometric analysis of magnetic resonance imaging. *Archives of Clinical Neuropsychology, 11,* 521–528.

Seshadri, S., Wolf, P. A., Beiser, A., Au, R., McNulty, K., White, R., et al. (1997). Lifetime risk of dementia and Alzheimer's disease: The impact of mortality on risk estimates in the Framingham Study. *Neurology, 49*(6), 1498–1504.

Seurinck, R., Vingerhoets, G., de Lange, F. P., & Achten, E. (2004). Does egocentric mental rotation elicit sex differences? *NeuroImage, 4,* 1440–1449.

Shallice, T. (1982). Specific impairments of planning. *Philosophical Transactions of the Royal Society of London B, 298,* 199–209.

Shallice, T. (2001). 'Theory of mind' and the prefrontal cortex. *Brain, 124,* 247–248.

Shallice, T., & Warrington, E. K. (1970). Independent functioning of verbal memory stores: A neuropsychological study. *Quarterly Journal of Experimental Psychology, 22,* 261–273.

Shallice, T., & Warrington, E. K. (1977). The possible role of selective attention in acquired dyslexia. *Neuropsychologia, 15,* 31–41.

Shaywitz, B. A., Shaywitz, S. E., Pugh, K. R., Constable, R. T., Skudlarski, P., Fulbright, R. K., et al. (1995). Sex differences in the functional organization of the brain for language. *Nature, 373*(6515), 607–609.

Shaywitz, B. A., Shaywitz, S. E., Pugh, K. R., Mencel, W. E., Fulbright, R. K., Skudlarski, P., et al. (2002). Disruption of posterior brain systems for reading in children with developmental dyslexia. *Society of Biological Psychiatry, 52,* 101–110.

Shaywitz, S., & Shaywitz, B. (1999). Dyslexia. In K. Swaiman & S. Ashwal (Eds.), *Pediatric neurology: Principles & practice* (Vol. 1, pp. 576–584). St. Louis, MO: Mosby.

Shaywitz, S. E., & Shawitz, B. A. (2005). Dyslexia (specific reading disability). *Biological Psychiatry, 57,* 1301–1309.

Shaywitz, S. E., Shaywitz, B. A., Fulbright, R. K., Skudlarski, P. M., Mencl, W. E., Constable, R. T., et al. (2003). Neural systems for compensation and persistence: Young adult outcome of childhood reasoning disability. *Biological Psychiatry, 54,* 25–33.

Shaywitz, S. E., Shaywitz, B. A., Pugh, K. R., Fulbright, R. K., Constable, R. T., Mencl, W. E., et al. (1998). Functional disruption in the organization of the brain for reading in dyslexia. *Proceedings of the National Academy of Sciences, 95,* 2636–2641.

Shaywitz, S. E., Shaywitz, B. A., Pugh, K. R., Fulbright, R. K., Skudlarski, P. M., Mencl, W. E., et al. (1999). Effect of estrogen on brain activation patterns in postmenopausal women during working memory tasks. *Journal of the American Medical Association, 281,* 1197–1202.

Sheppard, D. M., Bradshaw, J. L., Purcell, R., & Pantelis, C. (1999). Tourette's and comorbid syndromes: Obsessive compulsive and attention deficit hyperactivity disorder. A common etiology? *Clinical Psychology Review, 19,* 531–552.

Sherin, J. E., Shiromani, P., McCarley, R. W., & Saper, C. B. (1996). Ventrolateral preoptic neurons that innervate the tuberomammillary nucleus are activated during sleep. *Science, 271,* 216–219.

Sherwin, B. B., & Tulandi, T. (1996). "Add-back" estrogen reverses cognitive deficits induced by a gonadotropin releasing-hormone agonist in women with leiomyomata uteri. *Journal of Clinical Endocrinology and Metabolism, 81,* 2545–2549.

Shumaker, S. A., Legault, C., Kuller, L., Rapp, S. R., Thal, L., Lane, D. S., et al. (2004). Conjugated equine estrogens and incidence of probable dementia and mild cognitive impairment in postmenopausal women. *Journal of the American Medical Association, 291,* 2947–2958.

Shumaker, S. A., Legault, C., Rapp, S. R., Thal, L., Wallace, R. B., Ockene, J. K., et al. (2003). Estrogen plus progestin and the incidence of dementia and mild cognitive impairment in postmenopausal women. *Journal of the American Medical Association, 289,* 2651–2662.

Siegel, L. S. (2003). IQ-discrepancy definitions and the diagnosis of LD: Introduction to the special issue. *Journal of Learning Disabilities, 36,* 2–3.

Siegel-Hinson, R. I., & McKeever, W. F. (2002). Hemispheric specialization, spatial activity experience, and sex differences on tests of mental rotation ability. *Laterality: Asymmetries of Body, Brain, and Cognition, 7,* 59–74.

Sigman, M. (1994). What are the core deficits in autism? In S. H. Broman, & Grafman, J. (Eds.), *Atypical cognitive deficits in developmental disorders* (pp. 139–158). New York: Oxford University Press.

Silverstein, S. M., Como, P. G., Palumbo, D. R., West, L. L., & Osborn, L. M. (1995). Multiple sources of attentional dysfunction in adults with Tourette's syndrome: Comparison with attention deficit-hyperactivity disorder. *Neuropsychology, 9,* 157–164.

Singer, H. S., & Minzer, K. (2003). Neurobiology of Tourette's syndrome: Concepts of neuroanatomic localization and neurochemical abnormalities. *Brain Development, 25*(Suppl.), 70–84.

Sitaram, N., Moore, A. M., & Gillin, J. C. (1978). Experimental acceleration and slowing of REM ultradian rhythm by cholinergic agonist and antagonist. *Nature, 274,* 490–492.

Skottun, B. C., & Parke, L. A. (1999). The possible relationship between visual deficits and dyslexia: Examination of a critical assumption. *Journal of Disabilities, 32,* 2–5.

Smalley, S. L., Bailey, J. N., Palmer, C. G., Cantwell, D. P., McGough, J. J., Del'Homme, M. A., et al. (1998). Evidence that the dopamine D4 receptor is a susceptibility gene in attention deficit hyperactivity disorder. *Molecular Psychiatry, 3,* 427–430.

Smith, A. (1982). *Symbol Digit Modalities Test SDMT. Manual revised.* Los Angeles: Western Psychological Services.

Smith, D. V., & Vogt, M. B. (1997). The neural code and integrative processes of taste. In G. K. Beauchamp & L. Bartoshuk (Eds.), *Tasting and smelling.* San Diego, CA: Academic Press.

Smith, E. E., Marshuetz, C., & Geva, A. (2002). Working memory: Findings from neuroimaging and patient studies. In F. Boller, J. Grafman (Series Eds.), & J. Grafman (Vol. Ed.), *Handbook of neuropsychology. The frontal lobes* (Vol. 7, 2nd ed., pp. 55–72). New York: Elsevier.

Snead, O. C. (1995). Basic mechanisms of generalized absence seizures. *Annals of Neurology, 37,* 146–157.

Snowdon, D. A., Greiner, L. H., Kemper, S. J., Nanayakkara, N., & Mortimer, J. A. (1999). Linguistic ability in early life and longevity: Findings from the Nun Study. In J. M. Robine, B. Forette, C. Franceschi, & M. Allard (Eds.), *The paradoxes of longevity.* Berlin: Springer.

Snyder, A. Z., Petersen, S., Fox, P., & Raichle, M. E. (1989). PET studies of visual word recognition. *Journal of Cerebral Blood Flow and Metabolism, 9*(Suppl. 1), S576.

Soliveri, P., Brown, R. G., Jahanshahi, M., & Marsden, C. D. (1992). Procedural memory and neurological disease. *European Journal of Cognitive Psychology, 4,* 161–193.

Sommer, I. E. C., Aleman, A., Bouma, A., & Kahn, R. S. (2004). Do women really have more bilateral language representation than men? A meta-analysis of functional imaging studies. *Brain, 127,* 1845–1852.

Song, H. J., Stevens, C. F., & Gagge, F. H. (2002). Neural stem cells from adult hippocampus develop essential properties of functional CNS neurons. *Natural Neuroscience, 5,* 438–445.

Sowell, E. R., Thompson, P. M., Welcome, S. E., Henkenius, A. L., Toga, A. W., & Peterson, B. S. (2004). Cortical abnormalities in children and adolescents with attention deficit hyperactivity disorder. *Lancet, 362,* 1699–1707.

Sparks, B. F., Friedman, S. D., Shaw, D. W., Aylward, E. H., Echelard, D., Artru, A. A., et al. (2002). Brain structural abnormalities in young children witrh autism spectrum disorder. *Neurology, 59,* 184–192.

Spencer, T. J. (2002). Attention-deficit/hyperactivity disorder. *Archives of Neurology, 59,* 314–316.

Spiers, M. (1995). *The cognitive screening for medication self-management.* Unpublished test, Drexel University, Philadelphia, Pennsylvania.

Spiers, M. V., & Kutzik, D. M. (1995). Self-reported memory of medication use by the elderly. *American Journal of Health-System Pharmacy, 52,* 985–990.

Spiers, M. V., Pouk, J. A., & Santoro, J. M. (1994). Examining perspective-taking in the severely head-injured. *Brain Injury, 8,* 463–473.

Spreen, O., Risser, A. T., & Edgell, D. (1995). *Developmental neuropsychiatry.* New York: Oxford University Press.

Springer, J. A., Binder, J. R., Hammeke, T. A., Swanson, S. J., Frost, J. A., Bellgowan, P. S. F., et al. (1999). Language dominance in neurologically normal and epilepsy subjects. *Brain, 122,* 2033–2046.

Springer, S. P., & Deutsch, G. (1993). *Left brain, right brain* (4th ed.). New York: W. H. Freeman.

Squire, L. R. (1987). *Memory and brain.* New York: Oxford University Press.

Squire, L. R. (1994). Declarative and nondeclarative memory: Multiple brain systems supporting learning and memory. In D. L. Schacter & E. Tulving (Eds.), *Memory systems* (pp. 203–232). Cambridge, MA: MIT Press.

Squire, L. R., & Butters, N. (1992). *Neuropsychology of memory* (2nd ed.). New York: Guilford Press.

Squire, L. R., & Cohen, N. J. (1984). Human memory and Amnesia. In G. Lynch, J. L. McGaugh, & N. M. Weinberger (Eds.), *Neurobiology of learning and memory.* New York: Guilford Press.

Squire, L. R., & Knowlton, B. J. (2000). The medial temporal lobe, the hippocampus, and the memory systems of the brain. In M. S. Gazzaniga (Ed.), *The new cognitive neurosciences* (2nd ed., pp. 765–779). Cambridge, MA: MIT Press.

Stahl, S. M. (2000). *Essential psychopharmacology: Neuroscientific basis and practical application* (2nd ed.). Cambridge, United Kingdom: Cambridge Press.

Stebbins, G. T., Singh, J., Weiner, J., Wilson, R. S., Goetz, C. G., & Gabrieli, J. D. E. (1995). Selective impairments of memory functioning in unmedicated adults with Gilles de la Tourette's syndrome. *Neuropsychology, 9,* 329–337.

Stein, J. (2001). The sensory basis of reading problems. *Developmental Neuropsychology, 20,* 509–534.

Steinhausen, H. C., Willms, J., & Spohr, H. L. (1993). Long-term psychopathological and cognitive outcome of children with fetal alcohol syndrome. *Journal of the American Academy of Child and Adolescent Psychiatry, 32,* 990–994.

Steinmetz, H., Jancke, L., Kleinschmidt, A., Schlaug, G., Volkmann, J., & Huang, Y. (1992). Sex but no hand difference in the isthmus of the corpus callosum. *Neurology, 42,* 749–752.

Steinmetz, H., Staiger, J. F., Schlaug, G., Huang, Y., & Jancke, L. (1995). Corpus callosum and brain volume in women and men. *NeuroReport, 6,* 1002–1004.

Stevens, T., Livingston, G., Kitchen, G., Manela, M., Walker, Z., & Katona, C. (2002). Islington study of dementia subtypes in the community. *British Journal of Psychiatry, 180,* 270–276.

Stewart, B. (1995). American football. *American History, 30,* 29–69.

Stiles, J. (2000). Neural plasticity and cognitive development. *Developmental Neuropsychology, 18,* 237–272.

Stiles, J., Bates, E. A., Thal, D., Trauner, D., & Reilly, J. (1998). Linguistic, cognitive, and affective development in children with pre- and perinatal focal brain injury: A ten-year overview from the San Diego longitudinal project. In C. Rovee-Collier, L. P. Lipsitt, & H. Hayne (Eds.), *Advances in infancy research* (pp. 131–163). Stamford, CT: Ablex Publishing.

Strassburger, T. L., Lee, H. C., Daly, E. M., Szczepanik, J., Krasuski, J. S., Mentis, M. J., et al. (1997). Interactive effects of age and hypertension on volumes of brain structures. *Stroke, 28*(7), 1410–1417.

Streissguth, A. (1997). *Fetal alcohol syndrome.* Baltimore: Paul H. Brookes.

Streissguth, A. P., Barr, H. M., Bookstein, F. L., Sampson, P. D., & Carmichael Olson, H. (1999). The long-term neurocognitive consequences of prenatal alcohol exposure: A 14-year study. *Psychological Science, 10,* 186–190.

Streissguth, A. P., & Connor, P. D. (2001). Fetal alcohol syndrome and other effects of prenatal alcohol: Developmental cognitive neuroscience implications. In C. A. Nelson & M. Luciana (Eds.), *Handbook of developmental cognitive neuroscience* (pp. 505–518). Cambridge, MA: MIT Press.

Stroop, J. R. (1935). Studies of interference in serial verbal reactions. *Journal of Experimental Psychology: Learning Memory & Cognition, 18,* 643–662.

Stuss, D. T., & Benson, D. F. (1986). *The frontal lobes.* New York: Raven Press.

Stuss, D. T., Gallup, G. G., & Alexander, M. P. (2001). The frontal lobes are necessary for 'theory of mind.' *Brain, 124,* 279–286.

Suganthy, J., Raghuram, L., Antonisamy, B., Vettivel, S., Madhavi, C., & Koshi, R. (2003). Gender- and age-related differences in the morphology of the corpus callosum. *Clinical Anatomy, 16,* 396–403.

Sullivan, K., Winner, E., & Tager-Flusberg, H. (2003). Can adolescents with Williams syndrome tell the difference between lies and jokes? *Developmental Neuropsychology, 23,* 85–104.

Sutcliffe, J. S., & Nurmi, E. L. (2003). Genetics of childhood disorders: XLVII. Autism, part 6: Duplication and inherited susceptibility of chromosome 15q11-q13 genes in autism. *Journal of the American Child and Adolescent Psychiatry, 42,* 253–256.

Swanson, H. L., Mink, J., & Bocian, K. M. (1999). Cognitive processing deficits in poor readers with symptoms of reading disabilities and ADHD: More alike than different? *Journal of Educational Psychology, 91,* 321–333.

Swanson, H. L., Posner, M., Potkin, S., Bonforte, S., Youpa, D., Fiore, C., et al. (1991). Activating tasks for the study of visual-spatial attention in ADHD children: A cognitive anatomic approach. *Journal of Child Neurology, 6,* S119–S127.

Swanson, H. L., & Sachse-Lee, C. (2001). A subgroup analysis of working memory in children with reading disabilities: Domain-general or domain-specific deficiency? *Journal of Learning Disabilities, 34,* 249–263.

Swanson, J., Oosterlaan, J., Murias, M., Schuck, S., Flodman, P., Spence M. A., et al. (2000). Attention deficit/hyperactivity disorder children with a 7-repeat allele of the dopamine receptor D4 gene have extreme behavior but normal performance on critical neuropsychological tests of attention. *Procceedings of the National Academy of Sciences, 97,* 4754–4759.

Swanson, J., Posner, M. I., Cantwell, D., Wigal, S., Crinella, F., Filipek, P., et al. (2000). Attention-deficit/hyperactivity disorder: Symptom domains, cognitive processes, and neural networks. In R. Parasuraman (Ed.), *The attentive brain* (pp. 445–460). Cambridge, MA: MIT Press.

Swillen, A., Fryns, J. P., Kleczkowska, A., Massa, G., Vanderschueren-Lodeweyck, M., & Van den Berghe, H. (1993). Intelligence, behaviour and psychosocial development in Turner syndrome: A cross-sectional study of 50 preadolescent and adolescent girls 4–20 years. *Genetic Counseling, 4,* 7–18.

Szaflarski, J. P., Binder, J. R., Possing, E. T., McKiernan, K. A., Ward, B. D., & Hammeke, T. A. (2002). Language lateralization left-handed and ambidextrous people: FMRI data. *Neurology, 59,* 238–244.

Talland, G. A. (1965). *Deranged memory.* New York: Academic Press.

Tamm, L. Menon, V., & Reiss, A. L. (2003). Abnormal prefrontal cortex function during response inhibition in Turner syndrome: Functional magnetic resonance imaging evidence. *Society of Biological Psychiatry, 53,* 107–111.

Tanguay, P. E. (2000). Pervasive developmental disorders: A 10-year review. *Journal of the American Academy of Child and Adolescent Psychiatry, 39,* 1079–1095.

Teasdale, G., & Jennett, B. (1974). Assessment of coma and impaired consciousness. *Lancet, 2,* 81–84.

Teicher, M. H., Polcari, A., Anderson, C. M., Andersen, S. L., Glod, C. A., & Renshaw, P. (1996). Dose-dependent effects of methylphenidate on activity, attention, and magnetic imaging measures in children with ADHD [Abstract]. *Society for Neuroscience Abstracts, 22,* 1191.

Temple, C., & Marriott, A. J. (1998). Arithmetical ability and disability in Turner's syndrome: A cognitive neuropsychological analysis. *Developmental Neuropsychology, 14,* 47–67.

Temple, C. M., Carney, R. A., & Mullarkey, S. (1996). Frontal lobe function and executive skills in children with Turner's syndrome. *Developmental Neuropsychology, 12,* 343–363.

Terry, R. D., & Davies, P. (1980). Dementia of the Alzheimer type. *Annual Review of Neuroscience, 3,* 77–95.

Terry, R. D., Peck, A., DeTeresa, R., Schechter, R., & Horoupian, D. S. (1981). Some morphometric aspects of the brain in senile dementia of the Alzheimer type. *Annals of Neurology, 10,* 184–192.

Teuber, H. L. (1950). Neuropsychology. In M. R. Harrower (Ed.), *Recent advances in psychological testing* (pp. 30–52). Springfield, IL: Charles C. Thomas.

Teuber, H. L. (1959). Some alterations in behavior after cerebral lesions in man. In A. D. Bass (Ed.), *Evolution of nervous control.* Washington, DC: American Association for the Advancement of Science.

Teuber, H. L., Battersby, W. S., & Bender, M. B. (1960). *Visual field defects after penetrating missile wounds.* Cambridge, MA: Harvard University Press.

Thiele, E. A. (2003). Assessing the efficacy of antiepileptic treatments: the ketogenic diet. *Epilepsia, 44*(Suppl. 7), 26–29.

Thomsen, I. V. (1974). The patient with severe head-injury and his family: A follow-up study of 50 patients. *Scandinavian Journal of Rehabilitation Medicine, 6,* 180–183.

Tombaugh, T. (2003). The test of memory malingering (TOMM) in forensic psychology. *Journal of Forensic Neuropsychology, 2*(3/4), 69–96.

Tombaugh, T. N. (1996). *Test of Memory Malingering (TOMM).* New York: Multi-Health Systems Inc.

Toole, J. F. (1990). *Cerebrovascular diseases* (4th ed.). New York: Raven.

Tranel, D., & Eslinger, P. J. (2000). Effects of early onset brain injury on the development of cognition and behavior: Introduction to the special issue. *Developmental Neuropsychology, 18,* 273–280.

Träskmann, L., Asberg, M., Bertilsson, L., & Sjöstrand, L. (1981). Monoamine metabolites in CSF and suicidal behavior. *Archives of General Psychiatry, 38,* 631–636.

Tsatsanis, K. D., & Rourke, B. P. (1995). Conclusions and future directions. In B. P. Rourke (Ed.), *Syndrome of nonverbal learning disabilities: Neurodevelopmental manifestations* (pp. 476–496). New York: Guilford Press.

Tulving, E. (1972). Episodic and semantic memory. In E. Tulving & W. Donaldson (Eds.), *Organization of memory* (pp. 381–403). New York: Academic Press.

Tulving, E., Kapur, S., Craik, F. I. M., Moscovitch, M., & Houle, S. (1994). Hemisphere encoding/retrieval asymmetry in episodic memory: Positron emission tomography findings. *Proceedings of the National Academy of Sciences, 91,* 2016–2020.

Turner, H. H. (1938). A syndrome of infantilism, congenital webbed neck, and cubitus valgus. *Endocrinology, 23,* 566–574.

Tysvaer, A. T., Storli, O. V., & Bachen, N. I. (1989). Soccer injuries to the brain: A neurologic and electroencephalographic study of former players. *Acta Neurologica Scandinavica, 80,* 151–156.

Ullrich, O. (1930). Uber typicke kombinationsbilder multipler abartungen. *Zeitschrift fur kinderheilkunde, 49,* 271–276.

Ullsperger, M., & von Cramon, D. Y. (2004). Decision making, performance and outcome monitoring in frontal cortical areas. *Nature Neuroscience, 7,* 1173–1174.

Valenstein, E. S. (1973). *Brain control.* New York: Wiley.

Vallar, G., Sandroni, P., Rusconi, M. L., & Barbieri, S. (1991). Hemianopia, hemianesthesia, and spatial neglect: A study with evoked potentials. *Neurology, 41,* 1918–1922.

Van den Broeck, W. (2002). The misconception of the regression-based discrepancy operationalization in the definition and research of learning disabilities. *Journal of Learning Disabilities, 35,* 194–204.

van Goozen, S. H. (1994). *Male and female: Effects of sex hormones on aggression, cognition and motivation.* Amsterdam: University of Amsterdam Press.

van Goozen, S. H., Cohen-Kettenis, P. T., Gooren, L. J., Frijda, N. H., & van de Poll, N. E. (1995). Gender differences in behavior: Activating effects of cross-sex hormones. *Psychoneuroendocrinology, 20,* 343–363.

van Goozen, S. H. M., Gooren, L. J. G., Slabbekoorn, D., Sanders, G., & Cohen-Kettenis, P. T. (2002). Organizing and activating effects of sex hormones in homosexual transsexuals. *Behavioral Neuroscience, 116,* 982–988.

Van Hoesen, G., & Damasio, A. R. (1987). Neural correlates of cognitive impairment in Alzheimer's disease. In V. B. Brooks (Ed.), *Handbook of physiology: The nervous system* (Vol. V). Bethesda, MD: American Physiological Society.

Vanneste, J. A. L. (2000). Diagnosis and management of normal-pressure hydrocephalus. *Journal of Neurology, 247,* 5–14.

Van Raalte, J. L., & Brewer, B. W. (1996). *Exploring sport and exercise psychology.* Washington, DC: American Psychological Association.

van Veen, V., & Carter, C. S. (2002). The timing of action-monitoring processes in the anterior cingulate cortex. *Journal of Cognitive Neuroscience, 14,* 593–602.

Venneri, A., Cornoldi, C., & Caruit, M. (2003). Arithmetic difficulties in children with visuospatial learning disability (VLD). *Child Neuropsychology, 9,* 175–183.

Verrees, M., & Selman, W. R. (2004). Management of normal pressure hydrocephalus. *American Family Physician, 70,* 1071–1078.

Victor, M., & Ropper, A. H. (2001). *Adams and Victor's principles of neurology* (7th ed.). New York: McGraw-Hill.

Vilkki, J., & Laitinen, V. (1974). Differential effects of left and right ventrolateral thalamotomy on receptive and expressive verbal performances and face matching. *Neuropsychologia, 12,* 11.

Villardita, C., Smirni, P., LaPira, F., Zappala, G., & Nicoletti, F. (1982). Mental deterioration, visuoperceptive disabilities and constructional apraxia in Parkinson's disease. *Acta Neurologica Scandinavica, 66,* 112–120.

Vining, E. P. (1999). Clinical efficacy of the ketogenic diet. *Epilepsy Research, 37*(3), 181–190.

Virues-Ortega, J., Buela-Casal, G., Garrido, E., & Alcazar, B. (2004). Neuropsychological functioning associated with high-altitude exposure. *Neuropsychol Rev, 14*(4), 197–224.

Voeller, K. K. S. (1996). Brief report: Developmental neurobiological aspects of autism. *Journal of Autism and Developmental Disorders, 26,* 189–193.

Volkmar, F. R., & Klin, A. (2000). Diagnostic issues in Asperger syndrome. In A. Klin, F. R. Volkmar, & S. S. Sparrow (Eds.), *Asperger syndrome* (pp. 25–71). New York: Guilford Press.

Volkmar, F. R., Klin, A., Schultz, R., Bronen, R., Marans, W. D., Sparrow, S., et al. (1996). Asperger's syndrome. *Journal of the American Academy of Child and Adolescent Psychiatry, 35,* 118–123.

Volkmar, F. R., Lord, C., Bailey, A., Schultz, R. T., & Klin, A. (2004). Autism and pervasive developmental disorders. *Journal of Child Psychology and Psychiatry, 45,* 135–170.

Volterra, V., Caselli, M. C., Capirci, O., Tonucci, F., & Vicari, S. (2003). Early linguistic abilities of Italian children with Williams syndrome. *Developmental Neuropsychology, 23,* 35–59.

von Monakow, C. (1911). Lokalisation der Hirnfunktionen. *Journal of Psychiatry and Neurology, 17,* 185–200.

Von Senden, M. (1960). *Space and sight: The perception of space and shape in the congenitally blind before and after operation.* Urbana-Champaign, IL: Free Press of Illinois.

von Stockert, F. G. (1932). Subcortical dementia. *Archives of Psychiatry, 97,* 77–100.

Vonsattel, J. P. (1992). Neuropathology of Huntington's disease. In A. B. Joseph & R. R. Young (Eds.), *Movement disorders in neuropathology and neuropsychiatry* (pp. 186–194). Oxford, United Kingdom: Blackwell Scientific.

Vouloumanos, A., Kiehl, K. A., Werker, J. F., & Liddle, P. F. (2001). Detection of sounds in the auditory stream: Event-related fMRI evidence for differential activation to speech and nonspeech. *Journal of Cognitive Neuroscience, 13,* 994–1005.

Voyer, D. (1997). Scoring procedures, performance factors, and magnitude of sex differences in spatial performance. *American Journal of Psychology, 110,* 259–276.

Voyer, D., Rodgers, M. A., & McCormick, P. A. (2004). Timing conditions and the magnitude of gender differences on the Mental Rotations Test. *Memory and Cognition, 32,* 72–82.

Voyer, D., Voyer, S., & Bryden, M. P. (1995). Magnitude of sex differences in spatial abilities: A meta-analysis and consideration of critical variables. *Psychological Bulletin, 117,* 250–270.

Vuilleumier, P., Armony, J. L., Driver, J., & Dolan, R. J. (2001). Effects of attention and emotion on face processing in the human brain: An event-related fMRI study. *Neuron, 30,* 829–841.

Vygotsky, L. S. (1965). Psychology and localization of functions. *Neuropsychologia, 3,* 381.

Waber, D. P., Forbes, P. W., Wolff, P. H., & Weiler, M. D. (2004). Neurodevelopmental characteristics of children with learning impairments classified according to the double-deficit hypothesis. *Journal of Learning Disabilities, 37,* 451–461.

Wada, J., & Rasmussen, T. (1960). Intracarotid injection of sodium amytal for the lateralization of cerebral speech dominance: Experimental and clinical observations. *Journal of Neurosurgery, 17,* 266–282.

Wagar, B. M., & Thagard, P. (2004). Spiking Phineas Gage: A neurocomputational theory of cognitive-affective integration in decision making. *Psychological Review, 111,* 67–79.

Wager, T. D., Phan K. L., Liberzon, I., & Taylor, S. F. (2003). Valence, gender, and lateralization of functional brain anatomy in emotion: A meta-analysis of findings from neuroimaging. *NeuroImage, 19,* 513–531.

Waldman, I. D., Rowe, D. C., Abramowitz, A., Kozel, S. T., Mohr, J. H., Sherman, S. L., et al. (1998). Association and linkage of the dopamine transporter gene and attention-deficit hyperactivity in children: Heterogeneity owing to diagnostic subtype and severity. *American Journal of Human Genetics, 63,* 1767–1776.

Walker, J.E., & Kozlowski, G. P. (2005). Neurofeedback treatment of epilepsy. *Child and Adolescent Psychiatric Clinics of North America, 14,* 163–176, viii.

Walt, V. (2005, March 7). A land where girls rule in math. *Time, 165,* 56–57.

Walton, J. N. (1994). *Brain's diseases of the nervous system* (10th ed.). Oxford, United Kingdom: Oxford University Press.

Wang, A. T., Dapretto, M., Hariri, A. R., Sigman, M., & Bookheimer, S. Y. (2004). Neural correlates of facial affect processing in children and adolescents with autism spectrum disorder. *Journal of the American Child and Adolescent Psychiatry, 43,* 481–490.

Wang, L. N., Zhu, M. W., Gui, Q. P., & Li, X. H. (2003). [An analysis of the causes of dementia in 383 elderly autopsied cases]. *Zhonghua Nei Ke Za Zhi, 42*(11), 789–792.

Wang, Q. S., & Zhou, J. N. (2002). Retrieval and encoding of episodic memory in normal aging and patients with mild cognitive impairment. *Brain Research, 924*(1), 113–115.

Wang, W., Wu, S., Cheng, X., Dai, H., Ross, K., Du, X., et al. (2000). Prevalence of Alzheimer's disease and other dementing disorders in an urban community of Beijing, China. *Neuroepidemiology, 19*(4), 194–200.

Wapner, W., Judd, T., & Gardner, H. (1978). Visual agnosia in an artist. *Cortex, 14,* 343–364.

Wass, T. S., Persutte, W. H., & Hobbins, J. C. (2001). The impact of prenatal alcohol exposure on frontal cortex development in utero. *American Journal of Obstetrics and Gynecology, 185,* 737–742.

Wassertheil-Smoller, S., Hendrix, S., Limacher, M., Heiss, G., Kooperberg, C., Baird, A., et al. (2003). Effect of estrogen plus progestin on stroke in postmenopausal women. *Journal of the American Medical Association, 289,* 2673–2684.

Waterhouse, L., Fein, D., & Modahl, C. (1996). Autism. *Psychology Review, 103,* 457–489.

Wechsler, D. (1944). *The measurement of adult intelligence* (3rd ed.). Baltimore: Williams & Wilkins.

Wechsler, D. (1945). A standardized memory scale for clinical use. *Journal of Psychology, 19,* 87–95.

Wechsler, D. (1974). *Wechsler Intelligence Scale for Children–Revised.* New York: Psychological Corporation.

Wechsler, D. (1981). *Wechsler Adult Intelligence Scale–Revised.* New York: Psychological Corporation.

Wechsler, D. (1991). *Manual for the Wechsler Intelligence Scale for Children, Third Edition, WISC-III.* San Antonio, TX: Psychological Corporation.

Wechsler, D. (1997). *Wechsler Adult Intelligence Scale–III.* San Antonio, TX: The Psychological Corporation.

Wechsler, D. (2002). *Wechsler Primary and Preschool Scale–III.* San Antonio, TX: The Psychological Corporation.

Wechsler, D. (2003). *Wechsler Intelligence Scale for Children–IV.* San Antonio, TX: The Psychological Corporation.

Wehman, P. H. (1991). Cognitive rehabilitation in the workplace. In J. S. Kreutzer & P. H. Wehman (Eds.), *Cognitive rehabilitation for persons with traumatic brain injury.* Baltimore: Paul H. Brookes.

Weimar, C., Kurth, T., Kraywinkel, K., Wagner, M., Busse, O., Haberl, R. L., et al. (2002). Assessment of functioning and disability after ischemic stroke. *Stroke, 33*(8), 2053–2059.

Weinand, M. E., Hermann, B., Wyler, A. R., Carter, L. P., Oommen, K. J., Labiner, D., et al. (1994). Long-term subdural strip electrocorticographic monitoring of ictal deja vu. *Epilepsia, 35*(5), 1054–1059.

Weiss, G., & Hechtman, L. T. (1993). *Hyperactive children grown up* (2nd ed.). New York: Guilford Press.

Weiss, M., Tannock, R., Kratochvil, C., Dunn, D., Velez-Borras, J., Thomason, C., et al. (2005). A randomized, placebo-controlled study of once-daily atomoxetine in the school setting in children with ADHD. *Journal of the American Academy of Child and Adolescent Psychiatry, 44,* 647–655.

Weiss, S., Dunne, C., Hewson, J., Wohl, C., Wheatley, M., Peterson, A. C., & Reynolds, B. A. (1996). Multipotent CNS stem cells are present in the adult mammalian spinal cord and ventricular neuroaxis. *Journal of Neuroscience, 16,* 7599–7609.

Weiten, W. (1994). *Psychology: Themes and variations* (2nd ed.). Pacific Grove, CA: Brooks/Cole.

Weiten, W. (1998). *Psychology: Themes and variations* (4th ed.). Pacific Grove, CA: Brooks/Cole.

Wells, S. (1869). *How to read character: New illustrated handbook of phrenology and physiognomy.* New York: Fowler & Wells.

Welsh, M. C. (1991). Rule-guided behavior and self-monitoring on the Tower of Hanoi disk-transfer task. *Cognitive Development, 6,* 59–76.

Welsh, M. C., Pennington, B. F., & Groisser, D. B. (1991). A normative-developmental study of executive function: A window on prefrontal function in children. *Developmental Neuropsychology, 7,* 131–149.

Wenk, G. L. (2004). Functional neuroanatomy of learning and memory. In D. S. Charney & E. J. Nestler (Eds.), *Neurobiology of mental illness* (2nd ed., pp. 807–812). New York: Oxford University Press.

Wexler, A. (1995). *Mapping fate: A memoir of family, risk, and genetic research.* New York: Random House.

Whalley, L. J., Starr, J. M., Athawes, R., Hunter, D., Pattie, A., & Deary, I. J. (2000). Childhood mental ability and dementia. *Neurology, 55*(10), 1455–1459.

White, B. J. (1994). The Turner syndrome: Origin, cytogenetic variants, and factors influencing the phenotype. In S. H. Broman & J. Grafman (Eds.), *Atypical cognitive deficits in developmental disorders* (pp. 183–196). New York: Oxford University Press.

Whyte, J. (1986). Outcome evaluation in the remediation of attention and memory deficits. *Journal of Head Trauma Rehabilitation, 1,* 43–53.

Wilens, T. E., Biederman, J., Brown, S., Tanguay, S., Monuteaux, M. C., Blake, C., et al. (2002). Psychiatric comorbidity and functioning in clinically referred preschool children and school-age youths with ADHD. *Journal of the American Child and Adolescent Psychiatry, 41,* 262–268.

Wilkins, R. H., & Brody, I. A. (1970). Wernicke's sensory aphasia. *Archives of Neurology, 22,* 279.

Willerman, L., Schultz, R., Rutledge, N., & Bigler, E. (1992). Hemisphere size asymmetry predicts relative verbal and nonverbal intelligence differently in the sexes: An MRI study of structure-function relations. *Intelligence, 16,* 315–328.

Williams, J. C. P., Barratt-Boyes, B. G., & Lowe, J. B. (1961). Supravalvular aortic stenosis. *Circulation, 24,* 1311–1318.

Williams, R. L., & Karacan, I. (1978). *Sleep disorders: Diagnosis and treatment.* New York: Wiley.

Williams, R. W., & Herrup, K. (1988). The control of neuron number. *Annual Review of Neuroscience, 11,* 423–453.

Willis, K. E. (1993). Neuropsychological functioning in children with spina bifida and/or hydrocephalus. *Journal of Clinical Child Psychology, 22,* 247–265.

Wilson, S. A. K. (1912). Progressive lenticular degeneration: A familial nervous disease associated with cirrhosis of the liver. *Brain, 34,* 296–508.

Winson, J. (1972). Interspecies differences in the occurrence of theta. *Behavioral Biology, 7,* 479–487.

Witelson, S. F., Glezer, I. I., & Kigar, D. L. (1995). Women have greater density of neurons in posterior temporal cortex. *Journal of Neuroscience, 15,* 3418–3428.

Witelson, S. F., Kigar, D. L., & Harvey, T. (1999). The exceptional brain of Albert Einstein. *Lancet, 353,* 2149–2153.

Witol, A., & Webbe, F. (1993). Neuropsychological deficits associated with soccer play. *Archives of Clinical Neuropsychology, 9,* 204–205.

Wolfson, C., Wolfson, D. B., Asgharian, M., M'Lan, C. E., Ostbye, T., Rockwood, K., et al. (2001). A reevaluation of the duration of survival after the onset of dementia. *New England Journal of Medicine, 344*(15), 1111–1116.

Wood, F. B., & Grigorenko, E. L. (2001). Emerging issues in the genetics of dyslexia: A methodological preview. *Journal of Learning Disabilities, 34,* 503–511.

World Health Organization. (1992). *The ICD-10 classification of mental and behavioral disorders: Clinical descriptions and diagnostic guidelines.* Geneva, Switzerland: World Health Organization.

Wright, R. (1994). *The moral animal.* New York: Vintage.

Xu, Y., & Corkin, S. (2001). H. M. revisits the Tower of Hanoi puzzle. *Neuropsychology, 15,* 69–79.

Yaffe, K., Sawaya, G., Lieberburg, I., & Grady, D. (1998). Estrogen therapy in postmenopausal women. *Journal of the American Medical Association, 279,* 688–695.

Yeo, R. A., Hill, D. E., Campbell, R. A., Vigil, J., Petropoulos, H., Hart, B., et al. (2003). Proton magnetic resonance spectroscopy investigation of the right frontal lobe in children with attention-deficit/hyperactivity disorder. *Journal of the American Child and Adolescent Psychiatry, 42,* 303–310.

Yeterian, E. H., & Van Hoesen, G. W. (1978). Cortico-striate projections in the rhesus monkey: The organization of certain cortico-caudate connections. *Brain Research, 139,* 43–63.

Yücel, M., Stuart, G. W., Maruff, P., Velakoulis, D., Crowe, S. F., Savage, G., et al. (2001). Hemispheric and gender-related differences in the gross morphology of the anterior cingulate/paracingulate cortex in normal volunteers: An MRI morphometric study. *Cerebral Cortex, 11,* 17–25.

Zaidel, D., & Sperry, R. W. (1973). Performance on Raven's Colored Progressive Matrices Test by subjects with cerebral commissurotomy. *Cortex, 9,* 34.

Zald, D. H., & Kim, S. W. (2001). The orbitofrontal cortex. In S. P. Salloway, P. F. Malloy, & J. D. Duffy (Eds.), *The frontal lobes and neuropsychiatric illness* (pp. 33–70). Washington, DC: American Psychiatric Publishing.

Zametkin, A. J., Liebenauer, L. L., Fitzgerald, G. A., King, A. C., Minkunas, D. V., Herscovitch, P., et al. (1993). Brain metabolism in teenagers with attention-deficit hyperactivity disorder. *Archives of General Psychiatry, 50,* 333–340.

Zametkin, A. J., Nordahl, T. E., Gross, M., King, A. C., Semple, W. E., Rumsey, J., et al. (1990). Cerebral glucose metabolism in adults with hyperactivity of childhood onset. *New England Journal of Medicine, 323,* 1362–1365.

Zang, Y. F., Jin, Z., Weng, X. C., Zhang, L., Zeng, Y. W., Yang, L., et al. (2005). Functional MRI in attention-deficit hyperactivity disorder: Evidence for hypofrontality. *Brain and Development, 27,* 544–550.

Zangwill, O. L. (1960). *Cerebral dominance and its relation to psychological function.* Edinburgh, United Kingdom: Oliver & Boyd.

Zec, R. F. (1993). Neuropsychological functioning in Alzheimer's disease. In R. W. Parks, R. F. Zec, & R. S. Wilson (Eds.), *Neuropsychology of Alzheimer's disease and other dementias.* New York: Oxford University Press.

Zeki, S. (1992). *The visual image in mind and brain. Readings from Scientific American.* New York: W. H. Freeman.

Zihl, J. (1995). Eye movement patterns in hemianopic dyslexia. *Brain, 118,* 891–912.

Zillmer, E. A. (1991). Rorschach Interpretation Assistance Program-Version 2 Review. *Journal of Personality Assessment, 572,* 381–383.

Zillmer, E. A. (1995). The case of Aaron B. In D. L. Chute & M. E. Bliss (Eds.), *Exploring psychological disorders* (pp. 115–124). Pacific Grove, CA: Brooks/Cole.

Zillmer, E. A. (1996, November). Mind over matter: Brain research in the next millennium. Invited paper to Congressional staff on Capitol Hill, Washington, D.C.

Zillmer, E. A. (2003a). The neuropsychology of repeated 1- and 3-meter springboard diving among college athletes. *Applied Neuropsychology, 10*(1), 23–30.

Zillmer, E. A. (2003b, editor-special edition). Introduction to special issue on psychological and neuropsychological assessment in the forensic arena: Art or science? *Assessment, 10*(4), 318–320.

Zillmer, E. A. (2003c, editor-special edition). Sports-related concussions. *Applied Neuropsychology, 10*(1), 1–3.

Zillmer, E. A. (2004). National Academy of Neuropsychology: President's address. The future of neuropsychology. *Archives of Clinical Neuropsychology, 19*(6), 713–724.

Zillmer, E. A., Chelder, M. J., & Efthimiou, J. (1995). *Assessment of Impairment AIM Measure.* Philadelphia: Drexel University.

Zillmer, E. A., Fowler, P. C., Gutnick, H. N., & Becker, E. (1990). Comparison of two cognitive bedside screening instruments in nursing home residents: A factor analytic study. *Journal of Gerontology: Psychological Sciences, 45,* 69–74.

Zillmer, E. A., Fowler, P. C., Waechtler, C., Harris, B., & Khan, F. (1992). The effects of unilateral and multifocal lesions on the WAIS-R: A factor analytic study of stroke patients. *Archives of Clinical Neuropsychology, 7,* 29–41.

Zillmer, E. A., & Greene, H. (2006). Neuropsychological assessment in the forensic setting. In R. P. Archer (Ed.), *Clinical assessment instruments in forensic settings: Uses and limitations.* Mawah, NJ: Lawrence Erlbaum.

Zillmer, E. A., Harrower, M., Ritzler, B., & Archer, R. P. (1995). *The quest for the Nazi personality: A psychological investigation of Nazi war criminals.* Hillsdale, NJ: Erlbaum.

Zillmer, E. A., Lucci, K., Barth, J. T., Peake, T., & Spyker, D. (1986). Neurobehavioral sequelae of subcutaneous injection with metallic mercury. *Journal of Toxicology: Clinical Toxicology, 24,* 100–110.

Zillmer, E. A., Montenegro, L., Wiser, J., Barth, J. T., & Spyker, D. (1996). Neuropsychological sequelae in subacute home chlordane poisoning: Ten case studies. *Archives of Clinical Neuropsychology, 11,* 77–89.

Zillmer, E. A., & Passuth, P. M. (1989). Predicting functional ability from mental status among nursing home residents. *The Gerontologist, 29,* 142A.

Zillmer, E. A., & Perry, W. (1996). Cognitive-neuropsychological abilities and related psychological disturbance: A factor model of neuropsychological, Rorschach, and MMPI indices. *Assessment, 3,* 209–224.

Zillmer, E., Schneider, J., Tinker, J., & Kaminaris, C. (2006). A history of sports-related concussions: a neuropsychological perspective. In R. Echemendia (Ed.), *Sports neuropsychology: Assessment and management of traumatic brain injury.* New York: Guilford Press.

Zillmer, E. A., Ware, J. C., Rose, V., & Bond, T. (1989). An examination of the Symptom Checklist 90-Revised SCL-90-R in the assessment of personality function in sleep disorders. *Sleep Research, 18,* 189.

Zillmer, E. A., Ware, J. C., Rose, V., & Maximin, A. (1988). MMPI characteristics of patients with different severity of sleep apnea. *Sleep Research, 17,* 136.

Zillmer, E. A., & Wickramaserkera, I. (1987). Biofeedback and hypnotizability: Initial treatment considerations. *Clinical Biofeedback and Health, 10,* 51–57.

Zola-Morgan, S., & Squire, L. R. (1993). Neuroanatomy of memory. *Annual Review of Neuroscience, 16,* 547–563.

Zubenko, G. S., Moossy, J., Martinez, A. J., Rao, G. R., Kopp, U., & Hanin, I. (1989). A brain regional analysis of morphologic and cholinergic abnormalities in Alzheimer's disease. *Archives of Neurology, 46,* 634–639.

GLOSSARY

Ablation experiment   Developed by Pierre Flourens, and involved removing parts of the brain of pigeons and hens. Flourens reported that excising any part of the brain in birds led to generalized, not localized, disorders of behavior.

Absence seizures   Occur when the normally asynchronous waking state is abruptly interrupted by low-wave synchronous activity; characterized by synchronous bilateral spike-and-wave discharge.

Abulia   A syndrome similar to that of *akinetic mutism,* but of lesser severity. The syndrome is characterized by significant reduction in drive, interest, and spontaneous behavior. The syndrome is associated with medial damage to the frontal lobes.

Acceleration   The brain experiencing a significant physical force that propels it quickly, from stationary to moving.

Acetylcholine (ACh)   Also called *choline;* the first neurotransmitter to be identified; plays a prominent role in the peripheral nervous system, influencing motor control, and in autonomic nervous system functioning.

Achievement tests   Most influenced by past educational attainment; measures how well a subject has profited by learning and experience compared with others.

Achromatopsia   The complete loss of ability to detect color.

Acidophilic adenoma   A functioning type of pituitary tumor that usually appears in the anterior lobe of the pituitary gland. The acidophilic adenoma creates excessive secretion of growth hormones often resulting in giantism (excessive growth of hands and feet).

Acoustic neuroma   Progressively enlarging, benign tumor within the auditory canal arising from Schwann cells of the VIIIth cranial nerve.

Acquired sociopathy   See **Pseudopsychopathy.**

Action potential   An electrical potential across the neuron membrane. The action potential spreads down the axon as the voltage-controlled sodium channels open up sequentially, like falling dominoes.

Adrenocorticotropic hormone (ACTH)   A hormone secreted by the anterior pituitary gland that mediates the release of hormones from the adrenal cortex. Increased and decreased secretions of ACTH have been associated with a various disorders and disease states.

Affective significance of stimuli   The binding or attachment of emotion to novel and social stimuli.

Afferent nerves (sensory nerves)   Convey incoming messages from the sensory receptors to the central nervous system.

Agenesis   Complete or partial failure of an organ to develop.

Ageusia   Inability to recognize tastes.

Agnosia   An absence of knowing. The distinction between the ability to recognize an object and the inability to name it. Term first coined by Sigmund Freud.

Agyria, or **lissencephaly**   A congenital disorder in which the normal gyri and sulci of the brain fail to develop. Believed to occur between the third and fourth month of gestation.

Air encephalogram or **pneumoencephalography**   The radiographic visualization of the fluid-containing structures of the brain, the ventricles, and spinal column. It is similar to the X-ray, but it involves the withdrawal of cerebrospinal fluid by lumbar puncture, which is then replaced with a gas including air, oxygen, or helium.

Akinesia   A difficulty in initiating and maintaining behavior. Patients with akinesia may be extremely slow to start or perform a movement, may become rapidly fatigued when performing repetitive movements, or may have problems in performing simultaneous or sequential movements.

Akinetic mutism   A syndrome associated with medial frontal damage involving a loss of initiative, apathy, reduced verbal and motor behaviors, and profound indifference.

Akinetopsia   The specific inability to identify objects in motion.

Alcohol-related neurodevelopmental disabilities (ARND) See **Fetal alcohol effect.**

Alternating attention The ability to switch back and forth between tasks.

Alzheimer's disease (AD) An irreversible cortical dementia, not due to an identifiable cause, that is characterized by neuropathologic markers including neurofibrillary tangles and senile plaques.

Amino acids A group of neurotransmitters that plays a major role in the more basic type of neuronal transmission that depends on rapid communication among neurons.

Amygdala Literally "almond," because of its shape; has a specific role in fear conditioning and impacts the strength of stored memory.

Amyotrophic lateral sclerosis (ALS) Disease of the motor system in which people experience a gradual to total loss of muscle control and muscle function.

Anastomosis Communication between blood vessels by collateral channels. See **Collateral blood vessel.**

Androgen hormone Any steroid hormone, primarily produced by the testes, that has a "masculinizing" effect on development. Effects include the masculinization of the fetus, production of sperm, and development of secondary sexual characteristics.

Androgen insensitivity Refers to a set of genetic disorders resulting from mutation of the gene encoding for the androgen receptor. Affected males demonstrate varying degrees of under-development of male-sex physical characteristics.

Anencephaly A congenital condition characterized by a failure in development of the two hemispheres, mesencephalon, and diencephalon of the brain. The brain is represented by a vascular mass. The condition produces severe neurologic deficits and is incompatible with life.

Aneurysms Weak areas in the walls of an artery that cause the vessel to balloon.

Angiography X-raying blood vessels in the brain after introducing contrast material into the arterial or venous bloodstream. Angiography is the most useful technique for examining the blood supply to and from the brain.

Anomia Problems in word finding. Only a word or two, here and there, is lost, and the communication can proceed pretty much as normal. In more severe cases, most or all words can be lost.

Anopias Term for visual difficulties.

Anosmia Total loss of smell.

Anosognosia A term first coined by Babinski to indicate the inability or refusal to recognize that one has a particular disease or disorder.

Anoxia The complete cessation of oxygen supply to the brain. Anoxia often occurs with stroke or other severe traumas of the brain, such as are often seen in gunshot wounds to the head.

Anterior Toward the front or front end.

Anterior attention system (executive attention system) An attentional system of the brain mediating the voluntary control of attention that is supported by the frontal and medial cortices of the brain.

Anterior cerebral artery Resulting from half of the division of an internal carotid artery, it supplies the anterior medial portion of its corresponding cerebral hemisphere.

Anterior commissure Minor intercerebral fibers.

Anterior communicating artery Connects the left and right anterior cerebral arteries.

Anterograde amnesia The loss of memory for events after trauma or disease onset.

Anterograde degeneration The degeneration of the axon after the cell body has been damaged.

Anticholinergics Treatment for Parkinson's disease; act by blocking the action of acetylcholine.

Anton's syndrome Actual denial of cerebral blindness; a behavioral mirror of apperceptive agnosia.

Aortic arch Arises from the left ventricle of the heart.

Aphasia A disturbance of language usage or comprehension. It may involve the impairment of the power to speak, write, read, gesture, or comprehend spoken, written, or gestured language.

Apnea The cessation of airflow; literally means "a lack of breath."

Apperceptive visual agnosia A visual problem with object perception as the primary difficulty.

Apraxia An absence of action, but the term is most often used to describe a variety of missing or inappropriate actions that cannot be clearly attributed to primary motor deficits or the lack of comprehension or motivation. Thus, *apraxia* refers to an inability to perform voluntary actions despite an adequate amount of motor strength and control.

Arachnoid granulations Small "pockets" of cauliflower-like veins within the subarachnoid space, which serve as pathways for the subarachnoid cerebrospinal fluid to be absorbed and re-enter the venous circulation.

Arachnoid membrane A "spiderlike" avascular membrane of the meninges.

Arborization The sprouting and branching of dendrites during brain development.

Aristotle (Greek, 384–322 B.C.) a disciple of Plato; erroneously believed that the heart is the source of all mental processes. Aristotle argued that because the brain is bloodless, it fills the function of a "radiator," cooling hot blood ascending from the heart.

Arteriovenous malformations (AVM)   Abnormal, often redundant vessels that result in abnormal blood flow. Because AVMs have inherently weak vessel walls, they may lead to slow bleeding or inadequate distribution of blood in the regions surrounding the vessels.

Articulation   The ability to form phonetic sounds of vowels and consonants, which then are placed in different combinations to form words and sentences.

Articulatory phonologic loop   A working memory "slave system" that stores speech-based information and is important in the acquisition of vocabulary.

Ascending spinal-thalamic tract   Carries sensory information related to pain and temperature and runs in parallel to the spinal cord. It synapses over a wide region of the thalamus, primarily on the intralaminar and ventral posterior nuclei of the thalamus, and then to the somatosensory cortex.

Asociality   Denotes a lack of social interest and relatedness. This anomaly is hypothesized to be one of the mechanisms responsible for autistic behaviors.

Asperger's syndrome   A pervasive developmental disorder characterized by symptoms of autism, including impairments in social relatedness and atypical patterns of behavior, interest, or activity. However, in contrast with autism, impairment in language, adaptive skills (with the exception of social skills), and curiosity about the environment are not pronounced. The disorder tends to have a later age of onset than autism.

Association or polymodal areas   Brain regions involved in the integration of sensory information from different sensory cortices and linking the sensory cortices to the motor cortices. These associative cortices support complex mental and behavioral functions.

Associative visual agnosia   A visual problem having to do with difficulty in assigning meaning to an object.

Astereognosia   Inability to recognize an object by touch.

Astereognosis   See **Tactile agnosia.**

Astrocytes   Non-neural, star-shaped glia cells that are highly branched and occupy much space between neurons in the gray matter. Their multiple functions include supporting neurons by interweaving among nerve fibers, contributing to the metabolism of synaptic transmitters, and regulating the balance of ions. Astrocytes join together to provide a barrier between parts of the central nervous system (CNS) and non-CNS tissue.

Astrocytomas   A form of malignant tumors primarily composed of astrocytes, a type of glia cell.

Atharva-Veda   700 B.C. Indian text that proposed that the soul was nonmaterial and never died.

Atherosclerosis   A neuropathologic process characterized by irregularly distributed yellow fatty plaques in large and medium-sized arteries.

Atonia   Lack or reduction of muscle tone.

Atonic seizures   Are characterized by a sudden loss of muscle tone and may result in a fall. They last no longer than 15 seconds while the person remains conscious.

Atrial fibrillation   A disorder that upsets the heart's rhythm, which may cause it to not pump enough blood to meet the body's needs. A normal heart contracts and relaxes to a regular beat. In atrial fibrillation the heart contracts at a very irregular and sometimes very rapid rate, which results in an irregular heart rhythm.

Atrophy   Brain shrinkage.

Attention-deficit/hyperactivity disorder (ADHD)   A neuropsychological developmental disorder characterized by age-inappropriate inattention, impulsivity, and overactivity.

Aura   A neurologic event that occurs before the onset of a migraine or a seizure. The aura presents usually as a visual symptom including flashing lights, zigzag lines, or blurred or partial loss of vision.

Autism   Previously referred to as *infantile autism* or *Kanner's autism*. A pervasive developmental disorder, evident before age 3, involving impaired communication, socialization, and behavioral adaptation. Atypical behaviors, preoccupations, or interests are frequently evident. The cause of the disorder is unknown, and the prognosis is poor.

Autistic aloneness   A term proposed by Leo Kanner in his description of autistic children, referring to one of the central symptoms of the disorder, namely, the profound separation and disconnection of autistic individuals from other people.

Automatisms   Stereotyped hand movements or facial tics often seen during an absence seizure.

Autonomic nervous system (ANS)   Provides the "automatic" neural control of internal organs (such as heart, intestines). Most autonomic organs receive both sympathetic and parasympathetic input.

Autosomes   A non-sex chromosome. Humans generally have 22 pairs of autosomes in each cell of the body.

These chromosomes are involved in transmitting all genetic traits and conditions other than those that are sex-linked.

Axon   Extends from cell body. Its main function is to transmit information in the form of an action potential.

Babinski, Joseph   (1857–1932) Founder of British neurology.

Balint's syndrome   Related to damage of the parieto-occipital area of both hemispheres; includes visual agnosia together with other visuospatial difficulties such as misreaching and left-sided neglect.

Basal forebrain   Structure of the telencephalon, surrounding the inferior tip of the frontal horn; strongly interconnects with limbic structures; includes various structures such as the amygdala and the septum.

Basal ganglia   Also called the *basal nuclei;* deep nuclei of the telencephalon. Structures include the caudate nucleus, putamen, globus pallidus, substantia nigra, and subthalamic nuclei. Important relay stations in motor behavior (for example, the striato-pallido-thalamic loop). Coordinate stereotyped postural and reflexive motor activity.

Basal nuclei   See **Basal ganglia.**

Base rate   The frequency with which a pathologic condition is diagnosed in the population.

Basilar artery   Formed from a joining of the two vertebral arteries at the level of the brainstem.

Basolateral circuit   Anatomic circuit centered around the amygdala; its most likely role is in emotional processing.

Basophilic adenomas   A functioning type of tumor of the pituitary gland in the anterior lobe of the pituitary gland, which causes excessive secretion of adrenocorticotropic hormone, which can cause Cushing's syndrome.

Behavioral-adaptive scales   Tests that examine what an individual usually and habitually does, not what he or she can do. Such scales are most frequently used in evaluating the daily self-care skills of people who are quite impaired.

Benign   Describes cell growth that is usually surrounded by a fibrous capsule, is typically noninfiltrative (that is, noninvasive), and will not spread to other parts of the body.

Benton, Arthur   American neuropsychologist who pioneered the role of the right cerebral hemisphere in behavior.

Benzodiazepines   A family of sedating drugs used to treat anxiety and sleep disorders.

Beta-amyloid   Amino acid peptide protein core found in the center of senile plaques. Also written as *β-amyloid.*

Bipolar neurons   Neurons with two axons.

Blindsight   The ability in those with cortical blindness to indicate that a stimulus is present, that it has moved, or that it is in a certain location, even though they have no conscious ability to "see" in the conventional sense.

Blood–brain barrier   Affords protection from potentially harmful substances circulating in the body through the bloodstream. It bars certain drugs totally from the brain, and other substances require an active transport system across the blood–brain barrier.

Bradykinesia   A poverty of movement that is not only slowed but reduced in magnitude; negative motor symptom of Parkinson's disease.

Bradyphrenia   Extremely slow information processing speed characteristic of patients with subcortical dementias.

Brain   The anterior portion of the central nervous system located within the skull. It is continuous with the spinal cord and comprised of white/gray matter.

Brain abscesses   A "walled-off," localized pocket of pus within the brain often related to an infection.

Brain herniation   A pathologic process associated with increasing intracranial pressure that occurs in the cranium, which may result in a displacement and deformation of the brain.

Brain hypothesis   Suggests that the brain is the source of all behavior.

Brainstem   Evolutionary old brain structure involved in regulating brain activation. It emerges from the uppermost portion of the spinal cord and includes all the subdivisions below the telencephalon (that is, the diencephalon, the mesencephalon, the metencephalon, and the myelencephalon), except for the cerebellum.

Broca, Paul   (1824–1880) French anthropologist and scientist who advanced surgery, neuroanatomy, neurophysiology, and neuropathology.

Brodmann's areas   Cytoarchitectural scheme dividing the cortex into 52 sections.

Canalesthesia   The fragmentation of the processing of incoming information from the sensory modalities. The anomaly is believed to be one of the causative factors of autistic behaviors.

Cannon–Bard theory   Opposite of James–Lange theory. Walter Cannon, and later Philip Bard, argued the conscious emotional experience can be divorced from bodily sensation or expression. Although today most scientists agree that there is a correspondence between cognitive experience of emotion and sensory experience, types of emotion, emotional intensity, and individual variation appear to vary considerably.

Cardiac hypothesis Proposed that the heart was the seat of such emotions as love and anger.

Cataplexy The most debilitating of the narcolepsy symptoms; a brief episode of muscle weakness, actual paralysis, or both.

Catecholamines A class of neurotransmitters that includes dopamine and norepinephrine.

Caudal Toward the rear, away from the head.

Caudate nucleus Structure of the basal ganglia.

Cell doctrine A hypothesis that assumed the ventricles were the location of the mind. Today, the cell doctrine is known to be entirely inaccurate.

Central executive Concept from the theory of working memory in which the central executive is an attention-controlling system; supervises and coordinates slave systems and is the proposed deficit in Alzheimer's disease.

Central nervous system (CNS) The CNS includes the brain and the spinal cord. It is located within and protected by the bony cavities of the skull and the spine.

Central sleep apnea Apnea that occurs most often during rapid eye movement sleep in which disordered breathing is related to the brain failing to send the necessary signals to breathe. This may reflect brainstem abnormalities that manifest only during sleep.

Central sulcus Separates the frontal and parietal lobes.

Cerebellar peduncles Large neural tracts connecting the cerebellum to the midbrain.

Cerebellum Means "little brain"; sits posterior to the brainstem and inferior to the telencephalon, and functions in coordinating motor and sensory information.

Cerebral (or Sylvian) aqueduct A narrow channel passing through the midbrain connecting the third to the fourth ventricle.

Cerebral achromatopsia Total color blindness.

Cerebral hemispheres (cerebrum) Includes structures of the frontal, parietal, occipital, and temporal lobes; plays a role in higher cognitive functioning.

Cerebrospinal fluid (CSF) A protective fluid that surrounds and supports the brain and spinal cord.

Cerebrovascular accident (CVA) A technical term for stroke; describes a heterogeneous groups of vascular disorders associated with damage to the brain's blood vessels and decreased blood flow within and to the brain.

Cerebrum The largest part of the brain, consisting of the left and right hemisphere, and the corpus callosum. The cerebrum does not include the medulla, pons, and cerebellum.

Chemoreceptors Structures that respond to various chemicals on the surface of the skin and mucous membranes. They range from detecting levels of stomach acidity to skin irritations. Smell and taste are special examples of chemoreception and are discussed separately. Thermoreceptors detect heat and cold.

Chorea Twisting, writhing, undulating, grimacing movements of the face and body. Commonly associated with Huntington's disease.

Choroid plexus A highly vascularized network of small blood vessels that protrudes into the ventricles from the pia mater and secretes cerebrospinal fluid.

Chromophobic adenoma A functioning type of tumor of the pituitary gland localized in the anterior aspects of the pituitary gland that is often associated with hyperpituitarism or hypopituitarism.

Chromosomal disorders A disorder that is the consequence of either an abnormal number of chromosomes or some defect in the structure of the chromosome.

Cingulate gyrus A structure of the limbic system, the medial cortex surrounding the corpus callosum.

Cingulate motor area (CMA) or cingulate motor cortex Structures of the secondary motor cortex involved in higher order voluntary movement.

Cingulum A major intracerebral fiber.

Circadian rhythm Daily biorhythm oscillation of heightened and lowered brain arousal observed throughout the wake/sleep cycle.

Circle of Willis A spiderlike arterial structure formed by the anterior cerebral branches of the internal carotid artery and its connections, the anterior communicating artery, the posterior communicating artery, and the posterior cerebral branches of the basilar artery. It allows for a certain degree of redundancy among blood vessels and blood supply to the various areas of the brain.

Cisterns Cavities that are expansions of the subarachnoid space in the central nervous system.

Clonic Motoric jerking.

Closed head injuries A type of head injury that is associated with a blow to the head, but that does not penetrate the skull.

Dorsal simultagnosia   A visual disorder related to damage of the parieto-occipital area of both hemispheres. Even though parts of a picture may be recognized, the whole is not perceived.

Dorsolateral prefrontal cortex   This area is located, functionally, in the prefrontal cortex, which is responsible for orchestrating and organizing many functions of the brain. The dorsolateral prefrontal cortex is not a "movement center" in and of itself but is instrumental in deploying movement. Sensory information from the integrative association area of the parietal lobes is relayed to this motor planning area.

Double-deficit hypothesis   Poses that reading disorders can be traced to deficits in phonological processing and/or naming speed. The presence of both a deficit in phonological processing and slow naming speed is predictive of the most severe reading problem.

Double dissociation   A logical progression of scientific assumptions in localizing functional areas in the brain. For example, if symptom A appears with lesions in brain structure X, but not with those in Y, and symptom B appears with lesions of Y, but not of X, then those specific areas of the brain each have a specific function.

Down's syndrome   Also referred to as trisomy 21. A genetic disorder due to an extra chromosome on the 21st pair. The disorder is characterized by recognizable facial features, short stature, and mild to severe cognitive deficits.

Dura mater   "Tough mother"; a dense, inelastic, double-layered, vascularized membrane of the meninges that adheres to the inner surface of the skull.

Dysarthria   A specific motor apraxia involving the vocal musculature. People with dysarthria differ from pure aphasiacs, although the two conditions may occur together in that such patients know what they want to say but are unable to formulate words because of a problem with motor control.

Dyscalculia   A disorder of mathematics involving impaired ability to comprehend number concepts, spatially orient numbers, reason mathematically, or perform mathematical operations.

Dysgenesis   Abnormal or defective development of an organ.

Dysgraphia   An impairment of the ability to write or express oneself in writing. Deficits are evident in one or more of the following areas: (1) letter formation, speed of writing, and spatial organization of writing; (2) written expression; (3) mechanical knowledge of spelling, grammar, punctuation, and capitalization; and (4) organization and thematic construction of written expression.

Dysgeusia   Distorted taste sensation.

Dyskinesia   Uncontrolled involuntary movement.

Dyslexia   A developmental or acquired disorder of reading involving the disruption of one or more of the component skills of reading. Central reading skills include letter identification, phonologic awareness and processing, and decoding of the written word.

Dysosmia   Distorted smell sensation.

Dysphonia   Loss of vocal emotional expression resulting in a monotonous voice tone.

Echolalia   An atypical communication behavior characterized by the repetition or "echoing" of the words or phrases just spoken by another person. Often displayed by children with pervasive developmental disorders.

Ectopias   Also referred to as "brain warts." Small areas of abnormally placed brain neurons.

Edema   The swelling of the brain

Efferent nerves   Motor nerves carry outgoing signals for action from the central nervous system to the muscles.

Elastin   A protein within elastic fibers of connective tissue accounting for the elasticity of structures such as the skin, blood vessels, heart, lungs and tendons.

Electroconvulsive therapy (ECT)   Shock therapy; administering a large amount of electricity to the skull causing the collective firing of neurons: an induced seizure. ECT sometimes improves severe forms of depression within a few days. Although the mechanism is not clearly understood, therapists use ECT when it is important to intervene quickly to prevent the patient from acting on suicidal thoughts.

Electrocorticogram (ECoG)   A form of EEG in which electrodes are placed directly on the exposed cortex during surgery to isolate a precise location of brain pathology.

Electroencephalography (EEG)   One of the most widely used techniques in neurology. In EEG, the electrical activity of nerve cells of the brain are recorded through electrodes attached to various locations on the scalp.

Epileptogenic focus   The anatomic site of onset.

Embolism   Derived from Greek *embolos*, meaning "plug" or "wedge"; a type of occlusion of an artery in which the clot forms in one area of the body and travels through the arterial system to another area, in this case, the brain, where it becomes lodged and obstructs cranial blood flow. Approximately 14% of all CVAs are caused by an embolism.

Emotional perception   The ability to identify and comprehend the emotions of others from both verbal and nonverbal behavioral cues.

Encode attention   An element of attention that is involved in short-term or working memory.

Endorphins   The most prominent neuropeptide with opioid properties. Endorphins have received much scientific attention for their analgesic effects and their possible role in a pain-inhibiting neuronal system.

Endothelium   The layer of epithelial cells that line the blood vessels. When the endothelium is breached, the blood-clotting properties of the platelets are activated. They change shape and adhere to the vessel wall, each other, and red blood cells. If this occurs pathologically (that is, in a normal vessel), it leads to a thrombosis, ultimately occluding the vessel.

Engaging attention   The attentional operation of focusing, or centering of attention on a stimulus.

Enhanced computed transaxial tomography (CT)   A CT scan that involves the injection of a contrast agent to provide better visualization of brain structures, particularly bleeds.

Enuresis   The continuation of frequent bed-wetting beyond the age of 5 that is not a consequence of a physiological dysfunction.

Environmental dependency syndrome (stimulus-bound)   Neuropsychological syndrome characterized by an over-responsiveness to environmental stimuli due to a loss of inhibitory control, often as a consequence of bilateral frontal damage.

Ependymal glioma   A bulky, solid, firm vascular tumor of the fourth ventricle.

Epidural hematoma   Represents a bleed between the meninges and the skull and occurs in 1% to 3% of major closed head injuries. The cause of an epidural is most often related to the rupture of an artery.

Epidural space   The space between the two dural layers of the meninges.

Epilepsy   "Falling sickness"; a syndrome in which brain seizure activity is a primary symptom.

Epileptic syndrome   Most people with repeat seizures are considered to have an epileptic syndrome, which is more serious than a single seizure.

Episodic buffer   A component of Baddeley's working memory model that is hypothesized to temporarily maintain and integrate the information of different sensory inputs (visual and auditory) through its relationship with long-term memory.

Episodic memory   Individual episodes, usually autobiographical, that have specific spatial and temporal tags in memory.

Equipotentiality   Term first coined by Flourens to describe the notion that mental abilities depend on the brain functioning as a whole. Thus, the effects of brain injury are determined by the size of the injury rather than its location.

Evoked potential (EP)   Also called *event-related potentials (ERPs);* an electrophysiologic diagnostic test that involves the stimulation of specific sensory fibers, which, in turn, generate electrical activity along the central and peripheral pathways, as well as the specific primary receptive areas in the brain.

Excessive daytime sleepiness   Pathologic daytime sleepiness; the most frequent first sign in narcolepsy.

Excitatory postsynaptic potential (EPSP)   Depolarization that increases the probability of the postsynaptic cell to reach its threshold and fire.

Executive attention system   See **Anterior attention system.**

Executive functions   Higher order regulatory and supervisory functions that researchers believe are subserved, in part, by the frontal lobes. Cognitive operations such as planning, mental flexibility, attentional allocation, working memory, and inhibitory control are considered executive functions.

Executive planning   Higher order problem solving necessary for the generation and organization of behavior to achieve a goal. Executive planning requires the ability to anticipate change, respond objectively, generate and select alternatives, and sustain attention.

Explicit memory   Information that can be consciously recalled and verbalized.

Expressive aphasia   A disorder of speech output.

Extended paraphasia   See **Word salad.**

Extended selective attention   Overly extended attentional focus and an inappropriate delay in shifting attention. The anomaly is considered one of the causative factors in the symptoms of autism.

Extradural hematoma   Less frequent than the subdural hematoma, a bleed that occurs between the skull and the dura. Extradural hematomas are most likely caused by a tearing of the large middle meningeal arteries.

Extrapyramidal motor system   Responsible for stereotyped postural and reflexive motor activity. The system also acts to keep individual muscles ready to respond.

False positive   Also known as a *Type I error* or *false alarm*. Refers to a case in which a neuropsychological test erroneously indicates the presence of a pathologic condition.

Familial sinistrality   The degree of left-handedness within the nuclear and extended family.

Femorocerebral angiography   Angiography that introduces a catheter into the arterial system via the femoral artery.

Festinating gait   The rapid, shuffling gait characteristic of Parkinson's disease.

Fetal alcohol effect (FAE)   A developmental disorder that involves the cognitive and behavioral deficits associated with FAS, but without the physical stigmata of FAS. Also see **Fetal alcohol syndrome.**

Fetal alcohol syndrome (FAS)   A developmental disorder caused by the pregnant mother ingesting alcohol. The disorder is characterized by recognizable physical stigmata, neurologic abnormalities, and cognitive and behavioral impairments. Unlike many of the congenital disorders, FAS is preventable.

Fibers   See **Tracts.**

Finger agnosia   Inability to recognize or orient to one's own fingers.

Fissure   A very deep sulcus in the cortex.

Flicker fusion rate   Denotes the speed at which two separate visual images appear to fuse visually into a single image.

Flourens, Pierre   (French, 1794–1867) The foremost early advocate of an alternative to localization theories.

Fluent aphasia   A disorder of speech in which the patient remains able to talk, but his or her speech makes no sense, often sounding like some unknown foreign language.

Fluid functions   Believed to be culture-free and independent of learning. Problem solving and abstract reasoning are considered fluid functions.

Fluid intelligence   Novel reasoning and the efficiency of solving new problems or responding to abstract ideas.

Fluorescent in situ hybridization (FISH)   A laboratory technique in which a DNA probe is labelled with a fluorescent dye to detect chromosomal abnormalities.

Focus-execute attention   The ability to respond and pick out the important elements or "figure" of attention from the "ground" or background of external and internal stimulation. Also implies a measure of concentration or effortful processing.

Focused attention   A form of selective attention involving the restriction of attention to a specific feature, or set of features, to the exclusion of other features.

Fontanelles   Literally "small springs or fountains"; membranous gaps between the bony skull plates that are evident in newborns.

Foramen of Magendie   The middle opening, of three, of the membranous roof of the fourth ventricle, allowing the cerebrospinal fluid to flow outside the brain and recirculate.

Foramen magnum   The largest of the foramina; provides a large median opening in the occipital bone for the spinal cord to pass through to the brainstem.

Foramen of Monro   See **Interventricular foramen.**

Foramina   More-or-less symmetric orifices in the base of the skull that provide passage for nerves and blood vessels.

Foramina of Luschka   The two lateral openings, of three, of the membranous roof of the fourth ventricle, allowing the cerebrospinal fluid to flow outside the brain and recirculate.

Forebrain, or **prosencephalon**   The topmost division of the developing brain.

Fornix   A structure of the limbic system that contains nearly 1 million fibers; it rises out of the hippocampal complex and arches anteriorly under the corpus callosum. The fornix relays information to the mammillary bodies.

Fossae   Conspicuous ridges in the base of the skull that hold the brain in place.

Fragile X   A genetic disorder frequently associated with mental retardation and other cognitive deficits and distinctive physical features. The disorder is related to a compression or break of the X chromosome.

Freud, Sigmund   (Austrian, 1856–1939) Best known as the founder of psychoanalysis and the father of clinical psychology. Freud's initial love was neurology and investigating the secrets of the central nervous system.

Frontal lobe   One of the four cortical lobes; contains the primary motor cortex and the prefrontal lobe. Its functions are motor processing and executive, including planning, inhibition, and formulation of behavior.

Frontal operculum   Broca's area.

Functional systems   A concept first formulated by Luria in which behavior results from interaction among many areas of the brain.

Functioning adenomas   Pituitary tumors that play an "uninvited" role in the operation of the pituitary gland, often affecting the release of the gland's hormones.

Galen   (A.D. 129–201) Roman anatomist and physician who identified many of the major brain structures and described behavioral changes as a function of brain trauma.

Gall, Franz   (1758–1828) Austrian anatomist who postulated that mental faculties were innate and related to the topical structures of the brain.

Gamma-aminobutyric acid (GABA)   One of more than 20 amino acids, GABA is a neurotransmitter known to have strong inhibitory properties.

Ganglia (singular, *ganglion*)   A strategic collection of nerve cells in the peripheral nervous system.

Generalized seizure   A seizure caused by an abnormal rhythm of the entire brain; formally known as "grand mal"; bilaterally symmetric episodes characterized by a temporary lack of awareness, or what appears on observation to be a complete loss of consciousness.

Gerstmann-Straussler-Scheinker syndrome (GSS)   An extremely rare familial Creutzfeldt–Jakob disease variant that results in a "fatal insomnia."

Geschwind, Norman (1926–1984)   American neurologist who proposed that behavioral disturbances were based on the destruction of specific brain pathways that he called *disconnections.*

Gigantocellular tegmental field (GTF)   Located in the higher pons; appears to generate brain waves. Left unchecked, the neurons fire spontaneously, producing a high level of activity. One particular set of discharges is termed *PGO spikes* because they travel from the pons (P) to the lateral geniculate (G) nucleus of the thalamus and to the occipital (O) cortex.

Gilles de la Tourette syndrome   See **Tourette's syndrome.**

Glasgow Coma Scale (GCS)   A three-item scale often used in the medical setting to assess the severity of coma. The GCS ranges from 3 to 15 points, with lower scores indicating severe coma and higher scores suggesting a confusional state.

Glia   Greek meaning "glue"; glia cells outnumber neurons and provide supportive structure and metabolic function to the neuron.

Glioblastoma multiforme (GBM)   A particularly destructive and fatal glioma.

Gliomas   A type of brain tumor, gliomas are a relatively fast growing brain tumor that arises from supporting glia cells. Gliomas are the most common infiltrative brain tumor, which make up approximately 40% to 50% of all brain tumors. The term *glioma* is often used to describe all primary, intrinsic neoplasms of the brain and the spinal cord.

Globus pallidus   A structure of the basal ganglia.

Glutamate   One of more than 20 amino acids, glutamate is the major excitatory neurotransmitter of the brain.

Golgi, Camillo   (1843–1926) Italian physician who made the discovery in the early 1870s that silver chromate stained dead neurons black. This allowed people to visualize individual neurons for the first time.

Gonadotropins   Hormonal substances that stimulate the functions of the testes and ovaries.

Grading of tumors   A method of evaluating the malignant features of brain tumors. Grading is from 1 to 4, with a grade 1 tumor representing a slow-growing tumor accompanied by few neuropsychological deficits. Grades 2 and 3 represent intermediate rates of growth and neuropsychological dysfunction. Grade 4 tumors are fast growing and typically have a poor prognosis for recovery.

Grand mal seizure   Literally "big bad" seizure; consist of violent motoric abnormalities of stiffening and jerking episodes and the accompanying loss of consciousness.

Gray matter   Areas of the brain that are dense in cell bodies such as the cortex and that appear gray.

Gyri (singular, gyrus)   Ridges of the cortex between sulci.

Halstead–Reitan Neuropsychological Battery (HRNB)   The first neuropsychology laboratory in the United States was founded in 1935 by Ward Halstead at the University of Chicago. Halstead worked closely with neurosurgery patients and developed assessment devices that differentiated between patients with and without brain damage. Halstead later developed, with Ralph Reitan, the HRNB, which represented an empirical approach to the assessment of brain damage.

Hebb, Donald   Publisher of the classic *The Organization of Behavior: A Neuropsychological Theory.* This book brought much growth to the field of neuropsychology.

Hécaen, Henry French neuropsychologist (born 1912) who made important contributions to brain–behavior relations in health and disease, especially the role of the right hemisphere.

Hematoma The massive accumulation of blood within the cranium.

Hemianopia Also called *homonymous hemianopia;* half-blindness. Partial blindness on the same side, or visual field, of each eye. The partial blindness is not related to a malfunction of the eye, but to the brain connection to the occipital lobes. This problem is also attributed to unilateral damage to the right or left occipital lobes.

Hemiplegia The loss of voluntary movement to one side of the body, often as a result of stroke.

Hemispatial neglect A failure to attend to either the right or left visual field. Often associated with right, posterior brain damage.

Hemispheric asymmetry The differentiation in morphology and physiology of the brain between the right and left hemispheres.

Hemorrhage Type of stroke related to a significant bleed in the brain. Hemorrhages are the most severe form of stroke and often result in permanent brain damage or death.

Heraclitus Sixth century B.C. Greek philosopher who referred to the mind as an enormous space whose boundaries could never be reached.

Herpes encephalitis An infection that aggressively attacks the medial temporal and orbital frontal areas, resulting in the destruction of much of the limbic system, especially the hippocampus.

Heschl's gyrus A gyrus of the superior temporal lobes known as the *primary auditory cortex;* often larger in area in the right hemisphere because two gyri are often present. Plays a role in nonspeech and musical processing.

Hindbrain Also called *rhombencephalon;* the lower division of the developing brain.

Hippocampal commissure Minor intercerebral fibers.

Hippocampal formation A set of structures of the limbic system centered around the hippocampus; includes the hippocampus, dentate gyrus, and subiculum.

Hippocampus Anatomic brain structure of the limbic system thought to be involved in consolidating memory.

Hippocrates (460–377 B.C.) Greek physician who has been honored as the father of medicine, also shared the belief that the brain controlled all senses and movements. He was the first to recognize that paral-ysis occurred on the side of the body opposite the side of a head injury.

Homonymous Same-sided.

Homonymous hemianopia Same-sided half-blindness. Partial blindness on the same side, or visual field, of each eye. The partial blindness is not related to a malfunction of the eye, but to the brain connection to the occipital lobes. This problem is also attributed to unilateral damage to the right or left occipital lobes.

Horizontal plane A plane (*x*-axis) that shows the brain as seen from above or parallel to the ground.

Horseradish peroxidase (HRP) An enzyme, found in the roots of horseradish, that allows mapping of neuronal pathways using an axonal transport mechanism.

Human immunodeficiency virus (HIV) The HIV/ AIDS virus has a wide effect on the brain as it progressively destroys the immune system. The virus itself may have direct consequences for the brain. It also opens the brain to opportunistic infections and other diseases that can attack the brain.

Humors Medieval physicians believed that humors, body liquids, were influential in health and disease.

Huntington's disease (HD) Also called *Huntington's chorea.* A genetic, autosomal dominant progressive subcortical dementia that inflicts devastating motor impairment in the form of chorea, as well as cognitive decline on adults in the prime of their lives.

Hydrocephalus (HC) A condition in which the ventricles become abnormally enlarged, most often related to a problem with cerebrospinal fluid flow, production, or absorption.

Hyperacusis Abnormally high sound acuity that is often accompanied by low tolerance for loud sounds.

Hypercalcemia Elevated concentrations of calcium in the blood stream.

Hyperdensity Increased density of brain tissue that typically signals an abnormal density such as seen in tumor or bleeding.

Hyperlexia Early reading acquisition (decoding) without adequate comprehension. An anomaly exhibited by some children with developmental disorders, such as autism.

Hyperserotonemia Elevated or excessive levels of serotonin in the body.

Hypertonia Abnormally high muscle tone or strength.

Hypnagogic hallucinations Vivid, dreamlike intrusions into wakefulness; occur in the transition between wakefulness and sleep onset.

Hypodensity Low density of brain mass.

Hypogeusia Diminished taste sensitivity.

Hypokinesia   Reduced motor initiation; negative motor symptom of Parkinson's disease.

Hyposmia   Diminished smell sensation.

Hypothalamus   A structure of the diencephalon, part of the limbic system; considered instrumental in controlling the autonomic system. Activates, controls, and integrates the peripheral autonomic mechanisms, endocrine activity, and somatic functions, including body temperature, food intake, and development of secondary sexual characteristics.

Hypotonia   Abnormally low muscle tone or strength.

Hypoxia   The reduced oxygenation of brain. Hypoxia is typically not associated with cell death, but some possible interference in the functioning of the neuron. Hypoxia is usually related to inadequate breathing, such as experienced during sleep apnea, can occur at high altitude, or is related to carbon monoxide poisoning.

Ideomotor apraxia   See **Motor apraxia.**

Impact injury   A type of closed head injury in which the physical forces act on the brain tissue at the point of impact.

Impaired affective assignment   A failure to link the appropriate emotional meaning to both internal and external stimuli. Considered a key deficit of autism.

Implicit memory   Demonstrated by means whereby conscious awareness is not always necessary, such as implicit priming, skill learning, and conditioning.

Implicit priming   The phenomenon in which, if "primed" with three-letter word stems, people are more likely to complete the stem with a word they have already seen.

Infarction   A severe loss of blood caused by a blockage of an artery, often resulting in more lasting neuropsychological deficits.

Inferior   Toward the bottom, or below.

Inferior colliculi   Two elevations within the roof of the tectum, which serve as an important relay center for the auditory pathway.

Infiltrative tumors   Tumors that take over or infiltrate neighboring areas of the brain and destroy its tissue.

Inhibitory control   Inhibition of behavior through involuntary and voluntary neuropsychological processes. At a voluntary level, this capacity is considered an executive function and connotes the volitional capacity to withhold behavior, particularly when invoking environmental contingencies are evident.

Inhibitory postsynaptic potential (IPSP)   The presence of an ionic current flow that hyperpolarizes the postsynaptic neuron. As a result, a greater depolarization than normal is required for excitation and there is only a small probability that there will be an action potential.

Intelligence   The aggregate or global capacity involving an individual's ability to act purposefully, to think rationally, and to deal effectively with the environment.

Intelligence tests   Complex composite measures of verbal and performance abilities that are related partly to achievement (for example, factual knowledge) and partly to aptitude (for example, problem solving). Although there are well over 100 different tests of intelligence, the scales that David Wechsler developed have become widely used throughout the world and typically include a variety of scales measuring verbal-comprehension skills and tests tapping perceptual-organization abilities.

Intercerebral fibers   Connect structures between two hemispheres.

Interference control   The ability to screen or block out internal or external distractions that could intrude into and disrupt attentional focus.

Interictal   Between seizures.

Internal carotid arteries   Two of the four major arteries to the brain, supplying the anterior portions of the brain.

Interneurons   Neurons with short axons or no axons.

Interpretive hypotheses   Inferences about the patient's cognitive status that the neuropsychologist makes in the process of interpreting neuropsychological assessment data.

Interventricular foramen (foramen of Monro)   A small opening connecting the lateral ventricles.

Intracerebral   "Within the cerebrum" or brain.

Intracerebral fibers   Fibers that connect regions within one hemisphere.

Intracranial pressure (ICP)   Related to the presence of a bleed (or hemorrhage) within the cranium (skull) usually associated with the development of a space-occupying mass or pocket of blood, which may press on nearby brain structures, affecting their integrity.

Intraventricular hemorrhage (IVH)   Bleeding within the ventricles of the brain. A common cause of hydrocephalus in premature infants. Vessels in the area surrounding the ventricles rupture, and the blood and cellular debris obstruct the structures that allow for the reabsorption of the cerebrospinal fluid into the bloodstream.

Ions   Atoms or molecules that have acquired an electrical charge by gaining or losing one or more electrons. Four ions that are important in neuronal communication are sodium (NA⁺), potassium (K⁺), calcium (Ca⁺⁺), and chloride (Cl⁻).

Ipsilateral   On the same side.

Ischemia   A restriction or insufficiency of blood supply to an area of the brain, with possible damage or dysfunction depending on the duration of the ischemia. These events can also be short-lasting, with transient deficits.

Isochromosome   An abnormal karyotype characterized by identical arms on the X (female) chromosome. The chromosomal anomaly is associated with Turner's syndrome.

Jackson, Hughlings   British neurologist (1835–1911) who wrote on the integration of the localization and equipotentiality models of brain function. He suggested that behavior resulted from interactions among all areas of the brain, but that each area in the nervous system had a specific function that contributed to the overall system.

Jacksonian seizure   Involves motor areas; such events have been called marching seizures because they begin with jerking or tingling of a single body area and spread to other areas.

James–Lange theory of emotion   Promoted by American psychologist William James and Danish psychologist Carl Lange, postulating that emotion is consciously experienced as a reaction to physical sensory experience. In other words, we feel fear *because* our hearts are racing; we are sad *because* we are crying. Although critics saw this as an overstatement, the James–Lange theory did correctly insist that sensory and cognitive experiences were intimately entwined and could not be separated from each other.

Joint attention   The reciprocal attention evident in the interaction of individuals. Disruption of this interactional capacity of mother and child has been associated with autism.

Joint contractures   An abnormal shortening of the elastic tissue of a joint resulting in distortion or deformity.

Karyotype   A visual representation of an individual's chromosomes that displays the structural components and integrity of the chromosomes.

Kennard principle   A principle of neural recovery that bears the name of its originator, Margaret Kennard. The principle holds that earlier brain injury is associated with less impairment and better recovery of functions than injury occurring later in development. Subsequent clinical and experimental studies have not fully supported this principle.

Kinesthetic sense   A sense of one's physical body is supplied by a combination of vision, the vestibular organs, and the proprioceptive sense.

Kuru   A spongiform encephalopathy suffered by the Fore people of Papua New Guinea.

Lancisi, Giovanni   (1654–1720) Italian clinician who contributed greatly to the knowledge of aneurysm: abnormal blood-filled ballooning of an artery in the brain.

Lashley, Karl   (1890–1958) American neuropsychologist who was one of the first to combine behavioral sophistication in experiments with neurologic sophistication, thereby creating the field of experimental neuropsychology.

Lateral   Toward the side, away from the midline.

Lateral fissure   Separates the frontal and parietal lobes.

Lateralization   With *dominance,* refers to the differences in functional specialization between the two brain hemispheres.

Lesions   Derived from Latin *laesio,* meaning "to hurt"; any pathologic or traumatic discontinuity of brain tissue. Depending on their size and location, lesions result in minor or major behavioral effects.

Lewy bodies   Small, tightly packed granular structures with ringlike filaments, found within dying cells.

Lexicon store   A "storehouse" of words that an individual knows or understands.

Lezak, Muriel   American neuropsychologist who pioneered the assessment approach in clinical neuropsychology.

Limb-kinetic apraxia   A subtype of apraxia involving problems in executing precise, independent, or coordinated finger movements.

Limbic system   Includes the fornix; some brainstem areas, particularly the mammillary bodies of the hypothalamus; and specific basal forebrain structures, including the amygdala ("almond" because of its shape) and the septum.

Lissencephaly   See **Agyria.**

Localization theory   Assigns specific functions to particular places in the cerebral cortex.

Locus ceruleus   Located below the wall of the fourth ventricle, it has been implicated as an important norepinephrine pathway.

Longitudinal fissure   The space between the two hemispheres.

Long-term memory (LTM)   Theoretically of unlimited capacity and relatively permanent except for models suggesting that loss of information through forgetting is possible.

Lucid dreaming   The ability while dreaming to become conscious of that one is in a dream state.

Lumbar puncture   Also known as a *spinal tap;* a medical technique for collecting a specimen of cerebrospinal fluid surrounding the spinal cord for diagnostic study.

Luria, Alexander   (1902–1977) Russian neuropsychologist who was responsible for the most profound changes in the scientific understanding of the brain and mind.

Magnetic resonance imaging (MRI)   A visualization procedure that provides the most detailed images of brain structures. The advantage of functional MRI over other functional procedures, such as positron emission tomography, is that it provides good spatial resolution and images in short time periods, or "real time."

Magnetoencephalogram (MEG)   The magnetic equivalent of the electroencephalogram in which a three-dimensional magnetic field of the brain can then be calculated. Superconducting quantum interference device (SQUID) detects the small magnetic fields in the brain that are a marker of neural activity. A disadvantage of MEG is related to that it is expensive and not readily available for clinical applications.

Magnocellular visual system   One of the two visual systems that extends from the eyes to the visual cortex. It consists of large cells that are inferiorly located in the lateral geniculate bodies that are highly sensitive to movement, low contrast, and spatial location.

Magnus, Albertus   (German, ca. 1200–1280) De-emphasized the role of the ventricles in brain functioning.

Malignant tumors   Tumors whose cells invade other tissues and are likely to regrow or spread.

Malingering   The intentional exaggeration or presentation of neuropsychological symptoms.

Mammillary bodies   Two small nuclei on the floor of the posterior hypothalamus.

Masked facies   Used to describe the masklike expression of patients with Parkinson's disease.

Mass action   The extent to which behavioral impairments are directly proportional to the mass of the removed brain tissue.

Materialism   A theory that brain–behavior functions are produced by matter in motion, favoring a mechanistic view of the brain as a machine.

Mechanical receptors   Structures that transduce energy from touch, vibration, and the stretching and bending of skin, muscle, internal organs, and blood vessels.

Medial   Toward the middle/midline, away from the side.

Medial lemniscus   A white matter tract that courses through the contralateral side of the brainstem through the medulla, pons, and midbrain to be routed up through the thalamus (ventral posterior nucleus, VP) and on to the primary somatosensory cortex.

Medulla oblongata   Myelencephalon; a structure of the brainstem.

Medulloblastoma   A brain tumor seen most frequently in children; rapidly growing and very malignant; located in the inferior vermis close to the exit of cerebrospinal fluid from the fourth ventricle. This type of tumor accounts for about two thirds of all tumors in children and produces increased intracranial pressure caused by obstructive hydrocephalus.

Membrane potential   See **Resting potential.**

Meninges   Protective covering of the brain and spinal cord consisting of the pia mater, the arachnoid membrane, and the dura mater.

Meningiomas   Highly encapsulated, benign tumors that arise from the arachnoid layer of the meninges. Meningiomas represent approximately 15% of all brain tumors.

Meningitis   Inflammation of the meninges caused by bacterial infection or viral infection. It can progress quickly, within 24 hours, from a respiratory illness, with fever, headache, and a stiff neck, to changes in consciousness including stupor, coma, and death.

Mental rotation   Refers to the ability to mentally visualize and rotate forms, objects, or scenes in two- or three-dimensional space.

Mesencephalon   One of the five principal divisions of the brain, part of the brainstem.

Meta-analysis   A statistical technique designed to analyze the results from a number of different and independent studies. The technique allows for the identification of significant relationships and outcomes.

Metacognition   A higher order cognitive ability that enables an individual to examine and analyze the manner in which he or she thinks, solves problems, encodes and retrieves information, and performs cognitive operations.

Metacognitive awareness   An ability to monitor one's own behavior and performance.

Metastasis   A form of tumor spreading in which tissue from a malignant tumor "travels" to other organs in the body through the bloodstream. The capacity for metastasis is a characteristic of all malignant tumors. Metastatic brain tumors typically originate from sites other than the brain, most frequently the lung or the breast.

Metastatic tumors   Growths that arise secondarily to cancerous tumors that have their primary site in other parts of the body, such as the lungs, breasts, or the lymphatic system. The secondary growths arise because cancer cells from the primary neoplasm detach and travel to other sites through the blood system.

Metencephalon   One of the five principal divisions of the brain, part of the brainstem.

Microcephaly   A congenital disorder characterized by an abnormally small head in relation to the rest of the body. The head is more than two standard deviations below the average circumference for a child of a similar age and sex. The size of the brain is also subnormal, and the condition is associated with mental retardation.

Microglia   Small cells within the CNS that undergo rapid proliferation in response to tissue destruction, migrating toward the site of injured or dead cells, where they act as scavengers and metabolize tissue debris.

Micrographia   Small handwriting; a common motor symptom of Parkinson's disease.

Midbrain (mesencephalon)   The middle division of the developing brain.

Middle cerebral artery   Resulting from half of the division of an internal carotid artery, it supplies the lateral hemisphere and most of the basal ganglia of its corresponding cerebral hemisphere.

Migraine stroke   A rare type of stroke in which a transient ischemic attack, typically associated with classic migraine, is severe enough to cause a stroke.

Migratory process   A phase of prenatal central nervous system development characterized by the movement of neural cells along the wall of the neural tube to genetically predetermined locations.

Mild cognitive impairment (MCI)   Implies an intermediary, and perhaps transitional, stage between normal aging and dementia.

Mind-blindness   A neuropsychological deficit in which an animal's behavior suggests that it can "see" objects—that is, the test subjects do not bump into the object—but fail to recognize its significance (for example, as an object of fear).

Molecular cytogenic disorders   Disorders or diseases related to chromosome abnormalities (extra, missing, or rearranged).

Monopolar neurons   Unipolar neurons; neurons with a single axon.

Mosaic karyotypes   The presence of both structurally normal and abnormal female chromosomes that produces one form of Turner's syndrome.

Motor apraxia   Ideomotor apraxia; an inability to access a stored motor sequence or an inability to relay that information to the motor association areas. An example is the inability to show me how you would make a telephone call from beginning to end.

Motor neurons   Neurons responsible for contracting muscles or changing the activity of a gland.

Motor perseveration   The act of continuing in the same motor behavior, or constantly selecting it in the presence of other choices.

Move attention   A cognitive-attentional operation involving the shifting or movement of attentional focus from one stimuli to the next.

Multi-infarct dementia   A dementia caused by multiple small strokes or ischemic attacks.

Multipolar neurons   Neurons with more than two axons.

Munk, Hermann   (German, 1839–1912) Found that experimental lesions in the visual association cortex produced temporary mind-blindness in dogs.

Muscarinic choline   One of two main subtypes of acetylcholine, a neurotransmitter known to stimulate receptors.

Myelencephalon   One of the five principal divisions of the brain; part of the brainstem.

Myelin   A lipid sheath that surrounds and insulates the axons of the central and peripheral nervous systems. It serves to increase the speed of nerve conduction.

Myelin sheath   Fatty-type covering of axons that increases the speed of axonal transmission.

Myelin staining   Selectively dyes the sheaths of myelinated axons. As a result, white matter, which consists of myelinated axons, stains black, unlike other areas of the brain that consist mostly of cell bodies and nuclei.

Myoclonic seizures   Manifest in arrhythmic bursts of jerky motor movements that usually do not last more than a second and tend to occur in clusters over a short period.

Narcolepsy   A disorder that consists of irresistible daytime "sleep attacks"; a central nervous system disorder of the region of the brainstem that controls and regulates sleep and wakefulness. The primary symptom of this disorder is excessive daytime sleepiness.

Necrosis (or neuronal cell death)   A direct result of a critical interference with the cellular metabolism of the neuron. In general, a period of 4 to 6 minutes of anoxia may cause necrosis.

Neologism   Atypical language characterized by the generation or production of words that are meaningless.

Neoplasm   Literally "new tissue." The neurologic term for tumor.

Neostriatum   This structure, also known as the *striatal complex,* includes the caudate and putamen and receives projected information from cortical sensory areas. From the neostriatum, information is then funneled through the globus pallidus, then on to the thalamus, where it projects to the premotor and prefrontal areas.

Nerves   A large collection of axons located in the peripheral nervous system, primarily composed of white matter.

Neural tube   The embryonic tube that develops into the central nervous system, specifically the brain and spinal cord. The neural tube develops during the third week of gestation. Abnormalities in neural tube development can lead to congenital developmental disorders.

Neurofibrillary tangles   Excessive collections of tau proteins resembling entwined and twisted pairs of rope within the cytoplasm of swollen cell bodies in the brain. These are pathologic markers of Alzheimer's disease.

Neurogenesis   The congenital process by which the neurons of the brain develop.

Neurologic examination   A routine introductory evaluation performed by a neurologist—a physician who has specialized in evaluating and treating neurologic disorders. Although there are many variations, in principle, the neurologic examination involves a detailed history of the patient's medical history and a careful assessment of the patient's reflexes, cranial nerve functioning, gross movements, muscle tone, and ability to perceive sensory stimuli.

Neuromas   Tumors or new growths that are largely made up of nerve cells and nerve fibers.

Neuronal ectopias   Also known as "brain warts." An abnormal placement and development of neural cells often associated with a disruption of the migratory phase of brain development.

Neurons   Specialized nerve cells that allow complex information exchange.

Neuropsychological evaluation   Involves a detailed examination, often using standardized tests, to describe an individual's cognitive strengths and weaknesses. Often used in conjunction with other pertinent information, for diagnosis, patient management, intervention, rehabilitation, and discharge planning.

Neuropsychological tests   Traditionally defined as those measures that are sensitive indicators of brain functioning.

Neuropsychology   The study of the relations between brain functions and behavior; specifically, changes in thoughts and behaviors that relate to the structural or cognitive integrity of the brain.

Neurotransmitters   Chemicals that influence neuronal behavior.

Neurotrophins   Neuron-feeding nutrients.

Neurulation   The congenital process involving the formation and closure of the neural tube that subsequently develops into the brain and spinal cord.

Nicotinic choline   One of two main subtypes of acetylcholine, a neurotransmitter named after nicotine (from tobacco, *Nicotiana tabacum*), a bitter-tasting alkaloid that stimulates receptors.

Nissl, Franz   (1860–1919) German histologist who discovered in the 1880s that a simple dye can stain the cell bodies in neurons. The Nissl method is particularly useful for detecting the distribution of cell bodies in specific regions of the brain.

Nocioceptors   Derived from Latin *nocere,* meaning "to hurt." Receptors that serve as monitors to alert the brain to damage or threat of damage. They can be mechanical or chemical but are specifically activated by potentially damaging stimulation such as heat or cold, painful pressure or pricking, or chemical damage such as exposure to noxious chemicals.

Nocturnal myoclonus   Restless leg syndrome; twitching of muscles that occurs during non–rapid eye movement sleep. In severe cases, this will wake up the subject.

Nodes of Ranvier   Regular gaps along the axon where the myelin is interrupted.

Noncommunicating hydrocephalus   See **Obstructive hydrocephalus.**

Nondeclarative memory   Knowledge that is implicit and inaccessible to conscious recall or verbalization. This form of memory is demonstrated through performance (e.g., riding a bicycle).

Nonfluent aphasia   A difficulty in the flow of articulation, so that speech becomes broken or halting.

Nonfunctioning adenomas   Benign neoplasms of the pituitary gland.

Noninfiltrative tumors   Invasive tumors; encapsulated and differentiated (easily distinguished from brain tissue); cause dysfunction by compressing surrounding brain tissue.

Nonobstructive hydrocephalus   Also referred to as *communicating hydrocephalus.* A form of hydrocephalus produced by blockage that disrupts reabsorption of cerebrospinal fluid into the bloodstream.

Norepinephrine (NE)   A neurotransmitter that is important to the regulation of mood, memory, hormones (via the hypothalamus), cerebral blood flow, and motor behavior.

Normal distribution   A frequency distribution in which the values or scores group around a mean. In neuropsychological testing, many test scores display such distributions.

Normal-pressure hydrocephalus (NPH)   A neurologic condition involving ventricular enlargement in the absence of elevated intracranial pressure. Most frequently evident in older adults and characterized by a triad of progressive neurologic signs (postural imbalance, dementia, and urinary incontinence).

Normative data   These data compare the patient's score on a test to an expected score, or norm. The expected test score is determined from the performance of a normative sample of patients and control subjects.

NREM sleep (non–rapid eye movement sleep)   Includes sleep stages 1 through 4.

Nuclei (singular, nucleus)   A strategic collection of nerve cells in the central nervous system.

Nuclei of the raphe   A collection of neurons located throughout the midline of the brainstem; implicated in serotonin pathways.

Nucleus basalis of Meynert   Named after its discoverer; a collection of neurons implicated in Alzheimer's disease.

Nucleus reticularis thalami (NRT)   A group of neurons within the thalamus that regulates oscillatory behavior of the thalamocortical loop.

Object permanence   A cognitive capacity described by the developmental psychologist Jean Piaget, which is initially absent in the infant, but subsequently develops. The infant is unable to store in memory a representation of an object that is removed from view. In essence, what is out of sight is "out of mind."

Objective personality tests   Typically use the questionnaire technique of measurement (for example, true/false or multiple-choice questions).

Obsessive-compulsive disorder   A psychiatric disorder characterized by recurrent thoughts or images (obsessions) that are intrusive and anxiety producing which prompt or compel overt or mental behaviors (compulsions) to reduce this anxiety. Although obsessive-compulsive behaviors are viewed by the patient as irrational and excessive, this awareness does not alter the symptoms.

Obstructive hydrocephalus   Also referred to as *noncommunicating hydrocephalus.* A form of hydrocephalus produced by obstruction within the ventricular system of the brain. The obstruction can be a consequence of congenital malformation, tumors, or scarring.

Obstructive sleep apnea   Apnea that occurs most often during rapid eye movement sleep when either the upper airway collapses, not allowing air to pass, or the body weight of the patient on the chest compromises respiratory effort.

Occipital lobe   One of the four cortical lobes, primarily dedicated to visual processing.

Occipital notch   Sulci within the medial occipital lobe.

Occupational therapy   Rehabilitation specialty that focuses on improving self-care activities such as grooming, bathing, dressing, and feeding, as well as activities concerned with a person's occupation and avocation.

Oligodendrocytes   A type of non-neural cell; the projections of the surface membrane of each such cell fan out and coil around the axon of neurons in the central nervous system to form the myelin sheath.

Oligodendroglioma   A rare, slowly growing tumor that mostly affects young adults and is derived from and composed of oligodendrogliocytes.

Optic gliomas   A slowly growing glioma of the optic nerve or optic chiasm; associated with visual loss and loss of ocular movement.

Orientation   A patient's basic awareness of himself or herself in relation to the world around.

Orthotic   Customizable cognitive adjunct, such as a computer, used in rehabilitating people with brain injury.

Overcorrection   An aversive behavior modification technique that involves having a child practice a positive response that is incompatible with an inappropriate behavior. Overcorrection is particularly effective in reducing self-stimulating and other inappropriate behaviors.

Palilalia   Compulsive word or phrase repetition.

Pallidotomy   A surgical treatment for Parkinson's disease; in this technique, the ventral, or internal portion, of the globus pallidus is lesioned via heat coagulation of the neurons.

Papez circuit   Anatomic circuit centered around the hippocampus; plays a role in declarative memory processing.

Papillae   Bumps on which lie from one to several hundred taste buds consisting of between 50 to 150 taste receptor cells.

Paragrammatism   See **Word salad.**

Parahippocampal gyrus   Structure of the limbic system.

Parasympathetic nervous system   Division of the autonomic nervous system; functions to store energy by facilitating functions such as digestion through gastric and intestinal motility.

Parental imprinting disorders   Also known as genomic imprinting. A child receives two sets of chromosomes, one set from the mother, and the other from the father. The expression of the genes in each set is in accordance with the parent of origin. If the child receives both sets of chromosomes from the same parent, there will be a loss of expression of the genes of the other parent. This abnormal imprinting has been associated with several neurodevelopmental disorders.

Paresthesia   Spontaneous crawling, burning, or "pins and needles sensation."

Parietal lobe   One of the four cortical lobes, concerned with the integration of information from sensory areas.

Parkinson's disease (PD)   A progressive disease process characterized by a dopamine deficiency of the substantia nigra; results in resting tremors and allied motor symptoms; may cause a subcortical dementia.

Parkinsonism   A behavioral syndrome marked by motor symptoms including tremor, rigidity, and slowness of movement.

Partial seizure   A seizure caused by an abnormal rhythm confined to a particular brain area; also known as *focal seizures;* always begins as a local neuronal discharge; the most common type of seizure.

Parvocellular visual system   One of the two visual systems extending from the eyes to the visual cortex. It consists of small cells dorsally located in the lateral geniculate bodies that are sensitive to viewing stationary objects, high contrasts, and fine spatial details.

Pathognomonic signs   Neurologic symptoms from which a specific diagnosis can be made.

Pathways   See **Tracts.**

Pattern analysis   Examines the relations among the scores in a test battery.

Penetrating head injury   A type of head injury associated with a penetrating mechanism such as a bullet from a gun, a knife, or scissors.

Penfield, Wilder   Famous neurosurgeon who made advancements in the understanding of the relation between brain anatomy and behavior.

Peptides   A group of neurotransmitters, peptides are short chains of amino acid. More than 60 neuroactive peptides have been identified.

Perception   The process of "knowing"; depends on intact sensation.

Peripheral nervous system (PNS)   The PNS includes all the portions of the nervous system outside the central nervous system. The PNS consists of the somatic and the autonomic nervous systems.

Peripheral neuropathy   Peripheral nervous system dysfunction causing sensory loss (as in diabetes).

Personality tests   Measures of such characteristics as emotional states, interpersonal relations, and motivation.

Petit mal seizure   Literally "little bad" seizure; causes an altered state of consciousness but lacks the violent physical loss of control seen during the grand mal seizure.

Phantogeusia   Experience of a phantom or hallucinatory taste.

Phantom limb pain   A feeling of pain in a nonexistent limb.

Phantosmia   Experience of a phantom or hallucinatory smell.

Phenylketonuria (PKU)   A genetic disorder affecting the metabolism of phenylalanine. If untreated, mental retardation and other cognitive deficits can result. Dietary control, particularly if started early, can reduce or eliminate the negative effects of the disorder.

Phonemic paraphasias   Errors of word usage of similar-sounding words (for example, using the word *bark* for *tarp*).

Phonologic awareness   The awareness of and ability to differentiate between individual phonemes or speech sounds.

Phonologic processing   The application of codes for translating letters and letter sequences into the appropriate speech–sound equivalents. Deficits in this processing have been linked to dyslexia.

Phrenology   An obsolete theory proposing that if a given brain area was larger in an individual, then the corresponding skull at that point should be enlarged, indicating a well-developed area of the brain. Conversely, a depression signaled an underdeveloped area of the cortex. Phrenology involved, in its most popular form, the reading of cranial bumps to ascertain which of the cerebral areas were largest.

Physiatry The medical specialty of combining physical medicine and rehabilitation.

Physical therapy A rehabilitation specialty that focuses on improving motor control and physical functioning.

Pia mater Literally "pious mother"; a vascularized part of the meninges that directly adheres to the surface of the central nervous system.

Pinealoma A type of tumor of the pineal body.

Pituitary adenoma Tumors of the pituitary gland that are often classified into functioning (changing the secretion of the pituitary gland) and nonfunctioning (benign).

Pituitary stalk Also known as the infundibular stalk. It is the axon bundle extending from the hypothalamus to the posterior region of the pituitary. This connection mediates the release of oxytocin and antidiuretic hormone directly into the bloodstream.

Pituitary tumors Tumors that arise from the pituitary gland. It is traditional to divide pituitary tumors into functioning and nonfunctioning adenomas.

Planum temporale Region of the posterior surface of the temporal lobes between the Heschl's gyrus and the Sylvian fissure. The planum temporale of the left hemisphere is involved in mediating phonologic processing and language comprehension.

Plasticity Behavioral or neural ability to reorganize after brain injury.

Platelets Disk-shaped cells found in the blood of all mammals. They are important for their role in blood coagulation and are produced in large numbers in the bone marrow. From there they are released into the bloodstream, where they circulate for approximately 10 days.

Plato (Greek, 420–347 B.C.) Suggested that the soul can be divided into three parts: appetite, reason, and temper. Plato also discussed the concept of health as being related to the harmony between the body and the mind. Thus, he has been credited as being the first to propose the concept of mental health.

Pluripotentiality The multiple, functional role of the brain. That is, any given area of the brain can be involved in relatively few or relatively many behaviors.

Polymicrogyria A congenital disorder that can be traced to a disruption of the structure of the developing brain during the fifth to sixth month of gestation. As a consequence of this disruption, the gyri fail to develop appropriately. On inspection, the gyri are found to be small and crowded together. Learning disorders, mental retardation, epilepsy, and other neuropsychological anomalies are linked to the disorder.

Pons Metencephalon; a "bridge" resembling two bulbs, a structure of the brainstem.

Porencephaly A congenital disorder of brain formation in which cystic lesions are on the surface of the brain.

Positron emission tomography (PET) A visualization technique that tracks blood flow, which is associated with brain activity. It is mostly used to assess brain physiology, including glucose and oxygen metabolism, and the presence of specific neurotransmitters.

Posterior Toward the back or tail.

Posterior attention system One of the attentional systems of the brain that mediates visuospatial orienting and is supported by the parietal, midbrain, and thalamic regions.

Posterior cerebral arteries Formed by a division of the basilar artery.

Posterior communicating arteries Arise from the internal carotid arteries and connect the middle and posterior cerebral arteries.

Postictal phase Phase in which the person gradually emerges into full consciousness; follows the seizure episode.

Post-traumatic amnesia (PTA) A patient's memory of events surrounding an accident.

Pragmatics of language Aspects of language that extend beyond the literal.

Precursor or **progenitor cells** Early cells lining the neural tube that proliferate to create the neurons and glia cells of the brain.

Prefrontal motor cortex Section of the frontal lobe. This area is considered to be the "conductor" or "executor" of the brain. Also called *prefrontal cortex.*

Premorbid functioning The cognitive and neuropsychological status occurring before the development of disease or trauma.

Premotor area (PMA) See **Premotor cortex.**

Premotor cortex Also known as *premotor area.* Located in Brodmann's area 6 of the frontal lobes; receives neuronal input from posterior parietal areas, secondary somatosensory areas, and cerebellum; plays a role in motor planning and sequencing, and may aid in the procedural aspects of carrying out motor plans.

Prepotent response   A response that has been "primed" to occur through reinforcement, repeated use, habit, or reflex.

Prestriate cortex   See **Secondary association.**

Primary motor cortex   Part of the frontal lobe, concerned with the initiation, activation, and performance of motor activity.

Procedural memory   Memory that is usually implicit and is demonstrated via performance. Procedural memory's domain is that of rules and procedures rather than information that can be verbalized, although procedural memory has not been clearly operationally defined and includes a hodgepodge of tasks such as motor skill learning, mirror reading, and verbal priming.

Process approach   Also known as the "hypothesis approach"; based on the idea that each examination should be adapted to the individual patient. Rather than using a standard battery of tests, the neuropsychologist selects the tests and procedures for each examination, based on hypotheses made from impressions of the patient and from information available about the patient. As a result, each examination may vary considerably from patient to patient for length and test selection.

Prodromal phase   A phase before the seizure, in which an aura occurs; odd, transient symptoms such as nausea, dizziness, or numbness may occur, as well as sensory alterations or hallucinations in any sensory domain.

Progenitor cells   See **Precursor cells.**

Projection fibers   Neurons that connect sets of brain structures to each other (e.g. subcortical structures to the cortex and vice versa).

Projective personality test   Tests that rely on relatively ambiguous, vague, and unstructured stimuli, such as inkblots.

Proprioception   The position of the body in extrapersonal space. Sensory dysfunctions that result in proprioceptive disorders include altered sense of bodily sensation and bodily position.

Proprioceptive disorder   Loss of body position sense.

Proprioceptors   Derived from Latin *proprius,* meaning "one's own"; structures on skeletal muscles that detect movement via degree of stretch, angle, and relative position of limbs. Proprioceptors on the hands help identify the shapes of objects via touch.

Prosencephalon   See **Forebrain.**

Prosody   An aspect of speech that conveys meaning through intonation, tempo, pitch, word stress, fluency, and rhythm. It augments the meaning of spoken language and is important in communicating the emotional content of language.

Prosopagnosia   The special case of inability to recognize people by their faces.

Prospective memory   The intention to remember to perform an action in the future.

Prosthetic   Cognitive replacement, such as a computer, used in the rehabilitation of people with brain injury.

Proximal   Near the trunk or center, close to the origin of attachment.

Pruning   The process of eliminating excessive neurons and synapses in the developing brain. The elimination appears to reflect a purposeful "sculpting" of the brain to promote neural efficiency.

Pseudopsycopathy   Also known as "acquired sociopathy." The emergence of uninhibited and poorly modulated behavior, poor judgment and violation of social norms following orbitofrontal damage. Unlike the true psychopath or sociopath, the patient with orbitofrontal damage experiences remorse for inappropriate actions and does not demonstrate the intentional viciousness or planning with regard to committing antisocial acts.

Psychology   The study of describing, explaining, predicting, and modifying behavior.

Psychometrics   The science of measuring human traits or abilities. Concerned with the standardization of psychological and neuropsychological tests.

Psychomotor epilepsy   See **Temporal lobe epilepsy.**

Purkinje cells   A specific type of neuron that is found in the cerebellum. The dendrites characteristically spread out in one plane.

Putamen   Structure of the basal ganglia.

Pyramidal cells   A specific type of neuron that is found in all areas of the cerebral cortex. These cells have bodies that are pyramidal or conical in shape.

Pyramidal motor system   This system originates in the cerebral cortex and controls voluntary movement.

Pythagoras   (ca. 580–500 B.C.) Greek scholar who suggested that the brain is at the center of human reasoning and plays a central role in the "soul's life."

Receptive aphasia   A difficulty in auditory comprehension. Also see **Wernicke's aphasia.**

Receptor cells   Receptor cells detect numerous stimuli, including sight, sound, pressure, pain, chemical irritation, smell, and taste. Not technically neurons, although they create energy that is transduced into an electrical stimulus that is carried to neurons and then processed in the brain.

Receptor sites   Sites on the postsynaptic neuron to which neurotransmitters are delivered.

Reductionism   Investigating complex phenomena by dividing them into more easily understood components. Related to brain research, reductionists argue that behavior is no more than the results of chemical and structural relation among neurons.

Refractory period   A recovery period after a neuron has fired. During this period, which lasts one or more milliseconds, the neuron resists re-excitation and is incapable of firing.

Reliability   The stability or dependability of a test score as reflected in its consistency on repeated measurement of the same individual. A reliable test should produce similar findings on each administration.

REM sleep   Rapid eye movement sleep; state of sleep where dreams occur.

Remote memory   Memory for long-past events.

Response cost   A behavioral modification technique that involves removing or taking away an already present positive reinforcer contingent on the display of a specific undesirable behavior. The technique is used to inhibit or suppress a specific behavior.

Response inhibition   Three interrelated control processes: (1) stopping an ongoing response, (2) blocking or screening out distractions, and (3) restraining a response primed for release.

Resting potential   Membrane potential; a slight electrical imbalance between the inner and outer surfaces of the membrane caused by the separation of electrically charged ions.

Resting tremor   Rhythmic shaking that often occurs in one hand first; positive motor symptom of Parkinson's disease; characterized as "pill rolling."

Restitution   One of two primary approaches to brain injury rehabilitation; stresses the retraining of an impaired skill in the hope that the brain can rebuild axonal connections through retraining.

Reticular activating system (RAS)   Also called *reticular formation;* a neural network located within the lower brainstem transversing between the medulla and the midbrain. Functions in nonspecific arousal and activation, sleep and wakefulness.

Retrograde amnesia   In this disorder, the patient has no recollection of the interval preceding the injury; the loss of old memories before an event or illness.

Retrograde degeneration   The degeneration of the axon back to the cell body, once the axon has been damaged. This process may lead to cell death.

Rhinencephalon   Evolutionarily old "smell brain."

Rhombencephalon   See **Hindbrain.**

Rigidity   Tightening of muscles and joints; positive motor symptom of Parkinson's disease.

Ring X karyotypes   A relatively rare karyotype that is associated with one variant of Turner's syndrome. Mental retardation frequently occurs in this form of Turner's syndrome.

Röntgen, Wilhelm Conrad   (1845–1923) Physicist who made a remarkable discovery that an invisible ray that, unlike heat or light waves, could pass through wood, metal, and other materials. This ray, also called X-ray, gave rise to radiology.

Rostral   Toward the head.

Saccadic eye movements   Quick eye movements made when the eye moves from one point of fixation to the next.

Sagittal plane   Derived from Latin *sagitta,* meaning "arrow." A plane (*z*-axis) that shows the brain as seen from the side or perpendicular to the ground, bisecting the brain into right and left halves.

Savant skills   Extraordinary skills possessed by an individual who otherwise displays limited capacity. For example, the ability of a retarded child to mentally calculate complex square roots is a savant skill.

Schwann cells   Type of non-neural cells. The projections of the surface membrane of each of those cells fan out and coil around the axons of neurons in the peripheral nervous system to form myelin sheaths.

Secondarily generalized seizure   A simple seizure that crosses the corpus callosum and eventually involves the entire brain.

Secondary association   Prestriate cortex; processes primary features of visual information such as light wavelength, line orientation, and features of shape.

Secondary motor cortex   Functions in strategic planning of the specific aspects of movement. The intention to move is also a function of this area.

Seizures   Massive waves of synchronized nerve cell activation that can involve the entire brain. Seizures may have dramatic behavioral manifestations, including uncontrolled muscles contractions, changes in perception, and alterations in mood and consciousness.

Semantic memory   Memory for information and facts that have no specific time-tag reference.

Senile plaques   Also called *neuritic plaques.* Round aggregates of beta-amyloid that on disintegration leave holes and misshapen neurons where there once were active connections.

Sensation The elementary process when a stimulus has excited a receptor and results in a detectable experience in any sensory modality.

Sensitivity How sensitive a test is in measuring a particular neuropsychological construct.

Sensory association area An area of the cortex that functions to integrate information from different sensory areas.

Sensory neurons Neurons that respond directly to changes in light, touch, temperature, or odor.

Septum In general, refers to a thin plate of brain tissue separating two cavities or tissue areas. The septal area stretches between the fornix and the corpus callosum, forming one of the walls of the frontal horn of the lateral ventricle. The septal area interconnects with the hippocampus and the hypothalamus.

Serotonin A neurotransmitter that is involved in sleep, depression, memory, and other neurologic processes.

Sex chromosomes A chromosome that determines the sex of a person. Humans have two sex chromosomes, X and Y, with the former determining female sexual characteristics, and the latter, male sexual characteristics. A male is defined by the pairing of XY chromosomes, and a female, by the pairing of XX chromosomes.

Shifting attention An element of attention involving the movement of attentional focus from one stimuli or task to another.

Short-term memory (STM) Memory of limited capacity (7 ± 2 bits of information); degrades quickly over a matter of seconds if information is not held via a means such as rehearsal or transfer to long-term memory.

Shunt A medical procedure to drain excessive cerebrospinal fluid from the ventricular system to the stomach. The procedure is used with people who have acquired hydrocephalus.

Simple seizures Focal events that may involve sensorimotor expression or psychic expression (mood, emotion, altered consciousness).

Simulation A form of malingering in which the patient is faking or exaggerating an illness or the severity of the symptoms, usually to gain some secondary gain (such as attention, hospitalization, or a financial settlement).

Single-gene disorders A disease or disorder that is due to a mutation of a single gene. An example of a single gene disorder is Tay-Sachs disease.

Single-photon emission computed tomography (SPECT) A visualization technique that measures blood flow, a correlate of brain activity. Because it takes the radioactive tracer almost 2 days to be eliminated from the body, SPECT cannot be used to monitor the brain's mental activity "moment to moment."

Sleep apnea Derived from Greek *a pnoia,* meaning "negative breathing"; refers to breathing that is disturbed while sleeping and often completely stops for periods as long as a minute.

Sleep apnea syndrome A serious sleeping disorder resulting from frequent episodes of apnea.

Sleep paralysis Momentary paralysis on awakening or at sleep onset; the body is totally unable to move for seconds to minutes.

Social emotional learning disability Disturbed socioemotional behavior that is directly related to neuropsychological processing deficits and does not reflect a secondary reaction to a learning disability such as dyslexia.

Sodium–potassium pump An active transport system across the membrane of the axon that exchanges three sodium ions for every two potassium ions.

Somatic nervous system (SNS) That part of the peripheral nervous system that provides "voluntary" neural control with the external environment. Communicates with the central nervous system through spinal and cranial nerves.

Somatopic organization Organization that follows the distorted figure of the sensory homunculus mapped onto the primary somatosensory cortex, which represents the relative importance and distribution of touch in various areas of the body rather than the actual size of the body part.

Somatosensory cortex Structure found in the anterior portion of the parietal lobe, concerned with primary tactile sensory processing.

Somatosensory system Body system that involves two types of sensory stimulation, external and internal. The somatosensory system can monitor sensations such as cold and heat, whether the sensation comes from the handling of an ice cube or from a fever. So the system processes external stimulation of touch (pressure, shape, texture, heat) in recognizing objects by feel and is also concerned with the position of the body in extrapersonal space (proprioception).

Spatial perception Refers to the ability to mentally visualize forms, objects or scenes in two- or three-dimensional space.

Specificity   A factor in setting a cutoff score on a test. Neuropsychological tests with high specificity examine specific aspects of neuropsychological functions; that is, they are not correlated with other tests or factors.

Speech apraxia   See **Dysarthria.**

Speech therapy   A rehabilitation specialty that focuses on communication difficulties such as deficits in speech production, understanding speech, reading, and writing.

Spina bifida   A congenital developmental disorder characterized by an opening in the spinal cord, commonly found in the lower region of the cord. The disorder is a consequence of a failure of the posterior end of the neural tube to close during gestation.

Spinal cord   Part of the central nervous system that acts as the conduit for the majority of sensory and motor information to and from the body.

Spurzheim, Johann   (1776–1832) Austrian student of Gall; lectured extensively on phrenology in the United States.

Stable attention   An element of attention referring to the consistency of attentional performance over time.

Standard battery approach   In this approach, the same tests are given to all patients, regardless of the clinician's impression of the patient or the referral question. Typically, a technician gives the tests and administers them according to standardized rules of procedures.

Standardized test   A task or set of tasks administered under standard conditions. Designed to assess some aspect of a person's knowledge or skill. Standardized psychological tests typically yield one or more objectively obtained quantitative scores, which permit systematic comparisons to be made among different groups of individuals regarding some psychological or cognitive concept.

Stem cells   Undifferentiated cells; they do not yet have either an identified or specialized function. They eventually differentiate into the building blocks of tissues and organs.

Stenosis   Narrowing of an artery.

Striatal complex   This group of structures includes the caudate and putamen and receives projected information from cortical sensory areas. From the striatum, information then funnels through the globus pallidus, then on to the thalamus, where it projects to the premotor and prefrontal areas. Also see **Neostriatum.**

Striate cortex   A collection of brain structures involved in the motor system named after their striped or striated appearance. It is located in the most posterior aspect of the occipital lobes, but a major portion of it extends onto the medial portion of each hemisphere. Also see **Striatal complex.**

Striatum   A collection of brain structures (including the caudate nucleus and the putamen) involved in the motor system; named after their striped or striated appearance. It is located in the most posterior aspect of the occipital lobes, but a major portion of it extends onto the medial portion of each hemisphere.

Stroke   A neurologic event, also known as *cerebrovascular accident (CVA),* that always occurs in the brain and is the most common type of cerebrovascular disease.

Stuck-in-set perseveration   Maintenance of a problem-solving approach when changing demands signal the need for an altered or modified approach or response.

Subarachnoid hemorrhage   Occurs when a blood vessel on the surface of the brain bursts and blood flows into the small cavity that surrounds the brain, the subarachnoid space.

Subarachnoid space   Space containing cerebrospinal fluid; below the arachnoid membrane.

Subcallosal anterior cingulate   The subcallosal gyrus covers the inferior aspects of the rostrum of the corpus callosum. It continues posteriorly as the cingulate and parahippocampal gyrus. It is considered part of the limbic system of the brain.

Subcortical   Below the cortex.

Subcortical dementia   Dementia that primarily affects subcortical areas of the brain; characterized by slowness of cognitive processing, executive dysfunction, difficulty retrieving learned information, and abnormalities of mood and motivation; examples include Parkinson's, Huntington's, and Creutzfeldt–Jakob diseases.

Subdural hematoma   Bleeding into the subdural space; often encountered after a head injury.

Subdural space   The space between the dura and the arachnoid parts of the meninges.

Sublenticular nuclei   Nuclei of the extended amygdala, a forebrain continuum, that projects into the centromedial amygdala.

Substantia nigra   Structure of the basal ganglia. A collection of neurons and nuclei known to be important dopamine pathways.

Substitution   One of two primary approaches to brain injury; focuses on searching for adaptations to the person's environment in the context in which they will be used.

Subthalamic nucleus   Structure of the basal ganglia.

Sudden infant death syndrome (SIDS)   Death caused by the cessation of breathing during sleep.

Sulci (singular, sulcus)   Valleys formed by infolding of the cortex.

Superior   Toward the top or above.

Superior colliculi   Two elevations within the roof of the tectum functioning as important reflex centers for visual information.

Superior sagittal sinus   Large sinus of the brain.

Supplementary motor area   Located on the dorsal and medial portion of each frontal lobe; functions as a motor sequencer and planner. It receives input from the somatosensory strip and the basal ganglia.

Suprachiasmic nucleus (SCN)   A nucleus of the hypothalamus, hypothesized to be a biological clock that calibrates the sleep/wake cycle.

Supravalvar aortic stenosis (SVAS)   An acquired or congenital condition in which there is a narrowing of the aortic value impeding the flow of blood from the left ventricle to the arteries. The resulting cardiac problem can be life threatening.

Surface dyslexia   A developmental or acquired reading disorder characterized by impaired whole-word reading, but preserved phonological skills.

Sustained attention   The ability to maintain an effortful response over time. A form of attention involving the maintenance of attentional focus over time. Sometimes referred to as "time-on-task performance," or "behavioral persistence."

Sydenham's chorea (SC)   A neurologic movement disorder characterized by chorea of the face, neck, trunk, and limbs; diminished muscle tone and strength; and psychological disturbances, especially obsessive-compulsive behaviors. The disorder frequently affects children and adolescents after a streptococcal infection (a beta-hemolytic). It has been proposed that the disorder is caused by an abnormal autoimmune response to the streptococcal bacteria that reacts against the basal ganglia. The disorder often resolves spontaneously, and treatment is generally reserved for severe or chronic cases.

Sylvian aqueduct   See **Cerebral aqueduct.**

Sylvian fissure   The large fissure separating the frontal from the temporal and parietal lobes.

Sympathetic nervous system   Division of the autonomic nervous system that mobilizes the energy necessary for psychological arousal in response to, or anticipation of, a stressful event based on the "fight-or-flight" response. Sympathetic activation includes an increase in blood flow, blood pressure, heart rate, and sweating, and a decrease in digestion and sexual arousal.

Synapse   The tiny gap between the terminal button and the receptors of the two neurons. Neurons communicate through synapses. The anatomic location of this communication is known as the *synapse.*

Synaptic knobs   Ends of neurons that have characteristic swelling to increase the area of contact with the postsynaptic neuron.

Synaptic vesicles   Oval structures within the terminal that typically cluster close to the presynaptic membrane and where neurotransmitters are synthesized.

Synaptogenesis   The developmental process by which the synapses and dendrites of the brain form.

Tachyphemia   Segmented accelerated bursts of speech.

Tactile agnosia   Also called *astereognosis;* a disorder in which there is an inability to recognize objects by touch.

Tactile extinction/suppression/inattention   Suppression of touch sensation on one side of body.

Tardive dyskinesia   A disorder with Parkinson-like symptoms, including writhing movements of the mouth, face, and tongue, often develops in schizophrenics after long-term medication use.

Tectum   "Roof"; structure of the midbrain.

Tegmentum   "Covering"; a structure of the midbrain that surrounds the cerebral aqueduct.

Telencephalon   Also called the *endbrain;* one of the five principal divisions of the brain; consists of the two cerebral hemispheres, which are connected by a massive bundle of fibers, the corpus callosum.

Temporal lobe   One of the four cortical lobes, concerned with the reception and interpretation of auditory information; also plays a role in memory.

Temporal lobe (psychomotor) epilepsy   A form of seizure originating from the temporal lobe; emotional symptoms often present (such as changes in mood).

Tensile strength   The amount of physical, longitudinal stress that an axon can withstand before it ruptures.

Teratogen   Any agent that disrupts the normal development of the embryo and fetus.

Terminal buttons   Also called *axon terminals.* The site of interneuronal contact, where neurochemical information is transmitted from one neuron to another.

Teuber, Hans-Lukas   (American, 1916–1977) Credited for first using the term *neuropsychology* in a national forum during a presentation to the American Psychological Association in 1948.

Thalamus A structure of the diencephalon, an important sensory relay station.

Thalotomy A surgical treatment for Parkinson's disease and other disorders causing tremor; used to attack tremor by lesioning the thalamus.

Theory of mind The cognitive capacity to understand, attribute, and predict the mental state of others, and the relation of these mental states to behavior. Deficits in this capacity have been observed in autistic children and other developmental disorders.

Therapeutic recreation An approach to treatment that emphasizes the importance of recreational and leisure time activities in brain injury rehabilitation, to help in the "transfer" of learning. Therapeutic recreation also allows patients to begin socializing with each other in a structured, but less formal, atmosphere than that afforded in other therapy settings.

Thermoreceptors Receptors that serve as monitors to detect heat and cold throughout the body.

Thrombosis A type of occlusion in which a clot or thrombus (Greek meaning "clot") forms in an artery and obstructs blood flow at the site of its formation. This is the most common form of stroke and accounts for approximately 65% of all cerebrovascular accidents.

Tonic Motorically stiffened.

Tonotopic map Projected onto the auditory cortex in a manner similar to the retinopic mapping of the visual system. Because the cortical bands can respond to multiple frequencies, there is no strict one-to-one correspondence, but bands are more attuned to certain frequencies than others.

Tourette's syndrome A tic disorder defined by multiple involuntary motor and vocal tics. The disorder appears familial in origin. The cause is unclear, but dysfunction of the basal ganglia has been implicated. Also called *Gilles de la Tourette syndrome*.

Tracts Also known as *pathways* or *fibers*. Large collection of axons located in the central nervous system. Primarily composed of white matter.

Transduction Derived from Latin *transducere*, meaning "to lead across." An environmental stimulus activates a specific receptor cell, and this energy is transduced into an electrical stimulus, which is then carried to neurons to be processed by the brain.

Transient ischemic attack (TIA) A temporary (transient) lack of oxygen (ischemia) to the brain, which may cause a time-limited set of neuropsychological deficits. TIAs are technically not considered a stroke, because neuronal death typically does not occur.

Transtentorial herniation Associated with high intracranial pressure and generalized swelling of the brain. As a result, the brain is displaced downward.

Tremor Involuntary shaking, usually of a limb, tremors may be resting or occur with intentional movement.

Trephination An ancient procedure in which small holes were scraped or cut into the skull deliberately for either surgical or mystical reasons.

Tumor The morbid enlargement or new growth of tissue in which the multiplication of cells is uncontrolled and progressive. The tumor growth is often arranged in nonorganized ways, does not serve any functional purpose, and often grows at the expense of surrounding intact tissue.

Turner's syndrome (TS) A syndrome characterized by a failure to develop secondary sexual characteristics, short stature, webbed neck, and cubitus valgus. It is caused by an anomaly in the X chromosome (female).

Ultradian rhythm Ninety-minute cycles of heightened and lowered brain arousal observed throughout the wake/sleep cycle.

Ultrasonography A procedure for imaging the internal structures of the body by introducing and recording the reflection of high-frequency sound waves.

Utilization behavior A characteristic behavior of *environmental dependency syndrome* that involves the tendency to grasp and use objects that are within reach. The use of the object is in accordance with its function, but inappropriate for the situation. It is often associated with bilateral frontal damage.

Uvulopalatopharyngoplasty (UPPP) The removal of the uvula, the small, fleshy tissue hanging from the center of the soft palate, which may relax and sag, obstructing the upper airway. A surgical approach to the treatment of sleep apnea.

Validity The validity of a test is the meaningfulness of the test scores. Validity gauges whether a specific test really measures what it was intended to measure. There are different types of validity: construct, content, and criterion validity.

Vascular system The blood supply system of arteries and veins.

Ventral Toward the belly. The bottom of the brain is ventral in humans.

Ventricles Four interconnected, fluid-filled cavities in the brain.

Ventricular localization hypothesis   Theory that postulated that mental and spiritual processes were located in the ventricular chambers of the brain.

Ventricular system   Four interconnected, fluid-filled cavities in the brain.

Vermis   A structure of the cerebellum; two large, oval hemispheres connected by a single median portion.

Vertebral arteries   Two of the four major arteries to the brain, supplying the posterior portions of the brain.

Vertebral column   The bony structure that extends from the cranium to the coccyx and encloses the spinal cord.

Vesalius, Andreas   (1514–1564) Belgian-born anatomist who advanced neuroanatomy through continual dissections and careful scientific observations.

Vestigial ovarian streaks   A failure of gonadal development characteristic of Turner's syndrome. Reproductive cells are evident in the gonads of Turner's syndrome embryos but begin to deteriorate late in fetal development. By early childhood, the gonads consist only of fibrous streaks.

Vigilance attention system   One of the attentional systems of the brain that mediates sustained attention.

Visual agnosia   Inability to recognize a person or object by sight.

Visual cortex   The cerebral cortex of the occipital lobe of the brain that is responsible for vision.

Visual object agnosia   Failing to recognize objects at all, or in milder cases, confusing objects if they are observed from different angles or in different lighting conditions.

Visuospatial sketch pad   A working memory "slave system" that manipulates visual and spatial images.

Vitalism   A theory that suggests that behavior is only partly controlled by mechanical or logical forces.

Vocational inventories   Tests that measure opinions and attitudes indicating an individual's interest in different fields of work or occupational settings.

Wada technique   Also known as the *Wada test,* after its developer. Similar to the angiogram in that it places a catheter, typically in the left or right internal carotid artery. Then sodium amytal, a barbiturate, is injected, which temporarily anesthetizes one hemisphere. In this way, neuropsychologists can study the precise functions of one hemisphere whereas the other one "sleeps." Also called the *intracarotid sodium amytal procedure (IAP).*

Wada test   A technique for determining language lateralization and memory functions that involves anesthetizing one cerebral hemisphere, and then presenting cognitive tasks to the patient. The process is then repeated with the other hemisphere. Impaired performance of the cognitive tasks specific to the anesthetized hemisphere suggests the lateralization or presentation of language/memory functions in that hemisphere.

Wernicke, Carl   (German, 1848–1904) Announced that the understanding of speech was located in the superior, posterior aspects of the temporal lobe. Wernicke noted that a loss of speech comprehension due to damage in this area was not accompanied by any motor deficit; only the ability to understand speech was disrupted.

Wernicke's aphasia   Damage to the left hemisphere auditory processing areas results in the partial or total inability to decipher spoken words. This condition is also known as *receptive aphasia.*

Wernicke's area   A structure that includes the secondary auditory cortex and is located on the posterior aspect of the superior temporal gyrus. It is responsible for auditory processing of speech.

Wernicke–Korsakoff's syndrome   A disorder associated with memory function of the limbic system, typically observed in severe alcoholics who show multiple nutritional deficiencies. Such patients may develop a confusional state over time, as well as severe new-learning and motor difficulties.

White matter   Myelinated axons. Areas of the brain that are mostly made up of myelinated axons, such as neuronal tracts and pathways, which are characteristically white in appearance.

Williams syndrome (WS)   A neurodevelopmental disorder characterized by a recognizable pattern of dysmorphic facial features, cardiovascular and physical abnormalities, mental retardation, a specific cognitive profile, and a distinct personality.

Willis, Thomas   (1621–1675) English anatomist best known for his work on the blood circulation of the brain.

Word salad   Unconnected words and word sounds. This feature of Wernicke's aphasia is a deficit in placing words together in proper grammatical and syntactical form. This condition is more formally known as *paragrammatism* or *extended paraphasia,* and it is characterized by running speech that is logically incoherent, often sounding like an exotic foreign language.

Working memory   A concept introduced by Alan Baddeley, also referred to as *short-term memory,* or "working on memory." Working memory directs the temporary storage of information being processed in any range of tasks from reading to math to problem solving. It includes the concepts of the central executive, the articulatory phonologic loop, and the visuospatial sketch pad.

X-rays A type of light ray that is useful for clinical work of various parts of the body, because they show the presence and position of bones, fractures, and foreign bodies. A clinical disadvantage of X-rays, and specifically X-ray films of the brain, is that there is little differentiation between the brain structures and the cerebrospinal fluid, making the clinical use of this procedure ineffective.

Zangwill, Oliver (1913–1987) British neuropsychologist who contributed significantly to an understanding of the nature of neuropsychological deficits associated with unilateral brain disease or injury.

ANSWERS TO
CRITICAL THINKING QUESTIONS

CHAPTER 1

How does localization brain theory differ from equipotentiality brain theory? What are the lasting contributions of each theory?

Localization brain theory assumes that detailed brain processes in specific anatomic locations cause specific mental processes. Phrenology is a good example of localization theory. Equipotentiality brain theory assumes that the brain functions more or less as a unit. One proponent of equipotentiality brain theory is Flourens, who suggested that the entire brain is greater than the sum of its parts. The lasting contribution of localization theory is that, indeed, some brain functions appear to be localized to a specific brain region. For example, Broca's area specifically controls verbal motor output. However, many functions, such as thinking and problem solving, do not appear to have a strict or precise anatomic representation in the brain. The lasting contribution of equipotentiality theory is the idea that redundancy may be built into the brain and that if one area of the brain is damaged, another area may be able to compensate for the function.

Has the quest for the search of the organ of the soul been completed?

Yes and no. Yes, the search for the organ has been completed. There is no question that the healthy brain gives rise to the mind and the soul. The question that is not yet answered is, How exactly does the brain accomplish this? Much has been learned from recent research involving neuropsychology and modern imaging technology, but the precise mechanism—that is, how the soul arises from brain matter—has remained elusive.

Why is Luria's functional model of the brain such an important step in understanding brain functions?

Luria combined both the localization and equipotentiality approaches to neuropsychology into one model. As with equipotential theory, Luria regards behavior as the result of an interaction of many different areas of the brain. As with localization theory, Luria also assigns a specific role to each area of the brain. In Luria's functional model, each function depends on the interaction of specific brain systems. Luria suggests that behavior is the result of the brain operating as a whole. At the same time, each area within the brain has a specific role in the formation of behavior. The importance of any one area depends on the behavior to be performed. This model has been useful in rehabilitating patients with neuropsychological disorders, such as stroke and brain trauma, where one function may be damaged, but another function may compensate for the loss.

CHAPTER 2

What are the differences among electrical, magnetic, and metabolic technologies in imaging?

Electrical measures record the electrical activity of nerve cells of the brain through electrodes attached to various locations on the scalp. This procedure, known as *electroencephalography (EEG),* is most sensitive to the actual firing rate of large collections of neurons. Magnetic imaging measures the concentration of the hydrogen nucleus, which is present in high concentration in biologic systems and generates a small magnetic field. This procedure is known as *magnetic resonance imaging (MRI).* With MRI researchers can accurately calculate brain tissue densities and can generate a computer-constructed anatomic representation. The imaging of brain metabolism provides a completely different approach to the examination of the brain. For example, measuring glucose metabolism is a direct correlate of neuronal activity and can lead to a clearer understanding of the functioning brain. Medical technologies that use this approach are single-photon emission computed tomography (SPECT) and positron emission tomography (PET).

Why is co-registration, that is, the use of multiple assessments using different technologies, an important advancement in neuropsychology?

A major advancement in imaging technology has been to merge different assessment technologies, such as the anatomic detail of MRI with the ability of PET to localize function using the imaging of brain metabolism. Such co-registration of different approaches has resulted in multimodal approaches to neuroimaging, often providing new insights, as well as corroborating established findings.

Which medical technology to examine your brain would you volunteer for? Why?

We personally do not mind having our brains imaged using different technologies. A risk is always associated with this, however, namely, that some previously unknown pathology may be detected, but those chances are relatively small. The only other risk, then, is the inconvenience of an invasive procedure. On a continuum from least to most invasive, those procedures are (in our opinion): radiography, EEG, EP, MRI, MEG, SPECT, PET, EMG, lumbar puncture, and angiography. Because MRI is relatively noninvasive but allows for precise anatomic pictures of the brain, it would be the procedure we would volunteer for first.

Will neuropsychology be outdated by the increased use of sophisticated brain imaging technology? Why or why not?
No. Modern imaging technologies and the study of neuropsychology are compatible. Certainly, the advances in modern imaging technology have been spectacular in showing the anatomy of the brain. Furthermore, the domains previously held by neurologists and that by neuropsychologists are getting much closer, and both disciplines have much to learn from each other. But neuropsychologists are bringing special knowledge to the area of brain research and are participating in the research using this technology because of their expertise in the functional aspects of neuroanatomic structures, their knowledge of neuropsychological tests, and their background in scientific methodology and design. Thus, neuropsychologists play an important role in providing functional assessments of patients with brain injuries. Neuropsychologists also diagnose conditions (such as concussions) that are not easily detected using modern imaging technologies, and they evaluate a patient's potential for adapting to a specific neurologic disorder, their capacity to work, and their quality of life.

CHAPTER 3

Why are the concepts of reliability and validity so important in psychological and neuropsychological assessment?
If a test is not repeatable, it is not reliable and thus can provide no consistent score on a specific dimension. Think of weighing yourself on a scale that gives you a different weight every time you step on it. Such a scale could not be trusted, could it? Validity is important because it relates to the meaningfulness of a psychological test score. What if a psychological measure of depression does not really measure depression, but something else, such as stress? Such a scale would not be an appropriate measure of depression. Let us go back to the example of the scale. This time it is reliable. (Remember, if a test is not reliable, it cannot be valid.) A scale would not be a valid measure for anything other than estimating weight. For example, you would not use the scale to determine the room temperature. This is the assumption of validity, that is, whether a psychological or neuropsychological test measures what it is intended to measure.

What kinds of questions and tests do neuropsychologists use in a neuropsychological evaluation?
Neuropsychologists use primarily standardized tests and questions in a neuropsychological examination. That is, they may use specific tests and scales that have questions that every subject receives more or less in the same way. As a result, the neuropsychologist knows what it means if a person does not know the answer to a particular set of questions. Neuropsychologists use many different tests, tasks, puzzles, and questions to get an overview of an individual's cognitive strength and weaknesses. Thus, it is not uncommon to have a battery of tests that include measures of memory, attention, intelligence, personality functioning, and so on. The neuropsychologist uses a specific set of

procedures to answer the referral question. For example, he or she may treat a referral question about diagnosis differently from a referral question about employment capacity, in terms of selecting neuropsychological tests.

How are neuropsychology assessment procedures the same? How are they different?
All neuropsychological assessment procedures are similar in that the same rules of reliability and validity apply. Also, almost all neuropsychological tests are given in a standardized format and environment, and are administered to the patient individually. They are different in that they measure different aspects of behavior. Tests can measure memory, problem solving, and attention, to name just a few aspects. Some tests measure personality functioning, adaptive skills, intelligence, vocational skills, and educational attainment. These types of tests are strictly not neuropsychological tests, even though they depend on brain functioning, because they are not sensitive indicators of cortical dysfunction. A test is considered to be a neuropsychological test if a change in brain function systematically relates to a change in test behavior.

What sort of recommendations and treatments can neuropsychologists give to brain-impaired people that will be useful in their daily lives?
How to make recommendations to individuals about their everyday lives has become an important issue in neuropsychological assessment. This is important because many neuropsychological tests appear to be somewhat abstract on the surface. For example, a test of driving capacity has not been developed yet, so neuropsychologists rely on traditional measures of attention, memory, and eye-hand coordination to make inferences about whether a person with brain injury should be allowed to drive. In addition to driving, there are many instances in which neuropsychologists can help their patients regarding activities that have a cognitive component, but are performed almost every day. Those activities can range from balancing a checkbook, going shopping, and finding one's way around, to more basic activities such as getting dressed, taking a bath, or brushing one's teeth. Neuropsychologists can determine which everyday tasks patients with brain injuries may have problems performing. Neuropsychologists then recommend what task may be strengthened through rehabilitation or through compensation of other intact skills. For example, if a right hemisphere patient has trouble finding his or her way around a hospital and often gets lost, the patient may learn specific right/left directions and also compensate by learning to ask bystanders for directions. The patient may also rely on a notepad that always reminds him or her what the destination is. Thus, neuropsychologists play an important role in treating and rehabilitating patients with brain injuries.

How do the two major approaches (process and battery) to interpreting neuropsychological data differ?
The two approaches are different in a variety of ways (see Table 3.4); therefore, it is almost a philosophical difference in terms of neuropsychological assessment. The principal difference is that the battery approach is a standardized approach to assessment,

whereas the process approach is a clinical analysis of a patient. The former is akin to having a patient undergo a series of tests and standardized questions to understand his or her abilities and deficits. The latter is based on the idea that each patient's presentation is so unique that it is of most importance to understand the unique problems for which the patient is seeking treatment, and thus to tailor the examination to the individual. The standard battery approach has evolved through empirical analysis and the extensive testing history of psychological testing. The process approach has evolved in the clinical setting. Although proponents of the process approach would disagree with this conclusion, research supporting the process approach is not as robust as the empirical foundation of the standard battery approach. As with many issues that are so polarized, most neuropsychologists borrow certain aspects from each approach in their own approach to neuropsychological assessment.

CHAPTER 4

Will it be possible one day to "map" the circuits of the human brain?

Various "mapping systems" of the brain are discussed in the chapters that deal with brain anatomy. Mapping systems generally have focused on major structures of the brain as they pertain to function, or to various "architectural" layers of the brain and cortex. From these the correspondence of various structures with their functions has been demonstrated. However, here we are asking about mapping brain circuits that revolve around neuronal pathways and interconnections. As discussed in this chapter, there are billions of neurons and glial cells with multiple connections. It has been estimated that the human brain performs more than 1 quadrillion operations per second, which is more than a thousand times faster than the current supercomputers. The shear size and power of the human brain still makes it the most complex structure in the known universe. Attempts at mapping circuitry of simple organisms, such as the honeybee, have been accomplished. So is this just a matter of scale that computing power will one day be able to conquer? The answer to this question also lies in considering that there are vast individual differences in the way each person's brain is "wired," and that brain communication networks can modify themselves and change with experience, development, and learning. Mapping the circuitry of the human brain is not only extremely complex, it is a moving target.

Actor Christopher Reeve suffered a severe spinal cord injury and died without fulfilling his pledge to walk again. What is the outlook for other people with paralysis caused by spinal cord injury?

Not long ago, the traditional wisdom on neuronal damage to the spinal cord presumed that little healing occurs once a neuron in the brain or the spinal cord has been damaged. At best, the process called *collateral sprouting*, which occurs in nearby intact neurons, might facilitate a functional reorganization. The complexities involved in the regrowth of neurons and their millions

of projections to other neurons are daunting. All these connections can be lost within a split second due to brain trauma. The likelihood that these connections regrow spontaneously was thought to be quite small. Although Christopher Reeve never walked again, through intensive rehabilitation aimed at keeping his muscles toned and moving his limbs as he normally would in walking or cycling, he did recover some sensation even after 5 years. Was this actual neuronal repair, regrowth, or functional reorganization? The answer is unknown. However, it is now known that some function can return long after what was previously believed. In addition, current research in neuronal repair, either through stem cell research or in coaxing CNS neurons to act like PNS neurons, is promising. The current outlook is much more promising for people with paralysis caused by spinal cord injury.

Is it possible for a drug to be effective if it does not activate a naturally occurring brain chemical receptor?

The human brain is affected not only by internally produced chemical messengers, but also by externally originating chemicals that find their way to the synapse. The discovery that the brain has receptors for endogenous opiates, such as endorphins, which produce similar behavioral responses as external opiates, provides the fodder for this question. Why do substances such as caffeine, cocaine, nicotine, and alcohol affect the brain? The nervous system has specific receptor sites that bind drugs such as nicotine and opiate compounds. Others may work because they are a close enough mimic, or act as a blocking agent. Certain drugs, however, are totally barred from the brain, and other substances require an active transport system to cross the blood–brain barrier. In general, drugs at the synapse either increase or decrease the likelihood of neuronal transmission. Therefore, drugs can exert their actions in various ways, but it appears that brain receptors must react to them even if they are not perfect mimics.

What scientific and ethical questions will need to be resolved for research into neuronal repair and neurogenesis to be successful?

Scientifically, the primary question pertaining to neuronal repair is, "What is different about the growth and repair mechanisms between a CNS and a PNS neuron?" Current research suggests that some characteristics of myelin may be part of the issue, and much attention has focused on this. Interestingly, because myelin is an issue, research in multiple sclerosis and spinal cord injury may help to inform each other. One of the main questions pertaining to neurogenesis is, "What causes neurons to grow and die?" Both of these issues raise many other questions such as, "At what developmental stage do neurons decide to quit replicating?" and "What are the adaptive and maladaptive implications of naturally occurring and induced neurogenesis?" Ethically, for treatment of injury and disease, the questions revolve around a debate between the extent that science could be helpful in intervening to find cures for diseases and disorders against the issues of using embryonic stem cells to advance the research. Unfortunately, the debate is often framed as an "either/or" question. Scientists and the public will benefit from creative ways to solve this problem if informed solutions and ethical decision making is encouraged.

CHAPTER 5

Why is an understanding of the stages and processes of brain development important to the neuropsychologist?

The stages and processes of brain development are important to the neuropsychologist for a number of reasons. First, knowledge of the stages and timing of brain maturation allows for the identification of emerging cognitive-behavioral functions. Second, a recognized association exists between specific disorders and disruption/retardation at specific stages of brain development. For example, lissencephaly (absence of cortical sulci and gyri) is caused by disruption of neural cell migration during the 11th to 13th week of brain development. This knowledge can increase our understanding of the etiologies of the disorders and potentially shape preventive interventions. Third, knowledge of the relation between brain maturation and behavior provides a yardstick for determining whether the child's observed behaviors are consistent with healthy brain development. Fourth, studies of the interplay between environmental influences and brain development allow for a determination of conditions that support, enhance, or retard cognitive-behavioral development. Finally, knowledge of the stages and processes of brain maturation can prompt the development of restorative and rehabilitative interventions for treating those who have suffered early brain injury.

If a child was born without the telencephalon region of the brain, would the child be able to orient to visual and auditory stimuli, perform reflexive movements, and sit up? Explain why or why not.

Removal of the telencephalon would result in the loss of the following brain structures: cerebral cortex, basal ganglia, limbic system, and olfactory bulbs. Despite this loss, the child would be able to orient to visual and auditory stimuli, demonstrate reflexive movements, and sit up because of the preservation of subcortical and spinal structures and systems. For example, automatic orientation to visual and auditory stimuli is supported by the superior and inferior colliculi, respectively, of the midbrain. In addition, the child would be able to perform most elementary functions such as ambulation, eating, drinking, and sleeping. However, the ability to link automatic movements to voluntary movements and to respond flexibly and adaptively to environmental demands would be compromised. Furthermore, the ability to provide meaning, value, emotion, and voluntary intent to behavior would be lost.

To what extent can behavioral functions be localized to specific brain structures?

The structures presented in this chapter represent important topographic features on which the various processing systems of the brain depend. Aspects of behavior can be attributed directly to many of these structures. In general, the structures described in depth here, such as the brainstem structures, are responsible for rudimentary aspects of behavior. Many of the structures are necessary for sustaining life, for controlling wakefulness and

sleep, and for controlling other drive states. As a general rule, more basic and fundamental aspects of behavior are more easily traced to specific structures. In the following chapters it will become evident that as behavior becomes more complex, there is a move from specific structure-function correspondence to an emphasis on larger functional systems that subserve the complexities of human behavior.

What level of brain mapping is most useful to the neuropsychologist?

When it comes to understanding the relationship of the human brain to behavior, mapping at the level of the cell or the neuron is usually considered too minuscule to provide an accurate picture of the complexity of human behavior. Also, some functions are basic and automatic, and of less interest related to their psychological functions, such as the role of CSF as a waste product remover. Finally, understanding the complex organization of the brain, as a whole, would not provide useful information for neuropsychologists, who are often asked to respond to questions such as, "What effect does an injury to the basal ganglia have on behavior?" or "If a person has poor motor coordination, which areas of the brain are most likely to be affected?" In general, researchers tend to think of behavior related to its function, so it is most useful to consider the brain structures and systems that relate to that function. In this chapter, basic structures were presented with ties to function. However, in the following chapters, more complex functions such as visual perception or memory, as well as more complex and interconnected systems within the brain, emerge as the most useful level in describing most human behaviors.

CHAPTER 6

How would you explain the functional differences between the right and left hemispheres?

Several points should be made when describing the functional differences of the two brain hemispheres. First, although generalizations can be drawn, it is important to remember that there are notable exceptions. For example, although speech is generally considered to be lateralized to the left hemisphere, some individuals possess bilateral or right-lateralized speech. Second, hemispheric functional differences relate to the interaction of a number of variables to include the nature of the stimulus (e.g., visual vs auditory), mental computations required (e.g., detail vs global processing), routine or novel nature of processing demands, and manner of task presentation. Third, hemispheric function is rarely "either/or"; that is, both hemispheres function in a complementary manner to support a given function. For example, the left hemisphere is typically involved in the verbal aspects of speech, while the right hemisphere provides the affective or prosodic aspects to speech. Fourth, there are indications that the left hemisphere is more proficient in linear, sequential, and rule-bound processing, whereas the right hemisphere shows greater proficiency in holistic, simultaneous, and integrative performance. However, other conceptualizations provide equally meaningful descriptions of the functional differences of the hemispheres. Finally, we await further research to clarify the functioning of the brain as a whole, as well as the individual contributions of the respective hemispheres.

Are there adaptive reasons why the cerebral hemispheres would gravitate toward either a bilateral or asymmetric organization? Explain.

Although science does not provide a definitive answer to this issue, to approach this question it is important to think about what factors lead to differences in hemispheric organization. One of these factors is handedness. About 90% of the population is right-handed, with a tendency toward left hemisphere dominance for speech. Another factor is sex. Sex hormones affect brain organization starting during fetal development. Women tend to be more bilaterally organized than men. Considering these two factors, it is interesting to speculate whether, for example, men needed to have more lateralized brains for stereotypically "male" activities such as visuospatial abilities, and women needed to have more bilaterally organized brains for stereotypically "female" activities such as superior language function. And what advantages might right-handers have, if any?

What ecologic or evolutionary factors could account for the advantage of males in visuospatial abilities?

From an evolutionary perspective, a number of hypotheses have been posed to account for the advantage of male relative to female individuals in visuospatial abilities. Each of these hypotheses has met with criticism and countering interpretations. The hunter role of early man has been posed as a reason for the advanced visuospatial performance of the male sex. Specifically, the use of weapons (such as throwing a spear to kill game) is hypothesized to account for the visuospatial proficiency of the male sex. Another hypothesis that relates to the hunter role of early man proposes that the distances that hunters would have to travel in the pursuit of game would facilitate the development of visuospatial abilities. Similarly, wars throughout the ages (early clans through modern wars) have generally been fought by men, experiences that may have served to reinforce the development of spatial abilities. From an early age, male and female individuals encounter different socialization experiences regarding their roles as male or female. Male individuals are more likely to involve themselves in play involving active and spatially related activities. Whether this preference is solely a function of socialization continues to be an area of debate. However, it is clear, from a historical perspective, that the male sex has been expected to show more interest and involvement in play and work activities (e.g., sports, construction) that emphasize visuospatial abilities. Thus, male individuals have been provided greater exposure, experience, and training in visuospatial activities. As the distinction between male and female roles with regard to academic, vocational, athletic, and other life pursuits become less distinct (and limiting), it would be expected, from a socialization perspective, that the difference between male and female visuospatial abilities would be reduced or eliminated.

CHAPTER 7

In what ways do the study of sensory-perceptual and motor disorders inform us about intact brain functioning? In what instances might the study of damaged brains lead us astray?

The study of patients with damaged brains has provided important clues to the workings of brain systems. For example, by examining patients with lesions in Broca's or Wernicke's areas, or damage to area V4 (occipital cortex), functions of language and vision, respectively, have been mapped. However, this strategy can lead to erroneous information in that a lesioned area does not always "contain" the function, but it may, instead, act as a "cable" in the network that serves to join two or more functions.

Do conditions such as phantoms, neglect, and synesthesia represent altered states of consciousness? Explain.

Phantoms, such as phantom limbs, appear as sensory-perceptual "hallucinations." A neglect patient can show a total unawareness of the left side of the body and even deny the ownership of a limb. A synesthete can feel jaggedness when eating chocolate. These examples appear to be distortions from the "norm" of conscious awareness. Yet, these deviations of "reality testing" are not labeled as psychotic processes. Why not? Perhaps the most interesting fact here is the variations one can experience in conscious awareness. And for some, such as synesthetes, the melding of sensory perceptions may have constituted a "nornal" reality since birth.

Does intact motor processing require intact sensory-perceptual processing? Explain.

Consider the example of speech presented in this chapter. To what extent does speaking require the ability to understand speech? This chapter discusses the extent to which expressive speech is damaged in those with Wernicke's aphasia. Would this be more or less of a problem in a child who is born with a difficulty in understanding speech? Do you think this is the case in all sensory modalities? Can you think of any exceptions?

CHAPTER 8

What does the neuropsychology of sensory-perceptual processing have to contribute to the idea that there is an objective reality related to object perception?

This question is the fodder for philosophical debate. However, from a neuropsychological point of view, consider that the chapter began by saying, "The range of what humans can detect is unique to our species." The sensory detectors of other species may result in detection of different stimuli or experiences in a wider or narrower range than for humans. For example, many animals do not detect color, but can detect faint smells or have visual acuity that is far superior to humans. Whose actuality is real? Even if this question is limited to human experiences, consider that being "objective" implies being unbiased by personal experience. Sensory information comes in fragments; for example, an object's name, the intensity of pain, or the pleasantness of a smell must be attached at secondary and higher processing centers. At each level of processing, more aspects of interpretation are required. So, are there aspects of sensory perception where general agreement can constitute objective reality? Where would you draw a line between the seeming "realness" of sensation and the "personal experience" of perception?

How might it be possible to imagine or conjure up images in all sensory domains despite a lack of sensory input?

Although the mechanisms are not fully understood, it is known that one can have a sensory illusion or hallucination in any sensory domain. This most commonly occurs with psychiatric illnesses such as schizophrenia. In schizophrenia, the most common type of hallucination is auditory. This question also foreshadows a future discussion of consciousness to be presented in Chapter 16, which discusses seizures and epilepsy. Abnormal brain firing in regions concerned with sensory functioning often produces a sensory aura before a seizure. This may be an odd taste or smell, a tingling feeling in a part of the body, or unusual visual or auditory sensations. Thus, the brain can produce sensory "feeling" without external input. In the case of normal brain functioning, does this also happen? Take dreaming, for example. When you sleep, you conjure up visual images with your eyes closed. How does this happen? (Look ahead to Chapter 16.)

Can one be "conscious" in one sensory domain but not in another?

Yes. This chapter explores the example of neglect. Unilateral neglect is a condition in which the impaired individual loses "conscious awareness of an aspect of spatial or personal space despite adequately functioning sensory and motor systems." Also, in any type of agnosia, by definition, there is a "not knowing." Chapter 7 introduces this term and states that agnosia can occur in any sensory domain. Thus, for example, astereognosis is an inability to recognize or "know" objects by touch. Chapter 7 also discusses smell and taste agnosias. This chapter discusses language and vision. Although when discussing language we do not refer to a hearing agnosia but rather aphasia, the idea is the same. If damage occurs to a specific area, it is possible to lose conscious awareness in just one sensory domain while retaining a sense of meaning or awareness in the other sensory modalities.

CHAPTER 9

Do the higher cognitive functions discussed in this chapter represent more intelligent thought processes than those functions discussed in previous chapters? Explain.

The implication is that "higher" cognitive processes indicate the pinnacle of intellectual functioning, given that we often equate abstract and complex thought with the highest levels of human achievement. This may well be the case from the human point of view. Can you think of examples to dispute this statement from what you have read in previous chapters?

The memory, attention, and executive function systems interact. How would you explain this interaction?

Memory, attention, and executive function represent relatively distinct processes, although in some cases, disagreement exists whether a particular attentional or memory process is better classified as an executive function (e.g., working memory). Clearly, these processes are interrelated, but specifying the exact nature of this interrelation remains to be defined and specified. Nonetheless, some agreement exists that executive functions represent overarching controlling, organizing, integration, and supervisory computations. Attention and memory processes are subject to varying degrees of executive orchestration depending on the nature and type of attention and memory processes involved. From a neuroanatomic perspective, memory, attention, and executive functions are served by relatively distinct yet interconnected and overlapping neural systems. Furthermore, the interrelation of these functions is evident when one realizes that executive functions would be of little value if memory and attentional systems were not present. Jointly, attention, memory, and executive functions play a central role in thinking, reasoning, language, visuoconstruction skills, and sensorimotor and perceptual motor skills. Finally, attentional systems are necessary for the processing of relevant ongoing and novel events, memory systems for the symbolic maintenance of these experiences over time, and executive functions for the generation, guidance, and evaluation of behavior necessary to attain future goals (Eslinger, 1996).

Do disorders of executive functioning represent a greater disability for humans than sensory-perceptual and motor disorders? Why or why not?

Although some may answer unequivocally yes, it can also be argued that with sensory-perceptual and motor disorders, the building blocks of functioning may be so compromised that intact higher functions may not be able to be expressed adequately. What arguments can you make for each case?

Do emotions represent a higher cognitive function or a lower basic function? Explain.

In many ways, emotions represent the most basic of functions evolutionarily. Fear, anger, and other primary emotions are shared with the most primitive of creatures. We included emotions in the chapter on higher cognitive functioning because in humans, the interpretation and higher perception of emotions, particularly social emotions, by the cortex requires a high degree of cortical processing.

Are there advantages to multiple brain memory systems as contrasted to a single memory system?

Since it is highly unlikely that a single brain memory system could accommodate all the different types and processes of memory that have been identified, there are clear advantages to multiple brain memory systems. That is, differential memory systems allow for the support of a wide range of memory forms and computations. Furthermore, multiple memory systems are potentially an asset if an individual suffers injury to a neural network that supports a relatively specific memory system. Although this would result in the disruption of certain memory functions, other forms of memory supported by the uninjured memory systems would be preserved. Also, the knowledge of which memory systems are compromised and which are unimpaired provides the neuropsychologist with a framework for developing individualistic rehabilitation interventions.

CHAPTER 10

In light of the devastating effects of many of the genetic and chromosomal disorders, do you think that potential parents should seek genetic counseling before having children? Explain.

Genetic and chromosomal disorders can have devastating effects on the developing brain and other body systems of the child. Many of these disorders are not currently detectable before the child's conception, so genetic counseling would not necessarily prevent their occurrence. Fortunately, only a small percentage of children are afflicted. However, it is advisable that individuals with family histories of genetic/chromosomal disorders or of ethnic or regional origins often associated with specific disorders such as Tay-Sachs disease, seek genetic counseling.

In recent years, an increasing number of teratogens have been identified in the environment. Are our children at greater risk for brain anomalies than children of earlier generations? Why or why not?

An increasing number of teratogens have been identified, suggesting, at first glance, greater risk to our children. Although many of these teratogens have been present for years, the injurious effects to the unborn child have only recently been recognized. The identification of previously existing and new agents helps reduce birth defects by prompting appropriate control, avoidance, or elimination of these agents. Ideally, greater attention should be given to identifying and regulating potential teratogens before they are released into the environment. Unfortunately, identifying and regulating teratogens does not necessarily prevent their impact on our children. For example, the intrauterine teratogenic effects of alcohol have been documented for years; yet, children affected with FAS/FAE continue to be born.

What steps can be taken to prevent FAS?

The use of alcohol is an established fact in our society, and moderate use does not necessarily lead to deleterious effects. Unfortunately, some women fail to make the necessary modifications in drinking patterns when pregnant because they lack awareness or understanding of the potential effects of alcohol consumption on the developing child. In other cases, women continue drinking because alcohol consumption is a lifestyle preference or because they are struggling with alcoholism. Improving prevention would involve increasing public awareness of FAS, starting with early and appropriate education provided by medical agencies, schools, social agencies, and public health alerts. Women with chronic drinking problems require special attention because of difficulty in altering established drinking patterns. These individuals should be advised to forestall pregnancy until they can abstain from alcohol, and treatment options should be provided. If pregnancy has occurred, the risks of continued drinking to the fetus should be explained and treatment options quickly identified and provided.

What do the neuropsychological profiles associated with TS and WS tell us about the organization of the brain?

The studies of TS and WS have expanded our understanding of the organization of the brain. The relatively unique neurocognitive profiles of these two disorders suggest the following: (1) a number of cognitive functions are relatively independent of general cognitive ability, whereas others are strongly related to overall ability; (2) similar behaviors can be supported by different anatomic regions/circuitry; (3) the development of comparable skills and abilities by individuals with TS or WS are achieved by different processes; (4) there is significant intraindividual variability in the neurocognitive performance of individuals with TS and WS, indicating that factors other than genetic/chromosomal abnormalities affect performance outcomes; and (5) the neurocognitive profiles do not support a "modular" organization of the brain. For the latter, a modular view of brain organization proposes the presence of inborn, behaviorally designated, and independently functioning brain units. Injury to a given module results in the disruption of neurocognitive functions supported by that unit, while functions specific to other modules remain unaffected. In essence, the modular view of an injured brain is that of a normal brain with some "components" impaired and others preserved (Karmiloff-Smith, Brown, Grice, & Paterson, 2003). Several findings argue against the neurocognitive profiles of TS and WS as validating evidence for a modular conceptualization of brain functioning. First, the neurocognitive dissociations of TS and WS are "relative" and not "absolute." That is, preserved functions are "relative" rather than "absolute" strengths. For example, the language skills of a child with WS or TS may be more advanced than their visuoconstructive skills; however, both sets of skills are generally lower than those of typically developing children. A cognitive dissociation consistent with a modular conceptualization would predict that the aforementioned language skills would be unimpaired. Second, as noted earlier, similar neurocognitive behavior can be supported by different brain circuitry/regions and develop in different ways. Thus, neurocognitive behaviors are not localized to specific brain units or follow invariant steps or processes during their development.

CHAPTER 11

Why are the symptoms of NVLD and ADHD so often displayed by children exhibiting a wide range of developmental disorders?

As we have discussed, Rourke and associates hypothesize that white matter tissue damage causes NVLD. Insofar as white matter damage is evident across a number of developmental disorders, NVLD symptoms would be expected to occur, varying in number and intensity, depending on the extent and location of the impairment. Likewise, the functional neural systems that support attention and behavioral regulation are distributed throughout the brain, and accordingly, the injurious effects to different regions or circuits of the brain could result in behaviors of inattention, impulsivity, and overactivity. Thus, the symptoms of ADHD could potentially be evident across a variety of developmental disorders.

Can a child with autism or Asperger's syndrome develop normal social awareness and attachment? If so, how would this be accomplished?

A primary impairment of both autism and Asperger's syndrome is a significant deficit in social awareness and attachment. Unfortunately, these social deficits are rarely, if ever, fully resolved. Although therapists have used social skills training and other interventions, they have met little success. The amelioration of social impairments of autism and Asperger's syndrome is hampered by lack of understanding of the neuropsychological basis and determinants of social functioning. Specifically, neuropsychologists need to identify the developing relations of neural systems to special classes of social behavior (such as attachment), the effects of environmental influences on neural-social development, the causative factors specific to different types and forms of social impairments, and the malleability of and means of modifying neural-social behaviors necessary for altering social deficits. Once they gain this knowledge, people should be able to develop interventions necessary for the development of normal social relatedness and interaction.

How would you respond to the comment, "ADHD does not exist, it is merely a diagnosis to excuse lazy and undisciplined children?"

Some challenge the very existence of ADHD as an excuse for lazy and undisciplined children. To counter this challenge, cite the voluminous research that supports the existence of the disorder, the converging clinical and empirical studies that delineate the key symptoms and potential etiologies of the disorder, and the outcome studies that show significant improvement in regulatory control for children with ADHD who receive appropriate medical and psychological treatment. Finally, present specific because differences between the child who is exhibiting ADHD and one who is showing lazy and undisciplined behaviors.

As our understanding of the neural correlates of learning and neuropsychiatric disorders expands, what impact will this have on traditional psychological and educational treatment?

As researchers increasingly identify neural correlates of learning and neuropsychiatric disorders, significant changes will become evident in psychological and educational interventions. Although the potential changes are both numerous and unknown, several have been predicted. First, the discovery of genetic and chromosomal links to specific developmental disorders and accompanying neurogenetic interventions will enable children to be born relatively free of neuropsychological deficits. The need for traditional medical and psychological services specific to these disorders will be rendered virtually obsolete. Second, neurogenetic, molecular, and chemical advances will guide the development of medical interventions to repair and regenerate damaged brain tissue. In such cases, neuropsychological treatment will primarily focus on developing plans and interventions to enable parents and other caretakers to provide the experiences necessary to stimulate development and recovery of functions. Third, advances in the understanding of brain–behavior relations will encourage the development of increasingly complex neuropsychological models to predict appropriate

treatment options for specific brain disorders as affected by socioenvironmental factors, age, sex, health status, cognitive abilities, and other variables. Fourth, as understanding of brain–cognitive functioning expands, people will be able to develop specific educational strategies and interventions that will expand and maximize the learning of children, both disabled and nondisabled.

Does the finding that the symptoms of GTS often attenuate or resolve in later adolescence or early adulthood support a conceptualization of the disorder as a developmental lag? How do you account for individuals who do not show such improvement and struggle with GTS as a lifelong disorder?

The concept of developmental lag indicates a delay in the onset or rate of development of motor, communication, socialization, or other expected behaviors. The concept further assumes that a mature level of functioning ultimately will be achieved, and thus does not denote a disability. Clearly, the attenuation or resolution of GTS during late adolescence or early adulthood does not meet the standard of a slowly emerging or developing set of expected behaviors. Yet, inhibitory (motor) control is a developmental phenomenon that begins in infancy and continues to maturity in adolescence/adulthood. If research determines that tic behaviors are a function of a lag in the maturation of motor control, greater support will be provided for conceptualizing GTS as a developmental delay. However, the finding that a number of individuals with GTS do not show improvement with age, the complexity of behaviors that can constitute a "tic," the involuntary-voluntary quality of some tics, and the "waxing and waning" nature of tic behaviors argues against a simple causative explanation for GTS, such as developmental delay. The factors that determine whether an individual will or will not recover from GTS remain unclear. It is possible that there are yet to be identified subtypes of GTS that differ with regard to the progression and resolution of tic behaviors. Other factors that may affect the chronicity of GTS are tic severity, age at onset, presence of other comorbid conditions, and types and duration of treatment.

CHAPTER 12

What are the neurologic, behavioral, and emotional symptoms of a stroke?

The initial neurologic symptoms of stroke include a sudden headache, nausea, and loss of behavioral function, which may be relatively specific in nature. Because a stroke can affect many different areas of the brain, the neurologic symptoms may vary, but there can be an associated loss of consciousness. Behavioral symptoms relate to the precise area of the brain that has been affected. For those affected with left-hemisphere stroke, a common behavioral symptom is difficulty in understanding and expressing speech. Visual symptoms indicate posterior or basilar involvement, but a precise understanding of the behavioral symptoms is often not possible until a comprehensive neuropsychological evaluation is completed. Emotional symptoms can include depression for left-hemisphere stroke or irritability for right-hemisphere stroke. Again, a comprehensive neuropsychological evaluation may include a measure of emotional and personality functioning.

What are the major forms of treatment for stroke?

The acute treatment of the stroke patient involves medical stabilization and control of bleeding, through medication or surgery. Common medications include anticoagulants to dissolve blood clots or prevent clotting, vasodilators to dilate or expand the vessels, and blood pressure medication and steroids to control cerebral edema. Surgery can include clipping a bleeding aneurysm or evacuating blood to control the intracranial pressure often associated with a hemorrhage. Treatment for TIA symptoms is more difficult because of the ambiguous nature of the symptoms and is often restricted to pharmacologic intervention with anticoagulants. Long-term treatment of stroke patients may include intensive rehabilitation, including speech therapy, occupational training, and vocational training. Often, basic activities of daily living must be "relearned." Periodic re-evaluation by a neuropsychologist may determine treatment and rehabilitation progress and outcome.

Why do some stroke victims downplay their illness, whereas others go into a deep depression?

The symptoms of a right-hemisphere stroke are quite different from those of a left-hemisphere CVA because of the lateralization of many functions in the brain. A right-hemisphere stroke may result in a "lack of awareness" associated with poor insight and disinhibition. Patients with right brain damage tend to be unaware of their dysfunction associated with the consequences of the stroke. In fact, such patients often deny that there is anything wrong with them. Many patients with right brain damage display a range of emotions from indifference to euphoria. This contrasts with the depression that patients with left brain damage often show. Therefore, it is easy to assume that deficits from right brain damage are not as serious as those from left brain damage. As a result, right-hemisphere stroke patients may be blamed for being "rude," "disruptive," or "inappropriate" when they are actually exhibiting symptoms of right brain injury, including impulsivity, verbosity, inattention, and poor judgment. Obviously, these problems can be highly disruptive to the patient and family alike, often even exceeding the problems associated with left-hemisphere CVAs. Because right-hemisphere stroke patients and their families underestimate the severity of the condition, those patients are not diagnosed as rapidly as are left-hemisphere stroke patients.

Describe the most common neuropsychological deficits associated with stroke.

Almost always, neuropsychological disruption appears in stroke survivors; thus, neuropsychologists often evaluate stroke patients. Both the right and left hemispheres are associated with changes in motor and sensory functioning after a stroke. Those changes can be as benign as mild motor slowing to effects as debilitating as complete paralysis, particularly if there are lesions in the thalamic area or the motor and premotor area of the frontal lobes. Right-hemisphere stroke motor deficiencies, however, are generally less severe, because the nondominant left hand is not as important for skilled tasks. Deficits that affect the right cerebral artery involve areas responsible for spatial, rhythmic, and nonverbal processing. Right-hemisphere symptoms, although serious in the patient's overall functioning, can be less striking in the acute phase, particularly if they do not involve motor dysfunction. Research has shown consistently that patients with right-hemisphere stroke are hospitalized longer in rehabilitation facilities than are patients with left-hemisphere strokes. This fact is related to the pervasive deficits that right-hemisphere patients present with in the area of visuospatial abilities and the extended rehabilitation process that is required in rehabilitating these patients in areas of dressing, ambulating, and other self-care behaviors. The capacity to drive after a stroke continues to be one of the most sensitive issues facing health care workers, as well as the stroke patients and their families.

Would you want to know what type of cell a tumor arises from if one of your family members had brain cancer? Why? Should physicians routinely inform their patients of such medical details?

Yes, I (E.A.Z.) would like to know. The reason for knowing is that the more information the patient and family has, the easier it is to make personal decisions, such as estate management, issues of quality of life, and life expectancy. The specific type of brain tumor, and the type of cell it has arisen from, often signals a clear course of the disease. For example, the glioblastoma multiforme (GBM) is a particularly destructive and fatal glioma. Conversely, the presence of a meningioma often has little consequence to one's long-term well-being. Many physicians share detailed medical information with their patients and treat them as educated consumers. But many do not. My Aunt Edna died of a brain tumor, but the doctors never told her or her family what kind of tumor she had, even though clearly (to me) it was a GBM. As a result, the family had great hopes for her recovery, which unfortunately was not realistic; she passed away within 8 months. Would you like to know?

What is the neuropsychologist's role in diagnosing and treating patients with brain tumors? What is his or her role with the patient's family?

Since the advent of modern imaging technologies, neuropsychologists play only a minor role in the diagnosis of brain tumors. CT and MRI technology can often pinpoint the precise location and size of a brain tumor. If the tumor is thought to be fatal, neuropsychologists often provide counseling and education to patients with brain tumor and their families. If the brain tumor is operable and recovery is likely, neuropsychologists can provide a baseline assessment to which future evaluations (after surgery) can be compared. Treatment choices are complex and should have input from a team of oncologic professionals including neurosurgeon, oncologist-hematologist, radiation therapist, neuroradiologist, neurologist, and neuropsychologist. In general, neuropsychologists can play an important role in assessing brain tumor survivors and in providing rehabilitation care and intervention. As with other neurologic disorders, neuropsychologists can play an important role in helping people to understand the cognitive changes associated with brain tumor

How fluid are the boundaries between conscious and subconscious awareness?

This question concerns not only this chapter, but also ideas of conscious awareness, which have been presented throughout the book, as well as general ideas of consciousness debated in psychology. To approach this issue, first one must conceptualize and operationalize a definition of "conscious awareness" with particular attention to how conscious awareness is demonstrated. Must this always be in a verbal manner? Can one demonstrate awareness just through performance of an action? When one is in a state of consciousness, which is other than being "fully awake," what sense of awareness can there be? How does your knowledge of the functional and dysfunctional brain help to inform your ideas of consciousness?

How do REM sleep and dreaming change in people who have various neurologic disorders?

This issue presents an exciting and relatively underexplored area in neuropsychology. A number of case reports of people with abnormalities in dreaming from global cessation of dreaming, to decreased or odd qualities of dreaming, to problems in remembering dreams are in the literature. How do you think dreams of people with frontal lesions differ from those of people with parietal lesions? Do you think that people with motor problems will also have motor problems in their dreams?

In what ways might neuropsychology be able to contribute to treatments for people with sleep disorders or epilepsy?

If you consider the range of behavioral treatments of clinical psychology and the neuropsychological problems represented by the disorders presented in this chapter, you can see that a number of treatment strategies are possible. For example, memory and concentration problems are common in sleep apnea and, to a certain extent, in narcolepsy. Do you think strategies that aid memory will be useful for sleep apnea patients? Narcolepsy patients may have sleep attacks in response to emotional stimuli. Might relaxation techniques help them? With seizure patients, if auras are related to the foci of the seizure, might visualization techniques help to ward off visual auras, and therefore the seizure? What else can you think of? These areas are ripe for future investigation.

NAME INDEX

SUBJECT INDEX

Note: Page numbers in **boldface** type indicate pages on which terms are defined or introduced.

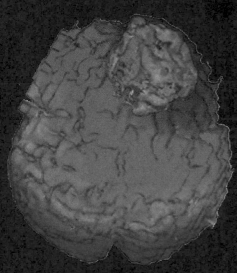

Figure 2.20 (Chapter 2)

Figure 2.20 (Chapter 2)

Sensory-evoked response examination with magnetic resonance imaging. With this technique, electrical activity and anatomic detail can be co-registered for clinical analysis. Image includes visualization of right frontal tumor. (Courtesy Dorota Kozinska, Ph.D., University of Warsaw, Warsaw, Poland.)

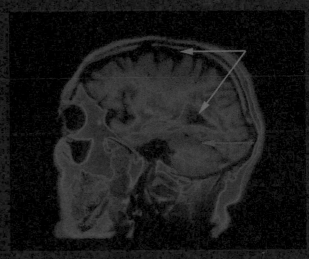

Figure 12.1 (Chapter 12)

Sagittal magnetic resonance imaging of brain with small stroke in the superior portion of the cerebellum (red arrow). Significant atrophy is associated with increased size of the lateral ventricles and intracranial space (blue arrows). (Courtesy Eric Zillmer.)

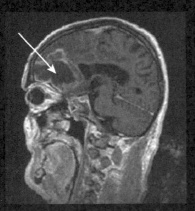

Figure 12.5 (Chapter 12)

Magnetic resonance imaging (MRI) examination of a patient with a cerebral glioma. The patient had suffered from increasing headaches for 6 weeks, memory impairment, and increasing paresis of the left side. Walking remained undamaged. MRI examination indicated a tumor 65 $\times$ 56 $\times$ 69 mm in size in the right frontal lobe. The tumor displaced the anterior part of the right lateral ventricle and moved a part of the corpus callosum to the left. (Courtesy Dorota Kozinska, University of Warsaw, Warsaw, Poland.)

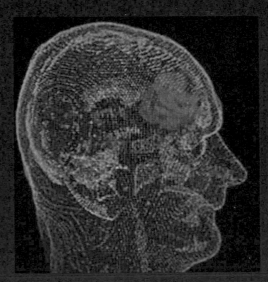

Figure 12.6 (Chapter 12)

Injected magnetic resonance imaging–visible dye amplifies boundaries of right frontal tumor, a glioma, in relation to cortex and scalp surfaces. (Courtesy Dorota Kozinska, University of Warsaw, Warsaw, Poland.)